Chemoinformatics in the Pharmaceutical Sciences

Chemoinformatics in the Pharmaceutical Sciences

Editor: Tosha McCallum

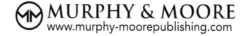
MURPHY & MOORE
www.murphy-moorepublishing.com

www.murphy-moorepublishing.com

MURPHY & MOORE

Cataloging-in-Publication Data

Chemoinformatics in the pharmaceutical sciences / edited by Tosha McCallum.
    p. cm.
Includes bibliographical references and index.
ISBN 978-1-63987-802-4
1. Cheminformatics. 2. Pharmacy. 3. Pharmacology. 4. Chemistry--Data processing.
5. Computational chemistry. 6. Chemistry--Information services. I. McCallum, Tosha.
RS418 .C443 2023
615.19--dc23

Murphy & Moore Publishing
1 Rockefeller Plaza,
New York City,
NY 10020, USA

ISBN 978-1-63987-802-4 (Hardback)

Contents

Preface...VII

Chapter 1   Chemoinformatics Strategies for Leishmaniasis Drug Discovery 1
Leonardo L. G. Ferreira and Adriano D. Andricopulo

Chapter 2   **Molecular Simulations of Carbohydrates with a Fucose-Binding**
Burkholderia ambifaria Lectin Suggest Modulation by
Surface Residues Outside the Fucose-Binding Pocket 12
Tamir Dingjan, Anne Imberty, Serge Pérez, Elizabeth Yuriev and Paul A. Ramsland

Chapter 3   **Bridging Molecular Docking to Molecular Dynamics in Exploring Ligand-Protein**
Recognition Process 28
Veronica Salmaso and Stefano Moro

Chapter 4   **Gossypol Inhibits Non-small Cell Lung Cancer Cells Proliferation by**
Targeting EGFR[L858R/T790M] 44
Yuwei Wang, Huanling Lai, Xingxing Fan, Lianxiang Luo, Fugang Duan, Zebo Jiang,
Qianqian Wang, Elaine Lai Han Leung, Liang Liu and Xiaojun Yao

Chapter 5   **Aromatic Rings Commonly Used in Medicinal Chemistry: Force Fields**
Comparison and Interactions with Water Toward the Design of
New Chemical Entities 52
Marcelo D. Polêto, Victor H. Rusu, Bruno I. Grisci, Marcio Dorn,
Roberto D. Lins and Hugo Verli

Chapter 6   **Identification of a Novel Protein Arginine Methyltransferase 5 Inhibitor in**
Non-small Cell Lung Cancer by Structure-Based Virtual Screening.....................72
Qianqian Wang, Jiahui Xu, Ying Li, Jumin Huang, Zebo Jiang, Yuwei Wang,
Liang Liu, Elaine Lai Han Leung and Xiaojun Yao

Chapter 7   **Discovery of Potent Disheveled/Dvl Inhibitors Using Virtual Screening**
Optimized with NMR-Based Docking Performance Index 82
Kiminori Hori, Kasumi Ajioka, Natsuko Goda, Asako Shindo, Maki Takagishi,
Takeshi Tenno and Hidekazu Hiroaki

Chapter 8   **Development of an Infrastructure for the Prediction of Biological Endpoints in**
Industrial Environments: Lessons Learned at the eTOX Project 96
Manuel Pastor, Jordi Quintana and Ferran Sanz

Chapter 9   **Structural Changes Due to Antagonist Binding in Ligand Binding Pocket of**
Androgen Receptor Elucidated Through Molecular Dynamics Simulations 104
Sugunadevi Sakkiah, Rebecca Kusko, Bohu Pan, Wenjing Guo, Weigong Ge,
Weida Tong and Huixiao Hong

Chapter 10   **Predicting Off-Target Binding Profiles with Confidence Using**
Conformal Prediction **117**
Samuel Lampa, Jonathan Alvarsson, Staffan Arvidsson Mc Shane, Arvid Berg,
Ernst Ahlberg and Ola Spjuth

Chapter 11   **Genotypic and Phenotypic Factors Influencing Drug Response in Mexican Patients**
with Type 2 Diabetes Mellitus..**130**
Hector E. Sanchez-Ibarra, Luisa M. Reyes-Cortes, Xian-Li Jiang,
Claudia M. Luna-Aguirre, Dionicio Aguirre-Trevino, Ivan A. Morales-Alvarado,
Rafael B. Leon-Cachon, Fernando Lavalle-Gonzalez, Faruck Morcos and
Hugo A. Barrera-Saldaña

Chapter 12   **Empirical Scoring Functions for Structure-Based Virtual Screening: Applications,**
Critical Aspects and Challenges..**141**
Isabella A. Guedes, Felipe S. S. Pereira and Laurent E. Dardenne

Chapter 13   **Using Machine Learning to Predict Synergistic Antimalarial**
Compound Combinations with Novel Structures..**159**
Daniel J. Mason, Richard T. Eastman, Richard P. I. Lewis, Ian P. Stott,
Rajarshi Guha and Andreas Bender

Chapter 14   **Molecular Connectivity Predefines Polypharmacology: Aliphatic Rings,**
Chirality and sp³ Centers Enhance Target Selectivity..**175**
Stefania Monteleone, Julian E. Fuchs and Klaus R. Liedl

Chapter 15   ***In Silico* Discovery of Plant-Origin Natural Product Inhibitors of Tumor Necrosis**
Factor (TNF) and Receptor Activator of NF-κB Ligand (RANKL).............................**184**
Georgia Melagraki, Evangelos Ntougkos, Dimitra Papadopoulou, Vagelis Rinotas,
Georgios Leonis, Eleni Douni, Antreas Afantitis and George Kollias

Chapter 16   **QSAR-Based Virtual Screening: Advances and Applications in Drug Discovery**...............................**196**
Bruno J. Neves, Rodolpho C. Braga, Cleber C. Melo-Filho, José Teófilo Moreira-Filho,
Eugene N. Muratov and Carolina Horta Andrade

Chapter 17   **Targets Fishing and Identification of Calenduloside E as Hsp90AB1: Design,**
Synthesis and Evaluation of Clickable Activity-Based Probe....................................**203**
Shan Wang, Yu Tian, Jing-Yi Zhang, Hui-Bo Xu, Ping Zhou, Min Wang,
Sen-Bao Lu, Yun Luo, Min Wang, Gui-Bo Sun, Xu-Dong Xu and Xiao-Bo Sun

Chapter 18   **Improving Docking Performance Using Negative Image-Based Rescoring** **217**
Sami T. Kurkinen, Sanna Niinivehmas, Mira Ahinko, Sakari Lätti,
Olli T. Pentikäinen and Pekka A. Postila

Permissions

List of Contributors

Index

Preface

The purpose of the book is to provide a glimpse into the dynamics and to present opinions and studies of some of the scientists engaged in the development of new ideas in the field from very different standpoints. This book will prove useful to students and researchers owing to its high content quality.

Chemoinformatics refers to the study of vast quantities of chemical information. It is also known as cheminformatics and chemical informatics. The link between chemical structure, chemical characteristics, and molecular activity can be examined using this data. It is done with the help of computers, software and simulations. Pharmaceutical companies employ these techniques to discover novel drugs. New drug development is a time-consuming procedure. Chemoinformatics has aided in speeding up the process of drug development. Some of the techniques used within this field are virtual screening, in silico ADMET and high throughput screening. This book aims to present researches in the area of chemoinformatics that have aided in the advancement of pharmaceutical sciences. It is a vital tool for all researching or studying this area of pharmaceutical science as it gives incredible insights with respect to recent trends.

At the end, I would like to appreciate all the efforts made by the authors in completing their chapters professionally. I express my deepest gratitude to all of them for contributing to this book by sharing their valuable works. A special thanks to my family and friends for their constant support in this journey.

Editor

Chemoinformatics Strategies for Leishmaniasis Drug Discovery

Leonardo L. G. Ferreira*† and Adriano D. Andricopulo*†

Laboratory of Medicinal and Computational Chemistry, Center for Research and Innovation in Biodiversity and Drug Discovery, São Carlos Institute of Physics, University of São Paulo, São Carlos, Brazil

*Correspondence:
Leonardo L. G. Ferreira
leonardo@ifsc.usp.br
Adriano D. Andricopulo
aandrico@ifsc.usp.br

† These authors have contributed
equally to this work

Leishmaniasis is a fatal neglected tropical disease (NTD) that is caused by more than 20 species of Leishmania parasites. The disease kills approximately 20,000 people each year and more than 1 billion are susceptible to infection. Although counting on a few compounds, the therapeutic arsenal faces some drawbacks such as drug resistance, toxicity issues, high treatment costs, and accessibility problems, which highlight the need for novel treatment options. Worldwide efforts have been made to that aim and, as well as in other therapeutic areas, chemoinformatics have contributed significantly to leishmaniasis drug discovery. Breakthrough advances in the comprehension of the parasites' molecular biology have enabled the design of high-affinity ligands for a number of macromolecular targets. In addition, the use of chemoinformatics has allowed highly accurate predictions of biological activity and physicochemical and pharmacokinetics properties of novel antileishmanial compounds. This review puts into perspective the current context of leishmaniasis drug discovery and focuses on the use of chemoinformatics to develop better therapies for this life-threatening condition.

Keywords: medicinal chemistry, ligand-based drug design, structure-based drug design, neglected tropical diseases, molecular modeling, leishmania

CURRENT PANORAMA OF LEISHMANIASIS

Leishmaniasis is a neglected tropical disease (NTD) that causes approximately 20,000 deaths each year. Nearly 300,000 new cases of the disease are registered annually, and over 1 billion people are exposed to the risk of infection[1]. The disease is caused by more than 20 species of Leishmania protozoan parasites that are transmitted to humans through the bites of female Phlebotomus and Lutzomyia sandflies. Leishmaniasis occurs in 98 tropical and subtropical countries encompassing the Mediterranean Basin, South-East Asia, Afro-Eurasia, East Africa, and the Americas. People who are exposed to adverse socioeconomic circumstances, malnutrition, poor housing, and unsanitary conditions are the main target of leishmaniasis (Hailu et al., 2016).

Although leishmaniasis is a curable condition, treatment depends on a variety of factors, including geographic region, clinical form of the disease and parasite species. The available chemotherapy consists of drugs that cause serious side effects, such as renal, pancreatic and hepatic toxicity, teratogenicity, and cardiac and gastrointestinal problems (Copeland and Aronson, 2015). The need for hospitalization, long-term and costly treatment, and drug resistance are additional drawbacks. To this list, one may add the difficulties in implementing the widespread use of the 2014-approved drug miltefosine due to problems of affordability and limited availability and accessibility (Sunyoto et al., 2018). Another current concern in endemic regions is the contingent of patients with leishmaniasis who are coinfected with the HIV virus. Lower cure rates are achieved

[1] http://www.who.int/leishmaniasis/en/

in these patients because both pathogens attack the immune system. Furthermore, this group is more vulnerable to the drug-associated adverse effects, which contribute to higher death rates (Abongomera et al., 2018). These drawbacks have driven the creation of robust worldwide efforts to pursue novel therapeutic options. This article provides a perspective on these efforts, focusing on recent advances that involve the use of chemoinformatics.

FROM TRIAL-AND-ERROR TO KNOWLEDGE-BASED DRUG DESIGN

Similar to most early NTD-focused research programs, drug discovery for leishmaniasis relied on trial-and-error strategies that were based solely on phenotypic screenings. This paradigm reflected the lack of a reasonable understanding of the molecular aspects of the *Leishmania* biology and the cellular processes involved in parasite–host interaction (Gilbert, 2013). This setting began to change when the outstanding findings from genome projects in the mid-2000s started to open an array of new opportunities in leishmaniasis drug discovery (Reguera et al., 2014). Simultaneously, novel collaborative networks were settled, incorporating pharmaceutical companies, and not-for-profit organizations, which, along with research and academic institutions, have brought previously unavailable technological and scientific developments to the field (Preston and Gasser, 2018). Since then, genomics, proteomics, and structural biology data have been made available via open-access NTD-focused databases, which have been essential to the use of chemoinformatics in leishmaniasis research. The Sanger Institute's GeneDB, for example, organizes the data of several *Leishmania* species and is a useful tool for searching particular gene sequences and investigating gene similarity and function (Logan-Klumpler et al., 2012). Another important virtual platform, the WHO's TDR Targets Database, is a chemogenomics resource that is focused on NTDs and connects information from diverse protein and small-molecule libraries (Magariños et al., 2012). In doing so, the TDR Targets Database algorithm generates privileged combinations of molecular targets and compounds to be considered for experimental studies. To this list, one may add LmSmdB, which is a database that simulates metabolic networks (Patel et al., 2016), and LeishMicrosatDB, which is a search engine for microsatellite sequences in *Leishmania* genomes (Dikhit et al., 2014). Resulting from these advances, more than 340 protein structures from *Leishmania* spp. are currently registered in the Protein Data Bank (PDB) (Berman et al., 2000). These data have been key to understanding the parasite's molecular machinery and interspecies variability, which are fundamental aspects to developing broad-spectrum drugs.

Taking advantage of this progress, researchers have increasingly engaged in research and development (R&D) organizational models that are characterized by well-structured worldwide collaboration networks, which are referred to as public-private-partnerships (PPPs) (Preston and Gasser, 2018). These initiatives have been pivotal to enhancing the research infrastructure of NTDs by providing state-of-the-art facilities

and technologies, high-quality compound libraries for screening and highly qualified human resources. One noteworthy example is the Drugs for Neglected Diseases Initiative's (DNDi) Lead Optimization Latin America (LOLA) consortium, which focuses on preclinical *in vitro* and *in vivo* efficacy, safety and pharmacokinetics assessment[2]. Experimental evaluation is routinely followed by chemoinformatics studies to identify structure-activity and structure-property relationships that guide the design of optimized compounds. The value of this type of initiative has been demonstrated by the successful development of several candidates that are currently undergoing advanced preclinical trials for leishmaniasis[3].

STRUCTURE- AND LIGAND-BASED STRATEGIES IN LEISHMANIASIS DRUG DISCOVERY

Technologies such as combinatorial chemistry and high-throughput screening (HTS) have enabled tests on large compound libraries that encompass a significant chemical diversity in short time scales (Folmer, 2016; Liu et al., 2017). Although these highly impactful approaches have enhanced the potential of the pharmaceutical industry to deliver better drugs in all therapeutic areas, they contributed to scale up the complexity of drug R&D. In this context, in which the outstanding demands for innovation are constantly challenged by significant attrition rates, the industry has put intensive effort into the integration of computational tools into the research pipeline (Rognan, 2017). Being cost-effective mainly in the early stages of discovery, this R&D setting is especially suited to clinical conditions, such as leishmaniasis, which have limited resources compared with mainstream therapeutic areas. Hence, given the ability of chemoinformatics to rapidly estimate ligand-receptor interactions and a number of physicochemical and pharmacokinetics properties, this approach has steadily grown as a key component of drug R&D (Ponder et al., 2014; Macalino et al., 2015).

Notwithstanding their broad diversity, chemoinformatics tools are generally classified into structure- and ligand-based drug design (SBDD and LBDD, respectively) approaches. SBDD methods consist of the use of the 3D coordinates of molecular targets to investigate and optimize ligand-receptor interactions (van Montfort and Workman, 2017). SBDD programs have revealed the 3D architecture of a variety drug targets, mainly by the use of techniques such as X-ray crystallography. By uncovering binding site attributes, such as shape and electronic distribution, SBDD efforts have been able to deliver ligands with accurately designed properties to achieve high-affinity interactions with their targets (Ferreira et al., 2015). This process is generally assisted by methods such as molecular docking and structure-based virtual screening (SBVS), whereby potential ligands can be evaluated as to their binding mode and energetics

[2]https://www.dndi.org/2013/media-centre/news-views-stories/news/first-early-stage-research-latin-america/

[3]https://www.dndi.org/diseases-projects/portfolio/

(**Figure 1A**). By examining these data along with experimental results, structure-activity relationships (SAR) can be derived and then used to optimize ligand-receptor affinity and other properties (dos Santos et al., 2018).

Some promising macromolecular targets have been investigated in leishmaniasis drug discovery. The most relevant are topoisomerases and proteases (mainly cysteine-proteases) (Ansari et al., 2017). Other important targets are tubulin, proteins of the folate metabolic route, kinases, phosphodiesterases, and enzymes that are involved in the trypanothione and purine salvage pathways (Ansari et al., 2017). Ligands belonging to a broad variety of chemical classes have been identified for these targets, providing high-quality data for drug design.

Ligand-based drug design studies can be performed without the receptor 3D structure. Instead, they require information on the structure, activity, and molecular properties of small molecules (Chen, 2013). These data are used to construct chemometric models that correlate molecular properties (molecular descriptors) with pharmacodynamics and pharmacokinetics parameters (target properties). In doing so, quantitative structure-activity and structure-property relationships (QSAR and QSPR, respectively) can be derived to identify molecular descriptors that are directly associated with the target property (Yousefinejad and Hemmateenejad, 2015). By providing this type of information, these models are useful for evaluating the target property and guiding the design of new compounds that have improved profiles (**Figure 1B**). Today, many free-access and commercial software programs that include well-validated QSAR and QSPR models are available for predicting a number of properties. They vary from online platforms that are very straightforward to use to packages that require local license installation.

The use of SBDD and LBDD methods in leishmaniasis drug discovery is an encouraging strategy that has advanced alongside the progress made in the NTD field (Njogu et al., 2016). Chemoinformatics studies have incorporated different SBDD workflows that focus on established and newly discovered molecular targets. On the other hand, the use of QSAR

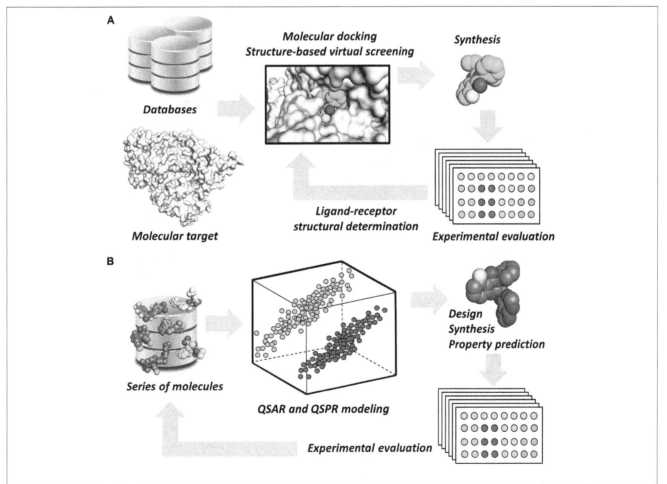

FIGURE 1 | Chemoinformatics strategies. **(A)** SBDD approaches using virtual screening and molecular docking. These methods are useful for revealing phenomena associated with intermolecular interactions and for improving parameters, such as ligand-receptor affinity. Active molecules can have their binding mode experimentally determined by techniques such as X-ray crystallography. **(B)** LBDD and the development of QSARs and QSPRs. These are broadly used for the design of novel compounds and for the prediction of pharmacodynamics and pharmacokinetics properties. The experimental data gathered from newly designed compounds can be added to the dataset to generate enriched models.

and QSPR models for predicting key pharmacodynamics and pharmacokinetics properties has also been noteworthy. The manipulation of this information, including genomics, metabolomics, structural, and small-molecule data, has been particularly useful for running metabolic network predictions for prospecting novel molecular targets and promising compounds and for proposing likely mechanisms of action. The next sections bring a perspective on a few recent cases using chemoinformatics, focusing on their contribution to the progress of leishmaniasis drug R&D.

Structure-Based Studies

Structure-based drug design efforts have prominently contributed to uncovering novel ligands for both well-established and newly discovered drug targets in *Leishmania* spp. One example is pteridine reductase 1 (PTR1), which is an enzyme involved in the pteridine salvage pathway and folate metabolism and a validated target in leishmaniasis drug discovery (Ong et al., 2011). This enzyme was explored in a study that reported on an SBDD strategy for designing novel inhibitors that combine the features of dihydropyrimidine and chalcone derivatives (Rashid et al., 2016). By using the crystallographic structure

of *L. major* PTR1, the authors proposed a series of analogs to achieve high-affinity interactions with the catalytic site of the enzyme. Molecular docking-guided structural modifications on the dihydropyrimidine and chalcone moieties and a reduction in the number of rotatable bonds led to the most active compounds against *L. major*. For example, compound **1** proved to be highly active against both *L. major* and *L. donovani* promastigotes, exhibiting a half-maximum inhibition concentration (IC_{50}) of 948 nM and 3 μM, respectively (**Figure 2A**). The predicted ligand-receptor binding energies were consistent with the *in vitro* antileishmanial activity values. These results demonstrate the suitability of these substituted dihydropyrimidines to be further investigated as potential agents against both visceral and cutaneous leishmaniasis.

Among *Leishmania* cysteine proteases, type B enzymes (CPB) have been recognized as key virulence factors whose activity is essential for parasite survival and the invasion of host cells (Casgrain et al., 2016). Within this group, the cathepsin-L-like endopeptidase CPB2.8 has emerged as a promising drug target in leishmaniasis. An article by De Luca et al. (2018) reported the discovery of a series of substituted benzimidazole derivatives that feature nanomolar affinity for *L. mexicana* CPB2.8 (K_i values

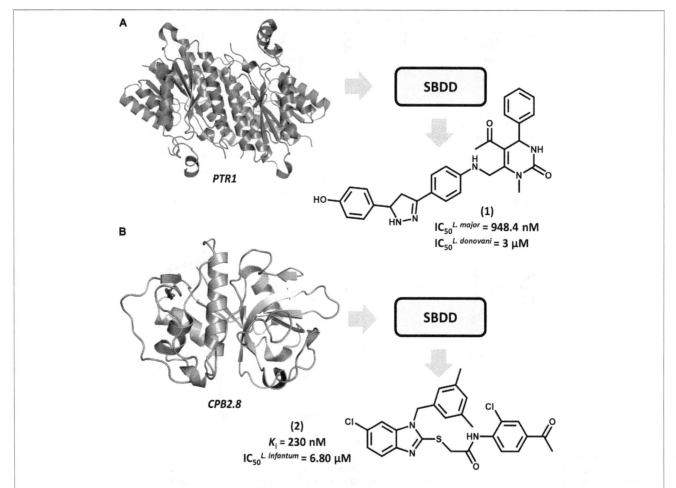

FIGURE 2 | SBDD in leishmaniasis drug discovery. **(A)** An SBDD approach using molecular docking on pteridine reductase 1 (PTR1) that led to the discovery of dihydropyrimidine **1** as a novel antileishmanial agent. **(B)** The design of the *L. infantum* cysteine-protease type 2 (CPB2.8) inhibitor **2** having antileishmanial activity.

ranging from 150 to 690 nM). A few analogs displayed interesting activity on *L. infantum* intracellular amastigotes, with the most potent one (**2**) yielding an IC_{50} of 6.8 µM (**Figure 2B**). Molecular docking studies were run to examine the binding mode of the compounds within the catalytic site of CPB2.8 and to rationalize the enzyme kinetics data. The administration, distribution, metabolism, excretion and toxicity (ADMET) were predicted to evaluate the drug-likeness of the series and hence, its suitability for further development. Compound **2** demonstrated a good bioavailability profile, which, along with the biochemical and biological results, rendered it a good candidate for future drug design efforts.

Type 2 NADH dehydrogenase (NDH2), a mitochondrial enzyme that catalyzes the electron transfer from NADH to ubiquinone, is an emerging drug target in leishmaniasis drug discovery (Marreiros et al., 2017). By constructing a homology model of the enzyme, Stevanović et al. (2018) conducted a pharmacophore-based virtual screening to find novel *L. infantum* NDH2 inhibitors. A group of 23 virtual hits were selected and

screened against the recombinant enzyme and subsequently tested for their activity on *L. infantum* whole cells. Out of this set, a 6-methoxy-quinalidine derivative (**3**, **Figure 3A**) proved to be the best NDH2 inhibitor (K_i = 8.9 µM). In addition, this compound exhibited nanomolar activity against both *L. infantum* axenic amastigotes (IC_{50} = 200 nM) and promastigotes (IC_{50} = 30 nM). These remarkable results make this novel quinalidine derivative a promising starting point for molecular optimization and *in vivo* studies for visceral leishmaniasis.

Ochoa et al. (2016) reported the use of the IBM World Community Grid to run an SBVS campaign on 53 different *Leishmania* proteins. First, molecular dynamics simulations were performed for this entire set, and then, distinct conformational states of each structure were selected for the SBVS effort. Approximately 2,000 conformations were selected and used to screen a database of 600,000 drug-like compounds, resulting in 1 billion protein-ligand complexes. A group of four proteins were observed engaging in high–affinity interactions with the database

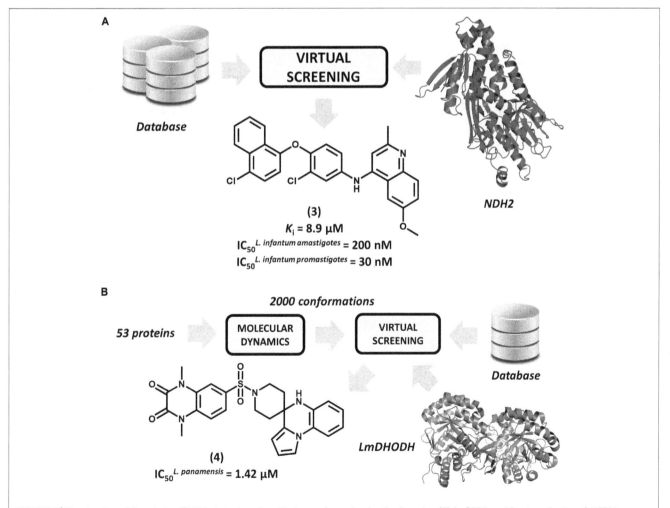

FIGURE 3 | Structure-based drug design (SBDD) strategies using virtual screening and molecular dynamics. **(A)** An SBDD workflow targeting type 2 NADH dehydrogenase (NDH2) resulting in the identification of compound **3**, a remarkably potent antileishmanial agent. **(B)** An SBDD strategy targeting diverse *Leishmania* proteins that led to the discovery of **4**, a novel compound having promising antileishmanial activity.

compounds, and the most favorable binding energy occurred in *L. major* dihydroorotate dehydrogenase (*Lm*DHODH). This enzyme catalyzes the oxidation of dihydroorotate, a key reaction in the pyrimidine synthesis pathway (Cordeiro et al., 2012). Ten top-scoring *Lm*DHODH inhibitors were selected and evaluated for their *in vitro* antileishmanial activity. Four molecules were active against *L. panamensis* intracellular amastigotes, with the most active one (**4**, **Figure 3B**) yielding a half maximal effective concentration (EC$_{50}$) of 1.42 µM, which is a value that is comparable to that of the reference drug amphotericin B. Furthermore, this compound showed no toxicity in human macrophages. This compound is a promising candidate for further development, and future investigations are expected to assess its efficacy in reducing *in vivo* parasite burden.

The enzyme topoisomerase 1 from *L. donovani* (*Ld*Top1) was selected as the molecular target in an SBDD study by Mamidala and coworkers (Mamidala et al., 2016). The enzyme catalyzes single-strand breaks in DNA, which enables the topological changes that are required during fundamental cellular processes such as gene replication and transcription (Pommier et al., 2016). The authors reported the discovery of a series of *Ld*Top1 inhibitors by using scaffold hopping and bioisosteric manipulations. The structure of known Top1 inhibitors such as camptothecin and edotecarin were used as the starting points for the molecular design. The outline of the compounds was guided by molecular docking runs using the X-ray structures of *Ld*Top1 and the human ortholog. Six compounds showed selective activity against *Ld*Top1 over the human enzyme, yielding EC$_{50}$ values from 1 to 30 µM (**5–10**, **Figure 4**). The best inhibitor (**5**, EC$_{50}$ = 3.51 µM) exhibited interesting biological activity against *L. donovani* promastigotes (IC$_{50}$ = 4.21 µM) and no toxicity against mammalian cells. The structure of the ternary complex **5**-*Ld*Top1-DNA, which was predicted by molecular docking, revealed key structural features to the design of novel analogs.

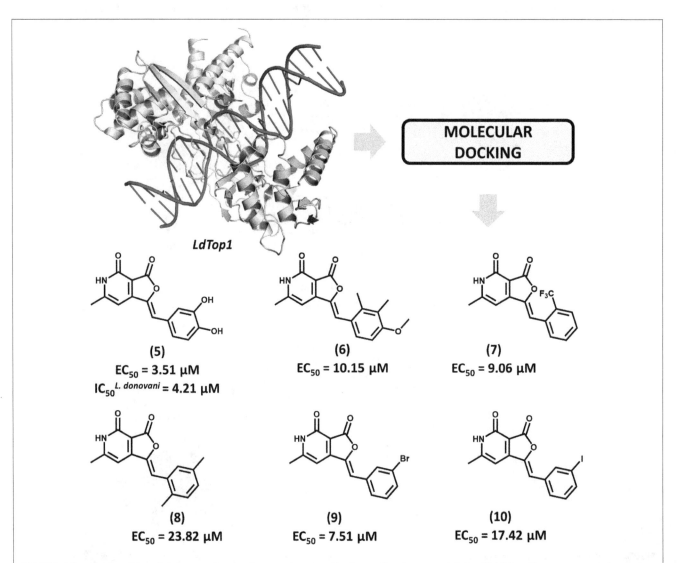

FIGURE 4 | Structure-based drug design approach to the discovery of a series of *L. donovani* topoisomerase 1 (*Ld*Top1) inhibitors. The strategy employing molecular docking led to the identification of compound **5** which shows suitable *in vitro* antiparasitic activity.

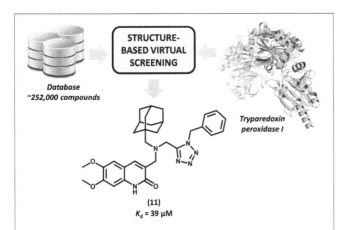

FIGURE 5 | Structure-based virtual screening that resulted in the first report of a series of non-covalent *L. major* tryparedoxin peroxidase I inhibitors. The molecular docking approach led to the identification of aliphatic adamantyl derivative **11** which shows suitable activity against the enzyme.

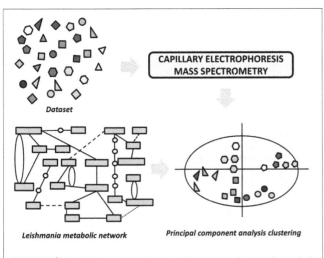

FIGURE 6 | Ligand-based approach to classify compounds according to their mechanism of action. The effects of the dataset compounds on *Leishmania* metabolism were analyzed by capillary electrophoresis–mass spectrometry, and the data were used in a principal component analysis (PCA). The PCA was able to cluster compounds according to the perturbation they caused in the parasite's metabolic network.

Considering the suitable antileishmanial activity and the lack of cytotoxicity, further studies on compound **5** would be useful for assessing other aspects, such as its pharmacokinetics profile.

Brindisi et al. (2015) reported for the first time the discovery of non-covalent tryparedoxin peroxidase inhibitors. Tryparedoxin peroxidase has been considered as a molecular target in SBDD studies since it reduces hydroperoxides produced by infected macrophages. This mechanism of detoxification is particularly attractive for drug design since it is unique to the parasite and essential for its survival (Fiorillo et al., 2012). By using the X-ray structure of *Leishmania major* tryparedoxin peroxidase I (*Lm*TXNPx), the authors run a molecular docking effort and selected a set of hits for experimental profiling. The docking

conformations were used for the design of a series of N,N-disubstituted 3-aminomethyl quinolones and some of them displayed activity against LmTXNPx. Forming a number of hydrogen bonds and hydrophobic contacts with the enzyme, the most potent compound (**11**, **Figure 5**), which has a bulky aliphatic adamantyl system, showed activity in the micromolar range (K_d = 39 μM). Calculation of physicochemical parameters demonstrated the drug-likeness of the designed series. In view of the activity and the drug-like properties of quinolone derivative **11**, this compound represents a suitable starting point for further studies aiming the development of novel drug candidates against leishmaniasis.

Ligand-Based Studies

A variety of LBDD approaches have been recently reported in leishmaniasis drug discovery. These studies are frequently conducted in combination with experimental protocols and SBDD methods. The main goals include the use of QSAR and QSPR models to predict activity and ADMET parameters and the search for novel compounds via ligand-based virtual screening (LBVS). One of these studies reports an approach to pursuing novel compounds based on their effects on cell metabolism (Armitage et al., 2018). A collection of structurally diverse compounds, including those enclosed in the Leishmania box (a set of 592 compounds identified in HTS campaigns at GSK) (Peña et al., 2015) was evaluated in axenic *L. donovani* amastigotes, and the resulting metabolic changes were examined by capillary electrophoresis–mass spectrometry (**Figure 6**). Next, a principal component analysis (PCA) was applied to generate a model that assorts these compounds according to their putative mode of action. The authors demonstrated structural patterns involved in the modulation of different metabolic pathways and additionally, the role of physicochemical properties in the stimulation of individual biochemical routes. The study is very interesting, as it enables the classification of compound databases according to the most likely mechanism of action and biological outcomes. It also provides a way to run mechanistic studies of compounds that are known to be active against *Leishmania* species, thus offering a guide for downstream experimental profiling.

With the aid of QSAR modeling, Bhagat and coauthors described the synthesis and *in vitro* evaluation of 26 aminophosphonate derivatives (Bhagat et al., 2014). Six compounds (**12–17**, **Figure 7A**) displayed activity on *L. donovani* promastigotes in the low micromolar range (IC_{50} from 7.10 to 8.95 μM) and cytotoxicity on J774 macrophages comparable to that of amphotericin B. The authors took the gathered data for the whole compound series to build Comparative Molecular Field Analysis (CoMFA) models that have high predictive ability (r^2_{pred} = 0.87) (Cramer et al., 1988). The models provided useful insights for future efforts on the optimization of this series. The CoMFA contour maps indicated that adding an electronegative group at the *para* position and a bulky electropositive substituent at the *meta* position in ring A would improve biological activity. Additionally, replacing ring B with substituted heterocyclic systems was stressed to be a worthwhile strategy for achieving more potent α-aminophosphonates as novel antileishmanial agents.

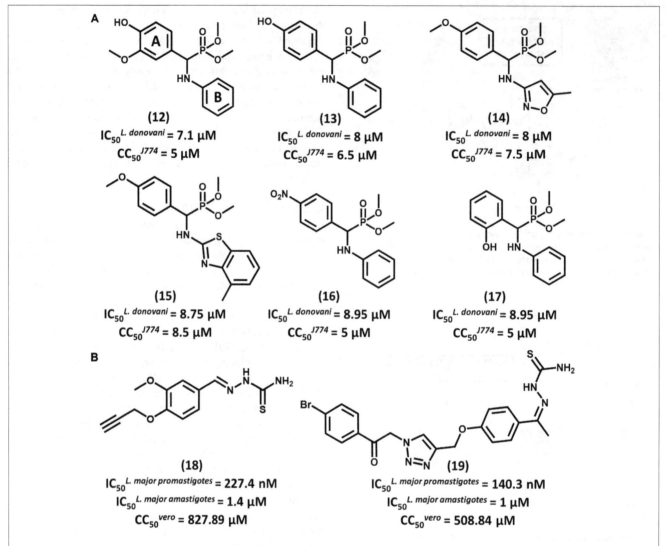

FIGURE 7 | (A) A series of aminophosphonate derivatives as novel compounds featuring antiparasitic activity against *L. donovani* promastigotes. The QSAR models assigned rings A and B as the most relevant sites for molecular modification. **(B)** Triazole and thiosemicarbazone hybrids **18** and **19** showed promising activity against *L. major* promastigotes and amastigotes.

In a recent study, Temraz et al. (2018) reported the design of 1,2,3-triazole and thiosemicarbazone hybrids as novel antileishmanial compounds and the calculation of their ADMET profile. Out of the 17 evaluated molecules, most of them exhibited biological activity that is comparable or superior to that of the reference drug miltefosine. The most promising analogs, **18** and **19**, exhibited IC_{50} values of 227.4 and 140.3 nM, respectively, on *L. major* promastigotes (**Figure 7B**). On amastigotes, IC_{50} values of 1.4 and 1 µM were obtained for compounds **18** and **19**, respectively. The folate pathway was proposed as the target metabolic route, since folic acid reversed the antiparasitic activity. Toxicity data on VERO cells showed a selectivity profile that was superior to that of miltefosine (SI > 3000). Additionally, compounds **18** and **19** demonstrated no acute toxicity in mice at doses up to 125 mg/kg (oral) and 75 mg/kg (parenteral). Calculation of ADMET parameters demonstrated the drug-likeness of these compounds and their agreement with Lipinski's

rule of five. Considering the activity, selectivity, physicochemical and ADMET data, these triazole and thiosemicarbazone hybrids consist of promising lead compounds to be further investigated.

Tetrahydro-β-carboline derivatives have recently been reported to have antileishmanial activity. In an investigation by Ashok et al. (2016) 16 analogs were designed, and most of them showed promising activity against *L. infantum* promastigotes (IC_{50} from 1.99 to 20.69 µM) and amastigotes (IC_{50} from 0.67 to 4.16 µM). Compound **20**, the most potent one ($IC_{50} = 0.67$ µM for amastigotes), showed activity comparable to that of amphotericin B ($IC_{50} = 0.32$ µM) and a selectivity index (SI) that is superior to 298 for the parasite over mammalian cells (**Figure 8A**). All compounds underwent QSPR studies for physicochemical profiling. Most analogs, including **20**, showed no violation of the Lipinski's rule of five, demonstrating that they are likely to have good bioavailability. Given the gathered activity, selectivity and physicochemical data, this series

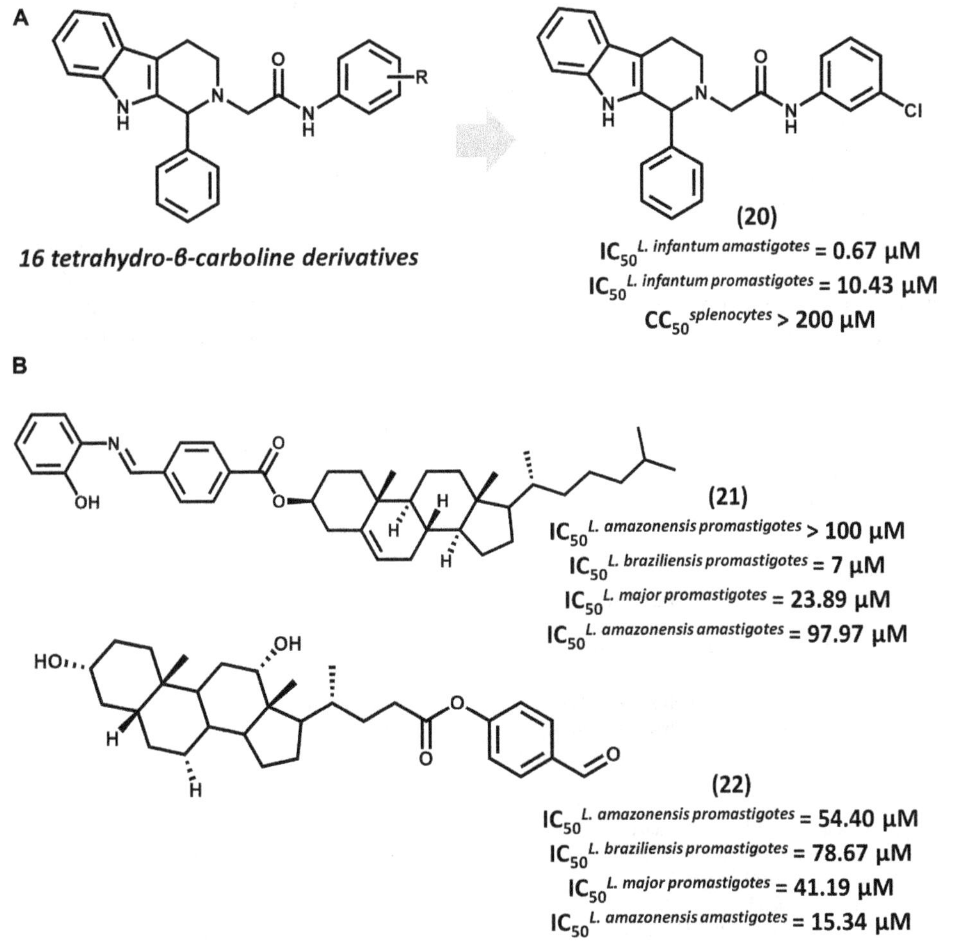

FIGURE 8 | (A) The synthesis of a series of 16 tetrahydro-β-carboline derivatives led to compound **20** having promising *in vitro* activity against *L. infantum* promastigotes and amastigotes. **(B)** Cholesterol and deoxycholic acid derivatives **21** and **22** feature suitable activity against several *Leishmania* species.

consists of appropriate starting points for further investigation. Additional studies would be highly desirable for evaluating the *in vivo* reduction in parasite burden and hence, the potential of this series as novel drug candidates for leishmaniasis.

Steroid derivatives were described as novel antileishmanial agents in a recent report by da Trindade Granato et al. (2018). Out of the 16 synthesized analogs, cholesterol derivative **21** and some deoxycholic acid (DOA) derivatives proved active against *Leishmania* promastigotes (**Figure 8B**). Most DOAs were active against *L. amazonensis* intracellular amastigotes and displayed low toxic effects to macrophages. DOA **22** showed the best antiparasitic activity (IC$_{50}$ = 15.34 μM) against amastigotes, which led to the investigation of its mechanism of action. Treatment of *L. amazonensis* with **22** led to the depolarization of the mitochondrial membrane potential and augmented reactive oxygen species (ROS) concentration, resulting in the arrest of the cell cycle. Estimation of ADMET properties revealed the suitability of **22** for oral administration. Additionally, the predictions indicated that this compound would have good blood-brain barrier permeation and would be susceptible to metabolic clearance by CYP3A4 enzymes. Further efforts to

improve the *in vitro* activity of **22** and evaluate its *in vivo* efficacy would be worthwhile.

CONCLUSION

A number of drug candidates are undergoing lead optimization studies and advanced *in vivo* preclinical profiling for leishmaniasis. Some of them could reach the clinical development phase, which have recently been filled by evaluations of different treatment regimens and combinations of previously approved drugs. Despite these advances and outcomes, it is prudent to adopt a conservative mindset given the long path that these compounds will have to take until potential approval and the high attrition rates that characterize pharmaceutical research. In this context, long-lasting efforts will be required to support state-of-the-art research programs that focus on the discovery of novel lead compounds for leishmaniasis. Such programs do exist today and have taken major advantage of the plentiful availability of data on *Leishmania*, as they move from trial-and-error to rational drug design. Current SBDD and LBDD campaigns have steadily contributed to rationalizing experimental data, thus providing effective insights into the design of optimized compounds. An important advance would be the validation of a higher number of molecular targets. Opportunely, some research centers have put intense efforts into this issue by developing large-scale chemical genomics and target deconvolution expertise. Regardless of the challenges ahead, chemoinformatics have been an important tool to prospect and profile promising compounds. This is corroborated by the findings discussed herein, which illustrate the rewarding integration of computational and experimental strategies in leishmaniasis drug R&D.

REFERENCES

Abongomera, C., Diro, E., de Lima Pereira, A., Buyze, J., Stille, K., Ahmed, F., et al. (2018). The initial effectiveness of liposomal amphotericin B (AmBisome) and miltefosine combination for treatment of visceral leishmaniasis in HIV co-infected patients in Ethiopia: a retrospective cohort study. *PLoS Negl. Trop. Dis.* 12:e0006527. doi: 10.1371/journal.pntd.0006527

Ansari, M. Y., Dikhit, M. R., Sahoo, G. C., Ali, V., and Das, P. (2017). Recent advancement and treatment of leishmaniasis based on pharmacoinformatics approach: current and future outlook. *Gene Rep.* 9, 86–97. doi: 10.1016/j.genrep.2017.09.003

Armitage, E. G., Godzien, J., Peña, I., López-Gonzálvez, Á., Angulo, S., Gradillas, A., et al. (2018). Metabolic clustering analysis as a strategy for compound selection in the drug discovery pipeline for Leishmaniasis. *ACS Chem. Biol.* 13, 1361–1369. doi: 10.1021/acschembio.8b00204

Ashok, P., Chander, S., Tejería, A., García-Calvo, L., Balaña-Fouce, R., and Murugesan, S. (2016). Synthesis and anti-leishmanial evaluation of 1-phenyl-2,3,4,9-tetrahydro-1H-β-carboline derivatives against *Leishmania infantum*. *Eur. J. Med. Chem.* 123, 814–821. doi: 10.1016/j.ejmech.2016.08.014

Berman, H. M., Westbrook, J., Feng, Z., Gilliland, G., Bhat, T. N., and Weissig, H. (2000). The protein data bank. *Nucleic Acids Res.* 28, 235–242. doi: 10.1093/nar/28.1.235

Bhagat, S., Shah, P., Garg, S. K., Mishra, S., Kaur, P. K., Singh, S., et al. (2014). α-Aminophosphonates as novel anti-leishmanial chemotypes: synthesis, biological evaluation, and CoMFA studies. *MedChemComm* 5, 665–670. doi: 10.1039/C3MD00388D

Brindisi, M., Brogi, S., Relitti, N., Vallone, A., Butini, S., Gemma, S., et al. (2015). Structure-based discovery of the first non-covalent inhibitors of Leishmania major tryparedoxin peroxidase by high throughput docking. *Sci. Rep.* 5:9705. doi: 10.1038/srep09705

Casgrain, P. A., Martel, C., McMaster, W. R., Mottram, J. C., Olivier, M., and Descoteaux, A. (2016). Cysteine peptidase B regulates *Leishmania mexicana* virulence through the modulation of GP63 expression. *PLoS Pathog.* 12:e1005658. doi: 10.1371/journal.ppat.1005658

Chen, C. Y. (2013). A novel integrated framework and improved methodology of computer-aided drug design. *Curr. Top. Med. Chem.* 13, 965–988. doi: 10.2174/1568026611313090002

Copeland, N. K., and Aronson, N. E. (2015). Leishmaniasis: treatment updates and clinical practice guidelines review. *Curr. Opin. Infect. Dis.* 28, 426–437. doi: 10.1097/QCO.0000000000000194

Cordeiro, A. T., Feliciano, P. R., Pinheiro, M. P., and Nonato, M. C. (2012). Crystal structure of dihydroorotate dehydrogenase from Leishmania major. *Biochimie* 94, 1739–1748. doi: 10.1016/j.biochi.2012.04.003

Cramer, R. D., Patterson, D. E., and Bunce, J. D. (1988). Comparative molecular field analysis (CoMFA). 1. Effect of shape on binding of steroids to carrier proteins. *J. Am. Chem. Soc.* 110, 5959–5967. doi: 10.1021/ja00226a005

da Trindade Granato, J., dos Santos, J. A., Calixto, S. L., da Silva, N. P., da Silva, Martins, J., et al. (2018). Novel steroid derivatives: synthesis, antileishmanial activity, mechanism of action, and in silico physicochemical and pharmacokinetics studies. *Biomed. Pharmacother.* 106, 1082–1090. doi: 10.1016/j.biopha.2018.07.056

AUTHOR CONTRIBUTIONS

All authors listed have made a substantial, direct and intellectual contribution to the work, and approved it for publication.

FUNDING

We gratefully acknowledge financial support from the São Paulo Research Foundation (FAPESP), grants 2013/07600-3 and 2013/25658-9, and the National Council for Scientific and Technological Development (CNPq), Brazil.

De Luca, L., Ferro, S., Buemi, M. R., Monforte, A. M., Gitto, R., Schirmeister, T., et al. (2018). Discovery of benzimidazole-based *Leishmania mexicana* cysteine protease CPB2.8ΔCTE inhibitors as potential therapeutics for leishmaniasis. *Chem. Biol. Drug Des.* 92, 1585–1596. doi: 10.1111/cbdd.13326

Dikhit, M. R., Moharana, K. C., Sahoo, B. R., Sahoo, G. C., and Das, P. (2014). LeishMicrosatDB: open source database of repeat sequences detected in six fully sequenced Leishmania genomes. *Database* 2014:bau078. doi: 10.1093/database/bau078

dos Santos, R. N., Ferreira, L. G., and Andricopulo, A. D. (2018). "Practices in molecular docking and structure-based virtual screening," in *Computational Drug Discovery and Design. Methods in Molecular Biology*, eds M. Gore and U. Jagtap (New York, NY: Humana Press), 31–50.

Ferreira, L. G., Dos Santos, R. N., Oliva, G., and Andricopulo, A. D. (2015). Molecular docking and structure-based drug design strategies. *Molecules* 20, 13384–13421. doi: 10.3390/molecules200713384

Fiorillo, A., Colotti, G., Boffi, A., Baiocco, P., and Ilari, A. (2012). The crystal structures of the tryparedoxin-tryparedoxin peroxidase couple unveil the structural determinants of Leishmania detoxification pathway. *PLoS Negl. Trop. Dis.* 6:e1781. doi: 10.1371/journal.pntd.0001781

Folmer, R. H. (2016). Integrating biophysics with HTS-driven drug discovery projects. *Drug Discov. Today* 21, 491–498. doi: 10.1016/j.drudis.2016.01.011

Gilbert, I. H. (2013). Drug discovery for neglected diseases: molecular target-based and phenotypic approaches. *J. Med. Chem.* 56, 7719–7726. doi: 10.1021/jm400362b

Hailu, A., Dagne, D. A., and Boelaert, M. (2016). "Leishmaniasis," in *Neglected Tropical Diseases-Sub-Saharan Africa*, eds J. Gyapong and B. Oatin (Berlin: Springer), 87–112. doi: 10.1007/978-3-319-25471-5_5

Liu, R., Li, X., and Lam, K. S. (2017). Combinatorial chemistry in drug discovery. *Curr. Opin. Chem. Biol.* 38, 117–126. doi: 10.1016/j.cbpa.2017.03.017

Logan-Klumpler, F. J., De Silva, N., Boehme, U., Rogers, M. B., Velarde, G., McQuillan, J. A., et al. (2012). GeneDB–an annotation database for pathogens. *Nucleic Acids Res.* 40, D98–D108. doi: 10.1093/nar/gkr1032

Macalino, S., Gosu, V., Hong, S., and Choi, S. (2015). Role of computer-aided drug design in modern drug discovery. *Arch. Pharm. Res.* 38, 1686–1701. doi: 10.1007/s12272-015-0640-5

Magariños, M. P., Carmona, S. J., Crowther, G. J., Ralph, S. A., Roos, D. S., Shanmugam, D., et al. (2012). TDR Targets: a chemogenomics resource for neglected diseases. *Nucleic Acids Res.* 40, D1118–D1127. doi: 10.1093/nar/gkr1053

Mamidala, R., Majumdar, P., Jha, K. K., Bathula, C., Agarwal, R., Chary, M. T., et al. (2016). Identification of *Leishmania donovani* Topoisomerase 1 inhibitors via intuitive scaffold hopping and bioisosteric modification of known Top 1 inhibitors. *Sci. Rep.* 6:26603. doi: 10.1038/srep26603

Marreiros, B. C., Sena, F. V., Sousa, F. M., Oliveira, A. S., Soares, C. M., Batista, A. P., et al. (2017). Structural and Functional insights into the catalytic mechanism of the Type II NADH:quinone oxidoreductase family. *Sci. Rep.* 7:42303. doi: 10.1038/srep42303

Njogu, P. M., Guantai, E. M., Pavadai, E., and Chibale, K. (2016). Computer-Aided drug discovery approaches against the tropical infectious diseases malaria, tuberculosis, Trypanosomiasis, and Leishmaniasis. *ACS Infect. Dis.* 2, 8–31. doi: 10.1021/acsinfecdis.5b00093

Ochoa, R., Watowich, S. J., Flórez, A., Mesa, C. V., Robledo, S. M., and Muskus, C. (2016). Drug search for leishmaniasis: a virtual screening approach by grid computing. *J. Comput. Aided Mol. Des.* 30, 541–552. doi: 10.1007/s10822-016-9921-4

Ong, H. B., Sienkiewicz, N., Wyllie, S., and Fairlamb, A. H. (2011). Dissecting the metabolic roles of pteridine reductase 1 in *Trypanosoma brucei* and Leishmania major. *J. Biol. Chem.* 286, 10429–10438. doi: 10.1074/jbc.M110.209593

Patel, P., Mandlik, V., and Singh, S. (2016). LmSmdB: an integrated database for metabolic and gene regulatory network in Leishmania major and *Schistosoma mansoni. Genom. Data* 7, 115–118. doi: 10.1016/j.gdata.2015.12.012

Peña, I., Pilar Manzano, M., Cantizani, K. A., Alonso-Padilla, J., and Bardera, A. I. (2015). New compound sets identified from high throughput phenotypic screening against three kinetoplastid parasites: an open resource. *Sci. Rep.* 5:8771. doi: 10.1038/srep08771

Pommier, Y., Sun, Y., Huang, S. N., and Nitiss, J. L. (2016). Roles of eukaryotic topoisomerases in transcription, replication and genomic stability. *Nat. Rev. Mol. Cell. Biol.* 17, 703–721. doi: 10.1038/nrm.2016.111

Ponder, E. L., Freundlich, J. S., Sarker, M., and Ekins, S. (2014). Computational models for neglected diseases: gaps and opportunities. *Pharm. Res.* 2, 271–277. doi: 10.1007/s11095-013-1170-9

Preston, S., and Gasser, R. B. (2018). Working towards new drugs against parasitic worms in a public-development partnership. *Trends Parasitol.* 34, 4–6. doi: 10.1016/j.pt.2017.07.005

Rashid, U., Sultana, R., Shaheen, N., Hassan, S. F., Yaqoob, F., Ahmad, M. J., et al. (2016). Structure based medicinal chemistry-driven strategy to design substituted dihydropyrimidines as potential antileishmanial agents. *Eur. J. Med. Chem.* 115, 230–244. doi: 10.1016/j.ejmech.2016.03.022

Reguera, R. M., Calvo-Álvarez, E., Alvarez-Velilla, R., and Balaña-Fouce, R. (2014). Target-based vs. phenotypic screenings in Leishmania drug discovery: a marriage of convenience or a dialogue of the deaf? *Int. J. Parasitol. Drugs Drug Resist.* 4, 355–357. doi: 10.1016/j.ijpddr.2014.05.001

Rognan, D. (2017). The impact of in silico screening in the discovery of novel and safer drug candidates. *Pharmacol. Ther.* 175, 47–66. doi: 10.1016/j.pharmthera.2017.02.034

Stevanović, S., Perdih, A., Senćanski, M., Glišić, S., Duarte, M., Tomás, A. M., et al. (2018). In Silico Discovery of a Substituted 6-Methoxy-quinalidine with Leishmanicidal Activity in *Leishmania infantum. Molecules* 23:772. doi: 10.3390/molecules23040772

Sunyoto, T., Potet, J., and Boelaert, M. (2018). Why miltefosine-a life-saving drug for leishmaniasis-is unavailable to people who need it the most. *BMJ Glob. Health* 3:e000709. doi: 10.1136/bmjgh-2018-000709

Temraz, M. G., Elzahhar, P. A., El-Din, A., Bekhit, A., Bekhit, A. A., Labib, H. F., et al. (2018). Anti-leishmanial click modifiable thiosemicarbazones: design, synthesis, biological evaluation and in silico studies. *Eur. J. Med. Chem.* 151, 585–600. doi: 10.1016/j.ejmech.2018.04.003

van Montfort, R. L. M., and Workman, P. (2017). Structure-based drug design: aiming for a perfect fit. *Essays Biochem.* 61, 431–437. doi: 10.1042/EBC20170052

Yousefinejad, S., and Hemmateenejad, B. (2015). Chemometrics tools in QSAR/QSPR studies: a historical perspective. *Chemometr. Intell. Lab. Syst.* 149, 177–204. doi: 10.1016/j.chemolab.2015.06.016

2

Molecular Simulations of Carbohydrates with a Fucose-Binding *Burkholderia ambifaria* Lectin Suggest Modulation by Surface Residues Outside the Fucose-Binding Pocket

Tamir Dingjan[1], Anne Imberty[2], Serge Pérez[3], Elizabeth Yuriev[1]* and Paul A. Ramsland[4, 5, 6, 7]*

[1] *Medicinal Chemistry, Monash Institute of Pharmaceutical Sciences, Monash University, Melbourne, VIC, Australia,* [2] *Centre de Recherches sur les Macromolécules Végétales, Centre National de la Recherche Scientifique UPR5301, Université Grenoble Alpes, Grenoble, France,* [3] *Département de Pharmacochimie Moléculaire, Centre National de la Recherche Scientifique, UMR5063, Université Grenoble Alpes, Grenoble, France,* [4] *School of Science, RMIT University, Melbourne, VIC, Australia,* [5] *Department of Surgery Austin Health, University of Melbourne, Melbourne, VIC, Australia,* [6] *Department of Immunology, Central Clinical School, Monash University, Melbourne, VIC, Australia,* [7] *Burnet Institute, Melbourne, VIC, Australia*

*Correspondence:
Elizabeth Yuriev
elizabeth.yuriev@monash.edu
Paul A Ramsland
paul.ramsland@rmit.edu.au

Burkholderia ambifaria is an opportunistic respiratory pathogen belonging to the *Burkholderia cepacia* complex, a collection of species responsible for the rapidly fatal cepacia syndrome in cystic fibrosis patients. A fucose-binding lectin identified in the *B. ambifaria* genome, BambL, is able to adhere to lung tissue, and may play a role in respiratory infection. X-ray crystallography has revealed the bound complex structures for four fucosylated human blood group epitopes (blood group B, H type 1, H type 2, and Le^x determinants). The present study employed computational approaches, including docking and molecular dynamics (MD), to extend the structural analysis of BambL-oligosaccharide complexes to include four additional blood group saccharides (A, Le^a, Le^b, and Le^y) and a library of blood-group-related carbohydrates. Carbohydrate recognition is dominated by interactions with fucose via a hydrogen-bonding network involving Arg15, Glu26, Ala38, and Trp79 and a stacking interaction with Trp74. Additional hydrogen bonds to non-fucose residues are formed with Asp30, Tyr35, Thr36, and Trp74. BambL recognition is dominated by interactions with fucose, but also features interactions with other parts of the ligands that may modulate specificity or affinity. The detailed computational characterization of the BambL carbohydrate-binding site provides guidelines for the future design of lectin inhibitors.

Keywords: blood group determinants, *Burkholderia ambifaria,* docking, fucose, molecular dynamics

INTRODUCTION

Cystic fibrosis morbidity is mostly due to respiratory infection by opportunistic pathogens (Lyczak et al., 2002; O'Sullivan and Freedman, 2009; Ciofu et al., 2013; Caverly et al., 2015). *Burkholderia cepacia* is one of the most dangerous pathogens isolated from cystic fibrosis patients; 20% of infected individuals succumb to a rapidly fatal pneumonia termed "cepacia syndrome" (Zahariadis et al., 2003; Blackburn et al., 2004; Lynch, 2009). Isolated *B. cepacia* strains have been classified into a steadily increasing number of species, referred to collectively as the *B. cepacia* complex (currently consisting of 20 species Vandamme et al., 1997; De Smet et al., 2015; Martinucci et al., 2016). Most members of the complex are resistant to multiple clinically used antibiotics, making the search for new therapeutics more urgent (Zhou et al., 2007; Loutet and Valvano, 2011; Podnecky et al., 2015). *Burkholderia ambifaria,* a member of the *B. cepacia* complex, has been isolated from both clinical and environmental samples (Coenye et al., 2001). In addition to infecting human respiratory tissue, *B. ambifaria* can colonize plant rhizospheres, where it promotes growth and protects against invading fungi (Li et al., 2002; Lee et al., 2006; Parra-Cota et al., 2014).

Previously, a carbohydrate-binding protein (named "BambL") was identified in the *B. ambifaria* genome; binding studies using human tissues suggest it may play a role in infection (Audfray et al., 2012). Opportunistic bacteria often adhere to tissues by binding to host carbohydrates using carbohydrate-recognizing proteins (lectins) displayed at the bacterial surface (Bavington and Page, 2005; Imberty and Varrot, 2008; Pieters, 2011; Audfray et al., 2013). Among the many carbohydrates present on human cells, fucose-bearing blood group determinants are often recognized by bacterial lectins (Lindén et al., 2008; Anstee, 2010; Holmner et al., 2010). In the cystic fibrosis respiratory epithelium, cell-surface carbohydrates, present on glycolipids, N-glycoproteins, and mucins, are more fucosylated than in healthy tissue (Rhim et al., 2001; Venkatakrishnan et al., 2015). This increased fucosylation may promote adhesion by fucose-recognizing pathogens (Stoykova and Scanlin, 2008; Audfray et al., 2013). Known cystic fibrosis pathogens *Pseudomonas aeruginosa, Burkholderia cenocepacia* and *Aspergillus fumigatus,* all have lectins that bind to fucosylated human blood group carbohydrates (Mitchell et al., 2002; Imberty et al., 2004; Sulak et al., 2010, 2011; Houser et al., 2013, 2015). Significantly, the *P. aeruginosa* lectins are strongly associated with respiratory tissue damage and bacterial load in a mouse model of lung injury, and treatment with monosaccharides, able to specifically inhibit lectin binding, reduces infection (Chemani et al., 2009). Similar effects have been reported in a human *P. aeruginosa* infection case study (von Bismarck et al., 2001) suggesting that interfering with lectin-carbohydrate interactions may offer a new frontier in anti-infective treatment (Sharon, 2006; Pera and Peters, 2014). Lectin inhibitor design begins with a thorough understanding

of the role of each functional group in the natively recognized carbohydrate (Ernst and Magnani, 2009).

The crystallographic structure of BambL has been solved, revealing a six-bladed β-propeller fold formed by three separate protomers (Audfray et al., 2012). Each subunit contains a single carbohydrate-binding site; upon oligomerization, three additional binding sites are formed at the interfaces between protomers, for a total of six binding sites in the β-propeller fold. The intra- and inter-protomeric sites have similar architectures and (for most blood group carbohydrates) similar binding properties. For this reason, the present work addresses interactions within the intra-protomeric site only. Crystal structures of BambL have also been obtained bound to multiple fucosylated human blood group tetrasaccharides: H type 1, H type 2, B type 2, and Le^x (PDB IDs: 3ZW2, 3ZZV, 3ZWE, and 3ZW1; Audfray et al., 2012; Topin et al., 2013; **Figure 1**). In each case, the carbohydrate is bound via a buried fucose residue, which participates in a network of hydrogen bonds within a tight fucose-binding pocket. Blood group carbohydrate binding specificity has also been determined by glycan array and affinity quantified by titration microcalorimetry: strongest affinity is for H type 2 tetrasaccharide (K_D 7.5 μM) and Le^y pentasaccharide (K_D 11.1 μM; Audfray et al., 2012). This binding preference indicates that BambL is more selective for blood and tissue carbohydrate determinants containing the type 2 epitope Fucα1-2Galβ1-4GlcNAc. Several of the blood group and tissue antigens recognized by BambL have not been structurally characterized in complex with the lectin (e.g., Le^y, Le^b, and A). Additionally, while existing crystal structures describe static recognition, the dynamic behavior of BambL complexes has not been described. The relative contributions of individual binding interactions to saccharide recognition is also unknown. Extending the structural analysis of BambL-blood group complexes to probe these aspects of recognition will enhance understanding of carbohydrate recognition and facilitate inhibitor design.

The goal of this computational study was to characterize BambL-saccharide binding modes and to inform future *in silico* or structure-based design of inhibitors for this bacterial lectin. We were interested in identifying lectin residues that are critical for ligand recognition and thus could be used as constraints in prospective virtual screening. In particular, we investigated whether the BambL binding site is restricted to recognizing fucose or is capable of engaging non-fucose saccharides using additional interactions. We first used docking and site mapping to study binding modes in complexes featuring A, B, O (H), and Lewis fucosylated carbohydrates and a library of blood-group-related saccharides. The dynamic behavior of these systems was then explored by molecular dynamics (MD) simulations. The recognition of fucose-containing saccharides by BambL is accomplished by a hydrogen-bonding network between fucose and Arg15, Glu26, Trp79, and to a lesser extent Ala38. A hydrophobic contact is made between the fucose non-polar face and the Trp79 imidazole. Additional hydrogen bonds outside the fucose-binding pocket to Asp30, Thr36, Trp74, and Tyr35 are formed in complex with multiple blood group and blood-group-related saccharides. Residues involved in these interactions are consistently engaged by blood-group-related saccharides,

---

Abbreviations: BambL, *Burkholderia ambifaria* lectin; H1, H type 1; H2, H type 2; Le^a, Lewis a; Le^b, Lewis b; Le^x, Lewis x; Le^y, Lewis y; MD, Molecular Dynamics; PDB, Protein Data Bank; vdW, van der Waals; RMSD, root mean square deviation

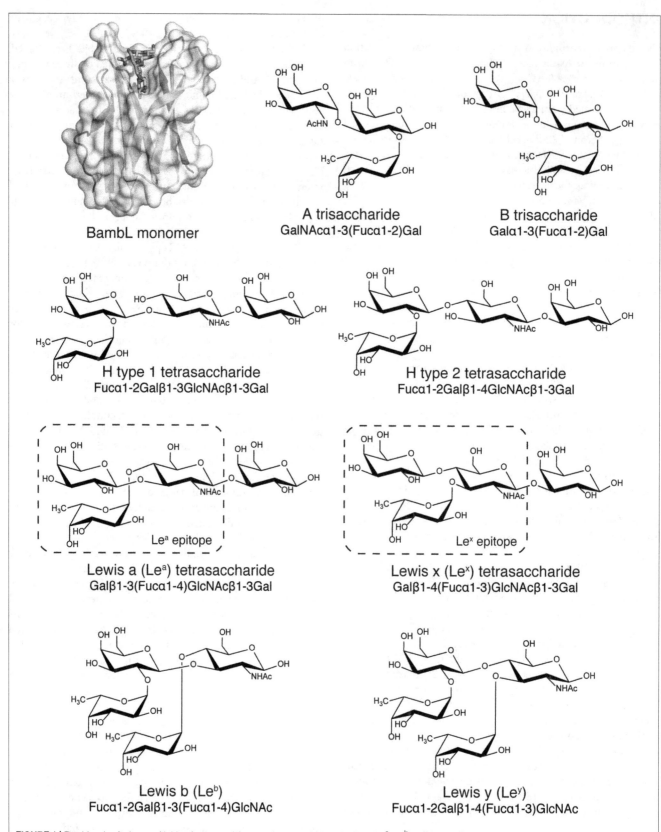

BambL monomer

A trisaccharide
GalNAcα1-3(Fucα1-2)Gal

B trisaccharide
Galα1-3(Fucα1-2)Gal

H type 1 tetrasaccharide
Fucα1-2Galβ1-3GlcNAcβ1-3Gal

H type 2 tetrasaccharide
Fucα1-2Galβ1-4GlcNAcβ1-3Gal

Le^a epitope

Lewis a (Le^a) tetrasaccharide
Galβ1-3(Fucα1-4)GlcNAcβ1-3Gal

Le^x epitope

Lewis x (Le^x) tetrasaccharide
Galβ1-4(Fucα1-3)GlcNAcβ1-3Gal

Lewis b (Le^b)
Fucα1-2Galβ1-3(Fucα1-4)GlcNAc

Lewis y (Le^y)
Fucα1-2Galβ1-4(Fucα1-3)GlcNAc

FIGURE 1 | BambL subunit shown with blood group and tissue antigen saccharides (A, B, H, Le^a, Le^b, Le^x, and Le^y) used for simulation. BambL structure from PDB ID: 3ZZV, with the intra-protomeric binding site and ligand shown.

suggesting they may be valuable interaction targets for BambL inhibitors.

MATERIALS AND METHODS

A single BambL subunit containing an intra-protomeric (Audfray et al., 2012) binding site was used in the below computational studies.

Blood-Group and Blood-Group-Related Carbohydrate Structure Generation

Low energy blood-group and blood-group-related carbohydrate structures were generated and simulation parameters produced using the GLYCAM web portal (Woods, 2005; Kirschner et al., 2008). The A and B determinants were modeled as trisaccharides for comparison to previous binding data for the soluble type A determinant (Audfray et al., 2012). The H type 1, H type 2, Le^a and Le^x determinants were modeled as tetrasaccharides for consistency to previously determined binding data (Audfray et al., 2012) and the Le^b and Le^y determinants were modeled as tetrasaccharides to encompass the entire epitope. The library of blood-group-related structures is shown in Supplementary Figure 1.

Docking

Docking experiments were performed using the docking program Glide 6.8 (Friesner et al., 2004, 2006; Halgren et al., 2004; Schrödinger, 2014a) available within the molecular modeling package Maestro (Schrödinger, 2014a,b). The BambL crystallographic complexes were downloaded from the Protein Data Bank, PDB (Berman et al., 2000), and the protein structures prepared using the Protein Preparation Wizard tool (Madhavi Sastry et al., 2013; Schrödinger, 2014b). During this step, structural details required for the docking calculation were specified. Double bond orders were applied for backbone carbonyl and aromatic side chain moieties, hydrogen atoms were added to the structure, water molecules removed, and disulfide bonds created between cysteine side chain sulfur atoms in close proximity. Missing atoms and side chains were added based on the protein's primary sequence using the Prime tool (Schrödinger, 2014c). To remove steric clashes between added hydrogen atoms, a minimization step was then conducted on hydrogen atoms only, using the OPLS2005 forcefield (Banks et al., 2005). A receptor grid was generated using default settings, with the binding site box centered on the crystallographic ligand. Ligands were docked into the receptor grid using Standard Precision mode with default settings. All carbohydrate atoms were treated flexibly during docking, including all glycosidic linkages and exocyclic groups. The lowest-energy docked poses were retained for MD simulation. Docked poses were filtered by glycosidic dihedral angle to exclude unfavorable high energy carbohydrate conformations. Cutoff values for dihedral filtering were chosen for each glycosidic linkage based on isoenergy contours previously calculated with the MM3 force field from Imberty et al. (1995). Conformations with dihedrals in the following ranges were removed from the analysis: Fucα1-2Gal $\varphi < -130°$ & $180° < \psi < 360°$; GalNAcα1-3Gal $\varphi > 240°$;

Galβ1-3GlcNAc $\varphi > 0°$ & $180° < \psi < -60°$. Thus, we have used energy maps to post-filter docked poses as a means of retaining reasonable conformations. These energy maps have been commonly used to evaluate carbohydrate conformations obtained from simulations and experimental work [for example Jackson et al. (2014) and Tempel et al. (2002)]. Hydrogen bonds and contacts were tallied using MDAnalysis (Michaud-Agrawal et al., 2011; distance = 3.0 Å, angle = 120).

Site Mapping

All BambL-blood group carbohydrate complexes were examined using LigPlot (Wallace et al., 1995; Laskowski and Swindells, 2011). Only poses that passed the glycosidic torsion filter requirements (see above), were used for site mapping, following a previously developed method (Yuriev et al., 2001; Agostino et al., 2009b, 2011, 2013; Dingjan et al., 2015a). In brief, each individual hydrogen bond made by a particular BambL residue was counted toward the hydrogen-bond tally. Non-polar vdW interactions between a specific BambL residue and a carbohydrate residue were counted as a single interaction toward the tally. The tallies were normalized to percentages of the total number of hydrogen bond or vdW interactions. Site maps were generated using residue inclusion cutoff values for lectin-carbohydrate complexes of 90% for hydrogen bonds, 0% for vdW interactions (Agostino et al., 2013). Site map images were rendered using PyMOL (Schrödinger, 2014d).

Molecular Dynamics

MD simulations were performed using Gromacs 5.0.4 (Berendsen et al., 1995; Van Der Spoel et al., 2005; Hess et al., 2008; Pronk et al., 2013). Proteins were parameterized using the AMBER99SB-ILDN (Lindorff-Larsen et al., 2010) forcefield. Carbohydrate topologies were generated using the GLYCAM06 (Kirschner et al., 2008) force field via the glycam.org web portal. The resulting AMBER-formatted topology was converted to GROMACS format using the "acpype" tool (Sousa da Silva and Vranken, 2012). The correctly formatted carbohydrate topology was then combined with the protein topology to describe the entire protein-carbohydrate system. Protein-carbohydrate docked complexes were placed in a rhombic dodecahedral box with a 10 Å minimum distance between solute and box wall, and subsequently solvated using the TIP3P water model. To maintain electrostatic neutrality, Na$^+$ and Cl$^-$ counterions were added by the *genion* module. To remove steric clashes between nearby atoms, the system contents were minimized using the steepest descent algorithm (maximum steps: 50,000). The positions and velocities of the solvent molecules and ions were then equilibrated at constant volume and temperature (NVT ensemble) using three restraint settings: with all protein heavy atoms restrained for 100 ps, then with only backbone atoms restrained for 100 ps (both at 10 K), followed by a 100 ps equilibration without restraints at 300 K. Finally, the pressure of the system was equilibrated for 300 ps without restraints at constant atmospheric pressure (NPT ensemble) at 310 K. During all equilibration steps, positional restraints were applied to protein residues using LINCS (Hess, 2007). The coordinates from the final equilibration step were used to begin production simulation, which was conducted for 400 ns.

For all MD simulations in the NPT ensemble, temperature was kept constant using the velocity rescaling thermostat coupled with a time constant of 0.1 ps. Pressure was held constant at 1 bar using the Parrinello-Rahman barometer, coupled with a time constant of 2 ps. Equations of motion were integrated using a leap-frog integrator with a 2 fs timestep. Long-range electrostatics were evaluated using the Particle Mesh Ewald method. Cutoff values for Coulomb and vdW interactions were set to 1.0 nm. Complexes with blood group carbohydrate ligands were simulated in triplicate, complexes with blood-group-related carbohydrate ligands were simulated in singlicate. Each replicate was commenced using randomized velocities, resulting in independent simulations with different initial velocities.

Analysis of MD Simulations

Hydrogen bonds in MD simulations were analyzed using the Baker-Hubbard method implemented in the MDTraj (McGibbon et al., 2015) software library. An occupancy value was assigned to each hydrogen bond by calculating the percentage of simulation frames in which the bond was present. Glycosidic dihedral angles were measured using MDTraj and compared to calculated isoenergy contours (see above). Carbohydrate ring conformations were analyzed using Best Four-Member Plane method from GLYCAM (Makeneni et al., 2014). CH-π interactions were represented by measuring a shortest distance from either of the fucose atoms C3, C4, C5, or C6 to atoms of the indole ring of Trp74. Atom labeling corresponds to the conventions of the PDB exchange dictionary (Berman et al., 2003).

RESULTS

Generation of BambL-Blood Group Complexes by Docking

To decide which of the crystallographic BambL receptor structures to use in this study, we compared complex structures predicted by re-docking with respective crystallographic complexes. The results of these cognate and cross-docking experiments are shown in **Table 1**, **Figure 2**. The Le[x] tetrasaccharide was poorly docked (RMSD > 2 Å) into all BambL structures. However, all four lectin structures afforded approximately equal performance when used as a receptor for the other three carbohydrate ligands: overall RMSD values of 1.09–2.62 and 0.14–0.56 Å for the buried fucose (Fucα1-2Gal) were observed. The crystallographic BambL structure from the PDB ID: 3ZZV complex was used as the receptor structure for site mapping and MD with all carbohydrates shown in **Figure 1**.

In a second step, all blood group saccharides were docked in BambL (PDB ID: 3ZZV) and the top docked poses were analyzed for structural features relevant to recognition (**Table 2**). In all cases except Le[x], the majority of binding interactions were made via a single buried fucose residue (**Figure 3**). The difucosylated Le[b] and Le[y] possess two fucose residues (Fucα1-2Gal and Fucα1-4GlcNAc in Le[b] or Fucα1-3GlcNAc in Le[y]) and therefore may occupy the fucose-binding pocket in two ways. Of the docked Le[b]

TABLE 1 | Top scoring docked pose characterization for BambL-blood group saccharide complexes.

| Ligand | RMSD of top docked pose to crystal structure (Å)[a] | | | |
	3ZWE (1.75 Å)	3ZW2 (1.60 Å)	3ZZV (1.68 Å)	3ZW1 (1.60 Å)
B[b]	**1.68 (0.42)**[c]	2.04 (0.25)	2.13 (0.36)	2.62 (0.28)
H1	1.80 (0.47)	**1.09 (0.29)**[c]	1.47 (0.14)	2.02 (0.27)
H2[b]	1.90 (0.39)	2.42 (0.39)	**1.56 (0.25)**[c]	1.52 (0.56)
Le[x]	9.47 (7.95)	4.61 (0.58)	6.94 (10.31)	**7.01 (0.32)**[c]

[a]The experimental resolution of each crystallographic BambL complex is shown in brackets beneath the PDB ID. RMSD values compare the ligand portion common between the docked and crystallographic ligand; RMSD values in brackets compare the fucose portion of the docked ligand to the fucose portion of the crystallographic ligand.
[b]Cross-docking performed using the ligands used in site mapping and molecular dynamics (**Figure 1**). Cognate docking performed using the ligand length present in the crystallographic complex.
[c]Values shown in bold indicate cognate docking experiments.

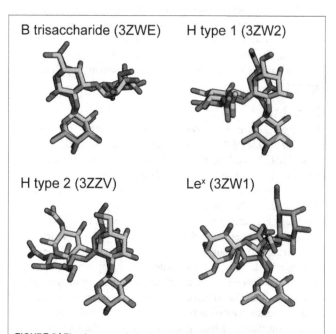

FIGURE 2 | Blood group carbohydrates docked into the BambL binding site of PDB ID: 3ZZV (orange), compared to their respective experimentally determined poses (green). The PDB IDs for experimental poses are indicated. For clarity, all carbohydrates are shown as the non-reducing-end trisaccharide without hydrogen atoms.

poses produced here, only the Fucα1-2Gal residue was predicted in the binding pocket. As for the docked Le[y] poses, all of the top 20 ranked poses positioned the Fucα1-2Gal residue in the pocket, with the exception of poses at rank 5 and 6 that predicted the Fucα1-3GlcNAc residue in the fucose binding pocket.

As expected, recognition of the buried fucose (Fucα1-2Gal) was governed by a conserved hydrogen-bonding network and a single hydrophobic stacking interaction (Supplementary Table 1). Rather than interacting via a buried fucose, the Le[x] top docked pose was placed "back-to-front" with the reducing end galactose in the fucose-binding pocket, and the fucose directed away from the protein.

TABLE 2 | Top scoring docked pose characterization for BambL-blood group saccharide complexes.

Ligand	Fucose RMSD (Å)[a]	Glycosidic dihedral angles[b]						Hydrogen bonds[c]	Docking score (kcal/mol)
		φ	ψ	φ	ψ	φ	ψ		
A tri	0.53	Fucα1-2Gal		GalNAcα1-3Gal				GalNAc2-H6O...Asp30-OD1	−5.848
		−106.8	55.9	81.3	76.8			GalNAc2-O4...Trp8-HE1	
B tri	0.24	Fucα1-2Gal		Galα1-3Gal				Gla3-H6O...Asp30-OD1	−5.890
		−107.9	63.9	49.5	45.8			Gla3-O3...Trp74-HE1	
H1	0.43	Fucα1-2Gal		Galβ1-3GlcNAc		GlcNAcβ1-3Gal		GlcNAc2-H4O...Asp30-OD2	−6.879
		−116.2	−129.6	−42.2	146.6	−106.1	159.2	GlcNAc2-O2N...Trp74-HE1	
H2	0.38	Fucα1-2Gal		Galβ1-4GlcNAc		GlcNAcβ1-3Gal		Gal1-H3O...Tyr35-O	−6.597
		−106.0	−88.0	−42.2	−91.8	−81.8	101.0	Gal1-H6O...Asp77-OD2	
								GlcNAc2-H6O...Gly76-O	
Le[a]	0.30	Fucα1-4GlcNAc		Galβ1-3GlcNAc		GlcNAcβ1-3Gal		Gal4-H2O...Asp30-OD2	−5.706
		−138.3	−147.3	−64.8	138.7	−68.1	96.6		
Le[x]	10.22	Fucα1-3GlcNAc		Galβ1-4GlcNAc		GlcNAcβ1-3Gal		Gal1-O5...Ala38-H	−5.786
		−76.4	151.5	−72.6	−112.7	−66.5	89.6	Gal1-O6...Trp79-HE1	
								Gal1-H6O...Glu26-OE1	
								Gal1-O4...Arg15-HH21	
								Gal1-H4O...Tyr35-OH	
								Fuc4-H2O...Asp30-OD2	
								Fuc4-H3O...Asp30-O	
								Gal3-H2O...Ser55-O	
								Gal3-O6...Thr11-HG1	
								Gal3-H6O...Ser13-OG	
Le[b]	0.38	Fucα1-2Gal		Fucα1-4GlcNAc		Galβ1-3GlcNAc		Fuc2-H2O...Asp30-OD1	−7.065
		−83.6	−98.8	−70.3	96.5	−39.5	166.6	Fuc2-O3...Trp8-HE1	
								GlcNAc1-O6...Trp74-HE1	
								GlcNAc1-H6O...Val57-O	
								GlcNAc1-HO1...Gly76-O	
Le[y]	0.33	Fucα1-2Gal		Fucα1-3GlcNAc		Galβ1-4GlcNAc		Fuc2-H2O...Asp30-OD2	−7.007
		−105.3	−138.3	−83.8	−51.3	−56.0	−103.7	GlcNAc1-H2N...Asp30-OD1	
								GlcNAc1-O1...Trp8-HE1	
								GlcNAc1-O6...Trp74-HE1	

[a] Calculated for buried fucose residue heavy atoms between crystallographic saccharide (PDB ID: 3ZZV) and docked ligand.
[b] Dihedral angles defined as: φ, O_5-C_1-O_1-C_x; ψ, C_1-O_1-C_x-C_{x+1}.
[c] Excluding hydrogen bonds involving the buried fucose residue.

Apart from interactions with the buried fucose residue, additional hydrogen bonds are made between non-fucose residues and amino acids in the four β-turn loops surrounding the fucose-binding pocket (**Table 2**). The most frequently participating residue, Asp30, interacts with non-fucose portions of multiple saccharides (B, H1, Le[a], Le[b], and Le[y]). The imidazole side-chain of Trp74 (which stacks against the buried fucose) also donates a hydrogen bond to non-fucose residues in several cases. In each case, the hydrogen bond is accepted by atoms in a similar location: two residues away from the buried fucose, at the GlcNAc 6-position (Le[b], Le[y]), Gal/GalNAc 3-position (A, B), or GlcNAc 2-position (H1). The presence of hydrogen bonds between non-fucose portions and loop residues suggests that BambL recognition may not rely solely on interactions with a single buried fucose.

Glycosidic dihedral angles in top docked poses lie close to global or secondary minima in previously calculated (Imberty et al., 1995) energy maps (see Supplementary Figures 2, 3). An exception is the Fucα1-2Gal linkage, which is positioned in between minima in the H type 1, H type 2, Le[b] and Le[y] top poses. In the A and B trisaccharide complexes, the Fucα1-2Gal linkage adopted the lowest energy conformation. These results agree with earlier BambL-blood group docking by Topin et al. (2013) in which top docked pose glycosidic linkages also occupied a range of energetic minima.

Site Mapping of BambL-Blood Group Complexes

Site mapping reveals binding site residues that are frequently involved in interactions throughout an ensemble of docked poses. Site maps for BambL-blood group complexes are shown in **Figure 4**. These maps are based on docking results for all carbohydrates shown in **Figure 1**. The BambL site maps agree

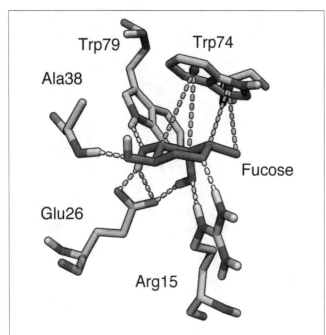

FIGURE 3 | Binding site interactions involving fucose in BambL-blood group saccharide docked poses. Hydrogen bonds shown as yellow dashes, hydrophobic interactions shown as teal dashes. Non-polar hydrogens omitted for clarity.

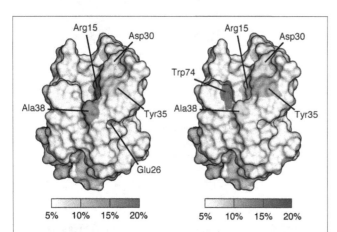

FIGURE 4 | Site maps of a BambL subunit showing binding site residues involved in docked pose interactions. Residues involved in 5% or fewer interactions are colored white; residues involved in 20% or greater interactions are colored red (for hydrogen bonding) or blue (for van der Waals). Residues with intermediate involvement are shaded according to the color scale.

with crystallographic complexes, identifying multiple residues in the fucose binding pocket known to interact with fucose in crystallographic structures (PDB IDs: 3ZW2, 3ZZV, 3ZWE, and 3ZW1; Audfray et al., 2012; Topin et al., 2013). Across the docked pose ensemble, hydrogen bonds were frequently formed to Arg15 (27.9%), Ala38 (11.6%), and Glu26 (13.7%), all located within the fucose-binding pocket. Surprisingly, Trp79 (4.9%), also in the crystallographic fucose pocket, was not often involved throughout the docked pose ensemble. van der Waals (vdW) interactions were frequently made with Trp74 (14.6%) in the

fucose pocket, in close agreement with crystallographic bound complexes. Site maps also revealed new interactions not seen in crystal structures, identifying hydrogen bonding to Asp30 (7.1%) and vdW interaction with Tyr35 (11.1%) as regularly occurring across all docked poses.

Molecular Dynamics Simulations of BambL-Blood Group Complexes

To investigate the dynamic behavior of BambL-blood group complexes, the lowest-energy poses generated by docking were simulated in explicit solvent. For difucosylated Le^b and Le^y, the lowest-energy poses with the Fucα1-2Gal residue in the fucose-binding pocket were used. The poorly docked Le^x complex was also simulated, but quickly dissociated from the protein or was unstable in the binding site (see Supplementary Figure 4). To probe the dynamic behavior of the Le^x binding interactions, the crystallographic complex was used instead (PDB ID: 3ZW1).

During MD simulations, all fucose-anchored blood group saccharides (A, B, H type 1, H type 2, Le^a, Le^b, Le^y) remained bound to BambL without dissociation for the entire duration (400 ns). Structural fluctuations in ligand RMSD were below 2 Å in all bound complexes, reflecting relatively small changes in ligand positions and geometries during the MD simulations (see Supplementary Figure 5). Carbohydrate ring conformations were found to generally adopt one of the two chair conformations ($^1C_4$ or $^4C_1$), while the GlcNAc rings in the H type 2, Le^a, and Le^x exhibited some variation (see Supplementary Figure 6). A similar hydrogen-bonding pattern was observed across all blood group simulations (**Figures 5, 6**), featuring interactions between the buried fucose residue and the fucose-binding pocket: Glu26 acidic group to O3 and O4 hydroxyl protons, Arg15 guanidinium to O4 and O5 oxygen atoms, and Trp79 indole to O3 oxygen atom. These hydrogen bonds were highly occupied (between 60 and 90% of simulation frames), with the exception of the Glu26 hydrogen bonds in the Le^b complex (50–60%). The high occupancy of these hydrogen bonds indicates the dominant role played by fucose in BambL-carbohydrate binding.

In addition to the above interactions, a low-occupancy (up to 30% of simulation frames) hydrogen bond was observed between the Ala38 backbone amide proton and the buried fucose 2-position hydroxyl oxygen atom. In contrast to the highly occupied hydrogen bonds, this interaction engages a backbone proton rather than a side-chain; combined with the low occupancy, this suggests a less significant contribution by this hydrogen bond to carbohydrate binding. Alongside hydrogen-bonding interactions, stacking of the fucose C3-C4-C5-C6 hydrophobic face against the Trp74 indole ring was consistently maintained during simulation (see Supplementary Figure 7).

Hydrogen bonds to non-fucose portions of the carbohydrate ligands were formed at low to moderate occupancies (20–50%) with fucose-binding residue Trp74 (Le^y: 44%, Le^a: 23%, Le^x: 22%) and surface residue Asp30 (B: 37%, H type 1: 44%, Le^b: 24%, Le^y: 31%).

Glycosidic linkage conformations explored during MD simulations occupy global, and occasionally secondary, minima

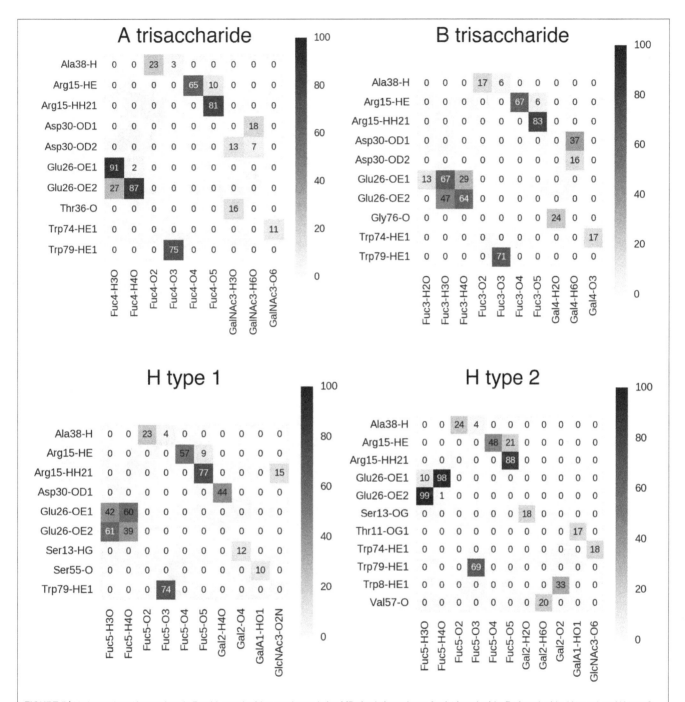

FIGURE 5 | Hydrogen bond interactions in BambL-saccharide complexes during MD simulations shown for A trisaccharide, B trisaccharide, H type 1 and H type 2 blood groups. Atoms are named to the conventions of the PDB exchange dictionary. Grid cells are colored and labeled by average occupancy from three replicate simulations. Occupancy values were calculated by dividing the number of frames in which the hydrogen bond exists by the total number of simulation frames.

(Figure 7). As observed in docking, the Fucα1-2Gal linkage is again an exception, adopting a position intermediate between the two minima for the entire duration of simulation in the H type 1, H type 2, Le^b and Le^y complexes. In the H type 1 and Le^b complexes, this linkage explores a narrower range of higher-energy conformations compared to H type 2 and Le^y. It is possible that this difference between the calculated energetic minima and the conformations observed in simulation

is due to the presence of the protein. Force field-based energy contours describe the energetic behavior of each linkage as an unbound disaccharide in vacuum (Imberty et al., 1995), while simulation of the bound complex introduces protein, water, and other saccharide units within the tri- or tetrasaccharide, all of which influence conformational behavior. A recent example of the influence of protein binding on carbohydrate conformation is the Le^x saccharide, which occupies well-characterized "closed"

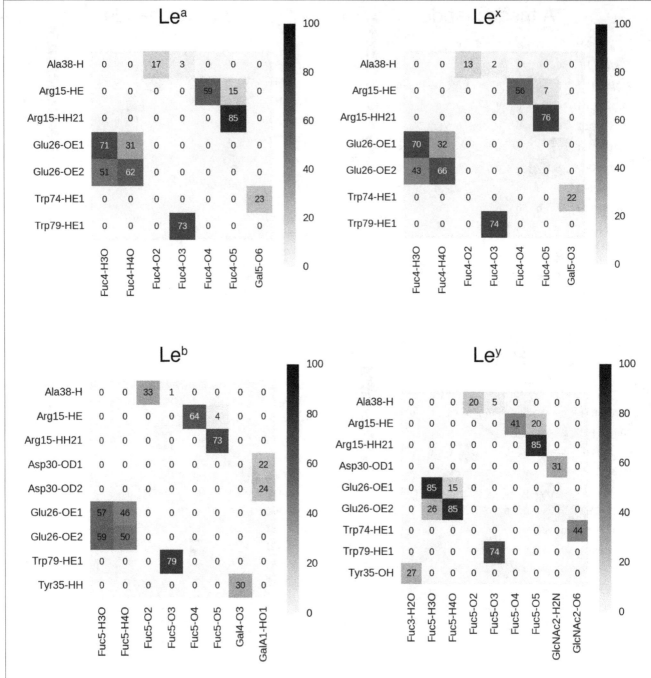

FIGURE 6 | Hydrogen bond interactions in BambL-saccharide complexes during MD simulations shown for Lewis group saccharides. Atoms are named to the conventions of the PDB exchange dictionary. Grid cells are colored and labeled by average occupancy from three replicate simulations. Occupancy values were calculated by dividing the number of frames in which the hydrogen bond exists by the total number of simulation frames.

conformations in solution and "open" conformations when bound to the RSL lectin (Topin et al., 2016; defined by the relative positions of the fucose and galactose rings). In the present study, the Le^x saccharide maintained an open conformation during MD simulation, corresponding to shapes "Open V" and "Open II" in the scheme defined by Topin et al. (2016) consistent with its continuous occupation of the binding site during simulation (see Supplementary Figure 8).

In the A and B trisaccharide simulations, the N-acetylgalactosamine and non-reducing end galactose move more freely than the saccharide occupying the same position in the other ligands. The Fucα1-2Gal glycosidic linkage in these two saccharides occupies two conformations, defined by variation in the ψ-angle between −60° and +100°. The A trisaccharide explores both, while the B trisaccharide only occupies the former conformation (**Figure 7**).

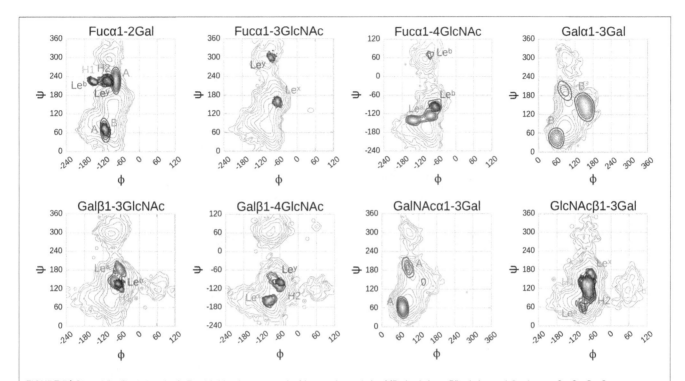

FIGURE 7 | Glycosidic dihedral angles in BambL-blood group saccharide complexes during MD simulations. Dihedrals are defined as: φ, O_5-C_1-O_1-C_x; ψ, C_1-O_1-C_x-C_{x+1}. Contour plots color coding: gray, calculated energy landscapes of constituting linkages; brown, A; light blue B; green H1; dark blue, H2; cyan Le^a; pink, Le^b; orange Le^x; red Le^y. Contour plot lines mark intervals of 1 kcal/mol.

Docking and MD Simulations of Complexes with Blood-Group-Related Carbohydrates

Interactions between BambL and blood group/tissue carbohydrates was mediated mainly via the single buried fucose, with occasional hydrogen bonds formed between non-fucose atoms and residues on loops surrounding the binding pocket. Identifying these non-fucose binding interactions may provide opportunities to improve inhibitor affinity for BambL beyond the current fucose-based inhibitors.

The potential for non-fucose binding interactions to form in BambL-saccharide complexes was explored by simulating complexes of 36 blood-group-related carbohydrates to the protein (i.e., a focused carbohydrate library). The related carbohydrates ranged in size from di- to heptasaccharides and were composed of fragments of blood group and tissue determinant carbohydrates and elongated versions of blood group carbohydrates bearing additional saccharides (for structures of all library members, see Supplementary Figure 1). Most of these structures contain fucose moieties and were expected to interact with BambL via the fucose-dominated mode observed in crystallographic structures. To explore how non-fucose residues (such as galactose and N-acetylgalactosamine) might occupy the fucose-binding site, a selection of di- and trisaccharides lacking fucose were also evaluated. Complexes with BambL were assembled by docking and simulated in explicit solvent for 400 ns.

Of the 36 complexes simulated, 28 remained stably engaged without dissociation of the ligand into bulk solvent. Multiple binding modes were observed among the stable complexes, exhibiting different hydrogen-bonding patterns (**Figure 8**). In some complexes (**2, 6, 34, 30**), very few hydrogen bonds were formed and were observed for only up to 30% of MD runs. These binding modes, while stable, did not feature significant hydrogen-bonding interactions with BambL.

In four cases (**5, 19, 18, 20**), the ligand was found to interact with the fucose-binding pocket via a non-fucose saccharide (galactose or N-acetylgalactosamine). While these non-fucose binding modes do include hydrogen bonds to the three fucose pocket residues (Arg15, Glu26, and Trp79), these interactions are not as highly occupied as those made by fucose-containing saccharides (**10, 9, 1, 17**). In non-fucose binding modes, hydrogen-bond occupancies over 70% were observed for only one or two interactions per ligand; for fucose-mediated binding, all three pocket residues are engaged more than 70% of the time.

The remaining 20 carbohydrates bound in a fucose-dominated manner, forming hydrogen bonds at over 70% occupancy between a fucose and all three residues of the fucose-binding pocket. In most cases, additional hydrogen bonds were formed with loop residues outside the fucose-binding pocket, with occupancies ranging from 10 to 90%. The highly stable (>70% occupancy) non-fucose hydrogen bonds involved residues Asp30 and Thr36, located on loop 4. The acidic sidechain of Asp30 projects toward the fucose-binding pocket, accepting hydrogen bonds from saccharides not directly bonded to the buried fucose. Thr36 is located further away from the fucose-binding pocket, and accepts hydrogen bonds via the

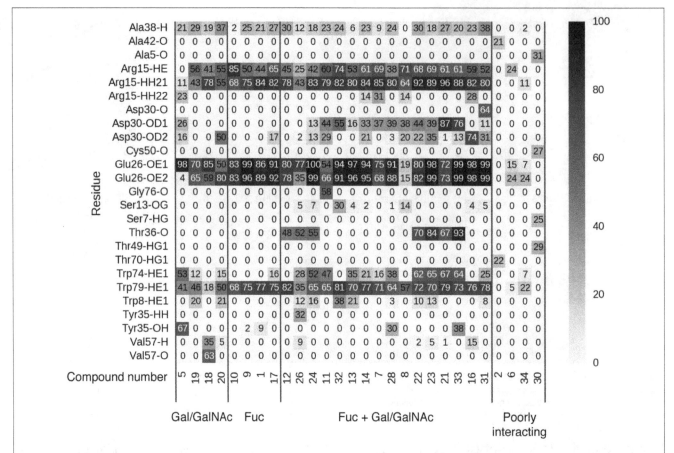

FIGURE 8 | Hydrogen bonding occupancy of blood-group-related saccharides during MD simulations. Saccharide names indicate the ligand moieties interacting with BambL during simulation.

backbone carbonyl oxygen atom. A less-occupied hydrogen bond (up to 67%) is formed to the indole nitrogen of Trp74, concurrent with hydrophobic stacking against a buried fucose. Finally, Tyr35 donates a hydrogen bond via the phenolic hydroxyl to compound **28** and **33** (and additionally to the non-fucose compound **5**). The fucose-dominated binding modes featuring highest occupancy of non-fucose hydrogen bonds involved carbohydrates **21** and **33**, illustrated in Supplementary Figure 9.

Combining all the BambL residues involved in hydrogen bonds to fucose and non-fucose saccharides presents a perspective of the target site that incorporates a wider view of BambL-saccharide recognition, considering multiple interaction points across the protein surface (**Figure 9**). This view of the BambL binding site presents opportunities for future inhibitor design to consider regions outside the fucose-binding pocket.

DISCUSSION

We have investigated the molecular aspects of carbohydrate recognition of the *B. ambifaria* lectin by computational methods: docking, site mapping, and MD. Molecular docking has been shown to be extremely useful for structural predictions, if not affinity calculations (Yuriev et al., 2015). However, docking carbohydrate ligands presents a number of challenges stemming from their extreme flexibility, a large number of hydroxyl groups, leading to the formation of (often) extensive hydrogen-bonding networks, and the formation of crucial CH/π stacking interactions between the C-H bonds of the carbohydrates (on their hydrophobic faces) and aromatic side chains of the protein (Agostino et al., 2009a, 2012a). Also, carbohydrate ligands are modular, and different residues (e.g., galactose vs. glucose) are able to establish highly similar interactions with the binding site. We have previously validated Glide and tested a range of other docking programs for structural prediction of carbohydrate complexes with antibodies (Agostino et al., 2009a, 2012b) and lectins (Agostino et al., 2011). We have demonstrated that, as the result of all the above-mentioned challenges, docking programs and scoring functions are not always able to predict the native binding pose faithfully as the top docked pose. To overcome this shortcoming and to harness the recognition information embedded in the docking output, we have developed a site mapping methodology that takes into account an ensemble of docked poses and identifies binding site residues critically involved in recognition of a ligand or ligand family (Yuriev et al., 2001, 2002; Agostino et al., 2013; Dingjan et al., 2015a).

In this study, docking with Glide produced reasonable top poses for a range of BambL complexes with blood group carbohydrates (**Table 2**). Using the BambL structure from PDB

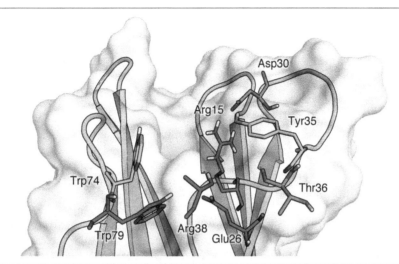

Method	Fucose-binding					Non-fucose-binding			
	Arg15	Glu26	Ala38	Trp74	Trp79	Asp30	Tyr35	Thr36	Trp74
Docking	HB	HB	HB	CH/π	HB	HB	-	-	HB
Site mapping	HB	HB	HB	CH/π	-	HB	CH/π	-	-
MD (blood group)	HB	HB	HB	CH/π	HB	HB	-	-	HB
MD (related)	HB	HB	-	CH/π	HB	HB	HB	HB	HB

FIGURE 9 | BambL binding site showing residues implicated in saccharide binding. Purple: Residues which form hydrogen bonds with the buried fucose saccharide. Orange: Residues which form hydrogen bonds with non-fucose saccharides. Green: Residues which participate in both hydrophobic and hydrogen bonding interactions.

ID: 3ZZV gave accurate complex prediction for the B, H type 1 and H type 2 saccharides and accurate fucose placement for the A, Le[a], Le[b], and Le[y] determinants. All these complexes featured a buried fucose residue (Fucα1-2Gal), providing the majority of hydrogen-bonding interactions, and conformational ranges reflective of predicted energetic minima (Imberty et al., 1995) and relevant experimental structures (Yuriev et al., 2005; Dingjan et al., 2015b). Notably, the distances between fucose carbon atoms and the geometric centers of the imidazole phenyl and pyrrole component ring systems of Trp74 (Supplementary Material, Table S1) are similar to reported geometries for fucose CH/π dispersion interactions of a closely related lectin, RSL (Wimmerova et al., 2012). As in the RSL-fucose complex, the C6 atom interacts with the pyrrole part of the imidazole ring (distance of 3.76 ± 0.3 Å), while C3 is further than 4 Å away. Unlike the RSL complex, C5 also interacts with the pyrrole ring (distance of 3.83 ± 0.1 Å), rather than the phenyl ring, which is further than 4 Å from the entire non-polar plane.

Detailed elaboration of structural aspects of molecular recognition requires expanding the single snapshot view afforded by crystal structures or top docked poses. To that effect, we have undertaken site mapping and MD investigations in order to identify BambL residues critical for recognition of blood group carbohydrates. The advantage of site mapping lies in its ability to consider alternative binding modes while MD also explicitly accounts for the role of water, mediating interactions of BambL to carbohydrates.

We have identified the atomic scale binding interactions that facilitate recognition of fucosylated human blood group saccharides by BambL. A network of hydrogen bonds combined with a single hydrophobic stacking interaction between the buried fucose and amino acids in the fucose-binding pocket account for the majority of binding interactions (**Figure 3**). These structural features of the fucose-driven recognition closely agree with experimental characterization of BambL-carbohydrate binding profile by glycan array, which has demonstrated a preference for short, fucose-bearing saccharides, with the fucose monosaccharide among the most highly ranked binders (Audfray et al., 2012). However, this fucose-driven recognition motif does not explain the specificity profile of BambL compared to other related fucose-binding lectins. Namely, the interactions between BambL and fucosylated saccharides are highly similar to those found in complexes featuring other six-bladed β-propeller fucose-binding lectins: found in fungi [*Aleuria aurantia* lectin, AAL (Fujihashi et al., 2003; Wimmerova et al., 2003); *Aspergillus fumigatus* lectin, AFL (Houser et al., 2013); *Aspergillus oryzae* lectin, AOL (Makyio et al., 2016)] and bacteria [*Ralstonia solanacearum* lectin, RSL (Kostlánová et al., 2005)]. Members of this lectin family bind fucose via the same interactions: hydrogen bonds between O2 and a backbone amide proton, O3 and indole nitrogen, O3 and O4 to a shared carboxylate moiety, and O4 and O5 to a shared guanidinium moiety. In a previous docking study of RSL-fucose recognition by Mishra et al. (2012) the same suite of interactions was reported.

Despite the common binding mode, these lectins prefer different blood group determinants: AAL exhibits broad specificity, while AFL prefers Le[y], and RSL prefers saccharides featuring Fucα1-2 and Fucα1-6 moieties (blood group A, B, and H and core of N-glycans). Varied blood group specificity has been proposed to arise from steric hindrance around the fucose-binding pocket, preventing strong binding to most branched carbohydrate structures (Fujihashi et al., 2003). Glycan array screening shows generally decreased binding to branched carbohydrates compared to mono- and disaccharides for these lectins, emphasizing the importance of steric effects (Houser et al., 2013). Additionally, the non-selective AAL lacks steric hindrance around the fucose-binding pocket: in a bound complex featuring the disaccharide Fucα1-6GlcNAcβ1-OMe, transferred NOE experiments confirmed conformational flexibility around the glycosidic linkage (Weimar and Peters, 1994). However, steric hindrance alone does not fully explain blood group selectivity in this lectin family. AFL binds the difucosylated Le[y] more strongly than the corresponding monofucosylated saccharide, H-type 2, despite similar steric complementarity to the binding site (Houser et al., 2013). We suggest that stabilizing interactions outside the fucose-binding pocket (as observed in simulations of BambL complexed with blood-group-related saccharides) play a role in saccharide binding in the 6-bladed β-propeller lectin family more generally.

Interactions with non-fucose residues are not as highly occupied as interactions with the fucose. However, they contribute to a wider view of BambL-carbohydrate recognition, considering multiple interaction points across the protein surface. They include hydrogen bonding to Asp30, Tyr35, Thr36, and Trp74 and hydrophobic contacts with Tyr35 (**Figure 9**). These contacts outside the fucose-binding pocket could be employed in future inhibitor design for BambL to address issues of opportunistic infections.

CONCLUSION

In summary, the present work details the recognition of fucosylated human blood group determinants by BambL,

quantifies the occupancy of hydrogen bonding interactions, and identifies opportunities for targeting residues outside the fucose-binding pocket. Recognition mainly involves the fucose monosaccharide through a network of highly occupied hydrogen-bonding interactions to Arg15, Glu26, and Trp79, and a lower occupancy interaction with Ala38. An additional stacking interaction between the fucose hydrophobic face and Trp74 is also highly occupied in MD simulations. Hydrogen bonds to non-fucose saccharides were formed in complexes with Le[y], Le[b], Le[a], H1, H2, and B trisaccharide and in multiple complexes involving blood-group-related saccharides. The most occupied interactions involved Asp30, Thr36, Trp74, and to a lesser degree Tyr35. Carbohydrate recognition by BambL is therefore proposed to be driven by interactions in the fucose-binding site and further stabilized by satellite interactions between non-fucose saccharides and surface residues outside the fucose-binding pocket. The analysis of carbohydrate recognition by BambL presented in this study lays the foundation for the development of fucomimetic molecules able to bind to BambL. Such molecules have potential as anti-adhesives for the treatment of *B. ambifaria* infection in cystic fibrosis patients.

AUTHOR CONTRIBUTIONS

Each author has contributed significantly to the submitted work. TD and EY conceived and designed the experiments. TD performed the experiments. TD, EY, and PR analyzed the data. TD, AI, SP, EY, and PR wrote the paper. All authors read and approved the final manuscript.

FUNDING

This work was supported by a Victorian Life Sciences Computation Initiative (VLSCI) grant number VR0250 on its Peak Computing Facility at the University of Melbourne, an initiative of the Victorian Government, Australia, and with the assistance of resources from the National Computational Infrastructure (NCI), which is supported by the Australian Government, and the Multi-modal Australian ScienceS Imaging and Visualization Environment (MASSIVE) via grant Y96. TD is supported by an Australian Postgraduate Award (APA) scholarship. AI and SP are supported by CNRS, Université Grenoble Alpes through Glyco@Alps (ANR-15-IDEX-02) and Labex ARCANE (ANR-11-LABX-0003-01). PR is supported by an RMIT University Vice Chancellor's Senior Research Fellowship.

REFERENCES

Agostino, M., Jene, C., Boyle, T., Ramsland, P. A., and Yuriev, E. (2009a). Molecular docking of carbohydrate ligands to antibodies: structural validation against crystal structures. *J. Chem. Inf. Model.* 49, 2749–2760. doi: 10.1021/ci900388a

Agostino, M., Mancera, R. L., Ramsland, P. A., and Yuriev, E. (2013). AutoMap: A tool for analyzing protein-ligand recognition using multiple ligand binding modes. *J. Mol. Graphics Modell.* 40, 80–90. doi: 10.1016/j.jmgm.2013.01.001

Agostino, M., Ramsland, P. A., and Yuriev, E. (2012a). "Docking of carbohydrates into protein binding sites," in *Structural Glycobiology*, eds E. Yuriev and P. A. Ramsland (Boca Raton, FL: CRC Press), 111–138.

Agostino, M., Sandrin, M. S., Thompson, P. E., Yuriev, E., and Ramsland, P. A. (2009b). *In silico* analysis of antibody-carbohydrate interactions and its application to xenoreactive antibodies. *Mol. Immunol.* 47, 233–246. doi: 10.1016/j.molimm.2009.09.031

Agostino, M., Yuriev, E., and Ramsland, P. A. (2011). A computational approach for exploring carbohydrate recognition by lectins in innate immunity. *Front. Immunol.* 2:23. doi: 10.3389/fimmu.2011.00023

Agostino, M., Yuriev, E., and Ramsland, P. A. (2012b). Antibody recognition of cancer-related gangliosides and their mimics investigated using in silico site mapping. *PLoS ONE* 7:e35457. doi: 10.1371/journal.pone.0035457

Anstee, D. J. (2010). The relationship between blood groups and disease. *Blood* 115, 4635–4643. doi: 10.1182/blood-2010-01-261859

Audfray, A., Claudinon, J., Abounit, S., Ruvoen-Clouet, N., Larson, G., Smith, D. F., et al. (2012). Fucose-binding lectin from opportunistic pathogen *Burkholderia ambifaria* binds to both plant and human oligosaccharidic epitopes. *J. Biol. Chem.* 287, 4335–4347. doi: 10.1074/jbc.M111.314831

Audfray, A., Varrot, A., and Imberty, A. (2013). Bacteria love our sugars: interaction between soluble lectins and human fucosylated glycans, structures, thermodynamics and design of competing glycocompounds. *C. R. Chim.* 16, 482–490. doi: 10.1016/j.crci.2012.11.021

Banks, J. L., Beard, H. S., Cao, Y., Cho, A. E., Damm, W., Farid, R., et al. (2005). Integrated modeling program, applied chemical theory (IMPACT). *J. Comput. Chem.* 26, 1752–1780. doi: 10.1002/jcc.20292

Bavington, C., and Page, C. (2005). Stopping bacterial adhesion: a novel approach to treating infections. *Respiration* 72, 335–344. doi: 10.1159/000086243

Berendsen, H. J. C., van der Spoel, D., and van Drunen, R. (1995). GROMACS: a message-passing parallel molecular dynamics implementation. *Comput. Phys. Commun.* 91, 43–56. doi: 10.1016/0010-4655(95)00042-E

Berman, H. M., Westbrook, J., Feng, Z., Gilliland, G., Bhat, T. N., Weissig, H., et al. (2000). The protein data bank. *Nucleic Acids Res.* 28, 235–242. doi: 10.1093/nar/28.1.235

Berman, H., Henrick, K., and Nakamura, H. (2003). Announcing the worldwide protein data bank. *Nat. Struct. Mol. Biol.* 10, 980–980. doi: 10.1038/nsb1203-980

Blackburn, L., Brownlee, K., Conway, S., and Denton, M. (2004). 'Cepacia syndrome' with *Burkholderia multivorans*, 9 years after initial colonization. *J. Cyst. Fibros.* 3, 133–134. doi: 10.1016/j.jcf.2004.03.007

Caverly, L. J., Zhao, J., and LiPuma, J. J. (2015). Cystic fibrosis lung microbiome: opportunities to reconsider management of airway infection. *Pediatr. Pulmonol.* 50, S31–S38. doi: 10.1002/ppul.23243

Chemani, C., Imberty, A., de Bentzmann, S., Pierre, M., Wimmerova, M., Guery, B. P., et al. (2009). Role of LecA and LecB lectins in *Pseudomonas aeruginosa*-induced lung injury and effect of carbohydrate ligands. *Infect. Immun.* 77, 2065–2075. doi: 10.1128/IAI.01204-08

Ciofu, O., Hansen, C. R., and Hoiby, N. (2013). Respiratory bacterial infections in cystic fibrosis. *Curr. Opin. Pulm. Med.* 19, 251–258. doi: 10.1097/MCP.0b013e32835f1afc

Coenye, T., Mahenthiralingam, E., Henry, D., LiPuma, J. J., Laevens, S., Gillis, M., et al. (2001). *Burkholderia ambifaria* sp nov., a novel member of the *Burkholderia cepacia complex* including biocontrol and cystic fibrosis-related isolates. *Int. J. Syst. Evol. Microbiol.* 51, 1481–1490. doi: 10.1099/00207713-51-4-1481

De Smet, B., Mayo, M., Peeters, C., Zlosnik, J. E. A., Spilker, T., Hird, T. J., et al. (2015). Burkholderia stagnalis sp. nov., and Burkholderia territorii sp. nov., two novel *Burkholderia cepacia complex* species from environmental and human sources. *Int. J. Syst. Evol. Microbiol.* 65, 2265–2271. doi: 10.1099/ijs.0.000251

Dingjan, T., Agostino, M., Ramsland, P. A., and Yuriev, E. (2015a). "Antibody-carbohydrate recognition from docked ensembles using the automap procedure," in *Carbohydrate-Based Vaccines*, ed B. Lepenies (New York, NY: Springer), 41–55. doi: 10.1007/978-1-4939-2874-3_4

Dingjan, T., Spendlove, I., Durrant, L. G., Scott, A. M., Yuriev, E., and Ramsland, P. A. (2015b). Structural biology of antibody recognition of carbohydrate epitopes and potential uses for targeted cancer immunotherapies. *Mol. Immunol.* 67, 75–88. doi: 10.1016/j.molimm.2015.02.028

Ernst, B., and Magnani, J. L. (2009). From carbohydrate leads to glycomimetic drugs. *Nat. Rev. Drug Disc.* 8, 661–677. doi: 10.1038/nrd2852

Friesner, R. A., Banks, J. L., Murphy, R. B., Halgren, T. A., Klicic, J. J., Mainz, D. T., et al. (2004). Glide: a new approach for rapid, accurate docking and scoring.

1. method and assessment of docking accuracy. *J. Med. Chem.* 47, 1739–1749. doi: 10.1021/jm0306430

Friesner, R. A., Murphy, R. B., Repasky, M. P., Frye, L. L., Greenwood, J. R., Halgren, T. A., et al. (2006). Extra precision Glide: docking and scoring incorporating a model of hydrophobic enclosure for protein–ligand complexes. *J. Med. Chem.* 49, 6177–6196. doi: 10.1021/jm051256o

Fujihashi, M., Peapus, D. H., Kamiya, N., Nagata, Y., and Miki, K. (2003). Crystal structure of fucose-specific lectin from Aleuria aurantia binding ligands at three of its five sugar recognition sites. *Biochemistry* 42, 11093–11099. doi: 10.1021/bi034983z

Halgren, T. A., Murphy, R. B., Friesner, R. A., Beard, H. S., Frye, L. L., Pollard, W. T., et al. (2004). Glide: a new approach for rapid, accurate docking and scoring. 2. enrichment factors in database screening. *J. Med. Chem.* 47, 1750–1759. doi: 10.1021/jm030644s

Hess, B. (2007). P-LINCS: a parallel linear constraint solver for molecular simulation. *J. Chem. Theory Comput.* 4, 116–122. doi: 10.1021/ct700200b

Hess, B., Kutzner, C., van der Spoel, D., and Lindahl, E. (2008). GROMACS 4: algorithms for highly efficient, load-balanced, and scalable molecular simulation. *J. Chem. Theory Comput.* 4, 435–447. doi: 10.1021/ct700301q

Holmner, Å., Mackenzie, A., and Krengel, U. (2010). Molecular basis of cholera blood-group dependence and implications for a world characterized by climate change. *FEBS Lett.* 584, 2548–2555. doi: 10.1016/j.febslet.2010.03.050

Houser, J., Komarek, J., Cioci, G., Varrot, A., Imberty, A., and Wimmerova, M. (2015). Structural insights into *Aspergillus fumigatus* lectin specificity: AFL binding sites are functionally non-equivalent. *Acta Crystallogr. D Biol. Crystallogr.* 71, 442–453. doi: 10.1107/S1399004714026595

Houser, J., Komarek, J., Kostlanova, N., Cioci, G., Varrot, A., Kerr, S. C., et al. (2013). A soluble fucose-specific lectin from *Aspergillus fumigatus* conidia - structure, specificity and possible role in fungal pathogenicity. *PLoS ONE* 8:e83077. doi: 10.1371/journal.pone.0083077

Imberty, A., and Varrot, A. (2008). Microbial recognition of human cell surface glycoconjugates. *Curr. Opin. Struct. Biol.* 18, 567–576. doi: 10.1016/j.sbi.2008.08.001

Imberty, A., Mikros, E., Koca, J., Mollicone, R., Oriol, R., and Perez, S. (1995). Computer simulation of histo-blood group oligosaccharides: energy maps of all constituting disaccharides and potential energy surfaces of 14 ABH and Lewis carbohydrate antigens. *Glycoconj. J.* 12, 331–349. doi: 10.1007/BF00731336

Imberty, A., Wimmerova, M., Mitchell, E. P., and Gilboa-Garber, N. (2004). Structures of the lectins from *Pseudomonas aeruginosa*: insights into the molecular basis for host glycan recognition. *Microbes Infect.* 6, 221–228. doi: 10.1016/j.micinf.2003.10.016

Jackson, T. A., Robertson, V., and Auzanneau, F. I. (2014). Evidence for two populated conformations for the Dimeric Le(X) and Le(A)Le(X) tumor-associated carbohydrate antigens. *J. Med. Chem.* 57, 817–827. doi: 10.1021/jm401576x

Kirschner, K. N., Yongye, A. B., Tschampel, S. M., González-Outeiriño, J., Daniels, C. R., Foley, B. L., et al., (2008). GLYCAM06: a generalizable biomolecular force field. *Carbohydrates. J. Comput. Chem.* 29, 622–655. doi: 10.1002/jcc.20820

Kostlánová, N., Mitchell, E. P., Lortat-Jacob, H., Oscarson, S., Lahmann, M., Gilboa-Garber, N., et al. (2005). The fucose-binding Lectin from *Ralstonia solanacearum*: a new type of β-propeller architecture formed by oligomerization and interacting with fucoside, fucosyllactose, and plant xyloglucan. *J. Biol. Chem.* 280, 27839–27849. doi: 10.1074/jbc.M505184200

Laskowski, R. A., and Swindells, M. B. (2011). LigPlot+: multiple ligand-protein interaction diagrams for drug discovery. *J. Chem. Inf. Model.* 51, 2778–2786. doi: 10.1021/ci200227u

Lee, C. H., Kim, M., Kim, H., Ahn, J. H., Yi, Y., Kang, K., et al. (2006). An antifungal property of *Burkholderia ambifaria* against phytopathogenic fungi. *J. Microbiol. Biotechnol.* 16, 465–468.

Li, W., Roberts, D. P., Dery, P. D., Meyer, S. L. F., Lohrke, S., Lumsden, R. D., et al. (2002). Broad spectrum anti-biotic activity and disease suppression by the potential biocontrol agent *Burkholderia ambifaria* BC-F. *Crop Prot.* 21, 129–135. doi: 10.1016/S0261-2194(01)00074-6

Lindén, S., Mahdavi, J., Semino-Mora, C., Olsen, C., Carlstedt, I., Borén, T., et al. (2008). Role of ABO secretor status in mucosal innate immunity and *H. pylori* Infection. *PLoS Pathog.* 4:e2. doi: 10.1371/journal.ppat.00 40002

Lindorff-Larsen, K., Piana, S., Palmo, K., Maragakis, P., Klepeis, J. L., Dror, R. O., et al. (2010). Improved side-chain torsion potentials for the Amber ff99SB protein force field. *Proteins* 78, 1950–1958. doi: 10.1002/prot. 22711

Loutet, S. A., and Valvano, M. A. (2011). Extreme antimicrobial Peptide and polymyxin B resistance in the genus burkholderia. *Front. Microbiol.* 2:59. doi: 10.3389/fmicb.2011.00159

Lyczak, J. B., Cannon, C. L., and Pier, G. B. (2002). Lung infections associated with cystic fibrosis. *Clin. Microbiol. Rev.* 15, 194–222. doi: 10.1128/CMR.15.2.194-222.2002

Lynch, J. P. III (2009). *Burkholderia cepacia* complex: impact on the cystic fibrosis lung lesion. *Sem. Resp. Crit. Care Med.* 30, 596–610. doi: 10.1055/s-0029-1238918

Madhavi Sastry, G., Adzhigirey, M., Day, T., Annabhimoju, R., and Sherman, W. (2013). Protein and ligand preparation: parameters, protocols, and influence on virtual screening enrichments. *J. Comput. Aided Mol. Des.* 27, 221–234. doi: 10.1007/s10822-013-9644-8

Makeneni, S., Foley, B. L., and Woods, R. J. (2014). BFMP: a method for discretizing and visualizing pyranose conformations. *J. Chem. Inf. Model.* 54, 2744–2750. doi: 10.1021/ci500325b

Makyio, H., Shimabukuro, J., Suzuki, T., Imamura, A., Ishida, H., Kiso, M., et al. (2016). Six independent fucose-binding sites in the crystal structure of *Aspergillus oryzae* lectin. *Biochem. Biophys. Res. Commun.* 477, 477–482. doi: 10.1016/j.bbrc.2016.06.069

Martinucci, M., Roscetto, E., Iula, V. D., Votsi, A., Catania, M. R., and De Gregorio, E. (2016). Accurate identification of members of the *Burkholderia cepacia* complex in cystic fibrosis sputum. *Lett. Appl. Microbiol.* 62, 221–229. doi: 10.1111/lam.12537

McGibbon, R. T., Beauchamp, K. A., Harrigan, M. P., Klein, C., Swails, J. M., Hernández, C. X., et al. (2015). MDTraj: a modern open library for the analysis of molecular dynamics trajectories. *Biophys. J.* 109, 1528–1532. doi: 10.1016/j.bpj.2015.08.015

Michaud-Agrawal, N., Denning, E. J., Woolf, T. B., and Beckstein, O. (2011). MDAnalysis: a toolkit for the analysis of molecular dynamics simulations. *J. Comput. Chem.* 32, 2319–2327. doi: 10.1002/jcc. 21787

Mishra, S. K., Adam, J., Wimmerova, M., and Koca, J. (2012). *In silico* mutagenesis and docking study of *Ralstonia solanacearum* RSL lectin: performance of docking software to predict saccharide binding. *J. Chem. Inf. Model.* 52, 1250–1261. doi: 10.1021/ci200529n

Mitchell, E., Houles, C., Sudakevitz, D., Wimmerova, M., Gautier, C., Perez, S., et al. (2002). Structural basis for oligosaccharide-mediated adhesion of *Pseudomonas aeruginosa* in the lungs of cystic fibrosis patients. *Nat. Struct. Biol.* 9, 918–921. doi: 10.1038/nsb865

O'Sullivan, B. P., and Freedman, S. D. (2009). Cystic fibrosis. *Lancet* 373, 1891–1904. doi: 10.1016/S0140-6736(09)60327-5

Parra-Cota, F. I., Pena-Cabriales, J. J., de los Santos-Villalobos, S., Martinez-Gallardo, N. A., and Delano-Frier, J. P. (2014). *Burkholderia ambifaria* and B. *caribensis* promote growth and increase yield in grain Amaranth (Amaranthus cruentus and A-hypochondriacus) by improving plant nitrogen uptake. *PLoS ONE* 9:14. doi: 10.1371/journal.pone.0088094

Pera, N. P., and Peters, R. J. (2014). Towards bacterial adhesion-based therapeutics and detection methods. *Med. Chem. Comm.* 5, 1027–1035. doi: 10.1039/C3MD00346A

Pieters, R. J. (2011). "The role of carbohydrates in bacterial infections," in *Carbohydrate Recognition,* eds B. Wang and G. J. Boons (Hoboken: John Wiley & Sons, Inc.), 93–106.

Podnecky, N. L., Rhodes, K. A., and Schweizer, H. P. (2015). Efflux pump-mediated drug resistance in Burkholderia. *Front. Microbiol.* 6:305. doi: 10.3389/fmicb.2015.00305

Pronk, S., Páll, S., Schulz, R., Larsson, P., Bjelkmar, P., Apostolov, R., et al. (2013). GROMACS 4.5: a high-throughput and highly parallel open source molecular simulation toolkit. *Bioinformatics* 29, 845–854. doi: 10.1093/bioinformatics/btt055

Rhim, A. D., Stoykova, L., Glick, M. C., and Scanlin, T. F. (2001). Terminal glycosylation in cystic fibrosis (CF): a review emphasizing the airway epithelial cell. *Glycoconj. J.* 18, 649–659. doi: 10.1023/A:1020815205022

Schrödinger (2014a). "Glide", in *Small-Molecule Drug Discovery Suite 2014-1, 6.2 Edn.* (New York, NY: Schrödinger, LLC)

Schrödinger (2014b). "Maestro," in *Schrödinger Release 2014-1, 9.7 Edn.* (New York, NY: Schrödinger, LLC).

Schrödinger (2014c). "Prime," in *Schrödinger Release 2014-1, 4.4 Edn.* (New York, NY: Schrödinger, LLC).

Schrödinger (2014d). *The PyMOL Molecular Graphics System, 1.8 Edn.* New York, NY: Schrödinger, LLC.

Sharon, N. (2006). Carbohydrates as future anti-adhesion drugs for infectious diseases. *Biochim. Biophys. Acta Gen. Subj.* 1760, 527–537. doi: 10.1016/j.bbagen.2005.12.008

Sousa da Silva, A., and Vranken, W. (2012). ACPYPE—AnteChamber PYthon Parser interfacE. *BMC Res. Notes* 5:367. doi: 10.1186/1756-0500-5-367

Stoykova, L. I., and Scanlin, T. F. (2008). Cystic fibrosis (CF), *Pseudomonas aeruginosa*, CFTR and the CF glycosylation phenotype: a review and update. *Curr. Org. Chem.* 12, 900–910. doi: 10.2174/138527208784892169

Sulak, O., Cioci, G., Delia, M., Lahmann, M., Varrot, A., Imberty, A., et al. (2010). A TNF-like trimeric lectin domain from *Burkholderia cenocepacia* with specificity for fucosylated human histo-blood group antigens. *Structure* 18, 59–72. doi: 10.1016/j.str.2009.10.021

Sulak, O., Cioci, G., Lameignere, E., Balloy, V., Round, A., Gutsche, I., et al. (2011). *Burkholderia cenocepacia* BC2L-C is a super lectin with dual specificity and proinflammatory activity. *PLoS Pathog.* 7:e1002238. doi: 10.1371/journal.ppat.1002238

Tempel, W., Tschampel, S., and Woods, R. J. (2002). The xenograft antigen bound to *Griffonia simplicifolia* lectin 1-B-4—X-ray crystal structure of the complex and molecular dynamics characterization of the binding site. *J. Biol. Chem.* 277, 6615–6621. doi: 10.1074/jbc.M109919200

Topin, J., Arnaud, J., Sarkar, A., Audfray, A., Gillon, E., Perez, S., et al. (2013). Deciphering the glycan preference of bacterial lectins by glycan array and molecular docking with validation by microcalorimetry and crystallography. *PLoS ONE* 8:e71149. doi: 10.1371/journal.pone.0071149

Topin, J., Lelimousin, M., Arnaud, J., Audfray, A., Pérez, S., Varrot, A., et al. (2016). The hidden conformation of Lewis x, a human histo-blood group antigen, is a determinant for recognition by pathogen lectins. *ACS Chem. Biol.* 11, 2011–2020. doi: 10.1021/acschembio.6b00333

Van Der Spoel, D., Lindahl, E., Hess, B., Groenhof, G., Mark, A. E., and Berendsen, H. J. C. (2005). GROMACS: fast, flexible, and free. *J. Comput. Chem.* 26, 1701–1718. doi: 10.1002/jcc.20291

Vandamme, P., Holmes, B., Vancanneyt, M., Coenye, T., Hoste, B., Coopman, R., et al. (1997). Occurrence of multiple genomovars of *Burkholderia cepacia* in cystic fibrosis patients and proposal of *Burkholderia multivorans* sp. nov. *Int. J. Syst. Bacteriol.* 47, 1188–1200. doi: 10.1099/00207713-47-4-1188

Venkatakrishnan, V., Thaysen-Andersen, M., Chen, S. C. A., Nevalainen, H., and Packer, N. H. (2015). Cystic fibrosis and bacterial colonization define the sputum N-glycosylation phenotype. *Glycobiology* 25, 88–100. doi: 10.1093/glycob/cwu092

von Bismarck, P., Schneppenheim, R., and Schumacher, U. (2001). Successful treatment of *Pseudomonas aeruginosa* respiratory tract infection with a sugar solution–a case report on a lectin based therapeutic principle. *Klin. Padiatr.* 213, 285–287. doi: 10.1055/s-2001-17220

Wallace, A. C., Laskowski, R. A., and Thornton, J. M. (1995). LIGPLOT—a program to generate schematic diagrams of protein ligand interactions. *Protein Eng.* 8, 127–134. doi: 10.1093/protein/8.2.127

Weimar, T., and Peters, T. (1994). *Aleuria aurantia* agglutinin recognizes multiple conformations of α-L-Fuc-(1→6)-β-D-GlcNAc-OMe. *Angew. Chem. Int. Ed. Engl.* 33, 88–91. doi: 10.1002/anie.199400881

Wimmerova, M., Kozmon, S., Necasova, I., Mishra, S. K., Komarek, J., and Koca, J. (2012). Stacking interactions between carbohydrate and protein quantified by combination of theoretical and experimental methods. *PLoS ONE* 7:e46032. doi: 10.1371/journal.pone.0046032

Wimmerova, M., Mitchell, E., Sanchez, J.-F., Gautier, C., and Imberty, A. (2003). Crystal structure of fungal lectin: six-bladed β-propeller fold and novel fucose recognition mode for *Aleuria aurantia* lectin. *J. Biol. Chem.* 278, 27059–27067. doi: 10.1074/jbc.M302642200

Woods, R. J. (2005). *GLYCAM Web* [Online]. Complex Carbohydrate Research Center, University of Georgia, Athens, G. A. Available Online at: http://www.glycam.com (Accessed June 1 2015).

Yuriev, E., Farrugia, W., Scott, A. M., and Ramsland, P. A. (2005). Three-dimensional structures of carbohydrate determinants of Lewis system antigens: implications for effective antibody targeting of cancer. *Immunol. Cell Biol.* 83, 709–717. doi: 10.1111/j.1440-1711.2005.01 374.x

Yuriev, E., Holien, J., and Ramsland, P. A. (2015). Improvements, trends, and new ideas in molecular docking: 2012–2013 in review. *J. Mol. Recognit.* 28, 581–604. doi: 10.1002/jmr.2471

Yuriev, E., Ramsland, P. A., and Edmundson, A. B. (2001). Docking of combinatorial peptide libraries into a broadly cross-reactive human IgM. *J. Mol. Recognit.* 14, 172–184. doi: 10.1002/jmr.533

Yuriev, E., Ramsland, P. A., and Edmundson, A. B. (2002). Recognition of IgG-derived peptides by a human IgM with an unusual combining site. *Scand. J. Immunol.* 55, 242–255. doi: 10.1046/j.0300-9475.2002.01 032.x

Zahariadis, G., Levy, M. H., and Burns, J. L. (2003). Cepacia-like syndrome caused by *Burkholderia multivorans*. *Can. J. Infect. Dis.* 14, 123–125. doi: 10.1155/2003/675159

Zhou, J., Chen, Y., Tabibi, S., Alba, L., Garber, E., and Saiman, L. (2007). Antimicrobial susceptibility and synergy studies of *Burkholderia cepacia* complex isolated from patients with cystic fibrosis. *Antimicrob. Agents Chemother.* 51, 1085–1088. doi: 10.1128/AAC.00954-06

3

Bridging Molecular Docking to Molecular Dynamics in Exploring Ligand-Protein Recognition Process

Veronica Salmaso and Stefano Moro*

Molecular Modeling Section, Department of Pharmaceutical and Pharmacological Sciences, University of Padova, Padova, Italy

Correspondence:
Stefano Moro
stefano.moro@unipd.it

Computational techniques have been applied in the drug discovery pipeline since the 1980s. Given the low computational resources of the time, the first molecular modeling strategies relied on a rigid view of the ligand-target binding process. During the years, the evolution of hardware technologies has gradually allowed simulating the dynamic nature of the binding event. In this work, we present an overview of the evolution of structure-based drug discovery techniques in the study of ligand-target recognition phenomenon, going from the static molecular docking toward enhanced molecular dynamics strategies.

Keywords: ligand-protein binding, molecular docking, molecular dynamics, enhanced sampling, protein flexibility, molecular recognition

INTRODUCTION

No protein is an island but exerts its function through the recognition of other molecular partners (Salmaso, 2018). Ligand-protein interactions are involved in many biological processes with consequent pharmaceutical implications. Thus, the scientific community has been putting a great effort into the investigation of the binding phenomenon during the years, leading to the proposal of several theories characterized by an increasing emphasis on the degree of flexibility of the ligand and protein counterparts.

The first explanation of binding was provided by Emil Fischer in 1894 (Fischer, 1894) with the "lock-key" model to interpret enzyme specificity: the ligand rigidly recognizes and occupies the protein binding site like a key to its lock, because of their native shape complementary. Since this model could not explain either the behavior of enzyme noncompetitive inhibition or allosteric modulation, different modifications have been proposed. Koshland (1958) introduced the "induced-fit" theory: according to his observations on enzyme-substrate interactions, the ligand is able to induce conformational changes to the protein, optimizing ligand-target interactions. Later works suggested that proteins naturally exist as an ensemble of conformations (Monod et al., 1965), described by an energy landscape (Frauenfelder et al., 1991), and ligands preferentially bind to one of them (Austin et al., 1975; Foote and Milstein, 1994). According to this interpretation of binding, known as "conformational selection," the ligand stabilizes one of the protein conformations with a consequent shift of the protein population equilibrium (Kumar et al., 2000). These two apparently contrasting theories have simply different ranges of applicability, and the descriptions they provide of molecular binding differ for the chronological sequence of events in which the binding process is decomposed (Kobilka and Deupi, 2007; Okazaki and Takada, 2008; Zhou, 2010). New theories are emerging, making a compromise between the aforementioned ones: according to the extended conformational selection model, for example, the conformational selection is followed by a conformational adjustment (induced fit) (Csermely et al., 2010).

The evolution of binding models has practical relevance besides an epistemological significance; the knowledge of ligand-target binding is at the basis of rational drug design but understanding this complex process on a mechanistic level may open new scenarios. In addition, to suggest ligand modification meant to optimize the final bound state, the medicinal chemist may look at kinetically relevant intermediate states and try to affect them.

COMPUTATIONAL METHODS TO STUDY LIGAND-PROTEIN BINDING

Since the 1980s, computer technologies have been applied to the drug discovery process (Van Drie, 2007), giving rise to Computer-Aided Drug Design (CADD). This technique earned soon great interest and deserved a cover article on October 5, 1981, Fortune magazine, entitled "Next Industrial Revolution: Designing Drugs by Computer at Merck" (Van Drie, 2007). CADD techniques are used principally for three reasons: virtual screening *hit/lead* optimization and design of novel compounds. In virtual screening a huge database of compounds is examined searching for binding capacity for a target and a subset of compounds is picked out and suggested for *in vitro* testing; the purpose is to increase the *hit* rate of novel drugs by reducing the number of compounds to test experimentally. The second application of CADD is the optimization of a *hit/lead* compound driven by the rationalization of a structure-activity relationship. After the individuation of key elements for binding, the design of new compounds can be attempted (Salmaso, 2018).

CADD methods may be classified as ligand-based (LB) and structure-based (SB), depending on the availability and employment of the target structure (Sliwoski et al., 2014). In the framework of CADD, structure-based drug design (SBDD) methods take advantage of the abundance of experimentally solved structures in the Protein Data Bank (Berman et al., 2000), which can possibly be used also as templates for homology models if the structure of interest is lacking. SBDD is based on the premise that the knowledge of the target structure can help to rationalize and optimize binding since ligand-target interactions are mediated by their complementarity. With the evolution of the binding models, it is clear that speaking of "target structure" is an approximation, given that proteins fluctuate among an ensemble of structures (Miller and Dill, 1997).

The possibility to predict ligand binding modes and to interpret binding processes is valuable to individuate, optimize and suggest novel ligands, and for this reason, the scientific community has been putting great efforts in developing new computational techniques.

In the following paragraphs, we will present an excursus over the main structure-based computational techniques employed in drug discovery. An urgency to simulate protein flexibility throughout binding has been experienced over the years, arising from the evolution of the binding models

from static to dynamic. The inclusion of flexibility features in conformational sampling entails an increase in the number of degrees of freedom of the system, and consequently in the computational effort. For this reason, the development of computational tools has been occurring in parallel and thanks to the continuous improvement of hardware technologies.

Molecular Docking

Molecular docking techniques aim to predict the best matching binding mode of a ligand to a macromolecular partner (here just proteins are considered). It consists in the generation of a number of possible conformations/orientations, i.e., poses, of the ligand within the protein binding site. For this reason, the availability of the three-dimensional structure of the molecular target is a necessary condition; it can be an experimentally solved structure (such as by X-ray crystallography or NMR) or a structure obtained by computational techniques (such as homology modeling) (Salmaso, 2018).

Molecular docking is composed mainly by two stages: an engine for conformations/orientations sampling and a scoring function, which associates a score to each predicted pose (Abagyan and Totrov, 2001; Kitchen et al., 2004; Huang and Zou, 2010). The sampling process should effectively search the conformational space described by the free energy landscape, where energy, in docking, is approximated by the scoring function. The scoring function should be able to associate the native bound-conformation to the global minimum of the energy hypersurface.

Scoring Functions

Scoring functions play the role of poses selector, used to discriminate putative correct binding modes and binders from non-binders in the pool of poses generated by the sampling engine.

There are essentially three types of scoring functions:

1. Force-field based scoring functions:

Force-field is a concept typical of molecular mechanics (see **Box 1**) which approximates the potential energy of a system with a combination of bonded (intramolecular) and nonbonded (intermolecular) components. In molecular docking, the nonbonded components are generally taken into account, with possibly the addition of the ligand-bonded terms, especially the torsional components. Intermolecular components include the van der Waals term, described by the Lennard-Jones potential, and the electrostatic potential, described by the Coulomb function, where a distance-dependent dielectric may be introduced to mimic the solvent effect. However, additional terms have been added to the force-field scoring functions, such as solvation terms (Brooijmans and Kuntz, 2003).

Examples of force field based scoring functions are GoldScore (Verdonk et al., 2003), AutoDock (Morris et al., 1998) (improved as a semiempirical version in AutoDock4, Huey et al., 2007), GBVI/WSA (Corbeil et al., 2012).

2. Empirical scoring functions:

These functions are the sum of various empirical energy terms such as van der Waals, electrostatic, hydrogen bond, desolvation, entropy, hydrophobicity, etc., which are weighted by coefficients optimized to reproduce binding affinity data of a training set by least squares fitting (Huang and Zou, 2010).

The LUDI (Böhm, 1994) scoring function was the first example of an empirical one. Other empirical scoring functions are GlideScore (Halgren et al., 2004; Friesner et al., 2006), ChemScore (Eldridge et al., 1997), PLANTS$_{CHEMPLP}$ (Korb et al., 2009).

3. Knowledge-based scoring functions:

Box 1 | Molecular mechanics.

Molecular mechanics is a method which approximates the treatment of molecules with the laws of classical mechanics, in order to limit the computational cost required for quantum mechanical calculations (Vanommeslaeghe et al., 2014). Atoms are considered as charged spheres connected by springs, neglecting the presence of electrons, in accordance with Born-Oppenheimer approximation (Born and Oppenheimer, 1927). The potential energy is approximated by a simple function which is called force-field; it is the sum of bonded (intramolecular) and nonbonded energy terms. The basic form of the function comprise bond stretching and bending described by harmonic potential, and torsional potential described by a trigonometric function, in the bonded portion. Nonbonded terms consist of van der Waals and Coulomb electrostatic interactions between couples of atoms.

As an example, these basic components of the CHARMM [78] force field are reported in the following equations

$$V = V_{bonded} + V_{nonbonded}$$

$$V_{bonded} = \sum_{bonds} K_b(b - b_0)^2 + \sum_{angles} K_\theta(\theta - \theta_0)^2$$
$$+ \sum_{dihedrals} K_\chi(1 + \cos(n\chi - \delta))$$

$$V_{nonbonded} = \sum_{\substack{nonbonded \\ pairs\ ij}} \frac{q_i q_j}{\varepsilon r_{ij}}$$
$$+ \sum_{\substack{nonbonded \\ pairs\ ij}} \varepsilon_{ij} \left[\left(\frac{R_{min,\ ij}}{r_{ij}} \right)^{12} - 2 \left(\frac{R_{min,\ ij}}{r_{ij}} \right)^6 \right]$$

where K_b, K_θ, and K_χ are the bond, angle and torsional force constants; b, θ and χ are bond length, bond angle and dihedral angle (those with the 0-subscript are the equilibrium values); n is multiplicity and δ the phase of the torsional periodic function; r_{ij} is the distance between atoms i and j; q_i and q_j are the partial charges of atoms i and j; ε is the effective dielectric constant; ε_{ij} is the Lennard-Jones well depth and $R_{min,ij}$ is the distance between atoms at Lennard-Jones minimum.

These terms may appear slightly different in different force-fields, and anharmonicity and cross-terms are generally added.

The parameters of the force field are obtained by fitting quantum mechanical or experimental values.

These methods assume that ligand-protein contacts statistically more explored are correlated with favorable interactions. Starting from a database of structures, the frequencies of ligand-protein atom pairs contacts are computed and converted into an energy component. When evaluating a pose, the aforementioned tabulated energy components are summed up for all ligand-protein atom pairs, giving the score of the pose.

DrugScore (Gohlke et al., 2000; Velec et al., 2005) and GOLD/ASP (Mooij and Verdonk, 2005) are examples of knowledge-based scoring functions.

Another strategy consists in the combination of multiple scoring functions leading to the so-called consensus scoring (Charifson et al., 1999).

In addition, new scoring functions have been developed: for example, based on machine learning technologies, interaction fingerprints and attempts with quantum mechanical scores (Yuriev et al., 2015).

Sampling

The first molecular docking algorithm was developed in the 1980s by Kuntz et al. (1982); the receptor was approximated by a series of spheres filling its surface clefts, and the ligand by another set of spheres defining its volume. A search was made to find the best steric overlap between binding site and receptor spheres, neglecting any kind of conformational movement.

This method belongs to the group of fully-rigid docking techniques, according to the classification which divides docking methods according to the degrees of flexibility of the molecules involved in the calculation Halperin et al., 2002 (**Figure 1**):

1. Rigid docking:

Both ligand and protein are considered rigid entities, and just the three translational and three rotational degrees of freedom are considered during sampling. This approximation is analogous to the "lock-key" binding model and is mainly used for protein-protein docking, where the number of conformational degrees of freedom is too high to be sampled. Generally, in these methods, the binding site and the ligand are approximated by "hot" points and the superposition of matching point is evaluated (Taylor et al., 2002).

2. Semi-flexible docking:

Just one of the molecules, the ligand, is flexible, while the protein is rigid. Thus, the conformational degrees of freedom of the ligand are sampled, in addition to the six translational plus rotational ones. These methods assume that a fixed conformation of a protein may correspond to the one able to recognize the ligands to be docked. This assumption, as already reported, is not always verified.

3. Flexible docking:

It is based on the concept that a protein is not a passive rigid entity during binding and considers both ligand and protein as flexible counterparts. Different methods have been introduced during the years, some rested on the induced fit binding model and others on conformational selection.

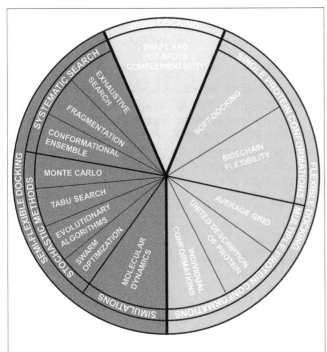

FIGURE 1 | Molecular docking techniques organized according to ligand-protein flexibility and conformational searching engines.

The great number of degrees of freedom introduced by flexible docking makes the potential energy surface to be a function of numerous coordinates. Consequently, the computational effort required to perform a docking calculation is augmented, but both sampling and scoring should be optimized to give a good balance between accuracy and speed. In fact, virtual screening campaign of millions of compounds depends on the velocity of docking calculations. For this reason, more and more improvements have been made in the development of the new algorithm, able to deeply search the phase space but not at the expense of velocity.

Semi-flexible Docking

Numerous docking algorithms have been developed since the 1980s. Often it is difficult to classify clearly each docking software, because different algorithms may be integrated into a multi-phase approach. However, docking algorithms can be classified as follows (Kitchen et al., 2004; Huang and Zou, 2010):

1. Systematic search techniques:

In a systematic search, a set of discretized values is associated with each degree of freedom, and all the values of each coordinate are explored in a combinatorial way (Brooijmans and Kuntz, 2003). These methods are subdivided into:

a. *Exhaustive search* - it is a systematic search in the strict sense since all the rotatable bonds of the ligands are examined in a systematic way. A number of constraints and termination criteria is generally established to limit the search space and to avoid a combinatorial explosion. The docking pipeline of the software Glide (Friesner et al., 2004; Halgren et al., 2004) involves a stage of the exhaustive search.

b. *Fragmentation* - the first implementation of ligand flexibility into docking was introduced by DesJarlais et al. (1986), who proposed a method made of fragmentation of the ligand, rigid docking of the fragments into the binding site, and subsequent linking of the fragments. In this way, partial flexibility is implemented at the joints between the fragments. Other methods, defined as incremental construction, dock one fragment first and then attach incrementally the others. Examples of methods utilizing fragmentation are FlexX (Rarey et al., 1996) and Hammerhead (Welch et al., 1996).

c. *Conformational Ensemble* - rigid docking algorithms can be easily enriched by a sort of flexibility if an ensemble of previously generated conformers of the ligand is docked to the target, in a sort of conformational selection fashion on the ligand counterpart. Examples are offered by FLOG (Miller et al., 1994), EUDOC (Pang et al., 2001), MS-DOCK (Sauton et al., 2008).

2. Stochastic methods:

Stochastic algorithms change randomly, instead of systematically, the values of the degrees of freedom of the system. The advantage of these techniques is the speed, so they could potentially find the optimal solution really fast. As a drawback, they do not ensure a full search of the conformational space, so the true solution may be missed. The lack of convergence is partially solved by increasing the number of iterations of the algorithm. The most famous stochastic algorithms are (Huang and Zou, 2010):

a. *Monte Carlo (MC) methods* - Monte Carlo methods are based on the Metropolis Monte Carlo algorithm, which introduces an acceptance criterion in the evolution of the docking search. In particular, at every iteration of the algorithm, a random modification of the ligand degrees of freedom is performed. Then, if the energy score of the pose is improved, the change is accepted, otherwise, it is accepted according to the probability expressed in the following equation:

$$P \sim exp\left[\frac{-(E_1 - E_0)}{k_B T}\right]$$

where E_1 and E_0 are the energy score before and after the modification, k_B the Boltzmann constant, and T the temperature of the system.

This is the original form of the Metropolis algorithm, but it is implemented in different variants within docking software. Some example are provided by the earlier versions of AutoDock (Goodsell and Olson, 1990; Morris et al., 1996), ICM (Abagyan et al., 1994), QXP (McMartin and Bohacek, 1997), MCDOCK (Liu and Wang, 1999), AutoDock Vina (Trott and Olson, 2010), ROSETTALIGAND (Meiler and Baker, 2006).

b. *Tabu search methods* - the aim of these algorithms is to prevent the exploration of already sampled zones of the conformational/positional space. Random modifications are performed on the degrees of freedom of the ligand at each iteration. The already sampled conformations are registered, and when a new pose is obtained, it is accepted only if not similar to any previously explored pose. PRO_LEADS (Baxter et al., 1998) and PSI-DOCK (Pei et al., 2006) are two examples of this category.

c. *Evolutionary Algorithms* (EA) - these algorithms are based on the idea of biological evolution, with the most famous Genetic Algorithms (GAs). The concept of the gene, chromosome, mutation, and crossover are borrowed from biology. In particular, the degrees of freedom are encoded into genes, and each conformation of the ligand is described by a chromosome (collection of genes), which is assigned a fitness score. Mutations and crossovers occur within a population of chromosomes, and chromosomes with higher fitness survive and replace the worst ones. The most famous examples are GOLD (Jones et al., 1995, 1997), AutoDock 3 & 4 (which implement a different version of GA, the Lamarckian GA) (Morris et al., 1998), PSI-DOCK (Pei et al., 2006), rDock (Ruiz-Carmona et al., 2014).

d. *Swarm optimization (SO) methods* - these methods take inspiration from swarm behavior. The sampling of the degrees of freedom of a ligand is guided by the information deposited by already sampling good poses. For example, PLANTS (Korb et al., 2006) adopts an ACO (Ant Colony Optimization) algorithm, which mimics the behavior of ants, who communicate the easiest way to reach a source of food through the deposition of pheromone. Here, each degree of freedom is associated with a pheromone. Virtual ants choose conformations considering the values of pheromones, and successful ants contribute to pheromone deposition.

Other examples of SOs are SODOCK (Chen et al., 2007), pso@autodock (Namasivayam and Günther, 2007), PSOVina (Ng et al., 2015).

3. Simulation methods:

The most famous example of this category is Molecular Dynamics, a method that describes the time evolution of a system. A wider explanation will be given in section Molecular Dynamics.

Energy minimization methods can be inserted in this category, but generally, they are not used as stand-alone search engines (Kitchen et al., 2004). Energy minimization is a local optimization technique, used to bring the system to the closest minimum on the potential energy surface.

Flexible Docking

Some attempts have been made to introduce protein flexibility into docking calculations. These methods take advantage of different degrees of approximation and can be divided into approaches that consider single protein or multiple protein conformations (Alonso et al., 2006).

1. Single Protein Conformation:

a. Soft docking:

This method, firstly described by Jiang and Kim (1991), consists of an implicit and rough treatment of protein flexibility. The van der Waals repulsion term employed in force field scoring functions is reduced, allowing small clashes that permit a closer ligand-protein packing. In this way, a sort of induced-fit is

simulated. As a drawback, this approach approximates just feeble protein movements and could implicate unreal poses (Apostolakis et al., 1998; Vieth et al., 1999).

b. Sidechain flexibility:

This strategy introduces alternative conformations for some protein side chains (Leach, 1994). This is generally done exploiting databases of rotamer libraries. Some docking methods, such as GOLD, sample some degrees of freedom within their own search engine. Obviously, considering side chain flexibility, huge conformational variations of the protein are neglected by these methods.

2. Multiple Protein Conformations:

Multiple experimental structures may be available for the same target. Moreover, an ensemble of protein conformations can be obtained via computational techniques, such as Monte Carlo or Molecular Dynamics simulations. The idea of multiple protein conformations docking is to take into account all the diverse structures, following different possible strategies:

a. Average grid:

The structures of the ensemble are used to construct a single average-grid, which can be either a simple or weighted average combination of them (Knegtel et al., 1997).

b. United description of the protein:

In this case, the structures do not collapse into an average grid but are used to construct the best performing "chimera" protein. For example, FlexE (Rarey et al., 1996) extracts the structurally conserved portions from the structures of the ensemble and uses them to construct an average rigid structure. This portion is fused to the flexible parts of the ensemble in a combinatorial fashion, giving a pool of "chimeras" that are used for docking.

c. Individual conformations:

The structures of the ensemble are considered as conformations that can possibly be bound by the ligand, so various docking runs are performed, evaluating the ligands of interest on all the target conformations (Huang and Zou, 2007). Moreover, a preliminary benchmark assessing the performance of different target structures in a cross-docking experiment may be employed to filter the ensemble of structures (Salmaso et al., 2016, 2018).

Among the drugs approved by the Food and Drug Administration, few examples of successful applications of CADD are available (Talele et al., 2010). Among them, the renin-inhibitor Aliskiren was developed by means of a combination of molecular modeling and crystallographic structure analysis (Wood et al., 2003). However, the binding of non-peptidomimetic ligands to renin has shown huge structural rearrangement of the protein (Teague, 2003), addressing the problem of considering protein flexibility in drug design campaigns. Recently, a comparative study evaluating the performance of ensemble docking and individual crystal structure docking has been proposed for renin (Strecker and Meyer, 2018). An ensemble of 4 crystal structures outperformed the mean results of individual crystal structures in terms of binding mode prediction and screening utility. The ensemble gave worse results than the best performing crystal structure, which though is not known a priori. Not as good results were obtained through a Molecular Dynamics ensemble when compared to crystallographic structures, as confirmed in other cases reported in the literature (Osguthorpe et al., 2012; Ganser et al., 2018). However, Molecular Dynamics has proven to be effective as a tool to explore molecular conformations and as a docking method itself, as reported in the following paragraphs.

Molecular Dynamics

Molecular dynamics (MD) is a computational technique which simulates the dynamic behavior of molecular systems as a function of time, treating all the entities in the simulation box (ligand, protein, as long as waters if explicit) as flexible (Salmaso, 2018).

It was developed to simulate simple systems, with the first application to study collisions among hard spheres, in 1957 (Alder and Wainwright, 1957). The first MD simulation of a biomolecule was accomplished in 1977 by McCammon et al. (McCammon et al., 1977); it was a 9.2 ps simulation of a 58-residues Bovine Pancreatic Trypsin Inhibitor (BPTI), performed in vacuum with a crude molecular mechanics potential.

Molecular dynamics compute the movements of atoms along time by the integration of Newton's equations of motions (classical mechanics), reported in the following equation (Leach, 2001; Adcock and McCammon, 2006).

$$\frac{d^2 r_i(t)}{dt^2} = \frac{F_i(t)}{m_i}$$

with $F_i(t)$ force exerted on atom i at time t, $r_i(t)$ vector position of the atom i at time t, m_i mass of the atom (**Figure 2**).

In particular, time is partitioned into time steps (δt), which are used to propagate the system forward in time. Several integration algorithms are available, which derive Newton's equations by a discrete-time numerical approximation. The velocity-Verlet integrator is reported in the following equations as an example to compute position and velocity of an atom i at the time step $t+\delta t$, starting from step t.

$$r_i(t + \delta t) = r_i(t) + v_i(t)\,\delta t + \frac{1}{2} a_i(t)\,\delta t^2$$

$$v_i(t + \delta t) = v_i(t) + \frac{1}{2}\left[a_i(t) + a_i(t + \delta t)\right]\delta t$$

where $r_i(t)$, $v_i(t)$ and $a_i(t)$ are respectively position, velocity and acceleration of atom i at time t, and $r_i(t+\delta t)$, $v_i(t+\delta t)$ and $a_i(t+\delta t)$ are respectively position, velocity and acceleration of atom i at time $t+\delta t$.

Acceleration is calculated from the forces acting on atom i according to Newton's second law, and forces are computed from the force field, according to the following equation:

$$a_i(t) = \frac{d^2 r_i(t)}{dt^2} = \frac{F_i(t)}{m_i} = -\frac{dV(r(t))}{m_i dr_i(t)}$$

where $V(r(t))$ is the potential energy function retrieved by the force field (see **Box 1**).

The most used force fields in molecular dynamics are CHARMM (MacKerell et al., 1998), AMBER (Cornell et al., 1995), OPLS (Jorgensen and Tirado-Rives, 1988) and GROMOS (Oostenbrink et al., 2004).

Molecular Dynamics and Exploration of the Phase Space

MD trajectories can be used as sampling engines; in fact, they produce protein conformations usable for Multiple Protein Conformations docking applications. In particular, McCammon et al. developed the so-called Relaxed-Complex Scheme (RCS), consisting in docking mini-libraries of compounds with AutoDock (Morris et al., 1998) against a large ensemble of snapshots derived from unliganded protein MD trajectories (Lin et al., 2002, 2003; Amaro et al., 2008). This approach is based on the conformational selection binding model, disregarding any influence of the ligand on the receptor. The application of the RCS to the UDP-galactose 4'-epimerase (TbGalE), for example, led to the identification of 14 low-micromolar inhibitors (Durrant et al., 2010). Another computational pipeline integrating MD simulations and virtual screening has proved to be effective: the coupling of MD, clustering, and choice of the target structure through fingerprints for ligand and proteins (MD-FLAP) improved VS performance (Spyrakis et al., 2015).

MD has further applications as a docking-coupled technique (Alonso et al., 2006) more anchored to the induced-fit model, as it can be used to assess stability (Sabbadin et al., 2014; Yu et al., 2018), to refine and to rescore docking poses (Rastelli et al., 2009).

The relevance of MD simulations as source of target conformational profusion can be exploited to retrieve insights into cryptic pockets or allosteric binding sites (Durrant and McCammon, 2011), as reported by Schame et al., who identified an alternative binding site, named "trench," close to the active site of the HIV-1 integrase (Schames et al., 2004). Moreover, simulations in the explicit solvent may give information on water molecules, that can be classified as "cold" or stable and "hot" or unstable (for a recent and comprehensive overview on the role of water in SBDD; see Spyrakis et al., 2017). In particular, MD may enable to individuate relevant water molecules, according to their order (Li and Lazaridis, 2003) and stationarity (Cuzzolin et al., 2018), and to estimate their contribution in modulating ligand binding (Bortolato et al., 2013; Betz et al., 2016).

All the aforementioned applications of MD are used as a complement to classic molecular docking techniques. however, the simulation of the complete binding process of a ligand, from the unbound state in bulk solvent to the bound state, be considered a fully-flexible docking in explicit solvent. The possibility to investigate the whole binding process could give insights into metastable states reached by the ligand during the simulation, alternative binding sites, the role of water during binding and conformational rearrangements preceding, concurrent or consecutive to binding.

However, the observation of a binding event during a classical MD simulation is very rare, raising the timescale problem. The timestep in molecular dynamics has to be compatible with the

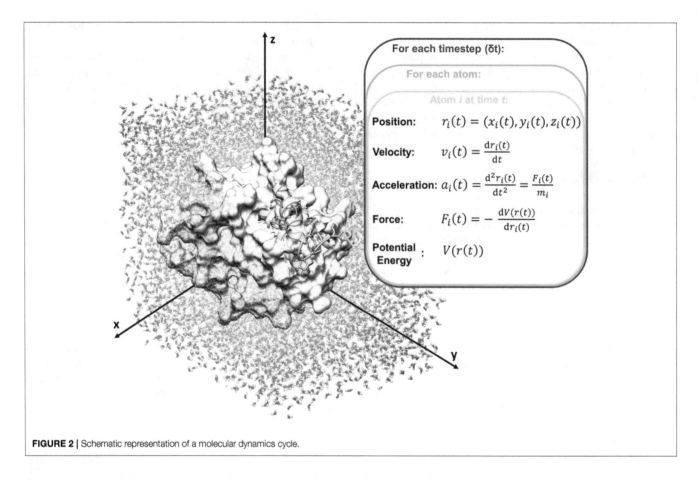

FIGURE 2 | Schematic representation of a molecular dynamics cycle.

fastest motion in the system; in particular, a timestep of 1–2 fs, corresponding to bond vibrations, has to be used. Thus, a high number of MD steps is required to simulate slow processes, such as large domain motions and binding (μs-ms) (Henzler-Wildman and Kern, 2007), making the computational effort really hard. In particular, slow timescale are linked to processes that require the overcoming of a high energy barrier (Henzler-Wildman and Kern, 2007), corresponding to low populated states in the conformational energy landscape; in this case the simulated system gets trapped in a local minimum, making classical MD inadequate to explore largely the conformational space.

Advances in Classical MD Simulations

In 1998 Duan and Kollman performed the first 1μs simulation of a protein in explicit solvent, observing the folding of a 36-residue villin headpiece subdomain from a fully unfolded state. This simulation was two orders of magnitude longer than a state-of-the-art simulation of that period, and it was made possible by advances in massively parallel supercomputers and efficient parallelized codes, but still required 2 months of CPU (Central Processing Units) time (Duan and Kollman, 1998).

Specialized informatic infrastructures have also been designed specifically for MD calculations; for example, a supercomputer named Anton was conceived as a "computational microscope" and was developed with the idea to reach previously inaccessible simulation timescales within a reasonable computation time (Shaw et al., 2008). This machine allowed Shaw et al. to

characterize the folding of FiP35 WW domain from a fully extended state in a 100 μs simulation and, in addition, to reach the millisecond timescale in a single simulation of BPTI in the folded-state (Shaw et al., 2010), followed recently by ubiquitin (Lindorff-Larsen et al., 2016). Moreover, with unbiased simulations in the order of ten microseconds, Shaw's group could simulate the complete binding process of beta blockers and agonists to the β_2-adrenergic receptor (Dror et al., 2011) and kinase inhibitors to Src kinase (Shan et al., 2011).

As a drawback, the utilization of supercomputer is an expense that not many research groups can afford. Fortunately, the recent years have been characterized by the development of code able to exploit the speed of GPUs (Graphics Processing Units), which has given access to tera-scale performances with the use of a common workstation, and a consequent relatively low cost (Van Meel et al., 2008; Friedrichs et al., 2009; Harvey et al., 2009; Nobile et al., 2017). The architecture of a GPU is meant to parallelize a computation over thousands of cores, with all cores executing the same instructions on different data ("Same Instruction Multiple Data," SIM) (Nobile et al., 2017). For this reason, together with few preliminary applications in the field of molecular docking (Korb et al., 2011; Khar et al., 2013), GPUs have been mainly exploited for MD simulations, which can be parallelized at the level of atoms. In fact, nowadays, simulations of hundreds of nanoseconds are easily performed, and reaching the microsecond timescale is an affordable issue on a GPU-equipped workstation (Harvey and De Fabritiis, 2012). In addition, cloud computing has been emerging nowadays, not just through the use of web-servers intended to make molecular modeling accessible to a community of non-developers users, but also with the provision of computation power scalable and on-demand (Ebejer et al., 2013). As an example, AceCloud is an on-demand service for MD simulations, which is accessed through an extension of the ACEMD MD code (Harvey and De Fabritiis, 2015).

Moreover, a paradigm shift seems to have been spreading, that is the possibility to simulate long processes using numerous trajectories shorter than the process itself instead of a single long trajectory. This idea has been exploited by the folding@home project, a worldwide distributed computing environment benefitting from the computers of private citizens, when not in use (Shirts and Pande, 2000). Since during a classical MD simulation, the system is stuck in a minimum, waiting for the fortunate event that triggers the overcoming of an energy barrier, the simulation of many trajectories in parallel would increase the probability to meet the lucky event. Thus, numerous simulations are started from the same initial condition and run in parallel on different computers, and when one escapes from the energy minimum, all the simulations are stopped and started from the new productive configuration (Pande et al., 2003).

The new paradigm has found its best application in the use of Markov State Models (MSMs) and adaptive sampling. In fact, MSMs are based on an ensemble view of the dynamics, from which statistical properties, such as the probability to occupy a state and the probability to jump from one state to another, are computed. The construction of a Markov model is made of the discretization and projection of a trajectory into microstates, and of a transition probability matrix $T(\tau)$ computation at a given time, the lag-time τ, chosen in a way that the transition is memory-less (Markovian). Each element $T_{ij}(\tau)$ of the transition matrix represents the conditional probability to find the system in state j at time $t + \tau$ while being in state i at time t. The transition matrix approximates the dynamic of the system and enables to extrapolate the free energy from the equilibrium probability distribution of the system and the timescale of the slowest processes, even if they are not directly explored. In a qualitative fashion, the MSM may individuate diverse metastable states and construct multi-states models of the processes (Prinz et al., 2011). As an example, an MSM was constructed on an aggregate of nearly 500 100 ns-trajectories describing benzamidine-trypsin binding (with 37% productive trajectories); this enabled to characterize the binding process individuating three transition states, and to estimate binding free energy with 1 kcal/mol difference from the experimental one (while a higher deviation from experiment was associated with the extrapolated k_{on} and k_{off}) (Buch et al., 2011). Moreover, the computation of MSM on the collected data can give a feedback about undersampled zones of the phase space, suggesting where to focus further simulation, adapting the sampling (adaptive sampling methods) and increasing the efficiency of simulations (Bowman et al., 2010; Doerr and De Fabritiis, 2014). Currently, the major difficulties of this technique are related to the trajectory partition into discrete states, the choice of the lagtime and sufficient sampling to guarantee statistical significance (Pande et al., 2010).

Several alternative techniques have been developed during the years to overcome the time limitation imposed by classical MD simulations. A first example consists of the Coarse-Grained MD simulations, in which groups of atoms are condensed into spheres, reducing the degrees of freedom of the system (Kmiecik et al., 2016). This simplifies the conformational landscape of the system, but, as a drawback, the information on the all-atom simulations, that are precious for drug-discovery aim, are lost.

Additional strategies consist of enhanced sampling techniques that apply a bias to molecular dynamics simulations to increase the accessible timescale, enabling the simulation of slow processes like binding, unbinding and folding processes in a reduced amount of time.

Enhanced Sampling Techniques

These methods add a bias force/potential to the system to increase the rate of escape from local minima, entailing an acceleration of conformational sampling. They have been conceived primarily to study either folding or binding or unbinding processes, sharing the underlying idea of enhancement of sampling and overcoming high energy barriers.

Enhanced sampling techniques can be divided into methods that make use of collective variables to introduce the bias and methods that do not (De Vivo et al., 2016) (**Figure 3**).

The employment of a collective variable (CV) is based on the idea that a complex system can be decomposed into one or a combination of reaction coordinates describing the process of interest. These coordinates are named as collective variables since it is assumed they can summarize the behavior of the entire system. After a careful choice of the CVs, the bias is added on these coordinates during the simulation enhancing sampling along the CVs. The phase space is reduced to the space of the collective variables, since the conformational space is projected to the selected CVs, with a consequent dimensional reduction of the free energy surface.

In the following paragraphs, few representative enhanced sampling techniques are reported as an example, focusing on their application in binding and unbinding and going toward a fully dynamic docking (De Vivo and Cavalli, 2017).

Collective variables-free methods

Replica Exchange Molecular Dynamics (REMD) This method adopts an increase in temperature to accelerate the conformational sampling. The first formulation of Replica Exchange MD (Sugita and Okamoto, 1999), also known as Parallel Tempering (PT), consists of the parallel simulation of a number of independent and simultaneous replicas of the same system, starting from the same configuration, but at different temperatures. At regular time intervals, two replicas characterized by neighbor temperatures are switched, or, in other terms, their temperatures are exchanged, with a probability determined by the energy (E) and temperature (T) of the system. In particular, the transition probability between simulations at temperature T_1 and T_2 is determined by the Metropolis criterion:

$$P(T_1 \rightarrow T_2) = \begin{cases} 1 & for \quad [\beta_2 - \beta_1](E_1 - E_2) \leq 0 \\ e^{-[\beta_2 - \beta_1](E_1 - E_2)} & for \quad [\beta_2 - \beta_1](E_1 - E_2) > 0 \end{cases}$$

where $\beta = 1/k_B T$ (with k_B the Boltzmann constant).

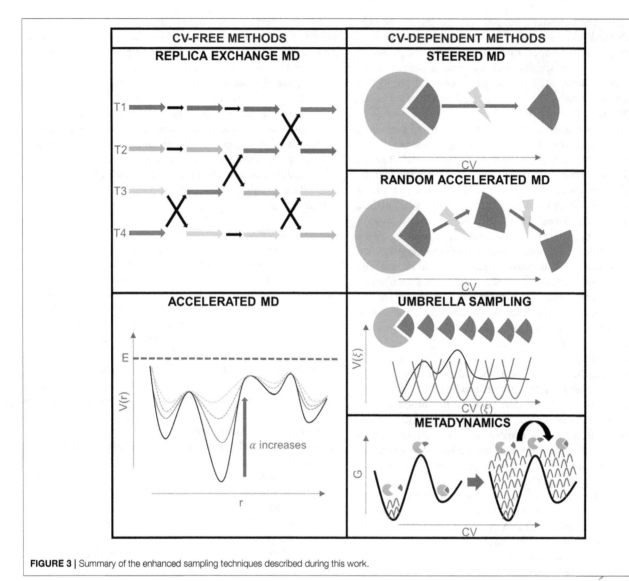

FIGURE 3 | Summary of the enhanced sampling techniques described during this work.

Temperatures are updated by rescaling the velocities of the parent simulations (v_1 and v_2 to v_1' and v_2') according to the following equation:

$$\begin{cases} v_1' = \sqrt{\frac{T_2}{T_1}} v_1 \\ v_2' = \sqrt{\frac{T_1}{T_2}} v_2 \end{cases}$$

The choice of the panel of temperatures is critical, and various strategies have been proposed to guide the selection (Patriksson and van der Spoel, 2008).

Further development of REMD has been introduced, such as the Hamiltonian Replica Exchange (H-REMD), where Hamiltonians are exchanged among replicas instead of temperatures (Fukunishi et al., 2002), and Replica Exchange with Solute Tempering, where a different treatment of the central group and the solvent buffer is performed (Liu et al., 2005). HREMD has been recently combined to conventional MD simulations using multi-ensemble Markov models (MEMMs) (Wu et al.,

2016) to investigate the multistate kinetics of Mdm2 and its inhibitor peptide PMI (Paul et al., 2017). An ensemble of 500 μs unbiased MD simulations conducted from different initial states, especially dissociated, were combined to HREMD simulations (6 simulations of 1 μs and with 14 replicas) to enhance sampling of rare dissociation events; the results were analyzed through the TRAMMBAR estimator, leading to the prediction of a residence time beyond the second timescale, despite a sub-millisecond simulation time. Moreover, the trajectories were furtherly analyzed to investigate the binding mechanism and binding-induced folding of PMI (Paul et al., 2018). It appeared that a multitude of parallel pathways is possible and that binding and folding are coupled, while not temporarily ordered and separated.

Accelerated Molecular Dynamics (aMD) Accelerated MD (aMD) facilitates the egress from a low energy basin by adding a bias potential function ($\Delta V(r)$) when the system is entrapped in an energy minimum. In particular, when the potential energy ($V(r)$) is lower than a certain cut-off (E), the bias is added giving a modified potential ($V^*(r)=V(r)+ \Delta V(r)$); otherwise the simulation continues in the true-unbiased potential ($V^*(r)=V(r)$).

The bias function is reported in the following equation:

$$\Delta V(r) = \frac{(E - V(r))^2}{\alpha + (E - V(r))}$$

where E is the potential energy cut-off and α is a tuning parameter determining the depth of the modified potential energy basin.

E has to be at least greater than V_{min} (the minimum potential energy, close to the starting configuration), while $\alpha = E - V_{min}$ will allow maintaining the underlying shape of the landscape (Hamelberg et al., 2004).

As an example, aMD showed qualitatively similar results to classical MD with fewer computational effort in the simulation of tiotropium-M$_3$ Muscarinic Acetylcholine Receptor binding: tiotropium was observed to recognize the extracellular vestibule of the receptor, as in a previously reported long (16 μs) classical MD simulation (Kruse et al., 2012), by accelerating the process of about one order of magnitude (three aMD replicas of 200 ns, 500 ns, and 1 μs) (Kappel et al., 2015).

Collective Variables-dependent methods

Steered Molecular Dynamics (SMD) Taking inspiration from atomic force microscopy experiments, in Steered MD (SMD) an external force is applied to a ligand to drive it out of the target binding site (Isralewitz et al., 1997, 2001; Izrailev et al., 1997). Other possibilities involve the application of forces on different CVs, such as nonlinear coordinates that can help to explore the conformational rearrangement of protein domains (Izrailev et al., 1999).

SMD gives insights into the ligand-target unbinding mechanism, which can be investigated through the dynamical evolution of the ligand-target pattern of interactions, as reported for a series of Cyclin-Dependent Kinase 5 (CDK5) inhibitors (Patel et al., 2014). In the same work, the second application of SMD in drug discovery is highlighted: since the bias force added during an SMD simulation is assumed to be related to the binding strength, the binding force profile can be used to discriminate binders from non-binders.

SMD relies on an a priori definition of the applied force direction, which can be fixed (for example a simple straight line) or can change during the simulation. The choice of the direction is not trivial, because a ligand may bump into obstructions during its way out of the protein, but a method evaluating the minimal steric hindrance has been reported (Vuong et al., 2015). Moreover, integration with the targeted molecular dynamics (TMD) are reported: in TMD a bias force is applied to conduct the system from an initial to a desired final configuration (Schlitter et al., 1993), leading to the individuation of a path that can be used as set of directions for an SMD simulation (Isralewitz et al., 2001).

Random Acceleration Molecular Dynamics (RAMD) Random Acceleration MD (RAMD), also defined Random Expulsion MD, is an extension of SMD, and, like this, was developed to study the egress of a ligand from its target binding site. It consists of the application of an artificial randomly-directed force on a ligand to accelerate its unbinding. In this way, in comparison with SMD, RAMD avoids the preliminary choice of the force direction; consequently, if some obstructions are found during the exit pathway, the escape direction is switched.

In particular, the direction of the force is chosen stochastically and maintained for a number of MD steps. If during this time interval the average velocity of the ligand is lower than a specified cut-off (or, in other terms, if the distance covered by the ligand is lower than a cut-off distance, r_{min}), meaning that probably a rigid obstruction has been met, a new force direction is assigned to allow the ligand to search for alternative exit pathways (Lüdemann et al., 2000).

As SMD, RAMD is predominantly used to simulate ligand unbinding from a molecular target. The egress of carazolol from β$_2$ Adrenergic Receptor was for example described thanks to an ensemble of RAMD simulations (100 simulation, with a variable length of maximum 1 ns): the extracellular surface opening of the receptor was individuated as the predominant exit root, entailing the rupture of a salt bridge linking extracellular loop 2 to transmembrane helix 7 (Wang and Duan, 2009).

Umbrella Sampling (US) Umbrella Sampling (US) (Torrie and Valleau, 1977) consists of restraining the system along one or a combination of CVs. Commonly, the range of interest of the CV is divided into windows, each characterized by a reference value of the CV (ξ_{ref}). The bias potential enhances sampling in each window by forcing the system to stay close to the respective CV reference value. The bias is a function of the reaction coordinate, and can have different shapes, but generally consists of a simple harmonic, as in the following equation:

$$V(\xi) = \frac{k}{2}(\xi - \xi_{ref})^2$$

Where k is the strength of the potential and ξ is the value of the CV.

The strength of the bias has to be high enough to let energy barriers crossing, but sufficiently low to enable the overlapping of system distributions of different windows, as required for post-processing analysis.

The aim of US is to force sampling in each window to collect sufficient statistics along with the whole reaction coordinate. Then the distribution of the system and consequently the free energy is calculated along the CV (Kästner, 2011). Different post-processing methods can be used to perform combination and analysis of the data coming from the different US windows; the most famous is umbrella integration (Kästner and Thiel, 2005), the weighted histogram analysis method (WHAM) (Kumar et al., 1992), and the more recent Dynamic Weighted Histogram Analysis (DHAM) (Rosta and Hummer, 2015), which can be used also to derive kinetic parameters.

Integrations of US with other enhanced sampling techniques are reported in the literature, such as the replica-exchange umbrella sampling method (REUS), where an umbrella potential is exchanged among replicas (Sugita et al., 2000; Kokubo et al., 2011). This technique was applied to the prediction of ligand-protein binding structures, starting from unbound initial states and employing as CV ξ the distance between the centers of mass of the ligand and of the backbone of two selected residues. This technique resulted to be effective in the prediction of the binding mode of a couple of ligands on p38 and JNK3 kinases (RMSD minor than 1.7 Å), and outperformed a cross-docking experiment, highlighting the importance of considering protein flexibility to accurately predict the coordinates of a complex (Kokubo et al., 2013).

Metadynamics Metadynamics (Laio and Parrinello, 2002) introduces a bias potential to the Hamiltonian of the system in the form of a Gaussian-shaped function of one or more CVs. In this case, the bias does not restrain or constrain the system, neither force the system along with a preferred direction in the CV space. The bias is used to keep the memory of the already explored zones of the phase space, and to discourage the system to visit them again (Laio and Gervasio, 2008).

At time t, the bias potential ($V_G(S,t)$) is reported in the following equation:

$$V_G(S,t) = \int_0^t dt' \, \omega \exp\left(-\sum_{i=1}^{d} \frac{\left(S_i(R) - S_i\left(R\left(t'\right)\right)\right)^2}{2\sigma_i^2}\right)$$

where $S(R)=(S_1(R),...,S_d(R))$ is a set of d CVs (which are functions of the coordinates R of the system), $S_i(R(t))$ is the value of the ith CV at time t, σ_i is the Gaussian width for the ith CV, and ω is the energy rate, given by:

$$\omega = \frac{W}{\tau_G}$$

with W the Gaussian height and τ_G the deposition rate.

Thus, the bias is "history-dependent," because it is the sum of the Gaussians that have already been deposited in the CV space during the time.

The free energy landscape is explored, starting from the bottom of a well, by a random walk; bias-Gaussians are deposited in the CV space with a given frequency, and at each iteration, the bias is given by the sum of the already deposited Gaussians. As time goes by, the system, instead of being trapped in the bottom of a well, is pushed out by the hill of deposited Gaussians and enters a new minimum. The process continues until all the minima are compensated by the bias potential (Barducci et al., 2011).

Metadynamics in this way enables to enhance sampling and to reconstruct the free energy surface; this can be used to explore binding/unbinding processes (Gervasio et al., 2005), and, with the application of funnel metadynamics (Limongelli et al., 2013), to the estimation of binding free energy.

Unfortunately, it may occur that the free energy surface is overfilled, but this has been partially solved by well-tempered metadynamics, in which the height of the added Gaussian is rescaled by the already deposited bias (Barducci et al., 2008). Another issue with metadynamics is the choice of the CVs, which should describe the slowest motions of the system and the initial-final-relevant intermediates. Moreover, a small number of CVs has to be used, and a good strategy is a combination with other techniques able to enhanced sampling along a great number of transverse coordinates (Barducci et al., 2011), such as with parallel tempering (Bussi et al., 2006). Using a well-tempered multiple-walker funnel-restrained metadynamics, the binding pathway of several ligands to 5 G-protein-coupled receptors (including X-ray crystal structures and homology models) has been recently explored, resulting in the prediction of

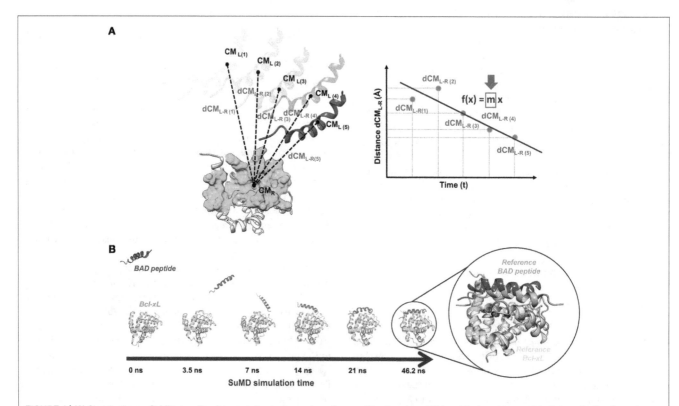

FIGURE 4 | (A) Sketch of a pepSuMD step: the distance between the centers of mass of the ligand (peptide) and the target is computed at regular time intervals during the SuMD step. The distance values are fitted by a line, whose slope (m) determines if the current SuMD step (m > 0) or a new one (m < 0) has to be simulated. **(B)** Representation of the binding pathway bringing BAD peptide to the Bcl-X$_L$ binding site, occurring in 46.2 ns. The superposition of the final pepSuMD state with the experimental structure (PDB ID: 1G5J, Petros et al., 2000) is reported on the right.

binding free energies with a root-mean-square error minor than 1 kcal mol^{-1} (Saleh et al., 2017).

Supervised Molecular Dynamics

In the last years, a new method, called Supervised Molecular Dynamics (SuMD), has been introduced to accelerate the binding process (Sabbadin and Moro, 2014; Cuzzolin et al., 2016). SuMD is distinguished from enhanced sampling simulations since it does not affect the energy profile of the system.

A SuMD simulation consists of a series of small MD windows (hundreds of picoseconds), called SuMD steps, where step $n+1$ is run after the evaluation of step n in terms of ligand-target approaching. During each SuMD step, the distance between the centers of mass of the ligand and of the target binding site (few selected residues) is computed; distance values are collected at regular intervals during the simulation and are fitted by a line (**Figure 4A**). If the slope of the line is negative, it means that the ligand is approaching the binding site, the SuMD step (step n) is considered productive, and a new step (step $n+1$) is started from the last coordinates and velocities of the current step. Otherwise, if the slope is positive, it means that the SuMD step is unproductive, thus the current SuMD step simulation is deleted and restarted from its initial coordinates (starting configuration of step n). The simulation is concluded after that the distance between the centers of mass of ligand and target fall under a certain cut-off. Finally, the consecutive SuMD steps are merged together providing the SuMD trajectory.

In this way, SuMD enables to observe a binding event in a reduced timescale, in the orders of tens to hundreds of nanoseconds, without the introduction of any energetic bias. Indeed, SuMD simply focuses sampling by the introduction of a tabu-like algorithm which favors the progress of a simulation toward productive events and avoids wasting simulation time in uninteresting portions of the search space.

Certainly, a single SuMD trajectory is not sufficient to explain the complex binding process, and the retrieval of thermodynamic quantities from a single simulation must be avoided. Nevertheless, a SuMD trajectory depicts one of the possible binding pathways leading a ligand to reach the target, so it can be useful to propose a mechanistic hypothesis.

The technique was first applied to Adenosine Receptors, where it facilitated the characterization of the binding pathways of several ligands toward the receptor, with the exploration of metabinding sites (Sabbadin and Moro, 2014; Sabbadin et al., 2015). In this context, SuMD can be useful in the interpretation of allosteric interactions (Deganutti et al., 2015) and has proved to be supportive to the identification of fragment-like positive allosteric modulators (Deganutti and Moro, 2017). In fact, SuMD turned out to be effective in simulating fragment compounds, as shown by the accurate prediction of the binding mode of a catechol fragment to human peroxiredoxin 5 (PRDX5), reaching a minimum RMSD of 0.7 Å from the crystallographic pose.

The applicability spectrum of SuMD has been furtherly enlarged, till the development of pepSuMD, a revised version of the technique able to simulate the binding pathway of a peptide ligand toward its protein binding site (Salmaso et al., 2017). The recognition process of the BAD peptide to Bcl-X$_L$ protein (**Figure 4B**) and of the p53 peptide to MDM2 has been recently reported, with the achievement of an RMSD less than 5 Å from the experimental conformation in tens of nanoseconds in both cases (46.2 and 23.40 ns, respectively). During the BAD/Bcl-X$_L$ simulation, the C-terminal helix explored different conformations, meaning that peptide and protein conformational rearrangements can be observed during a SuMD simulation when occurring in the same time scale of the SuMD-accelerated binding.

CONCLUSIONS AND PERSPECTIVES

In this review, an excursus over some relevant computational techniques in drug discovery has been performed, highlighting how protein flexibility has been introduced into the simulations during the years. Starting from simple rigid docking strategies justified by the lock-key model, it was soon necessary to consider conformational degrees of freedom of ligands during docking. Experimental data proving the existence of different conformations of protein structures has made the molecular models to face the problem of interpreting and simulating conformational transitions of macromolecules.

From rough attempts to include protein flexibility during classical molecular docking, the development of hardware technologies and of novel MD computational techniques has been allowing more and more to simulate huge conformational movements. The possibility to simulate contemporary folding and binding phenomena can be exploited to answer the long-standing debate about "induced-fit" and "conformational selection" binding models, by giving a mechanistic interpretation of binding pathways.

Moreover, some of the enhanced sampling techniques are no more an exclusive methodological exercise, but has become within reach of many research groups, whit a consequent real applicability in drug discovery.

AUTHOR CONTRIBUTIONS

VS and SM devised the organization, the main conceptual ideas, proof outline and wrote the review. The content of the present work has been largely taken from the PhD thesis entitled Exploring protein flexibility during docking to investigate ligand-target recognition written by VS under the supervision of SM.

ACKNOWLEDGMENTS

MMS lab is very grateful to Chemical Computing Group, OpenEye, and Acellera for the scientific and technical partnership. MMS lab gratefully acknowledges the support of NVIDIA Corporation with the donation of the Titan Xp GPU used for this research.

REFERENCES

Abagyan, R., and Totrov, M. (2001). High-throughput docking for lead generation. *Curr. Opin. Chem. Biol.* 5, 375–382. doi: 10.1016/S1367-5931(00)00217-9

Abagyan, R., Totrov, M., and Kuznetsov, D. (1994). ICM? A new method for protein modeling and design: applications to docking and structure prediction from the distorted native conformation. *J. Comput. Chem.* 15, 488–506. doi: 10.1002/jcc.540 150503

Adcock, S. A., and McCammon, J. A. (2006). Molecular dynamics: survey of methods for simulating the activity of proteins. *Chem. Rev.* 106, 1589–1615. doi: 10.1021/cr040426m

Alder, B. J., and Wainwright, T. E. (1957). Phase transition for a hard sphere system. *J. Chem. Phys.* 27, 1208–1209. doi: 10.1063/1.1743957

Alonso, H., Bliznyuk, A. A., and Gready, J. E. (2006). Combining docking and molecular dynamic simulations in drug design. *Med. Res. Rev.* 26, 531–568. doi: 10.1002/med.20067

Amaro, R. E., Baron, R., and McCammon, J. A. (2008). An improved relaxed complex scheme for receptor flexibility in computer-aided drug design. *J. Comput. Aided Mol. Des.* 22, 693–705. doi: 10.1007/s10822-007-9159-2

Apostolakis, J., Pluckthun, A., and Caflisch, A. (1998). Docking small ligands in flexible binding sites. *J. Comput. Chem.* 19, 21–37. doi: 10.1002/(SICI)1096-987X(19980115)19:1<21::AID-JCC2>3.0.CO;2-0

Austin, R. H., Beeson, K. W., Eisenstein, L., Frauenfelder, H., and Gunsalus, I. C. (1975). Dynamics of ligand binding to myoglobin. *Biochemistry* 14, 5355–5373. doi: 10.1021/bi00695a021

Barducci, A., Bonomi, M., and Parrinello, M. (2011). Metadynamics. *WIREs Comput. Mol. Sci.* 1, 826–843. doi: 10.1002/wcms.31

Barducci, A., Bussi, G., and Parrinello, M. (2008). Well-tempered metadynamics: a smoothly converging and tunable free-energy method. *Phys. Rev. Lett.* 100:020603. doi: 10.1103/PhysRevLett.100.020603

Baxter, C. A., Murray, C. W., Clark, D. E., Westhead, D. R., and Eldridge, M. D. (1998). Flexible docking using tabu search and an empirical estimate of binding affinity. *Proteins* 33, 367–382. doi: 10.1002/(SICI)1097-0134(19981115)33:3<367::AID-PROT6>3.0.CO;2-W

Berman, H. M., Westbrook, J., Feng, Z., Gilliland, G., Bhat, T. N., Weissig, H., et al. (2000). The protein data bank. *Nucleic Acids Res.* 28, 235–242. doi: 10.1093/nar/28.1.235

Betz, M., Wulsdorf, T., Krimmer, S. G., and Klebe, G. (2016). Impact of surface water layers on protein–ligand binding: how well are experimental data reproduced by molecular dynamics simulations in a thermolysin test case?. *J. Chem. Inf. Model.* 56, 223–233. doi: 10.1021/acs.jcim.5b00621

Böhm, H. J. (1994). The development of a simple empirical scoring function to estimate the binding constant for a protein-ligand complex of known three-dimensional structure. *J. Comput. Aided Mol. Des.* 8, 243–256. doi: 10.1007/BF00126743

Born, M., and Oppenheimer, R. (1927). Zur quantentheorie der molekeln. *Ann. Phys.* 389, 457–484. doi: 10.1002/andp.19273892002

Bortolato, A., Tehan, B. G., Bodnarchuk, M. S., Essex, J. W., and Mason, J. S. (2013). Water network perturbation in ligand binding: adenosine A(2A) antagonists as a case study. *J. Chem. Inf. Model.* 53, 1700–1713. doi: 10.1021/ci4001458

Bowman, G. R., Ensign, D. L., and Pande, V. S. (2010). Enhanced modeling via network theory: adaptive sampling of Markov state models. *J. Chem. Theory Comput.* 6, 787–794. doi: 10.1021/ct900620b

Brooijmans, N., and Kuntz, I. D. (2003). Molecular recognition and docking algorithms. *Annu. Rev. Biophys. Biomol. Struct.* 32, 335–373. doi: 10.1146/annurev.biophys.32.110601.142532

Buch, I., Giorgino, T., and De Fabritiis, G. (2011). Complete reconstruction of an enzyme-inhibitor binding process by molecular dynamics simulations. *Proc. Natl. Acad. Sci. U.S.A.* 108, 10184–10189. doi: 10.1073/pnas.1103547108

Bussi, G., Gervasio, F. L., Laio, A., and Parrinello, M. (2006). Free-energy landscape for beta hairpin folding from combined parallel tempering and metadynamics. *J. Am. Chem. Soc.* 128, 13435–13441. doi: 10.1021/ja062463w

Charifson, P. S., Corkery, J. J., Murcko, M. A., and Walters, W. P. (1999). Consensus scoring: a method for obtaining improved hit rates from docking databases of three-dimensional structures into proteins. *J. Med. Chem.* 42, 5100–5109. doi: 10.1021/jm990352k

Chen, H.-M., Liu, B.-F., Huang, H.-L., Hwang, S.-F., and Ho, S.-Y. (2007). SODOCK: swarm optimization for highly flexible protein-ligand docking. *J. Comput. Chem.* 28, 612–623. doi: 10.1002/jcc.20542

Corbeil, C. R., Williams, C. I., and Labute, P. (2012). Variability in docking success rates due to dataset preparation. *J. Comput. Aided Mol. Des.* 26, 775–786. doi: 10.1007/s10822-012-9570-1

Cornell, W. D., Cieplak, P., Bayly, C. I., Gould, I. R., Merz, K. M., Ferguson, D. M., et al. (1995). A second generation force field for the simulation of proteins, nucleic acids, and organic molecules. *J. Am. Chem. Soc.* 117, 5179–5197. doi: 10.1021/ja00124a002

Csermely, P., Palotai, R., and Nussinov, R. (2010). Induced fit, conformational selection and independent dynamic segments: an extended view of binding events. *Trends Biochem. Sci.* 35, 539–546. doi: 10.1016/j.tibs.2010.04.009

Cuzzolin, A., Deganutti, G., Salmaso, V., Sturlese, M., and Moro, S. (2018). AquaMMapS: an alternative tool to monitor the role of water molecules during protein-ligand association. *ChemMedChem* 13, 522–531. doi: 10.1002/cmdc.201700564

Cuzzolin, A., Sturlese, M., Deganutti, G., Salmaso, V., Sabbadin, D., Ciancetta, A., et al. (2016). Deciphering the complexity of ligand-protein recognition pathways using supervised molecular dynamics (SuMD) simulations. *J. Chem. Inf. Model.* 56, 687–705. doi: 10.1021/acs.jcim.5b00702

De Vivo, M., and Cavalli, A. (2017). Recent advances in dynamic docking for drug discovery. *WIREs Comput. Mol. Sci.* 7:e1320. doi: 10.1002/wcms.1320

De Vivo, M., Masetti, M., Bottegoni, G., and Cavalli, A. (2016). Role of molecular dynamics and related methods in drug discovery. *J. Med. Chem.* 59, 4035–4061. doi: 10.1021/acs.jmedchem.5b01684

Deganutti, G., Cuzzolin, A., Ciancetta, A., and Moro, S. (2015). Understanding allosteric interactions in G protein-coupled receptors using supervised molecular dynamics: a prototype study analysing the human A3 adenosine receptor positive allosteric modulator LUF6000. *Bioorg. Med. Chem.* 23, 4065–4071. doi: 10.1016/j.bmc.2015.03.039

Deganutti, G., and Moro, S. (2017). Supporting the identification of novel fragment-based positive allosteric modulators using a supervised molecular dynamics approach: a retrospective analysis considering the human A2A adenosine receptor as a key example. *Molecules* 22:818. doi: 10.3390/molecules22050818

DesJarlais, R. L., Sheridan, R. P., Dixon, J. S., Kuntz, I. D., and Venkataraghavan, R. (1986). Docking flexible ligands to macromolecular receptors by molecular shape. *J. Med. Chem.* 29, 2149–2153. doi: 10.1021/jm00161a004

Doerr, S., and De Fabritiis, G. (2014). On-the-fly learning and sampling of ligand binding by high-throughput molecular simulations. *J. Chem. Theory Comput.* 10, 2064–2069. doi: 10.1021/ct400919u

Dror, R. O., Pan, A. C., Arlow, D. H., Borhani, D. W., Maragakis, P., Shan, Y., et al. (2011). Pathway and mechanism of drug binding to G-protein-coupled receptors. *Proc. Natl. Acad. Sci. U.S.A.* 108, 13118–13123. doi: 10.1073/pnas.1104614108

Duan, Y., and Kollman, P. A. (1998). Pathways to a protein folding intermediate observed in a 1-microsecond simulation in aqueous solution. *Science* 282, 740–744. doi: 10.1126/science.282.5389.740

Durrant, J. D., and McCammon, J. A. (2011). Molecular dynamics simulations and drug discovery. *BMC Biol.* 9:71. doi: 10.1186/1741-7007-9-71

Durrant, J. D., Urbaniak, M. D., Ferguson, M. A., and McCammon, J. A. (2010). Computer-aided identification of Trypanosoma brucei uridine diphosphate galactose 4'-epimerase inhibitors: toward the development of novel therapies for African sleeping sickness. *J. Med. Chem.* 53, 5025–5032. doi: 10.1021/jm100456a

Ebejer, J.-P., Fulle, S., Morris, G. M., and Finn, P. W. (2013). The emerging role of cloud computing in molecular modelling. *J. Mol. Graph. Model.* 44, 177–187. doi: 10.1016/j.jmgm.2013.06.002

Eldridge, M. D., Murray, C. W., Auton, T. R., Paolini, G. V., and Mee, R. P. (1997). Empirical scoring functions: I. The development of a fast empirical scoring function to estimate the binding affinity of ligands in receptor complexes. *J. Comput. Aided Mol. Des.* 11, 425–445. doi: 10.1023/A:1007996124545

Fischer, E. (1894). Einfluss der configuration auf die wirkung der enzyme. *Ber. Dtsch. Chemischen Ges.* 27, 2985–2993. doi: 10.1002/cber.18940270364

Foote, J., and Milstein, C. (1994). Conformational isomerism and the diversity of antibodies. *Proc. Natl. Acad. Sci. U.S.A.* 91, 10370–10374. doi: 10.1073/pnas.91.22.10370

Frauenfelder, H., Sligar, S. G., and Wolynes, P. G. (1991). The energy landscapes and motions of proteins. *Science* 254, 1598–1603. doi: 10.1126/science.1749933

Friedrichs, M. S., Eastman, P., Vaidyanathan, V., Houston, M., Legrand, S., Beberg, A. L., et al. (2009). Accelerating molecular dynamic simulation on graphics processing units. *J. Comput. Chem.* 30, 864–872. doi: 10.1002/jcc.21209

Friesner, R. A., Banks, J. L., Murphy, R. B., Halgren, T. A., Klicic, J. J., Mainz, D. T., et al. (2004). Glide: a new approach for rapid, accurate docking and scoring. 1. Method and assessment of docking accuracy. *J. Med. Chem.* 47, 1739–1749. doi: 10.1021/jm0306430

Friesner, R. A., Murphy, R. B., Repasky, M. P., Frye, L. L., Greenwood, J. R., Halgren, T. A., et al. (2006). Extra precision glide: docking and scoring incorporating a model of hydrophobic enclosure for protein-ligand complexes. *J. Med. Chem.* 49, 6177–6196. doi: 10.1021/jm0512560

Fukunishi, H., Watanabe, O., and Takada, S. (2002). On the hamiltonian replica exchange method for efficient sampling of biomolecular systems: application to protein structure prediction. *J. Chem. Phys.* 116:9058. doi: 10.1063/1.1472510

Ganser, L. R., Lee, J., Rangadurai, A., Merriman, D. K., Kelly, M. L., Kansal, A. D., et al. (2018). High-performance virtual screening by targeting a high-resolution RNA dynamic ensemble. *Nat. Struct. Mol. Biol.* 25, 425–434. doi: 10.1038/s41594-018-0062-4

Gervasio, F. L., Laio, A., and Parrinello, M. (2005). Flexible docking in solution using metadynamics. *J. Am. Chem. Soc.* 127, 2600–2607. doi: 10.1021/ja0445950

Gohlke, H., Hendlich, M., and Klebe, G. (2000). Knowledge-based scoring function to predict protein-ligand interactions. *J. Mol. Biol.* 295, 337–356. doi: 10.1006/jmbi.1999.3371

Goodsell, D. S., and Olson, A. J. (1990). Automated docking of substrates to proteins by simulated annealing. *Proteins* 8, 195–202. doi: 10.1002/prot.340080302

Halgren, T. A., Murphy, R. B., Friesner, R. A., Beard, H. S., Frye, L. L., Pollard, W. T., et al. (2004). Glide: a new approach for rapid, accurate docking and scoring. 2. Enrichment factors in database screening. *J. Med. Chem.* 47, 1750–1759. doi: 10.1021/jm030644s

Halperin, I., Ma, B., Wolfson, H., and Nussinov, R. (2002). Principles of docking: an overview of search algorithms and a guide to scoring functions. *Proteins* 47, 409–443. doi: 10.1002/prot.10115

Hamelberg, D., Mongan, J., and McCammon, J. A. (2004). Accelerated molecular dynamics: a promising and efficient simulation method for biomolecules. *J. Chem. Phys.* 120, 11919–11929. doi: 10.1063/1.1755656

Harvey, M. J., and De Fabritiis, G. (2012). High-throughput molecular dynamics: the powerful new tool for drug discovery. *Drug Discov. Today* 17, 1059–1062. doi: 10.1016/j.drudis.2012.03.017

Harvey, M. J., and De Fabritiis, G. (2015). Acecloud: molecular dynamics simulations in the cloud. *J. Chem. Inf. Model.* 55, 909–914. doi: 10.1021/acs.jcim.5b00086

Harvey, M. J., Giupponi, G., and Fabritiis, G. D. (2009). ACEMD: accelerating biomolecular dynamics in the microsecond time scale. *J. Chem. Theory Comput.* 5, 1632–1639. doi: 10.1021/ct9000685

Henzler-Wildman, K., and Kern, D. (2007). Dynamic personalities of proteins. *Nature* 450, 964–972. doi: 10.1038/nature06522

Huang, S.-Y., and Zou, X. (2007). Ensemble docking of multiple protein structures: considering protein structural variations in molecular docking. *Proteins* 66, 399–421. doi: 10.1002/prot.21214

Huang, S.-Y., and Zou, X. (2010). Advances and challenges in protein-ligand docking. *Int. J. Mol. Sci.* 11, 3016–3034. doi: 10.3390/ijms11083016

Huey, R., Morris, G. M., Olson, A. J., and Goodsell, D. S. (2007). A semiempirical free energy force field with charge-based desolvation. *J. Comput. Chem.* 28, 1145–1152. doi: 10.1002/jcc.20634

Isralewitz, B., Gao, M., and Schulten, K. (2001). Steered molecular dynamics and mechanical functions of proteins. *Curr. Opin. Struct. Biol.* 11, 224–230. doi: 10.1016/S0959-440X(00)00194-9

Isralewitz, B., Izrailev, S., and Schulten, K. (1997). Binding pathway of retinal to bacterio-opsin: a prediction by molecular dynamics simulations. *Biophys. J.* 73, 2972–2979. doi: 10.1016/S0006-3495(97)78326-7

Izrailev, S., Crofts, A. R., Berry, E. A., and Schulten, K. (1999). Steered molecular dynamics simulation of the Rieske subunit motion in the cytochrome bc(1) complex. *Biophys. J.* 77, 1753–1768. doi: 10.1016/S0006-3495(99)77022-0

Izrailev, S., Stepaniants, S., Balsera, M., Oono, Y., and Schulten, K. (1997). Molecular dynamics study of unbinding of the avidin-biotin complex. *Biophys. J.* 72, 1568–1581. doi: 10.1016/S0006-3495(97)78804-0

Jiang, F., and Kim, S. H. (1991). "Soft docking": matching of molecular surface cubes. *J. Mol. Biol.* 219, 79–102. doi: 10.1016/0022-2836(91)90859-5

Jones, G., Willett, P., and Glen, R. C. (1995). Molecular recognition of receptor sites using a genetic algorithm with a description of desolvation. *J. Mol. Biol.* 245, 43–53. doi: 10.1016/S0022-2836(95)80037-9

Jones, G., Willett, P., Glen, R. C., Leach, A. R., and Taylor, R. (1997). Development and validation of a genetic algorithm for flexible docking. *J. Mol. Biol.* 267, 727–748. doi: 10.1006/jmbi.1996.0897

Jorgensen, W. L., and Tirado-Rives, J. (1988). The OPLS [optimized potentials for liquid simulations] potential functions for proteins, energy minimizations for crystals of cyclic peptides and crambin. *J. Am. Chem. Soc.* 110, 1657–1666. doi: 10.1021/ja00214a001

Kappel, K., Miao, Y., and McCammon, J. A. (2015). Accelerated molecular dynamics simulations of ligand binding to a muscarinic G-protein-coupled receptor. *Q. Rev. Biophys.* 48, 479–487. doi: 10.1017/S0033583515000153

Kästner, J. (2011). Umbrella sampling. *WIREs Comput. Mol. Sci.* 1, 932–942. doi: 10.1002/wcms.66

Kästner, J., and Thiel, W. (2005). Bridging the gap between thermodynamic integration and umbrella sampling provides a novel analysis method: "Umbrella integration". *J. Chem. Phys.* 123:144104. doi: 10.1063/1.2052648

Khar, K. R., Goldschmidt, L., and Karanicolas, J. (2013). Fast docking on graphics processing units via Ray-Casting. *PLoS ONE* 8:e70661. doi: 10.1371/journal.pone.0070661

Kitchen, D. B., Decornez, H., Furr, J. R., and Bajorath, J. (2004). Docking and scoring in virtual screening for drug discovery: methods and applications. *Nat. Rev. Drug Discov.* 3, 935–949. doi: 10.1038/nrd1549

Kmiecik, S., Gront, D., Kolinski, M., Wieteska, L., Dawid, A. E., and Kolinski, A. (2016). Coarse-grained protein models and their applications. *Chem. Rev.* 116, 7898–7936. doi: 10.1021/acs.chemrev.6b00163

Knegtel, R. M., Kuntz, I. D., and Oshiro, C. M. (1997). Molecular docking to ensembles of protein structures. *J. Mol. Biol.* 266, 424–440. doi: 10.1006/jmbi.1996.0776

Kobilka, B. K., and Deupi, X. (2007). Conformational complexity of G-protein-coupled receptors. *Trends Pharmacol. Sci.* 28, 397–406. doi: 10.1016/j.tips.2007.06.003

Kokubo, H., Tanaka, T., and Okamoto, Y. (2011). Ab initio prediction of protein-ligand binding structures by replica-exchange umbrella sampling simulations. *J. Comput. Chem.* 32, 2810–2821. doi: 10.1002/jcc.21860

Kokubo, H., Tanaka, T., and Okamoto, Y. (2013). Prediction of protein-ligand binding structures by replica-exchange umbrella sampling simulations: application to kinase systems. *J. Chem. Theory Comput.* 9, 4660–4671. doi: 10.1021/ct4004383

Korb, O., Stützle, T., and Exner, T. E. (2006). "PLANTS: application of ant colony optimization to structure-based drug design," in *Ant Colony Optimization and Swarm Intelligence*, eds M. Dorigo, L. M. Gambardella, M. Birattari, A. Martinoli, R. Poli, and T. Stützle (Berlin; Heidelberg: Springer), 247–258.

Korb, O., Stützle, T., and Exner, T. E. (2009). Empirical scoring functions for advanced protein-ligand docking with PLANTS. *J. Chem. Inf. Model.* 49, 84–96. doi: 10.1021/ci800298z

Korb, O., Stützle, T., and Exner, T. E. (2011). Accelerating molecular docking calculations using graphics processing units. *J. Chem. Inf. Model.* 51, 865–876. doi: 10.1021/ci100459b

Koshland, D. E. (1958). Application of a theory of enzyme specificity to protein synthesis. *Proc. Natl. Acad. Sci. U.S.A.* 44, 98–104. doi: 10.1073/pnas.44.2.98

Kruse, A. C., Hu, J., Pan, A. C., Arlow, D. H., Rosenbaum, D. M., Rosemond, E., et al. (2012). Structure and dynamics of the M3 muscarinic acetylcholine receptor. *Nature* 482, 552–556. doi: 10.1038/nature10867

Kumar, S., Ma, B., Tsai, C. J., Sinha, N., and Nussinov, R. (2000). Folding and binding cascades: dynamic landscapes and population shifts. *Protein Sci.* 9, 10–19. doi: 10.1110/ps.9.1.10

Kumar, S., Rosenberg, J. M., Bouzida, D., Swendsen, R. H., and Kollman, P. A. (1992). THE weighted histogram analysis method for free-energy calculations on biomolecules. I. The method. *J. Comput. Chem.* 13, 1011–1021. doi: 10.1002/jcc.540130812

Kuntz, I. D., Blaney, J. M., Oatley, S. J., Langridge, R., and Ferrin, T. E. (1982). A geometric approach to macromolecule-ligand interactions. *J. Mol. Biol.* 161, 269–288. doi: 10.1016/0022-2836(82)90153-X

Laio, A., and Gervasio, F. L. (2008). Metadynamics: a method to simulate rare events and reconstruct the free energy in biophysics, chemistry and material science. *Rep. Prog. Phys.* 71:126601. doi: 10.1088/0034-4885/71/12/126601

Laio, A., and Parrinello, M. (2002). Escaping free-energy minima. *Proc. Natl. Acad. Sci. U.S.A.* 99, 12562–12566. doi: 10.1073/pnas.202427399

Leach, A. R. (1994). Ligand docking to proteins with discrete side-chain flexibility. *J. Mol. Biol.* 235, 345–356. doi: 10.1016/S0022-2836(05)80038-5

Leach, A. R. (2001). *Molecular Modelling: Principles and Applications*. illustrated. Pearson Education. Available online at: https://books.google.it/books/about/Molecular_Modelling.html?id=kB7jsbV-uhkC&redir_esc=y

Li, Z., and Lazaridis, T. (2003). Thermodynamic contributions of the ordered water molecule in HIV-1 protease. *J. Am. Chem. Soc.* 125, 6636–6637. doi: 10.1021/ja0299203

Limongelli, V., Bonomi, M., and Parrinello, M. (2013). Funnel metadynamics as accurate binding free-energy method. *Proc. Natl. Acad. Sci. U.S.A.* 110, 6358–6363. doi: 10.1073/pnas.1303186110

Lin, J.-H., Perryman, A. L., Schames, J. R., and McCammon, J. A. (2002). Computational drug design accommodating receptor flexibility: the relaxed complex scheme. *J. Am. Chem. Soc.* 124, 5632–5633. doi: 10.1021/ja0260162

Lin, J.-H., Perryman, A. L., Schames, J. R., and McCammon, J. A. (2003). The relaxed complex method: accommodating receptor flexibility for drug design with an improved scoring scheme. *Biopolymers* 68, 47–62. doi: 10.1002/bip.10218

Lindorff-Larsen, K., Maragakis, P., Piana, S., and Shaw, D. E. (2016). Picosecond to millisecond structural dynamics in human ubiquitin. *J. Phys. Chem. B* 120, 8313–8320. doi: 10.1021/acs.jpcb.6b02024

Liu, M., and Wang, S. (1999). MCDOCK: a Monte Carlo simulation approach to the molecular docking problem. *J. Comput. Aided Mol. Des.* 13, 435–451. doi: 10.1023/A:1008005918983

Liu, P., Kim, B., Friesner, R. A., and Berne, B. J. (2005). Replica exchange with solute tempering: a method for sampling biological systems in explicit water. *Proc. Natl. Acad. Sci. U.S.A.* 102, 13749–13754. doi: 10.1073/pnas.0506346102

Lüdemann, S. K., Lounnas, V., and Wade, R. C. (2000). How do substrates enter and products exit the buried active site of cytochrome P450cam? 1. Random expulsion molecular dynamics investigation of ligand access channels and mechanisms. *J. Mol. Biol.* 303, 797–811. doi: 10.1006/jmbi.2000.4154

MacKerell, A. D., Bashford, D., Bellott, M., Dunbrack, R. L., Evanseck, J. D., Field, M. J., et al. (1998). All-atom empirical potential for molecular modeling and dynamics studies of proteins. *J. Phys. Chem. B* 102, 3586–3616. doi: 10.1021/jp973084f

McCammon, J. A., Gelin, B. R., and Karplus, M. (1977). Dynamics of folded proteins. *Nature* 267, 585–590. doi: 10.1038/267585a0

McMartin, C., and Bohacek, R. S. (1997). QXP: powerful, rapid computer algorithms for structure-based drug design. *J. Comput. Aided Mol. Des.* 11, 333–344. doi: 10.1023/A:1007907728892

Meiler, J., and Baker, D. (2006). ROSETTALIGAND: protein-small molecule docking with full side-chain flexibility. *Proteins* 65, 538–548. doi: 10.1002/prot.21086

Miller, D. W., and Dill, K. A. (1997). Ligand binding to proteins: the binding landscape model. *Protein Sci.* 6, 2166–2179. doi: 10.1002/pro.5560061011

Miller, M. D., Kearsley, S. K., Underwood, D. J., and Sheridan, R. P. (1994). FLOG: a system to select "quasi-flexible" ligands complementary to a receptor of known three-dimensional structure. *J. Comput. Aided Mol. Des.* 8, 153–174.

Monod, J., Wyman, J., and Changeux, J. P. (1965). ON THE NATURE OF ALLOSTERIC TRANSITIONS: A PLAUSIBLE MODEL. *J. Mol. Biol.* 12, 88–118. doi: 10.1016/S0022-2836(65)80285-6

Mooij, W. T., and Verdonk, M. L. (2005). General and targeted statistical potentials for protein-ligand interactions. *Proteins* 61, 272–287. doi: 10.1002/prot.20588

Morris, G. M., Goodsell, D. S., Halliday, R. S., Huey, R., Hart, W. E., Belew, R. K., et al. (1998). Automated docking using a Lamarckian genetic algorithm and an empirical binding free energy function. *J. Comput. Chem.* 19, 1639–1662. doi: 10.1002/(SICI)1096-987X(19981115)19:14<1639::AID-JCC10>3.0.CO;2-B

Morris, G. M., Goodsell, D. S., Huey, R., and Olson, A. J. (1996). Distributed automated docking of flexible ligands to proteins: parallel applications of AutoDock 2.4. *J. Comput. Aided Mol. Des.* 10, 293–304. doi: 10.1007/BF00124499

Namasivayam, V., and Günther, R. (2007). pso@autodock: a fast flexible molecular docking program based on Swarm intelligence. *Chem. Biol. Drug Des.* 70, 475–484. doi: 10.1111/j.1747-0285.2007.00588.x

Ng, M. C., Fong, S., and Siu, S. W. (2015). PSOVina: the hybrid particle swarm optimization algorithm for protein-ligand docking. *J. Bioinform. Comput. Biol.* 13:1541007. doi: 10.1142/S0219720015410073

Nobile, M. S., Cazzaniga, P., Tangherloni, A., and Besozzi, D. (2017). Graphics processing units in bioinformatics, computational biology and systems biology. *Brief Bioinform.* 18, 870–885. doi: 10.1093/bib/bbw058

Okazaki, K., and Takada, S. (2008). Dynamic energy landscape view of coupled binding and protein conformational change: induced-fit versus population-shift mechanisms. *Proc. Natl. Acad. Sci. U.S.A.* 105, 11182–11187. doi: 10.1073/pnas.0802524105

Oostenbrink, C., Villa, A., Mark, A. E., and van Gunsteren, W. F. (2004). A biomolecular force field based on the free enthalpy of hydration and solvation: the GROMOS force-field parameter sets 53A5 and 53A6. *J. Comput. Chem.* 25, 1656–1676. doi: 10.1002/jcc.20090

Osguthorpe, D. J., Sherman, W., and Hagler, A. T. (2012). Exploring protein flexibility: incorporating structural ensembles from crystal structures and simulation into virtual screening protocols. *J. Phys. Chem. B* 116, 6952–6959. doi: 10.1021/jp3003992

Pande, V. S., Baker, I., Chapman, J., Elmer, S. P., Khaliq, S., Larson, S. M., et al. (2003). Atomistic protein folding simulations on the submillisecond time scale using worldwide distributed computing. *Biopolymers* 68, 91–109. doi: 10.1002/bip.10219

Pande, V. S., Beauchamp, K., and Bowman, G. R. (2010). Everything you wanted to know about Markov State Models but were afraid to ask. *Methods* 52, 99–105. doi: 10.1016/j.ymeth.2010.06.002

Pang, Y.-P., Perola, E., Xu, K., and Prendergast, F. G. (2001). EUDOC: a computer program for identification of drug interaction sites in macromolecules and drug leads from chemical databases. *J. Comput. Chem.* 22, 1750–1771. doi: 10.1002/jcc.1129

Patel, J. S., Berteotti, A., Ronsisvalle, S., Rocchia, W., and Cavalli, A. (2014). Steered molecular dynamics simulations for studying protein-ligand interaction in cyclin-dependent kinase 5. *J. Chem. Inf. Model.* 54, 470–480. doi: 10.1021/ci4003574

Patriksson, A., and van der Spoel, D. (2008). A temperature predictor for parallel tempering simulations. *Phys. Chem. Chem. Phys.* 10, 2073–2077. doi: 10.1039/b716554d

Paul, F., Noé, F., and Weikl, T. R. (2018). Identifying conformational-selection and induced-fit aspects in the binding-induced folding of PMI from Markov state modeling of atomistic simulations. *J. Phys. Chem. B.* 122, 5649–5656. doi: 10.1021/acs.jpcb.7b12146

Paul, F., Wehmeyer, C., Abualrous, E. T., Wu, H., Crabtree, M. D., Schöneberg, J., et al. (2017). Protein-peptide association kinetics beyond the seconds timescale from atomistic simulations. *Nat. Commun.* 8:1095. doi: 10.1038/s41467-017-01163-6

Pei, J., Wang, Q., Liu, Z., Li, Q., Yang, K., and Lai, L. (2006). PSI-DOCK: towards highly efficient and accurate flexible ligand docking. *Proteins* 62, 934–946. doi: 10.1002/prot.20790

Petros, A. M., Nettesheim, D. G., Wang, Y., Olejniczak, E. T., Meadows, R. P., Mack, J., et al. (2000). Rationale for Bcl-xL/Bad peptide complex formation from structure, mutagenesis, and biophysical studies. *Protein Sci.* 9, 2528–2534. doi: 10.1110/ps.9.12.2528

Prinz, J.-H., Wu, H., Sarich, M., Keller, B., Senne, M., Held, M., et al. (2011). Markov models of molecular kinetics: generation and validation. *J. Chem. Phys.* 134:174105. doi: 10.1063/1.3565032

Rarey, M., Kramer, B., Lengauer, T., and Klebe, G. (1996). A fast flexible docking method using an incremental construction algorithm. *J. Mol. Biol.* 261, 470–489. doi: 10.1006/jmbi.1996.0477

Rastelli, G., Degliesposti, G., Del Rio, A., and Sgobba, M. (2009). Binding estimation after refinement, a new automated procedure for the refinement and rescoring of docked ligands in virtual screening. *Chem. Biol. Drug Des.* 73, 283–286. doi: 10.1111/j.1747-0285.2009.00780.x

Rosta, E., and Hummer, G. (2015). Free energies from dynamic weighted histogram analysis using unbiased Markov state model. *J. Chem. Theory Comput.* 11, 276–285. doi: 10.1021/ct500719p

Ruiz-Carmona, S., Alvarez-Garcia, D., Foloppe, N., Garmendia-Doval, A. B., Juhos, S., Schmidtke, P., et al. (2014). rDock: a fast, versatile and open source program for docking ligands to proteins and nucleic acids. *PLoS Comput. Biol.* 10:e1003571. doi: 10.1371/journal.pcbi.1003571

Sabbadin, D., Ciancetta, A., Deganutti, G., Cuzzolin, A., and Moro, S. (2015). Exploring the recognition pathway at the human A2A adenosine receptor of the endogenous agonist adenosine using supervised molecular dynamics simulations. *Medchemcomm* 6, 1081–1085. doi: 10.1039/C5MD00016E

Sabbadin, D., Ciancetta, A., and Moro, S. (2014). Bridging molecular docking to membrane molecular dynamics to investigate GPCR-ligand recognition: the human A2A adenosine receptor as a key study. *J. Chem. Inf. Model.* 54, 169–183. doi: 10.1021/ci400532b

Sabbadin, D., and Moro, S. (2014). Supervised molecular dynamics (SuMD) as a helpful tool to depict GPCR-ligand recognition pathway in a nanosecond time scale. *J. Chem. Inf. Model.* 54, 372–376. doi: 10.1021/ci40 0766b

Saleh, N., Ibrahim, P., Saladino, G., Gervasio, F. L., and Clark, T. (2017). An efficient metadynamics-based protocol to model the binding affinity and the transition state ensemble of G-protein-coupled receptor ligands. *J. Chem. Inf. Model.* 57, 1210–1217. doi: 10.1021/acs.jcim.6b00772

Salmaso, V. (2018) *Exploring Protein Flexibility During Docking to Investigate ligand-Target Recognition.* Ph.D. thesis, University of Padova, Padova.

Salmaso, V., Sturlese, M., Cuzzolin, A., and Moro, S. (2016). DockBench as docking selector tool: the lesson learned from D3R grand challenge 2015. *J. Comput. Aided Mol. Des.* 30, 773–789. doi: 10.1007/s10822-016-9966-4

Salmaso, V., Sturlese, M., Cuzzolin, A., and Moro, S. (2017). Exploring protein-peptide recognition pathways using a supervised molecular dynamics approach. *Structure* 25, 655.e2–662.e2. doi: 10.1016/j.str.2017.02.009

Salmaso, V., Sturlese, M., Cuzzolin, A., and Moro, S. (2018). Combining self- and cross-docking as benchmark tools: the performance of DockBench in the D3R grand challenge 2. *J. Comput. Aided Mol. Des.* 32, 251–264. doi: 10.1007/s10822-017-0051-4

Sauton, N., Lagorce, D., Villoutreix, B. O., and Miteva, M. A. (2008). MS-DOCK: accurate multiple conformation generator and rigid docking protocol for multi-step virtual ligand screening. *BMC Bioinformatics* 9:184. doi: 10.1186/1471-2105-9-184

Schames, J. R., Henchman, R. H., Siegel, J. S., Sotriffer, C. A., Ni, H., and McCammon, J. A. (2004). Discovery of a novel binding trench in HIV integrase. *J. Med. Chem.* 47, 1879–1881. doi: 10.1021/jm0341913

Schlitter, J., Engels, M., Krüger, P., Jacoby, E., and Wollmer, A. (1993). Targeted molecular dynamics simulation of conformational change-application to the T ↔ R transition in insulin. *Mol. Simul.* 10, 291–308. doi: 10.1080/08927029308022170

Shan, Y., Kim, E. T., Eastwood, M. P., Dror, R. O., Seeliger, M. A., and Shaw, D. E. (2011). How does a drug molecule find its target binding site? *J. Am. Chem. Soc.* 133, 9181–9183. doi: 10.1021/ja202726y

Shaw, D. E., Chao, J. C., Eastwood, M. P., Gagliardo, J., Grossman, J. P., Ho, C. R., et al. (2008). Anton, a special-purpose machine for molecular dynamics simulation. *Commun. ACM* 51, 91–97. doi: 10.1145/1364782.1364802

Shaw, D. E., Maragakis, P., Lindorff-Larsen, K., Piana, S., Dror, R. O., Eastwood, M. P., et al. (2010). Atomic-level characterization of the structural dynamics of proteins. *Science* 330, 341–346. doi: 10.1126/science.1187409

Shirts, M., and Pande, V. S. (2000). COMPUTING: screen savers of the world unite!. *Science* 290, 1903–1904. doi: 10.1126/science.290.5498.1903

Sliwoski, G., Kothiwale, S., Meiler, J., and Lowe, E. W. (2014). Computational methods in drug discovery. *Pharmacol. Rev.* 66, 334–395. doi: 10.1124/pr.112.007336

Spyrakis, F., Ahmed, M. H., Bayden, A. S., Cozzini, P., Mozzarelli, A., and Kellogg, G. E. (2017). The roles of water in the protein matrix: a largely untapped resource for drug discovery. *J. Med. Chem.* 60, 6781–6827. doi: 10.1021/acs.jmedchem.7b00057

Spyrakis, F., Benedetti, P., Decherchi, S., Rocchia, W., Cavalli, A., Alcaro, S., et al. (2015). A pipeline to enhance ligand virtual screening: integrating molecular dynamics and fingerprints for ligand and proteins. *J. Chem. Inf. Model.* 55, 2256–2274. doi: 10.1021/acs.jcim.5b00169

Strecker, C., and Meyer, B. (2018). Plasticity of the binding site of renin: optimized selection of protein structures for ensemble docking. *J. Chem. Inf. Model.* 58, 1121–1131. doi: 10.1021/acs.jcim.8b00010

Sugita, Y., Kitao, A., and Okamoto, Y. (2000). Multidimensional replica-exchange method for free-energy calculations. *J. Chem. Phys.* 113, 6042–6051. doi: 10.1063/1.1308516

Sugita, Y., and Okamoto, Y. (1999). Replica-exchange molecular dynamics method for protein folding. *Chem. Phys. Lett.* 314, 141–151. doi: 10.1016/S0009-2614(99)01123-9

Talele, T. T., Khedkar, S. A., and Rigby, A. C. (2010). Successful applications of computer aided drug discovery: moving drugs from concept to the clinic. *Curr. Top. Med. Chem.* 10, 127–141. doi: 10.2174/156802610790232251

Taylor, R. D., Jewsbury, P. J., and Essex, J. W. (2002). A review of protein-small molecule docking methods. *J. Comput. Aided Mol. Des.* 16, 151–166. doi: 10.1023/A:1020155510718

Teague, S. J. (2003). Implications of protein flexibility for drug discovery. *Nat. Rev. Drug Discov.* 2, 527–541. doi: 10.1038/nrd1129

Torrie, G. M., and Valleau, J. P. (1977). Nonphysical sampling distributions in Monte Carlo free-energy estimation: umbrella sampling. *J. Comput. Phys.* 23, 187–199. doi: 10.1016/0021-9991(77)90121-8

Trott, O., and Olson, A. J. (2010). AutoDock Vina: improving the speed and accuracy of docking with a new scoring function, efficient optimization, and multithreading. *J. Comput. Chem.* 31, 455–461. doi: 10.1002/jcc.21334

Van Drie, J. H. (2007). Computer-aided drug design: the next 20 years. *J. Comput. Aided Mol. Des.* 21, 591–601. doi: 10.1007/s10822-007-9142-y

Van Meel, J. A., Arnold, A., Frenkel, D., Portegies Zwart, S. F., and Belleman, R. G. (2008). Harvesting graphics power for MD simulations. *Mol. Simul.* 34, 259–266. doi: 10.1080/08927020701744295

Vanommeslaeghe, K., Guvench, O., and MacKerell, A. D. (2014). Molecular mechanics. *Curr. Pharm. Des.* 20, 3281–3292. doi: 10.2174/13816128113199990600

Velec, H. F. G., Gohlke, H., and Klebe, G. (2005). DrugScore(CSD)-knowledge-based scoring function derived from small molecule crystal data with superior recognition rate of near-native ligand poses and better affinity prediction. *J. Med. Chem.* 48, 6296–6303. doi: 10.1021/jm050436v

Verdonk, M. L., Cole, J. C., Hartshorn, M. J., Murray, C. W., and Taylor, R. D. (2003). Improved protein-ligand docking using GOLD. *Proteins* 52, 609–623. doi: 10.1002/prot.10465

Vieth, M., Hirst, J. D., Kolinski, A., and Brooks, C. L. III. (1999). Assessing energy functions for flexible docking. *J. Comput. Chem.* 19, 1612–1622.

Vuong, Q. V., Nguyen, T. T., and Li, M. S. (2015). A new method for navigating optimal direction for pulling ligand from binding pocket: application to ranking binding affinity by steered molecular dynamics. *J. Chem. Inf. Model.* 55, 2731–2738. doi: 10.1021/acs.jcim.5b00386

Wang, T., and Duan, Y. (2009). Ligand entry and exit pathways in the beta2-adrenergic receptor. *J. Mol. Biol.* 392, 1102–1115. doi: 10.1016/j.jmb.2009.07.093

Welch, W., Ruppert, J., and Jain, A. N. (1996). Hammerhead: fast, fully automated docking of flexible ligands to protein binding sites. *Chem. Biol.* 3, 449–462. doi: 10.1016/S1074-5521(96)90093-9

Wood, J. M., Maibaum, J., Rahuel, J., Grütter, M. G., Cohen, N.-C., Rasetti, V., et al. (2003). Structure-based design of aliskiren, a novel orally effective renin inhibitor. *Biochem. Biophys. Res. Commun.* 308, 698–705. doi: 10.1016/S0006-291X(03)01451-7

Wu, H., Paul, F., Wehmeyer, C., and Noé, F. (2016). Multiensemble Markov models of molecular thermodynamics and kinetics. *Proc. Natl. Acad. Sci. U.S.A.* 113, E3221–E3230. doi: 10.1073/pnas.1525092113

Yu, J., Ciancetta, A., Dudas, S., Duca, S., Lottermoser, J., and Jacobson, K. A. (2018). Structure-guided modification of heterocyclic antagonists of the P2Y14 receptor. *J. Med. Chem.* 61, 4860–4882. doi: 10.1021/acs.jmedchem.8b00168

Yuriev, E., Holien, J., and Ramsland, P. A. (2015). Improvements, trends, and new ideas in molecular docking: 2012-2013 in review. *J. Mol. Recognit.* 28, 581–604. doi: 10.1002/jmr.2471

Zhou, H.-X. (2010). From induced fit to conformational selection: a continuum of binding mechanism controlled by the timescale of conformational transitions. *Biophys. J.* 98, L15–L17. doi: 10.1016/j.bpj.2009.11.029

4

Gossypol Inhibits Non-small Cell Lung Cancer Cells Proliferation by Targeting EGFR$^{L858R/T790M}$

Yuwei Wang[1], Huanling Lai[1], Xingxing Fan[1], Lianxiang Luo[1], Fugang Duan[1], Zebo Jiang[1], Qianqian Wang[1], Elaine Lai Han Leung[1,2,3*], Liang Liu[1*] and Xiaojun Yao[1*]

[1] State Key Laboratory of Quality Research in Chinese Medicine, Macau University of Science and Technology, Macau, China, [2] Department of Thoracic Surgery, Guangzhou Institute of Respiratory Health and State Key Laboratory of Respiratory Disease, The First Affiliated Hospital of Guangzhou Medical University, Guangzhou, China, [3] Respiratory Medicine Department, Taihe Hospital, Hubei University of Medicine, Hubei, China

*Correspondence:
Elaine Lai Han Leung
lhleung@must.edu.mo
Liang Liu
lliu@must.edu.mo
Xiaojun Yao
xjyao@must.edu.mo

Background: Overexpression of epidermal growth factor receptor (EGFR) has been reported to be implicated in the pathogenesis of non-small cell lung cancer (NSCLC). Several EGFR inhibitors have been used in clinical treatment of NSCLC, but the emergence of EGFR$^{L858R/T790M}$ resistant mutation has reduced the efficacy of the clinical used EGFR inhibitors. There is an urgent need to develop novel EGFR$^{L858R/T790M}$ inhibitors for better NSCLC treatment.

Methods: By screening a natural product library, we have identified gossypol as a novel potent inhibitor targeting EGFR$^{L858R/T790M}$. The activity of gossypol on NSCLC cells was evaluated by cell proliferation, cell apoptosis and cell migration assays. Kinase activity inhibition assay and molecular docking were used to study the inhibition mechanism of gossypol to EGFR$^{L858R/T790M}$. Western blotting was performed to study the molecular mechanism of gossypol inhibiting the downstream pathways of EGFR.

Results: Gossypol inhibited the cell proliferation and cell migration of NSCLC cells, and induced caspase-dependent cell apoptosis of NSCLC cells by upregulating the expression of pro-apoptotic protein BAD. Molecular docking revealed that gossypol could bind to the kinase domain of EGFR$^{L858R/T790M}$ with good binding affinity through hydrogen bonds and hydrophobic interactions. Gossypol inhibited the kinase activity of EGFR$^{L858R/T790M}$ with EC$_{50}$ of 150.1 nM. Western blotting analysis demonstrated that gossypol inhibited the phosphorylation of EGFR and its downstream signal pathways in a dose-dependent manner.

Conclusion: Gossypol inhibited cell proliferation and induced apoptosis of NSCLC cells by targeting EGFR$^{L858R/T790M}$. Our findings provided a basis for developing novel EGFR$^{L858R/T790M}$ inhibitors for treatment of NSCLC.

Keywords: gossypol, molecular docking, NSCLC, EGFR, TKI

INTRODUCTION

Non-small cell lung cancer (NSCLC) accounts for approximately 85-90% of lung cancers, which has proven to be difficult to be treated due to poorly understood the pathogenesis (Oyewumi et al., 2014; Siegel et al., 2017). Conventional treatment strategies are used for NSCLC including surgical operation, radiotherapy and chemotherapy (Scott et al., 2007; Onishi et al., 2011;

Uzel and Abacıoğlu, 2015). In addition, tyrosine kinase-based inhibitors (TKIs) molecular-targeted therapy are also employed to the treatment of NSCLC patients with EGFR mutations. Overexpression of EGFR has been reported and implicated in the pathogenesis of NSCLC, which account for more than 60% of NSCLC (Ohsaki et al., 2000). Therefore, it is increasing in clinic application as molecular targets for NSCLC patients with EGFR mutation.

The role of aberrant activation of the EGFR in NSCLC is well-documented (Sordella et al., 2004; Tracy et al., 2004; Gazdar and Minna, 2005; Sharma and Settleman, 2007; Sharma et al., 2007). The most common activating mutations, including point mutation L858R in exon 21 and deletions within exon 19 (del746-750) (Riely et al., 2006; Sharma et al., 2007), promote EGFR-driven cell proliferation and survival. Both first and second generation EGFR-targeted TKIs (gefitinib and erlotinib) targeting those activating mutants have been demonstrated to have a remarkable clinical response in the treatment of EGFR-mutated NSCLC (Lynch et al., 2004; Paez et al., 2004; Jackman et al., 2009; Rosell et al., 2009; Sequist et al., 2010). Although the early clinical results of first-generation EGFR inhibitors are impressive, unfortunately, most NSCLC patients with activating mutations eventually develop acquired resistance to EGFR inhibitors within several months. The most common mechanism of acquired resistance is the secondary T790M (gatekeeper residue Thr790 to methionine within the EGFR kinase domain) point mutation in exon 20 that occurs with an EGFR mutation (e.g., L858R), which accounts for approximately 60% in these acquired resistances (Balak et al., 2006; Kosaka et al., 2006; Yu et al., 2013). To overcome the acquired resistance to first-generation TKIs, several second- and third-generation EGFR TKIs [such as EKB-569 (Kwak et al., 2005), BIBW2992 (Li et al., 2008) and PF00299804 (Engelman et al., 2007)] have been developed. However, these agents still display limited clinical benefit for NSCLC patients with T790M mutation owing to dose-limiting toxicities (Oxnard et al., 2011; Miller et al., 2012). Recently, third-generation covalent EGFR inhibitor osimertinib (Ward et al., 2013; Cross et al., 2014) has been developed as mutant-selective EGFR inhibitor that specifically targeting EGFR$^{L858R/T790M}$ mutation. However, the effective treatment of patients that harbor the EGFR T790M drug resistance mutation with osimertinib is limited by the emergence of new drug resistances to the tyrosine kinase inhibitor therapy (Thress et al., 2015; Büttner et al., 2017). C797S mutation was reported to be a major mechanism for resistance to third generation EGFR TKIs (Yu et al., 2015). In addition to C797S mutation, other rare tertiary EGFR mutations have also been reported, including novel solvent front mutations (G796S/R), hinge pocket mutations of the leucine residue at position 792 (L792F/H), binding interference at position 798 (L798I), and steric hindrance at position 718 (L718Q) (Bersanelli et al., 2016; Chabon et al., 2016; Chen et al., 2017; Ou Q. et al., 2017; Ou S.-H.I. et al., 2017). With the emergence of resistance mechanisms, there is an urgent need to discover a novel class of EGFR inhibitors that effectively inhibits drug-resistant EGFR$^{L858R/T790M}$ mutation.

Natural products have been widely regarded as a pivotal source of leading compounds for drug development, recently, several natural products have been identified targeting EGFR$^{L858R/T790M}$ to overcome resistance. (Jung et al., 2015; Xiao et al., 2016). In our previous studies, we have successfully identified several small molecules from natural products library that could inhibit the growth of gefitinib resistant NSCLC via different mechanisms. (Fan et al., 2015; Li et al., 2017). These compounds demonstrated significant anti-proliferative effects on a variety of NSCLC cell lines, including those with T790M and L858R/T790M mutations. In this study, we identified a small molecule gossypol from cottonseed, as a potent inhibitor targeting EGFR$^{L858R/T790M}$. Gossypol and its derivatives exert antitumor effects on different cancer types *in vitro* and *in vivo*, including breast cancer (Xiong et al., 2017), colon cancer (Lan et al., 2015), chronic myeloid leukemia (Goff et al., 2013) and prostate cancer (Volate et al., 2010) by targeting MDM2, VEGFR, Bcl-2 and p53. Herein, the results from our work proved that gossypol could inhibit the proliferation of NSCLC cells by targeting EGFR$^{L858R/T790M}$. Gossypol also inhibited the phosphorylation of EGFR and suppressed the phosphorylation of extracellular signal–regulated protein kinase (ERK) and AKT. These results indicated that gossypol could be developed as a new potent EGFR$^{L858R/T790M}$ inhibitor and could inhibit the proliferation of NSCLC.

RESULTS AND DISCUSSION

Gossypol Inhibits Cell Proliferation in NSCLC Cells

To identify potent small molecule inhibitor of EGFR$^{L858R/T790M}$, we screened a natural products library with 235 compounds. We evaluated the anti-proliferative effect of each compound on H1975 cell line harboring EGFR$^{L858R/T790M}$. Gossypol was identified and chosen for further mechanistic investigation due to its significantly anti-proliferative ability. H1975 cells were treated with an increasing concentration of gossypol for 72 h, and then cell viability was determined based on standard MTT assay protocol. As shown in **Figure 1**, the growth of H1975 cells were obviously inhibited by the treatment of gossypol in a dose-dependent manner, with 50% inhibition concentration (IC$_{50}$) of 10.89 ± 0.84 μM. In addition, we have tested the cytotoxicity effect of gossypol on human normal lung fibroblast cell line CCD19 (IC$_{50}$ is 14.89 ± 1.12 μM) and human NSCLC cell line H358 with EGFR^{WT} (IC$_{50}$ is 35.26 ± 1.09 μM) (the corresponding results can be seen in Supplementary Figure S1). Afatinib was used as positive control (IC$_{50}$ = 170.4 ± 1.1 nM). The structure and corresponding cytotoxicity of gossypol were showed in **Figure 1**. We also examined the effect of gossypol on cell colony formation (**Figure 2A**), in accordance with the cell cytotoxicity, gossypol significantly inhibited the colony formation capacity in a dose-dependent manner in H1975 cell line. Collectively, these results suggested that gossypol could inhibit the proliferation of H1975 cell line.

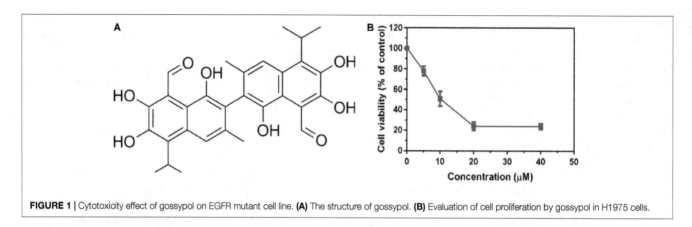

FIGURE 1 | Cytotoxicity effect of gossypol on EGFR mutant cell line. **(A)** The structure of gossypol. **(B)** Evaluation of cell proliferation by gossypol in H1975 cells.

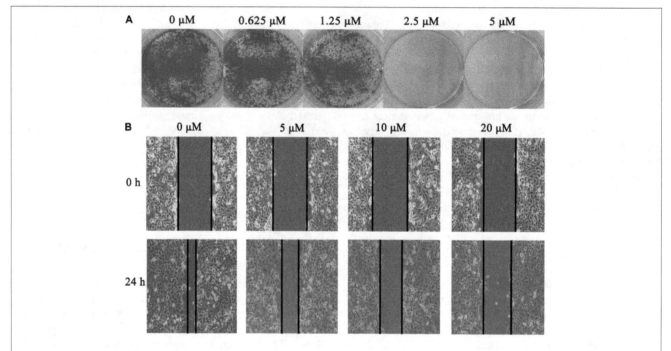

FIGURE 2 | Effect of gossypol on H1975 cell line. **(A)** Colony formation of H1975 cells was monitored after gossypol (0–5 μM) treatment for 14 days, and photomicrographs of crystal violet stained colonies were depicted. **(B)** H1975 cells were treated with 0, 5, 10, and 20 μM for 24 h, and were analyzed for wound healing.

Gossypol Induces Cell Apoptosis in NSCLC Cells

To investigate whether the induction of apoptosis also contributed to gossypol-mediated growth inhibition of H1975 cells, Annexin V-FITC/PI staining assay was employed to analyze the number of apoptotic cells after treatment with gossypol using a flow cytometer. As shown in **Figures 3A,B**, gossypol induced cell apoptosis on H1975 cell line with a concentration-dependent manner.

Bcl-2 family members play key roles in the regulation of apoptotic progress. To understand how gossypol induced apoptosis, we next examined whether gossypol could alter the expression of apoptotic proteins in H1975 cells. As shown in **Figure 3C** and Supplementary Figure S4, treatment with gossypol for 24 h remarkably upregulated the expression level

of proapoptotic protein Bad in a concentration-dependent manner. Moreover, we also observed that gossypol induced PARP cleavage, a hallmark of caspase-dependent apoptosis, in accordance with the expression level of cleaved caspase-3. Therefore, these results suggested that gossypol induced caspase-dependent apoptotic cell death by upregulating the expression of pro-apoptotic protein Bad in NSCLC cells.

Gossypol Inhibits the Cell Migration of H1975 Cell Line

The effect of gossypol on H1975 cell migration capability was estimated by a wound-healing assay. In the wound-healing assay (see **Figure 2B**), cells treated with gossypol reduced the rate of wound healing along with the increasing of treatment concentration, which was significantly lower than the untreated

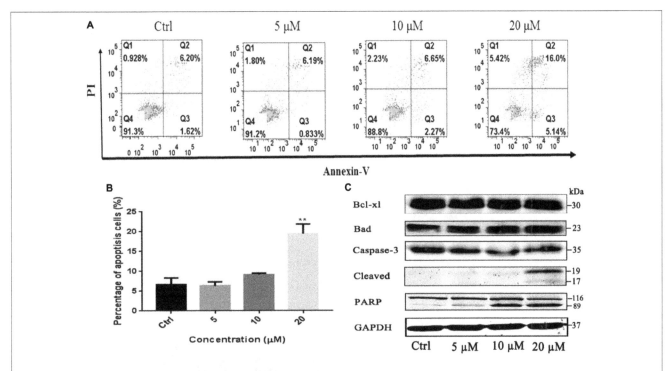

FIGURE 3 | Apoptosis effect of Gossypol on H1975 cells. Flow cytometric analysis of cell apoptosis with gossypol at different concentrations (0, 5, 10, and 20 μM) for 24 h was determined. **(A)** Flow cytometry analysis of the apoptosis levels of h1975 cells after treatment with gossypol for 24 h. **(B)** Data from **(A)** were statistically analyzed. Mean ± SE. **$P < 0.01$. **(C)** Western blot analysis of apoptotic markers of H1975 cells after treatment of gossypol for 24 h.

cells following incubation. These results demonstrated that gossypol inhibited the migration ability of H1975 cell lines in a dose-dependent manner.

Gossypol Inhibits the Activity of Tyrosine Kinase

To assess the kinase inhibition activities of gossypol, we performed a kinase inhibition profile assay of gossypol against recombinant human EGFR$^{L858R/T790M}$. The selected compound gossypol exhibited inhibitory activity, which effectively inhibited the enzymatic activity of EGFR$^{L858R/T790M}$ with an EC$_{50}$ value of 150 ± 30.7 nM (see Supplementary Figure S2). Besides, gossypol also inhibited the enzymatic activity of EGFR^{WT} with an EC$_{50}$ value of 252.9 ± 26.9 nM, higher than that to EGFR$^{L858R/T790M}$ (the corresponding results can be seen in Supplementary Figure S2). Afatinib was used as positive control (EC$_{50} = 9.6 \pm 2.9$ nM). The effect of gossypol on cells is very complicated, and it is still difficult to distinguish which part is caused by EGFR targeting. To ensure the consistency of the experimental results, we conducted the entire ELISA enzyme inhibiting assay at the same time. Therefore, EGFR^{WT} could be used as control to compare with EGFR$^{L858R/T790M}$.

Molecular Docking Predicts the Potential Binding of Gossypol to EGFR

Molecular docking calculation was performed to gain insight into the binding mode between gossypol and EGFR$^{L858R/T790M}$. The molecular docking results (see **Figure 4** and Supplementary Figure S3) proved that gossypol could be docked into the kinase domain mainly composed of hydrophobic residues of C-helix and A-loop with a docking score of -6.42 ± 0.24 kcal/mol. Five hydrogen bonds were formed between gossypol and the carbonyl group of Q791, amino group of M793, hydroxyl group of T854 and amino group of K875. In addition, the hydrophobic contacts formed between gossypol and surrounded residues, including L718, M790, F723, F858, L792, L844, and M793, which also contributed to the interaction between gossypol and EGFR$^{L858R/T790M}$. Therefore, the above results suggested that gossypol could bind to EGFR$^{L858R/T790M}$.

Gossypol Effectively Suppresses Phosphorylation of EGFR as Well as Its Downstream Signaling Pathway

To determine whether gossypol could inhibit the expression level of EGFR in cells, we investigated the effect of gossypol on the phosphorylation of EGFR in NSCLC cells. H1975 cells were treated with gossypol (0–20 μM) for 24 h. Western blot analysis showed that gossypol inhibited the phosphorylation of EGFR (Tyr 1068) in a concentration dependent manner (see **Figure 5**). To explore the detailed anti-cancer mechanism of gossypol, we further evaluated the downstream pathways of EGFR, including ERK and AKT signaling pathways. Treatment with gossypol also inhibited the phosphorylation of AKT and ERK in a concentration-dependent manner, consistent with the tendency of phosphorylation level of EGFR. Thus, our results indicated that gossypol

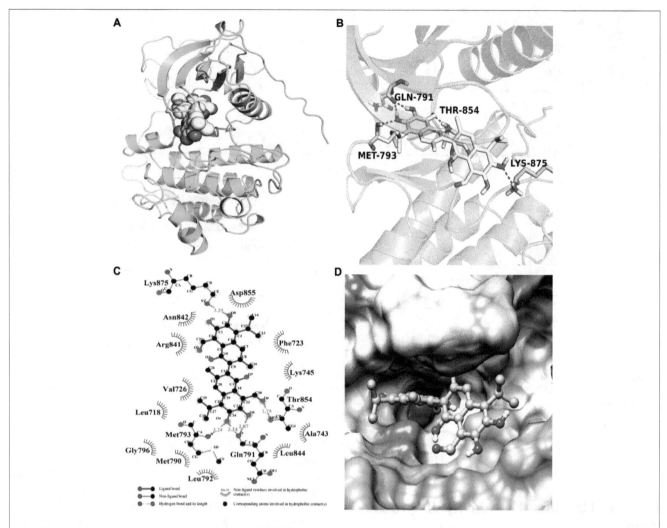

FIGURE 4 | The binding mode between gossypol and EGFR$^{L858R/T790M}$ protein. **(A)** The 3D structure of EGFR$^{L858R/T790M}$. **(B)** Gossypol was docked into the EGFR kinase domain, showing interactions between gossypol and key residues. **(C)** A two-dimensional interaction map of gossypol and EGFR. **(D)** The hydrophobic surface of EGFR$^{L858R/T790M}$.

could suppress the phosphorylation of EGFR and its downstream AKT and ERK signaling pathways, resulting in induction of apoptosis and proliferation inhibition of H1975 cells.

CONCLUSION

In this study, by screening a natural products library, we have identified that gossypol was a potential anticancer agent targeting EGFR$^{L858R/T790M}$. Our results proved that gossypol inhibited the proliferation and induced apoptosis of human NSCLC cell line harboring EGFR$^{L858R/T790M}$. Moreover, gossypol decreased the phosphorylation level of EGFR and its downstream signaling pathways AKT and ERK. Overall, our findings indicate that gossypol is a novel potent EGFR$^{L858R/T790M}$ inhibitor, which may serve as a useful therapeutic agent against NSCLC harboring EGFR$^{L858R/T790M}$ mutation.

MATERIALS AND METHODS

Reagents

Gossypol was purchased from Selleck Ltd., which was dissolved in dimethyl sulfoxide (DMSO) to form a 20 mM stock solution. Fetal bovine serum (FBS), antibiotics and RPMI medium were purchased from Gibco (Carlsbad, CA, United States). RIPA lysis buffer and antibodies Bad, Bcl-XL, PARP, Cleaved Caspase-3, anti-p-EGFR (1068), anti-p-extracellular signal-regulated kinase 1/2 (Erk1/2) (Thr202/Tyr204), anti-p-Akt (Ser473), anti-Erk1/2, anti-Akt, anti-PERK, and anti-EGFR were purchased from Cell Signaling Technology (Beverly, MA, United States). Anti-GAPDH was purchased from Santa Cruz (Dallas, TX, United States).

Cell Culture

The human NSCLC cell line H1975 was purchased from the American Type Culture Collection (ATCC) (Manassas, VA,

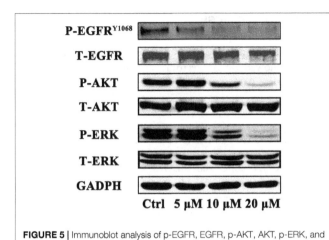

FIGURE 5 | Immunoblot analysis of p-EGFR, EGFR, p-AKT, AKT, p-ERK, and ERK in H1975 cell after treatment with gossypol for 24 h. GAPDH was used as a loading control.

United States). Cells were cultured in RPMI1640 medium supplemented with 10% FBS, 100 U/ml penicillin and 100 μg/ml streptomycin. All the cells were cultured at 37°C in a humidified atmosphere containing 5% CO_2.

Cell Proliferation Assay

Cell viability was evaluated by using the standard 3-(4,5-dimethylthiazol-2-yl)-2,5-diphenyltetrazolium bromide MTT assay. Briefly, 3×10^3 cells per well were plated in 96-well plates and cultured overnight for cell adhesion. The cells were treated with DMSO or various concentrations of gossypol for 72 h. Subsequently, 10 μL MTT was added into each well and incubated for 4 h, and then the dark blue crystals were dissolved with 100 μl of the resolved solution (99% DMSO). Finally, the absorbance at 570 nm was measured by microplate reader (Tecan, Morrisville, NC, United States). The cell viability was calculated relative to controls, with results based on at least three independent experiments. Cells treated with the vehicle (DMSO) alone served as a control.

Colony Formation Assay

Briefly, H1975 cells were seeded in 6-well plates (1000 cells/well), after attachment overnight, cells were exposed to various concentration of gossypol with medium changes every 3 days until visible colonies formed. The colonies were washed with cold PBS, then fixed in 4% paraformaldehyde (PFA) for 15 min, and then stained with 0.5% crystal violet (1% PFA, 0.5% crystal violet, and 20% methanol in ddH$_2$O) for 20 min. The colonies were photographed.

Apoptosis Analysis Assay

NSCLC cells were plated on 6-well plate with cell density of 2×10^5 cells per well and cultured overnight for adhesion. Subsequently, the cells were treated with different concentrations of gossypol for 24 h. After treatment, the cells were harvested by trypsin digestion and washed twice with ice-cold PBS, and resuspended in 100 μl 1 $\times$ binding buffer. Next, 4 μl of propidium iodide (PI, 1 mg/ml) and 1 μl Annexin-V fluorescein

dye were added to the solution and mixed well at room temperature in the dark for 15 min. After that, the cells were resuspended in 300 μl of 1 $\times$ binding buffer from BD Biosciences (San Jose, CA, United States). The percentage of apoptotic cells was quantitatively measured using a BD FACSAria III flow cytometer from BD Bioscience (San Jose, CA, United States).

Enzyme-Linked Immunosorbent Assay (ELISA)

The kinase activity was evaluated with ELISA assay based on the kinase domain of dual-mutant EGFR (EGFR$^{L858R/T790M}$) recombinant human protein (Peng et al., 2014). Briefly, 20 μg/mL Poly (Glu, Tyr) 4:1 (Sigma, St. Louis, MO, United States) was precoated in 96-well plates as substrate. Active kinases were added and incubated with indicated gossypol in 1 $\times$ reaction buffer containing 5 μmol/L ATP at 37°C for 1 h. Then, the wells were washed with PBS and then incubated with an anti-phosphotyrosine (PY99) antibody (Santa Cruz Biotechnology, Santa Cruz, CA, United States) followed by a horseradish peroxidase (HRP)-conjugated secondary antibody. The wells were read with a multiwell spectrophotometer (VERSAmax^{TM}, Molecular Devices, Sunnyvale, CA, United States) at 492 nm. The inhibitory rate (%) was calculated with the following formula: [1−(A$_{492}$ treated/A$_{492}$ control)] $\times$ 100%, and responding EC$_{50}$ values were calculated from the fitting inhibitory curves.

Molecular Docking

The X-ray structure of EGFR$^{L858R/T790M}$ with a resolution of 2.5 Å complexed with diaminopyrimidine derivative was retrieved from the Protein Data Bank [PDB ID code 4RJ8 (Hanan et al., 2014)] for docking with gossypol. Molecular structures were prepared using the standard procedure from the Protein Preparation Wizard module in Schrödinger 2015. The docking grid box was defined using the Receptor Grid Generation tool in Glide by centering on native ligand in the EGFR$^{L858R/T790M}$ structure. The structure of gossypol was derived from the PubChem database[1], which was imported to the LigPrep module (Version 2.3, Schrödinger, LLC, New York, NY, United States) based on OPLS-2005 force field (Kaminski et al., 2001). The ionized state was assigned by using Epik (Version 2.0, Schrödinger, LLC, New York, NY, United States) at a pH value of 7.0 ± 2.0. Gossypol was docked into the kinase domain of the EGFR$^{L858R/T790M}$ using the Glide (Version 5.5, Schrödinger, LLC, New York, NY, United States) with the extra precision (XP) scoring mode. In the process of molecular docking, 5000 poses were generated during the initial phase of the docking calculation. The best binding pose for Gossypol was conserved for the further analysis.

Western Blot Analysis

Preparation of whole-cell protein lysates for western blot analysis was conducted as follows. After treatment, cells were lysed in RIPA lysis buffer (150 mmol/L NaCl, 50 mmol/L Tris–HCl, pH 8.0,1% Triton X-100, 0.1% SDS, and 1% deoxycholate)

---

[1]http://pubchem.ncbi.nlm.nih.gov

containing protease inhibitor cocktail from Roche (Basel, Lewes, United Kingdom) for 15 min on ice and then boiled for 10 min. The concentration of total protein was determined with a Bio-Rad DCTM Protein Assay Kit (Bio-Rad, Hercules, CA, United States). Equal amounts of total protein (30 μg) protein lysate were loaded and separated by 10% SDS–polyacrylamide gel electrophoresis and then transferred to a nitrocellulose (NC) membrane from Millipore (Billerica, MA, United States). The membranes were blocked with 5% milk without fat in 1 × TBST for 2 h at room temperature, and then incubated with various primary antibodies, including phospho-AKT, phospho-ERK, t-AKT, t-ERK, phospho-EGFR (Tyr1068), t-EGFR at 1:1000 dilutions and anti-GADPH antibody at a 1:800 dilution overnight at 4°C. After washing the membranes in TBST three times (5 min per time), secondary fluorescent antibodies, either anti-rabbit or anti-mouse secondary antibodies depending on the source of the primary anti-bodies, were added to the membrane at 1:10,000 dilutions at room temperature for 2 h. GAPDH was used as the loading control and for normalization. The signal intensity of the membranes was detected using an LI-COR Odessy scanner (Belfast, ME, United States).

Statistical Analysis

The results were expressed as mean values ± standard error (mean ± SE). Statistical analysis was performed using one-way ANOVA followed by Bonferroni's post-tests. Significance was accepted at $P < 0.05$.

AUTHOR CONTRIBUTIONS

EL, LL, and XY conceived this research, led the project, and revised the manuscript. YW, HL, XF, FD, ZJ, QW, and LL carried out the experiments and analyzed the data. YW and XY wrote the manuscript. All authors reviewed the manuscript.

FUNDING

This work was supported by Macau Science and Technology Development Fund (Project Nos. 082/2013/A3, 086/2015/A3, 082/2015/A3, 005/2014/AMJ, and 046/2016/A2).

REFERENCES

Balak, M. N., Gong, Y., Riely, G. J., Somwar, R., Li, A. R., Zakowski, M. F., et al. (2006). Novel D761Y and common secondary T790M mutations in epidermal growth factor receptor–mutant lung adenocarcinomas with acquired resistance to kinase inhibitors. *Clin. Cancer Res.* 12:6494. doi: 10.1158/1078-0432.CCR-06-1570

Bersanelli, M., Minari, R., Bordi, P., Gnetti, L., Bozzetti, C., Squadrilli, A., et al. (2016). L718Q mutation as new mechanism of acquired resistance to AZD9291 in EGFR-mutated NSCLC. *J. Thoracic Oncol.* 11, e121–e123. doi: 10.1016/j.jtho.2016.05.019

Büttner, R., Wolf, J., Thomas, R. K., and Sos, M. L. (2017). Resistance mechanisms to AZD9291 and rociletinib—response. *Clin. Cancer Res.* 23, 3967–3968. doi: 10.1158/1078-0432.CCR-17-0948

Chabon, J. J., Simmons, A. D., Lovejoy, A. F., Esfahani, M. S., Newman, A. M., Haringsma, H. J., et al. (2016). Circulating tumour DNA profiling reveals heterogeneity of EGFR inhibitor resistance mechanisms in lung cancer patients. *Nat. Commun.* 7:11815. doi: 10.1038/ncomms11815

Chen, K., Zhou, F., Shen, W., Jiang, T., Wu, X., Tong, X., et al. (2017). Novel mutations on EGFR Leu792 potentially correlate to acquired resistance to osimertinib in advanced NSCLC. *J. Thoracic Oncol.* 12, e65–e68. doi: 10.1016/j.jtho.2016.12.024

Cross, D. A. E., Ashton, S. E., Ghiorghiu, S., Eberlein, C., Nebhan, C. A., Spitzler, P. J., et al. (2014). AZD9291, an irreversible EGFR TKI, overcomes T790M-mediated resistance to EGFR inhibitors in lung cancer. *Cancer Discov.* 4, 1046–1061. doi: 10.1158/2159-8290.CD-14-0337

Engelman, J. A., Zejnullahu, K., Gale, C.-M., Lifshits, E., Gonzales, A. J., Shimamura, T., et al. (2007). PF00299804, an irreversible pan-ERBB inhibitor, is effective in lung cancer models with EGFR and ERBB2 mutations that are resistant to gefitinib. *Cancer Res.* 67, 11924–11932. doi: 10.1158/0008-5472.CAN-07-1885

Fan, X. X., Yao, X. J., Xu, S. W., Wong, V. K., He, J. X., Ding, J., et al. (2015). (Z)3,4,5,4'-trans-tetramethoxystilbene, a new analogue of resveratrol, inhibits gefitinb-resistant non-small cell lung cancer via selectively elevating intracellular calcium level. *Sci Rep* 5, 16348. doi: 10.1038/srep16348

Gazdar, A. F., and Minna, J. D. (2005). Inhibition of EGFR signaling: all mutations are not created equal. *PLoS Med* 2:e377. doi: 10.1371/journal.pmed.0020377

Goff, D. J., Court Recart, A., Sadarangani, A., Chun, H.-J., Barrett, C. L., Krajewska, M., et al. (2013). A Pan-BCL2 Inhibitor Renders Bone-Marrow-Resident Human Leukemia Stem Cells Sensitive to Tyrosine Kinase Inhibition. *Cell Stem Cell* 12, 316–328. doi: 10.1016/j.stem.2012.12.011

Hanan, E. J., Eigenbrot, C., Bryan, M. C., Burdick, D. J., Chan, B. K., Chen, Y., et al. (2014). Discovery of Selective and Noncovalent Diaminopyrimidine-Based Inhibitors of Epidermal Growth Factor Receptor Containing the T790M Resistance Mutation. *J. Med. Chem.* 57, 10176–10191. doi: 10.1021/jm501578n

Jackman, D. M., Miller, V. A., Cioffredi, L. A., Yeap, B. Y., Janne, P. A., Riely, G. J., et al. (2009). Impact of epidermal growth factor receptor and KRAS mutations on clinical outcomes in previously untreated non-small cell lung cancer patients: results of an online tumor registry of clinical trials. *Clin. Cancer Res.* 15, 5267–5273. doi: 10.1158/1078-0432.CCR-09-0888

Jung, S. K., Lee, M.-H., Lim, D. Y., Lee, S. Y., Jeong, C.-H., Kim, J. E., et al. (2015). Butein, a novel dual inhibitor of MET and EGFR, overcomes gefitinib-resistant lung cancer growth. *Mol. Carcinog.* 54, 322–331. doi: 10.1002/mc.22191

Kaminski, G. A., Friesner, R. A., Tirado-Rives, J., and Jorgensen, W. L. (2001). Evaluation and reparametrization of the OPLS-AA force field for proteins via comparison with accurate quantum chemical calculations on peptides. *J. Phys. Chem. B* 105, 6474–6487. doi: 10.1021/jp003919d

Kosaka, T., Yatabe, Y., Endoh, H., Yoshida, K., Hida, T., Tsuboi, M., et al. (2006). Analysis of epidermal growth factor receptor gene mutation in patients with non-small cell lung cancer and acquired resistance to gefitinib. *Clin. Cancer Res* 12, 5764–5769. doi: 10.1158/1078-0432.CCR-06-0714

Kwak, E. L., Sordella, R., Bell, D. W., Godin-Heymann, N., Okimoto, R. A., Brannigan, B. W., et al. (2005). Irreversible inhibitors of the EGF receptor may circumvent acquired resistance to gefitinib. *Proc. Natl. Acad. Sci. U.S.A.* 102, 7665–7670. doi: 10.1073/pnas.0502860102

Lan, L., Appelman, C., Smith, A. R., Yu, J., Larsen, S., Marquez, R. T., et al. (2015). Natural product (-)-gossypol inhibits colon cancer cell growth by targeting RNA-binding protein Musashi-1. *Mol. Oncol.* 9, 1406–1420. doi: 10.1016/j.molonc.2015.03.014

Li, D., Ambrogio, L., Shimamura, T., Kubo, S., Takahashi, M., Chirieac, L. R., et al. (2008). BIBW2992, an irreversible EGFR/HER2 inhibitor highly effective in preclinical lung cancer models. *Oncogene* 27, 4702–4711. doi: 10.1038/onc.20 08.109

Li, X., Fan, X. X., Jiang, Z. B., Loo, W. T., Yao, X. J., Leung, E. L., et al. (2017). Shikonin inhibits gefitinib-resistant non-small cell lung cancer by inhibiting TrxR and activating the EGFR proteasomal degradation pathway. *Pharmacol. Res.* 115, 45–55. doi: 10.1016/j.phrs.2016.11.011

Lynch, T. J., Bell, D. W., Sordella, R., Gurubhagavatula, S., Okimoto, R. A., Brannigan, B. W., et al. (2004). Activating mutations in the epidermal growth factor receptor underlying responsiveness of non–small-cell lung cancer to gefitinib. *N. Engl. J. Med.* 350, 2129–2139. doi: 10.1056/NEJMoa040938

Miller, V. A., Hirsh, V., Cadranel, J., Chen, Y.-M., Park, K., Kim, S.-W., et al. (2012). Afatinib versus placebo for patients with advanced, metastatic non-small-cell lung cancer after failure of erlotinib, gefitinib, or both, and one or two lines of chemotherapy (LUX-Lung 1): a phase 2b/3 randomised trial. *Lancet Oncol.* 13, 528–538. doi: 10.1016/S1470-2045(12)70087-6

Ohsaki, Y., Tanno, S., Fujita, Y., Toyoshima, E., Fujiuchi, S., Nishigaki, Y., et al. (2000). Epidermal growth factor receptor expression correlates with poor prognosis in non-small cell lung cancer patients with p53 overexpression. *Oncol. Rep.* 7, 603–610. doi: 10.3892/or.7.3.603

Onishi, H., Shirato, H., Nagata, Y., Hiraoka, M., Fujino, M., Gomi, K., et al. (2011). Stereotactic body radiotherapy (SBRT) for operable stage I non–small-cell lung cancer: can SBRT be comparable to surgery? *Int. J. Radiat. Oncol. Biol. Phys.* 81, 1352–1358. doi: 10.1016/j.ijrobp.2009.07.1751

Ou, Q., Wu, X., Bao, H., Tong, X., Wang, X., Zhang, X., et al. (2017). Investigating novel resistance mechanisms to third generation EGFR TKI osimertinib in non-small cell lung cancer patients using next generation sequencing. *J. Clin. Oncol.* 35, 2572–2572.

Ou, S.-H. I., Cui, J., Schrock, A. B., Goldberg, M. E., Zhu, V. W., Albacker, L., et al. (2017). Emergence of novel and dominant acquired EGFR solvent-front mutations at Gly796 (G796S/R) together with C797S/R and L792F/H mutations in one EGFR (L858R/T790M) NSCLC patient who progressed on osimertinib. *Lung Cancer* 108, 228–231. doi: 10.1016/j.lungcan.2017.04.003

Oxnard, G. R., Arcila, M. E., Chmielecki, J., Ladanyi, M., Miller, V. A., and Pao, W. (2011). New strategies in overcoming acquired resistance to epidermal growth factor receptor tyrosine kinase inhibitors in lung cancer. *Clin. Cancer Res.* 17, 5530–5537. doi: 10.1158/1078-0432.CCR-10-2571

Oyewumi, M. O., Alazizi, A., Wehrung, D., Manochakian, R., and Safadi, F. F. (2014). Emerging lung cancer therapeutic targets based on the pathogenesis of bone metastases. *Int. J. Cell Biol.* 2014:236246. doi: 10.1155/2014/236246

Paez, J. G., Jänne, P. A., Lee, J. C., Tracy, S., Greulich, H., Gabriel, S., et al. (2004). EGFR mutations in lung cancer: correlation with clinical response to Gefitinib therapy. *Science* 304, 1497–500. doi: 10.1126/science.1099314

Peng, T., Wu, J.-R., Tong, L.-J., Li, M.-Y., Chen, F., Leng, Y.-X., et al. (2014). Identification of DW532 as a novel anti-tumor agent targeting both kinases and tubulin. *Acta Pharmacol. Sin.* 35, 916–928. doi: 10.1038/aps.2014.33

Riely, G. J., Politi, K. A., Miller, V. A., and Pao, W. (2006). Update on epidermal growth factor receptor mutations in non-small cell lung cancer. *Clin. Cancer Res.* 12, 7232. doi: 10.1158/1078-0432.CCR-06-0658

Rosell, R., Moran, T., Queralt, C., Porta, R., Cardenal, F., Camps, C., et al. (2009). Screening for epidermal growth factor receptor mutations in lung cancer. *N. Engl. J. Med.* 361, 958–967. doi: 10.1056/NEJMoa0904554

Scott, W. J., Howington, J., Feigenberg, S., Movsas, B., and Pisters, K. (2007). Treatment of non-small cell lung cancer stage I and stage II: ACCP evidence-based clinical practice guidelines (2nd Edition). *Chest* 132, 234S–242S. doi: 10.1378/chest.07-1378

Sequist, L. V., Besse, B., Lynch, T. J., Miller, V. A., Wong, K. K., Gitlitz, B., et al. (2010). Neratinib, an irreversible pan-ErbB receptor tyrosine kinase inhibitor: results of a phase II trial in patients with advanced non-small-cell lung cancer. *J. Clin. Oncol.* 28, 3076–3083. doi: 10.1200/JCO.2009.27.9414

Sharma, S. V., Bell, D. W., Settleman, J., and Haber, D. A. (2007). Epidermal growth factor receptor mutations in lung cancer. *Nat. Rev. Cancer* 7, 169–181. doi: 10.1038/nrc2088

Sharma, S. V., and Settleman, J. (2007). Oncogene addiction: setting the stage for molecularly targeted cancer therapy. *Genes Dev.* 21, 3214–3231. doi: 10.1101/gad.1609907

Siegel, R. L., Miller, K. D., and Jemal, A. (2017). Cancer statistics, 2017. *CA Cancer J. Clin.* 67, 7–30. doi: 10.3322/caac.21387

Sordella, R., Bell, D. W., Haber, D. A., and Settleman, J. (2004). Gefitinib-sensitizing EGFR mutations in lung cancer activate anti-apoptotic pathways. *Science* 305, 1163–1167. doi: 10.1126/science.1101637

Thress, K. S., Paweletz, C. P., Felip, E., Cho, B. C., Stetson, D., Dougherty, B., et al. (2015). Acquired EGFR C797S mutation mediates resistance to AZD9291 in non-small cell lung cancer harboring EGFR T790M. *Nat. Med.* 21, 560–562. doi: 10.1038/nm.3854

Tracy, S., Mukohara, T., Hansen, M., Meyerson, M., Johnson, B. E., and Jänne, P. A. (2004). Gefitinib induces apoptosis in the EGFRL858R non-small-cell lung cancer cell line H3255. *Cancer Res.* 64, 7241–7244. doi: 10.1158/0008-5472.CAN-04-1905

Uzel, E. K., and Abacıoğlu, U. (2015). Treatment of early stage non-small cell lung cancer: surgery or stereotactic ablative radiotherapy? *Balkan Med. J.* 32, 8–16. doi: 10.5152/balkanmedj.2015.15553

Volate, S. R., Kawasaki, B. T., Hurt, E. M., Milner, J. A., Kim, Y. S., White, J., et al. (2010). Gossypol induces apoptosis by activating p53 in prostate cancer cells and prostate tumor-initiating cells. *Mol. Cancer Ther.* 9, 461–470. doi: 10.1158/1535-7163.MCT-09-0507

Ward, R. A., Anderton, M. J., Ashton, S., Bethel, P. A., Box, M., Butterworth, S., et al. (2013). Structure- and reactivity-based development of covalent inhibitors of the activating and gatekeeper mutant forms of the epidermal growth factor receptor (EGFR). *J. Med. Chem.* 56, 7025–7048. doi: 10.1021/jm400822z

Xiao, X., He, Z., Cao, W., Cai, F., Zhang, L., Huang, Q., et al. (2016). Oridonin inhibits gefitinib-resistant lung cancer cells by suppressing EGFR/ERK/MMP-12 and CIP2A/Akt signaling pathways. *Int. J. Oncol.* 48, 2608–2618. doi: 10.3892/ijo.2016.3488

Xiong, J., Li, J., Yang, Q., Wang, J., Su, T., and Zhou, S. (2017). Gossypol has anti-cancer effects by dual-targeting MDM2 and VEGF in human breast cancer. *Breast Cancer Res.* 19:27. doi: 10.1186/s13058-017-0818-5

Yu, H. A., Arcila, M. E., Rekhtman, N., Sima, C. S., Zakowski, M. F., Pao, W., et al. (2013). Analysis of tumor specimens at the time of acquired resistance to EGFR-TKI therapy in 155 patients with EGFR-mutant lung cancers. *Clin. Cancer Res.* 19, 2240–22407. doi: 10.1158/1078-0432.CCR-12-2246

Yu, H. A., Tian, S. K., Drilon, A. E., Borsu, L., Riely, G. J., Arcila, M. E., et al. (2015). Acquired resistance of egfr-mutant lung cancer to a t790m-specific egfr inhibitor: emergence of a third mutation (c797s) in the egfr tyrosine kinase domain. *JAMA Oncology* 1, 982–984. doi: 10.1001/jamaoncol.2015.1066

Aromatic Rings Commonly Used in Medicinal Chemistry: Force Fields Comparison and Interactions with Water Toward the Design of New Chemical Entities

Marcelo D. Polêto[1], Victor H. Rusu[2], Bruno I. Grisci[3], Marcio Dorn[3], Roberto D. Lins[4] and Hugo Verli[1]*

[1] Grupo de Bioinformática Estrutural, Centro de Biotecnologia, Universidade Federal do Rio Grande do Sul, Porto Alegre, Brazil, [2] Swiss National Supercomputing Centre, Lugano, Switzerland, [3] Instituto de Informática, Universidade Federal do Rio Grande do Sul, Porto Alegre, Brazil, [4] Instituto Aggeu Magalhães, Fundação Oswaldo Cruz, Recife, Brazil

*Correspondence:
Hugo Verli
hverli@cbiot.ufrgs.br

The identification of lead compounds usually includes a step of chemical diversity generation. Its rationale may be supported by both qualitative (SAR) and quantitative (QSAR) approaches, offering models of the putative ligand-receptor interactions. In both scenarios, our understanding of which interactions functional groups can perform is mostly based on their chemical nature (such as electronegativity, volume, melting point, lipophilicity etc.) instead of their dynamics in aqueous, biological solutions (solvent accessibility, lifetime of hydrogen bonds, solvent structure etc.). As a consequence, it is challenging to predict from 2D structures which functional groups will be able to perform interactions with the target receptor, at which intensity and relative abundance in the biological environment, all of which will contribute to ligand potency and intrinsic activity. With this in mind, the aim of this work is to assess properties of aromatic rings, commonly used for drug design, in aqueous solution through molecular dynamics simulations in order to characterize their chemical features and infer their impact in complexation dynamics. For this, common aromatic and heteroaromatic rings were selected and received new atomic charge set based on the direction and module of the dipole moment from MP2/6-31G* calculations, while other topological terms were taken from GROMOS53A6 force field. Afterwards, liquid physicochemical properties were simulated for a calibration set composed by nearly 40 molecules and compared to their respective experimental data, in order to validate each topology. Based on the reliance of the employed strategy, we expanded the dataset to more than 100 aromatic rings. Properties in aqueous solution such as solvent accessible surface area, H-bonds availability, H-bonds residence time, and water structure around heteroatoms were calculated for each ring, creating a database of potential interactions, shedding light on features of drugs in biological solutions, on the structural basis for bioisosterism and on the enthalpic/entropic costs for ligand-receptor complexation dynamics.

Keywords: drug design, GROMOS, aromatic rings, functional groups, interactions

1. INTRODUCTION

The development of a drug is a multi step process, usually starting with the identification of hit compounds. The challenging task of optimizing these compounds into leads and finally into drugs is commonly facilitated by computer aided drug design (CADD) techniques (Anderson, 2003; Sliwoski et al., 2013; Bajorath, 2015). With the growing information on protein structure on the last years, structure based drug design (SBDD) has become a significant tool for hit discovery (Anderson, 2003; Lounnas et al., 2013; Lionta et al., 2014). When structural information of the receptor is absent, molecular fingerprints of approved drugs are also used to search for new ligands in a process also known as ligand based drug design (LBDD) (Lee et al., 2011). Nevertheless, there are still considerable challenges associated to the predictiveness of ligand potency and affinity via computational methods (Paul et al., 2010; Csermely et al., 2012).

In general, optimization of lead compounds is based in qualitative or quantitative structure-activity relationships (SAR or QSAR, respectively) (Shahlaei, 2013). These relationships are usually based in molecular descriptors to predict ligand pharmacodynamics and pharmacokinetics, such as $\log P$ to access lipophilicity, $\log S$ to access solubility or pKa to access the ionic state of a compound, along with other topological, geometrical and physicochemical descriptors (Danishuddin and Khan, 2016). While some correlations have reasonable power of predictiveness, many descriptors have no biological meaning and can mislead the optimization process. As highlighted by Hopkins et al. (2014), high-throughput screening methods have been linked to the rise of hits with inflated physicochemical properties during the optimization process (Keserü and Makara, 2009). Also, recent reviews have shown an increase of molar mass in the recent medicinal chemistry efforts (Leeson and Springthorpe, 2007) and many authors correlate this strategy with the likelihood of poor results of such compounds (Gleeson, 2008; Waring, 2009, 2010; Gleeson et al., 2011).

Many chemical moieties are regularly used in medicinal chemistry to produce chemical diversity (Bemis and Murcko, 1996; Welsch et al., 2010; Taylor et al., 2014), a practice well-known as fragment based drug design (FBDD), and its use for pharmacophore modeling and to prevent high toxicity is not recent (Gao et al., 2010). Particularly, aromatic rings are extensively used in drugs due to their well known synthetic and modification paths (Aldeghi et al., 2014). For example, at least, one aromatic ring can be found in 99% of a database containing more than 3,500 evaluated by the medicinal chemistry department of Pfizer, AstraZeneca (AZ) and GlaxoSmithKlin (GSK) (Roughley and Jordan, 2011). Still, little is known about their chemical features in biological solution, such as H-bonds availability, lifetime of H-bonds, solvent accessibility, and conformational ensemble. In this sense, molecular dynamics (MD) simulations can provide useful information with atomistic resolution and access the aforementioned features of chemical groups in water, providing fundamental data to drive medicinal chemistry approaches.

Still, dynamical properties of chemical moieties in biological solution are usually neglected in drug design and very difficult

to access (Ferenczy and Keseru, 2010; Reynolds and Holloway, 2011; Hopkins et al., 2014). Even though MD simulations have been used in medicinal chemistry to generate different receptor conformers and to validate binding poses predicted by docking (Zhao and Caflisch, 2015; Ganesan et al., 2017), simulations of free ligand in solution is rarely used to access the conformational ensemble and energies associated with solvation due to the challenge on solving conformational flexibility and internal energies (Butler et al., 2009; Blundell et al., 2016). When solvated, the enthalpic and entropic costs of disrupting a H-bond or dismantling the entire solvation shell of a ligand can be the determinant step to provide the proper energy of binding (Biela et al., 2012; Blundell et al., 2013; Mondal et al., 2014). Yet, free-energy of binding is often predicted via geometrical or alchemical transformations (Zwanzig, 1954; Aqvist et al., 1994; Woo and Roux, 2005; Gumbart et al., 2013), alongside with recent developments in funnel metadynamics (Limongelli et al., 2013). More recently, thermodynamical features of ligands have been experimentally investigated in order to enhance binding and efficiency (Freire, 2009; Ferenczy and Keseru, 2010; Reynolds and Holloway, 2011). Ligand features such as H-bonds lifetime, effects of vicinity in H-bonds availability and strength, accessible surface area and water structure around binding sites can provide substantial information for designing new molecular entities (Blundell et al., 2016).

Different force fields have been used for drug design purposes, such as MMF94 (Halgren, 1996), OPLS-AA (Jorgensen et al., 1996), and GAFF (Wang et al., 2004). While these force fields parameterized their electrostatic terms using *ab initio* calculations, the GROMOS force fields (derived from the Groningen Molecular Simulation package) used free-energy of solvation as target (Daura et al., 1998; Oostenbrink et al., 2004) to empirically assign atomic partial charges. Thus, in this work, we have chosen the GROMOS force field to simulate the dynamical behavior of 103 aromatic rings (including a calibration subset of 42 molecules) mostly commonly used in drug design and their interactions with solvent in order to access thermodynamical properties in solution. These interactions, in turn, offer a reference for future rational drug design studies, as describe in details how several functional groups interact with their surroundings.

2. METHODS
2.1. Selection of Rings

A series of 103 aromatic rings commonly used in drug design were selected for this study (Broughton and Watson, 2004; Jordan and Roughley, 2009; Welsch et al., 2010; Taylor et al., 2014, 2017). Among them, a calibration set of 42 molecules (**Table 1**), for which physical-chemical properties are known, were selected from the benchmark developed by Caleman et al. (2012). Briefly, both works of Taylor et al. (2014, 2017) employed a detailed search of substructure frequencies from FDA Orange Book and cross referenced with ChEMBL, DrugBank, Nature, Drug Reviews, the FDA Web site, and the Annual Reports in Medicinal Chemistry; the work of Broughton and Watson (2004) employed search of substructure frequencies in MDL Drug Data

TABLE 1 | Charge groups (colored) and aromatic rings used as calibration set in this work.

[1] Benzene [2] Furan [3] Tiophene [4] Pirrole [5] Pyridine [6] Pyrimidine [7] Fluorobenzene [8] 1,2-difluorobenzene [9] 1,3-difluorobenzene

[10] 1,2,3,4-tetrafluorobenzene [11] 1,2,3,5-tetrafluorobenzene [12] Phenol [13] Toluene [14] Nitrobenzene [15] 2-Chloroaniline [16] Benzenethiol [17] Benzonitrile [18] Trifluoromethylbenzene

[19] 2-methylpyridine [20] 3-methylpyridine [21] 4-methylpyridine [22] Benzaldehyde [23] Methoxybenzene [24] Phenilmethanol [25] 2-methylphenol [26] 3-methylphenol [27] 4-methylphenol

[28] 1-phenilethanone [29] Methylbenzoate [30] Methyl-2-hidroxybenzoate [31] Ethenylbenzene [32] Ethylbenzene [33] 1,2-dimethylbenzene [34] 1,2,4-trimethylbenzene [35] (1-methylethyl)-benzene [36] 1,2-dimethoxybenzene

[37] 2,4,6-trimethylpyridine [38] Aniline [39] Quinoline [40] Isoquinoline [41] 1-chloronaphtalene [42] Phenoxybenzene

Report database by using a "Phase II" keyword; and the work of Welsch et al. (2010) have pinpointed privileged scaffolds from natural-products works throughout literature.

2.2. Topology Construction

Structures for these aromatic rings were built using Avogadro (Hanwell et al., 2012). Molecular mechanical (MM) topological parameters as bonds, angles, and Lennard-Jones parameters were taken from GROMOS53A6 (Oostenbrink et al., 2004). Due to the well–known good performance of MP2 methods for small aromatic rings (Li et al., 2015; Matczak and Wojtulewski, 2015), atomic partial charges were based on quantum mechanical (QM) calculations using MP2 theory (Møller and Plesset, 1934), 6-31G* (Petersson et al., 1988) basis set and implicit solvent *Polarizable Continuum Model* (PCM) (Mennucci and Tomasi, 1997) followed by a RESP fitting (Bayly et al., 1993). The so obtained partial charges were adjusted in the MM to reproduce the QM dipole moment of the ring. The angle θ formed between the QM and MM model dipole moment vectors was monitored through an in house script to make sure the angle had the lowest value possible, guaranteeing the conservation of the QM dipole moment direction. For our calibration set, the module of

the MM partial charges were adjusted to better reproduce the physicochemical properties of the organic liquids. Following the philosophy of charge group assignment, groups were limited, at maximum, to the atoms at the *ortho* position on each ring. In more complex substitution patterns, a superimposition of two charge groups was required to correctly describe the chemical group. In such cases, the Coulombic terms of the overlapping atoms were adjusted to correctly describe the direction of the total dipole moment of the ring. For molecules containing linear constraints (benzonitrile), *virtual sites* were added in order to preserve the total moment of inertia and mass, thus preserving the linearity of these groups (Feenstra et al., 1999).

2.3. New Torsional Potentials

The quantum mechanical torsional profile of every dihedral angle was calculated using Gaussian (Frisch et al., 2016) (RRID:SCR_014897). Molecular structures were built using Avogadro (Hanwell et al., 2012) and their geometry were optimized using Hartree-Fock method (Fock, 1930; Hartree and Hartree, 1935) and basis set 3-21G* (Dobbs and Hehre, 1986). Afterwards, the *Scan* routine was used to calculate the total energy of the molecule conformation for each dihedral orientation, adopting a *tight* convergence criteria, with geometric optimization, MP2/6-31G* and steps of 30°. In order to calculate the torsional profile for molecular mechanics model, dihedral orientations were kept fixed during minimization using restraint forces for the same angles evaluated by quantum calculations. Both profiles were submitted to the Rotational Profiler server (Rusu et al., 2014) to obtain appropriate sets of classical mechanics parameters that provided a better fitting to the QM-obtained torsional profile.

2.4. General Simulation Settings

All simulations were carried out using the GROMACS 5.0.7 package (Abraham et al., 2015) (RRID:SCR_014565). In order to create parameters compatible with the GROMOS family, we have followed previous literature (Daura et al., 1998; Schuler et al., 2001; Oostenbrink et al., 2004) settings: twin-range scheme was used with short- and long-range cutoff distances of 0.8 and 1.4 nm, respectively. Also, the reaction-field method was applied to correct the effects of electrostatic interactions beyond the long-range cutoff distance (Barker and Watts, 1973; Tironi et al., 1995), using the dielectric constant as ε_{RF} for organic liquid simulations and $\varepsilon_{RF} = 62$ for simulations in water (Heinz et al., 2001; Oostenbrink et al., 2004). The LINCS algorithm (Hess et al., 1997; Hess, 2008) was used to constrain all covalent bonds, using a cubic interpolation, a Fourier grid of 0.12 nm and timestep of 2 fs. Configurations were saved at every 2 ps for analysis.

2.4.1. Organic Liquids Simulations

In order to build the organic liquid systems, cubic boxes of $2 \times 2 \times 2$ nm were created, each with a single organic molecule. A total of 125 of these boxes were stacked, forming an unique box with conventional periodic boundary conditions treatment of $10 \times 10 \times 10$ nm which was simulated under high pressure (100 bar) to induce liquid phase. The systems were then simulated and equilibrated at 1 bar. Afterwards, the boxes were staggered to obtain systems with 1000 molecules in liquid phase and simulated at 1 bar until the total energy drift converged to values below 0.5 J/(mol×ns×Degrees of Freedom). Such criterion is necessary to make sure that the fluctuating properties could be accurately calculated (Caleman et al., 2012). All simulations were carried out with Berendsen pressure and temperature coupling algorithm due to their efficiency in molecular relaxations (Berendsen et al., 1984), using $\tau_T = 0.2$ ps and $\tau_P = 0.5$ ps. When available, experimental values of isothermal compressibility and dielectric constant were used as an additional parameter for liquid simulations. Otherwise, the compressibility of the most chemically similar molecule was used. The experimental dielectric constants from each liquid were also used as parameters in the simulations (Oostenbrink et al., 2004).

In order to calculate the densities of liquids (ρ), simulations at constant pressure were carried out for 10 ns and ρ were calculated using block averages of 5 blocks. Enthalpy of vaporization (ΔH_{vap}) were calculated by block averaging the same 10 ns of liquid simulation to obtain $E_{pot}(l)$ and another 100 ns of gas phase simulation using a stochastic dynamics integrator (SD)

(Van Gunsteren and Berendsen, 1988) with a single molecule in vacuum, to obtain $E_{pot}(g)$ as the equation:

$$\Delta H_{vap} = (E_{pot}(g) + k_B T) - E_{pot}(l) \tag{1}$$

Aiming to calculate the dielectric constant (ε), the simulation of the liquid boxes from which ρ were obtained were extended up to 60 ns. Convergence calculations of ε were done using running averages and ε were evaluated only after convergence. In order to calculate thermal expansion coefficients (α_P) and classic isobaric heat capacities (C_{Pcla}), three constant pressure simulations were carried out for 5 ns each, with temperatures T, T+10K, and T-10K, for each liquid. The calculations of α_P and C_{Pcla} were done using the finite difference method (Kunz and van Gunsteren, 2009):

$$\alpha_P \approx \frac{1}{V}\left(\frac{\partial V}{\partial T}\right)_P \approx -\frac{\ln\langle\rho\rangle_{T_2} - \ln\langle\rho\rangle_{T_1}}{T_2 - T_1} \tag{2}$$

and:

$$C_P \approx \left(\frac{\partial U}{\partial T}\right)_P \approx \frac{\langle U\rangle_{T_2} - \langle U\rangle_{T_1}}{T_2 - T_1} \tag{3}$$

In order to calculate isothermal compressibilities (κ_T), three constant volume simulations were carried out for 5 ns each, with pressures 1, 0.9, and 1.1 bar. The calculations of κ_T was also done using the finite difference method:

$$\kappa_T \approx \frac{1}{V}\left(\frac{\partial V}{\partial P}\right)_T \approx -\frac{\ln\rho_2 - \ln\rho_1}{\langle P\rangle_{\rho_2} - \langle P\rangle_{\rho_1}} \tag{4}$$

2.4.2. Solvation Free Energy Simulations

Simulations in water were carried out to evaluate the solvation free energies (ΔG_{hyd}) of 30 molecules at 1 bar and 298 K. Each aromatic ring (solute) was centered into a cubic box with appropriate dimensions to reproduce the density of SPC water models (0.997 g/cm^3). In free-energy calculations using thermodynamic integration (TI) method, a coupling parameter λ is used to perturb solute-solvent interactions.

$$\Delta G_{sim} = \int_0^1 \left\langle\frac{\partial H}{\partial\lambda}\right\rangle_\lambda d\lambda \tag{5}$$

in which H is the Halmiltonian, $\lambda = 0$ refers to the state in which the solute fully interacts with the solvent and $\lambda = 1$ refers to the state in which the solute-solvent interactions do not exist. In our setup, Coulombic interactions were decoupled first, and the Lennard-Jones interactions after, using a soft-core potential to avoid issues related to strong Lennard-Jones interactions (Beutler et al., 1994). A soft-core power was set to 1 and α_{LJ} set to 0.5, following recommendations of Shirts and Pande (2005). Both interactions were decoupled using λ values: 0, 0.02, 0.04, 0.07, 0.1, 0.15, 0.2, ..., 0.8, 0.85, 0.9, 0.93, 0.96, 0.98, 1, totalizing 50 λ simulations.

Our simulation protocol consisted of an initial steepest-descent minimization, followed by a L-BFGS minimization until a maximum force of 10 kJ/(mol^{-1} nm^{-1}) was reached.

TABLE 2 | Dataset of aromatic rings evaluated in this work. Heteroatoms are highlighted in colors.

[43] Imidazole	[44] Thiazole	[45] Benzopyrrole	[46] Tetrazole	[47] Naphtalene	[48] Benzeimidazole	[49] 7,8-dihydro-1H-purine	[50] 1,2,4 - Triazole	[51] Quinazoline
[52] 1H-pyrimidin-2-one	[53] 4-quinolone	[54] Isoxazole	[55] Uracil	[56] Pyrazole	[57] Pyrazine	[58] 1,8-naphthyridin-4(1H)-one	[59] Xanthine	[60] 1,2-dihydro-3H-1,2,4-triazol-3-one
[61] 1,3,4 - Thiadiazole	[62] Indoxazine	[63] 3,9-dihydro-6H-purin-6-one	[64] Benzofuran	[65] Indazole	[66] Benzothiophene	[67] Chromen-4-one	[68] 1,4-naphthoquinone	[69] 1,2,3 - Triazole
[70] Pyridazine	[71] Triazine	[72] Quinoxaline	[73] Oxazole	[74] Isothiazole	[75] 1,3,4 - Oxadiazole	[76] 1,2,4 - Oxadiazole	[77] 1,2,5 - Oxadiazole	[78] 9H-purine
[79] 1,3-Thiazol-2-amine	[80] Cytosine	[81] Adenine	[82] 5-methylindole	[83] 3-methyl-1H-indole	[84] Paraxanthine	[85] Theophylline	[86] Theobromine	[87] 1H-tetrazole-5-thiol
[88] 3-methylisoxazole	[89] 5-methylisoxazole	[90] Methylimidazole	[91] 2-Methylimidazole	[92] Guanine	[93] 1-Methylindole	[94] Chlorobenzene	[95] 1,2-dichlorobenzene	[96] 1,3-dichlorobenzene
[97] 1,2,3,4-tetrachlorobenzene	[98] 1,2,3,5-tetrachlorobenzene	[99] 2-pyridone	[100] 1,3,5-triazin-2(1H)-one	[101] Phenoxazine	[102] 7H-purine	[103] 1,4-benzodioxine		

After, initial velocities were assigned and the systems were equilibrated for 100 ps using a NVT ensemble at each λ. The systems were subjected to another 100 ps of equilibration on a NPT ensemble, using the Parrinello-Rahman pressure coupling algorithm (Parrinello and Rahman, 1981), a $\tau_t = 5$ ps time constant for coupling and a compressibility of 4.5×10^5 bar^{-1}. Finally, production simulations were done using the Langevin integrator (Van Gunsteren and Berendsen, 1988) to sample the $\langle \partial H / \partial \lambda \rangle_\lambda$ until convergence. Therefore, simulations time varied between 1 and 5 ns. In addition, the last frame of the production phase of each λ was used as input for the next subsequent λ.

2.4.3. Simulation of Rings in Water

After an extensive comparison of simulated and experimental physicochemical properties of our calibration set and consequent validation, the same strategy of topological construction was applied to other 61 rings commonly used in drug design (**Table 2**)

for which experimental properties are not available, totalizing 103 aromatic rings in this study. Hence, in order to evaluate chemical features and interactions of aromatic rings with their surroundings, a total set of 103 aromatic was simulated in water, including all 42 molecules present in the calibration set (**Table 1**). Each solute was placed in a cubic box with a distance of 1.0 nm to its edges. The boxes were then filled with SPC water model and minimized long enough eliminate any possible clashes until convergence at a maximum force of 0.1 kJ/mol×nm. After, the system was equilibrated in a NVT ensemble at 298.15 K using the Nosé-Hoover algorithm (Nosé, 1984) for temperature coupling. Production runs of 250 ns were carried out with temperature and pressure coupling handled by V-rescale (Bussi et al., 2007) and Parrinelo-Rahman (Parrinello and Rahman, 1981) algorithms, using $\tau_T = 0.1$ ps and $\tau_P = 2.0$ ps. The GROMACS tools *hbond*, *rdf*, and *sorient* were used to calculate H-bonds related properties and solvation structure around the heteroatom using a block-averaging approach over 5 box of 50 ns.

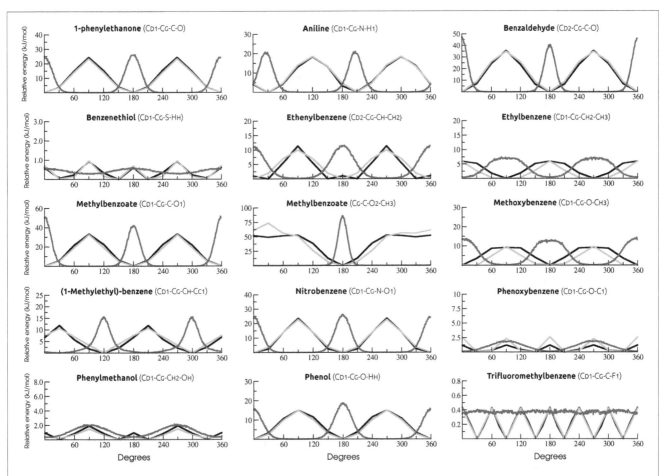

FIGURE 1 | Evaluation of torsional parameters and dihedral distribution. QM and adjusted MM torsional profiles are shown in black and green, respectively. In red, the dihedral distribution during simulations.

3. RESULTS

3.1. New Torsional Profiles

In order to accurately describe the torsional angles of the selected aromatic rings, a total of 15 new dihedral potentials were derived by fitting the MM profiles to the corresponding QM-calculated ones (Table S1). Fittings were conducted using the Rotational Profiler server (Rusu et al., 2014). For all cases, the use of new parameters yield almost identical values of minimum and barrier amplitudes to those calculated by QM (**Figure 1**). Dihedral distribution throughout simulations was also evaluated.

3.2. Physical-Chemical Properties

In order to validate our strategy of topology building, boxes of organic liquids were simulated to obtain physical-chemical properties for each compound. Reference experimental values (Table S2) were used to calculate the absolute error of each property and to guide adjustments on the coulombic terms in order to mitigate deviations. We have calculated the θ angle between QM and MM dipole moments and the final version of our calibration set (**Table 1**) yielded an average θ angle of 2.5° ± 6.1°, suggesting that our MM models conserve the direction of

the QM dipole moment, preserving the electrostatic potential of each molecule.

Following the GROMOS philosophy (Oostenbrink et al., 2004; Horta et al., 2016), density (ρ), enthalpy of vaporization (ΔH_{vap}), and free energy of solvation (ΔG_{hyd}) were used as targets for the parametrization, while isothermal coefficient (α_P), isothermal compressibility (κ_T), dielectric constant (ε), and classic isobaric heat capacity ($C_{P\text{cla}}$) were calculated as benchmarks for GROMOS performance and compared with the results obtained in Caleman et al. (2012) and Horta et al. (2016) (**Table 3**). Linear regression between experimental and simulated values were calculated in order to access the prediction power of the employed strategy (**Figure 2**). The equations further reported were calculated excluding outliers (values higher than 2 standard deviations).

Regarding the targeted properties, our calibration set yielded the equations $y = 0.9118x + 0.1001$ for density, $y = 1.0699x - 1.6491$ for enthalpy of vaporization and $y = 0.8676x + 0.8929$ for free energy of solvation, with correlation coefficients of $R = 0.92$, $R = 0.96$, and $R = 0.89$, respectively. In terms of average deviation (AVED), our calibration set overestimates ρ in 0.008 g/cm³, ΔH_{vap} in 1.51 kJ/mol and underestimates ΔG_{hyd} in 3.35

TABLE 3 | Average deviation between experimental and simulated physicochemical properties of aromatic rings evaluated in our calibration set. Simulated GAFF and OPLS-AA values were obtained from Caleman et al. (2012) and 2016H66 values from Horta et al. (2016). Density (ρ) in g/cm^3, enthalpy of vaporization (ΔH_{vap}) in kJ/mol, thermal expansion coefficient (α_P) in 10^{-3}/K, isothermal compressibility (κ_T) in 1/GPa, dielectric constant (ε), classic isobaric heat capacity (Cp_{cla}) in J/mol×K, and free-energy of solvation (ΔG_{hyd}) in kJ/mol.

Properties	Force field	Statistical N	Average Dev.	St. Dev.	R coefficient
ρ	This work	42	0.008	0.051	0.92
	2016H66	6	0.016	0.019	0.99
	GAFF	40	−0.008	0.045	0.93
	OPLS-AA	40	0.001	0.025	0.98
ΔH_{vap}	This work	42	1.514	4.457	0.96
	2016H66	6	2.257	6.758	0.96
	GAFF	40	2.298	5.419	0.88
	OPLS-AA	40	3.243	5.216	0.90
Cp_{cla}	This work	42	88.201	33.440	0.77
	2016H66	6	98.712	35.232	0.63
	GAFF	37	133.884	40.225	0.84
	OPLS-AA	37	129.397	35.330	0.91
α_P	This work	42	0.146	0.210	0.82
	2016H66	6	0.171	0.148	0.91
	GAFF	40	0.224	0.220	0.58
	OPLS-AA	40	0.155	0.210	0.64
κ_T	This work	42	0.046	0.500	0.70
	2016H66	6	0.276	0.279	0.71
	GAFF	40	0.054	0.150	0.77
	OPLS-AA	40	−0.016	0.130	0.78
ε	This work	42	−4.523	5.650	0.65
	2016H66	6	−2.217	2.515	0.89
	GAFF	29	−4.254	2.740	0.97
	OPLS-AA	33	−4.564	5.600	0.72

kJ/mol. Without the outliers, the AVED for ΔG_{hyd} improves to 2.83 kJ/mol.

Non-targeted properties were calculated to evaluate how they behaved in our simulations. Linear regressions yielded equations $y = 0.93825x + 0.1406$ for α_P (R = 0.82), $y = +0.90079x − 0.0140$ for κ_T (R = 0.70), $y = 0.2581x + 1.8961$ for ε (R = 0.65), and $y = 0.8989x + 100.5$ for Cp_{cla} (R = 0.77). In terms of AVED, α_P is overestimated in 0.14 10^{-3}/K and κ_T is overestimated in 0.0465 1/GPa. As expected (Caleman et al., 2012; Horta et al., 2016), ε is poorly described due to the lack of polarization effects, resulting in a underestimation of −4.52 in the dielectric constant. On other hand, Cp_{cla} was overestimated by 88.2 J/mol×K, a behavior aligned with recent works in literature (Caleman et al., 2012; Horta et al., 2016). Individual AVED and absolute errors can be found in Tables S4, S5 in Supplementary Material, along with experimental properties in Table S3.

3.3. Interactions in Water

In order to quantitatively evaluate the behavior of heteroaromatic rings in water and their interactions with the aqueous

surrounding, some properties were calculated throughout 250 ns of simulation. From these calculations, we were capable to assess the average H-bond ($Aver_{HB}$) of each heteroatom along with its residence time (τ_{HB}), lifetime ($lifetime_{HB}$), the free-energy of breakage of a H-bond (ΔG_{HB}), and the percentage of simulation time that a given heteroatom was involved in, at least, one H-bond (*Percent*). We were also capable to obtain the optimal binding distance between an heteratom and water (OBD_{HB}), along with the coordination number (CN_{HB}) at the OBD_{HB} and the average orientation of water molecules surrounding the heteroatom. These data are compiled in **Tables 4, 5**.

4. DISCUSSION

4.1. Topology Building Strategy

The accurate description of organic compounds' chemical diversity, mainly in the context of drugs and medicinal chemistry, is a challenging task in molecular mechanics since it must be described as broadly as possible by the force field fragments. However, the most common sets of MM parameters

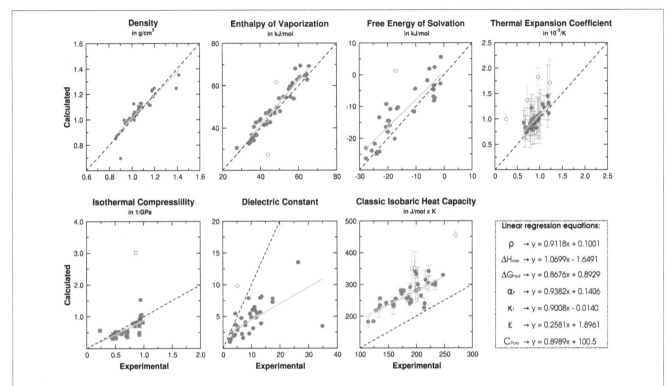

FIGURE 2 | Correlation between experimental and calculated physical-chemical properties of organic liquids for 42 aromatic compounds on the calibration set. Standard deviations are shown as bars, linear regressions are shown as green and empty dots represent outliers.

employed in biomolecules simulations are usually centered on the monomeric constituents of biopolymers and lipids, while parameters for synthetic compounds, as well as other common non-polymeric biological molecules (e.g., natural products), must be included from specific calculations or external sets of parameters.

In this sense, a proper description of torsional terms will impact directly the dynamical behavior of these small molecules, even considering that, when evaluating ligand-receptor complexes, the influence of these terms might be mitigated due to the ligand movement restriction inside the binding pocket. Still, accommodation of flexible docking derived poses, fine tunning of induced fit, and characterization of ligands conformational induction vs. selection (with potential inferences of the entropic costs of binding) require dihedrals potentials specifically adjusted to organic compounds. Hence, new parameters were generated in this work exclusively for 15 dihedrals in aromatic rings in our calibration set (**Figure 1**). In general, our results revealed that our MM parameters yielded a good description of the QM torsional profile, with the exceptions of [16] tiophenol, [42] phenoxybenzene, [24] phenylmethanol, and [18] trifluoromethylbenzene. For these molecules, the distribution profile was almost evenly spread, most likely due to the low energy barrier (below 2.5 kJ/mol), indicating that transient states are commonly achieved during our simulations in SPC water model. Simulations of these particular molecules in vacuum revealed little influence of water solvation in the dihedral profile (data not shown).

In another sense, the choice of an atomic charge set for ligands can drastically impact thermodynamical binding properties such as complexation free-energy and desolvation. Therefore, we employed in this work a dipole moment based strategy to describe the Coulombic contribution using physicochemical properties of organic liquids as target. The prediction power of our strategy was compared to recent comparisons of aromatic compounds in liquid phase (Caleman et al., 2012; Horta et al., 2016) and summarized in **Table 3**. In general, our calibration set yielded similar or lower average deviations than benchmarks made with OPLS-AA, GAFF, and 2016H66 sets for all physicochemical properties evaluated in this work. The main difference was in terms of Cp_{cla}, for which GAFF and OPLS-AA overestimate nearly 40 J/mol×K more than our parameters. Still, all four parameters sets overestimates Cp_{cla}. In addition, the GROMOS53A5 force field was designed to reproduce physicochemical properties, and later on adjusted to reproduce free energy of solvation and hydration (GROMOS53A6) (Oostenbrink et al., 2004). The average deviation on density, enthalpy of vaporization and free-energy of solvation of GROMOS53A5 were 0.0389 g/cm³, −0.4 and 3.8 kJ/mol, respectively. These values are very similar to our results, as shown in **Table 3**, reiterating the quality of our parameters.

It is important to mention that the employed benchmark set was built using the same Lennard-Jones parameters used in the benzene ring of phenylalanine in GROMOS53A6. While GROMOS53A6 produces a $\Delta G_{hyd} = 0.0$ kJ/mol for benzene

TABLE 4 | Properties of heteroaromatic rings in water. Average H-bonds ($Aver_{HB}$), H-bond residence time (τ_{HB}) is ps, H-bond lifetime ($lifetime_{HB}$) in 1/ps, free-energy of H-bond breakage (ΔG_{HB}) in kJ/mol, percentage of simulation with at least one formed H-bond (*Percent.*), coordination number of water (*CN*), optimal binding distance with water (OBD_{HB}) in nm, and overall water orientation around the heteroatom (*Orientation*).

Molecule	Atom	$Aver_{HB}$	τ_{HB}	$lifetime_{HB}$	ΔG_{HB}	Percent	CN	OBD_{HB}	Orientation
Water	**Ow**	1.73 ± 0.62	2.11 ± 0.02	0.47 ± 0.00	6.38 ± 0.03	98.58	4.11 ± 2.83	0.18 ± 0.00	Undefined
	OH[1]	0.87 ± 0.35	1.80 ± 0.03	0.55 ± 0.01	5.98 ± 0.05	86.25	4.11 ± 2.83	0.18 ± 0.00	O-oriented
	OH[2]	0.86 ± 0.35	1.83 ± 0.03	0.54 ± 0.01	6.03 ± 0.04	86.07	4.11 ± 2.83	0.18 ± 0.00	O-oriented
Phenol	**O**	1.10 ± 0.62	1.61 ± 0.03	0.62 ± 0.01	5.70 ± 0.04	85.96	1.46 ± 1.03	0.18 ± 0.00	Undefined
	OH	0.96 ± 0.20	9.49 ± 0.18	0.11 ± 0.00	10.11 ± 0.05	96.04	0.90 ± 0.01	0.17 ± 0.00	O-oriented
Phenylmethanol	**O**	1.42 ± 0.58	2.58 ± 0.03	0.39 ± 0.00	6.88 ± 0.02	96.51	2.68 ± 1.59	0.18 ± 0.00	Undefined
	OH	0.95 ± 0.24	5.37 ± 0.06	0.19 ± 0.00	8.70 ± 0.03	94.25	1.13 ± 0.01	0.17 ± 0.00	O-oriented
2-methylphenol	**O**	1.04 ± 0.59	1.88 ± 0.04	0.53 ± 0.01	6.09 ± 0.05	84.80	1.05 ± 0.00	0.18 ± 0.00	Undefined
	OH	0.95 ± 0.23	9.46 ± 0.17	0.11 ± 0.00	10.10 ± 0.04	94.53	0.87 ± 0.01	0.17 ± 0.00	O-oriented
3-methylphenol	**O**	1.08 ± 0.61	1.74 ± 0.02	0.58 ± 0.01	5.90 ± 0.03	85.83	1.43 ± 1.00	0.18 ± 0.00	Undefined
	OH	0.96 ± 0.19	10.12 ± 0.19	0.10 ± 0.00	10.27 ± 0.05	96.30	0.90 ± 0.01	0.17 ± 0.00	O-oriented
4-methylphenol	**O**	1.08 ± 0.61	1.73 ± 0.02	0.58 ± 0.01	5.89 ± 0.03	85.70	1.10 ± 0.01	0.18 ± 0.00	Undefined
	OH	0.96 ± 0.20	10.00 ± 0.21	0.10 ± 0.00	10.24 ± 0.05	96.21	0.90 ± 0.01	0.17 ± 0.00	O-oriented
Benzenethiol	**S**	0.67 ± 0.65	0.38 ± 0.01	2.63 ± 0.05	2.13 ± 0.04	57.29	0.81 ± 0.17	0.23 ± 0.00	Undefined
	SH	0.77 ± 0.43	1.00 ± 0.02	1.00 ± 0.02	4.52 ± 0.05	76.38	2.08 ± 0.02	0.23 ± 0.00	O-oriented
Aniline	**N**	0.93 ± 0.58	1.64 ± 0.02	0.61 ± 0.01	5.75 ± 0.03	79.89	1.01 ± 0.01	0.19 ± 0.00	Undefined
	NH[1]	0.63 ± 0.49	1.15 ± 0.03	0.87 ± 0.02	4.87 ± 0.06	62.48	1.25 ± 0.38	0.22 ± 0.00	O-oriented
	NH[2]	0.63 ± 0.50	0.99 ± 0.02	1.01 ± 0.02	4.51 ± 0.04	62.05	1.39 ± 0.25	0.23 ± 0.00	O-oriented
2-chloroaniline	**N**	0.86 ± 0.50	2.29 ± 0.04	0.44 ± 0.01	6.59 ± 0.05	79.39	0.92 ± 0.00	0.19 ± 0.00	Undefined
	NH[1]	0.51 ± 0.51	1.00 ± 0.03	1.00 ± 0.03	4.53 ± 0.06	50.60	1.33 ± 0.14	0.23 ± 0.00	O-oriented
	NH[2]	0.56 ± 0.51	0.87 ± 0.03	1.15 ± 0.04	4.18 ± 0.09	55.20	3.82 ± 5.29	0.23 ± 0.01	O-oriented
	Cl	0.24 ± 0.45	0.32 ± 0.08	3.26 ± 0.68	1.66 ± 0.56	22.67	18.94 ± 10.05	0.36 ± 0.00	Undefined
Pyridine	**N**	1.41 ± 0.71	1.33 ± 0.02	0.75 ± 0.01	5.24 ± 0.03	91.46	1.59 ± 0.01	0.20 ± 0.00	Undefined
Pyrimidine	**N[1]**	1.06 ± 0.68	0.91 ± 0.02	1.10 ± 0.02	4.30 ± 0.05	80.71	1.23 ± 0.01	0.20 ± 0.00	Undefined
	N[2]	0.98 ± 0.68	0.81 ± 0.02	1.24 ± 0.03	4.00 ± 0.06	76.96	1.17 ± 0.01	0.20 ± 0.00	Undefined
2-methylpyridine	**N**	1.52 ± 0.70	1.74 ± 0.04	0.57 ± 0.01	5.90 ± 0.06	93.96	1.68 ± 0.00	0.20 ± 0.00	Undefined
3-methylpyridine	**N**	1.43 ± 0.71	1.34 ± 0.04	0.74 ± 0.02	5.26 ± 0.07	91.65	1.61 ± 0.01	0.20 ± 0.00	Undefined
4-methylpyridine	**N**	1.46 ± 0.71	1.44 ± 0.04	0.69 ± 0.02	5.44 ± 0.07	92.57	1.62 ± 0.01	0.20 ± 0.00	Undefined
2,4,6-trimethylpyridine	**N**	0.36 ± 0.53	0.36 ± 0.04	2.79 ± 0.31	2.00 ± 0.28	33.67	24.48 ± 3.47	0.42 ± 0.09	Undefined
Quinoline	**N**	1.64 ± 0.68	2.00 ± 0.05	0.50 ± 0.01	6.25 ± 0.06	96.10	1.78 ± 0.01	0.19 ± 0.00	Undefined
Isoquinoline	**N**	1.26 ± 0.68	1.22 ± 0.04	0.82 ± 0.02	5.02 ± 0.07	88.67	1.43 ± 0.01	0.20 ± 0.00	Undefined
Benzonitrile	**N**	1.63 ± 0.72	1.30 ± 0.01	0.77 ± 0.01	5.17 ± 0.02	95.50	1.88 ± 0.01	0.19 ± 0.00	Undefined
Furan	**O**	0.42 ± 0.57	0.29 ± 0.01	3.41 ± 0.07	1.49 ± 0.05	37.99	31.54 ± 2.60	0.46 ± 0.01	Undefined
Tiophene	**S**	0.15 ± 0.37	0.25 ± 0.03	4.07 ± 0.49	1.07 ± 0.32	14.03	18.25 ± 5.37	0.37 ± 0.00	Undefined
Pyrrole	**NH**	0.92 ± 0.29	3.80 ± 0.06	0.26 ± 0.00	7.84 ± 0.04	91.73	0.38 ± 0.00	0.18 ± 0.00	O-oriented
	N	0.74 ± 0.67	1.33 ± 0.03	0.75 ± 0.02	5.23 ± 0.06	60.90	0.62 ± 0.01	0.23 ± 0.00	Undefined
Fluorobenzene	**F[1]**	0.30 ± 0.49	0.30 ± 0.03	3.35 ± 0.32	1.54 ± 0.24	27.84	13.84 ± 5.27	0.36 ± 0.01	Undefined

(Continued)

TABLE 4 | Continued

Molecule	Atom	$Aver_{HB}$	τ_{HB}	$lifetime_{HB}$	ΔG_{HB}	Percent	CN	OBD_{HB}	Orientation
1,2-difluorobenzene	F[1]	0.24 ± 0.45	0.33 ± 0.07	3.14 ± 0.61	1.74 ± 0.49	22.91	12.15 ± 2.45	0.37 ± 0.01	Undefined
	F[2]	0.24 ± 0.45	0.34 ± 0.07	3.08 ± 0.64	1.79 ± 0.51	22.90	13.31 ± 3.02	0.37 ± 0.01	Undefined
1,3-difluorobenzene	F[1]	0.23 ± 0.45	0.36 ± 0.10	2.91 ± 0.58	1.94 ± 0.59	22.23	14.99 ± 5.60	0.36 ± 0.01	Undefined
	F[3]	0.23 ± 0.45	0.32 ± 0.04	3.20 ± 0.36	1.66 ± 0.29	22.22	11.70 ± 1.33	0.36 ± 0.00	Undefined
1,2,3,4-tetrafluorobenzene	F[1]	0.17 ± 0.38	0.36 ± 0.08	2.88 ± 0.61	1.97 ± 0.53	16.08	12.99 ± 3.94	0.37 ± 0.01	Undefined
	F[2]	0.18 ± 0.40	0.42 ± 0.15	2.66 ± 0.78	2.22 ± 0.79	17.44	12.72 ± 2.45	0.37 ± 0.01	Undefined
	F[3]	0.18 ± 0.40	0.33 ± 0.04	3.11 ± 0.45	1.74 ± 0.34	17.31	13.89 ± 3.36	0.37 ± 0.01	Undefined
	F[4]	0.16 ± 0.38	0.43 ± 0.21	2.72 ± 0.83	2.20 ± 0.98	16.05	11.25 ± 1.36	0.36 ± 0.00	Undefined
1,2,3,5-tetrafluorobenzene	F[1]	0.17 ± 0.39	0.37 ± 0.10	2.84 ± 0.64	2.01 ± 0.61	16.51	12.34 ± 3.05	0.36 ± 0.01	Undefined
	F[2]	0.16 ± 0.37	0.48 ± 0.25	2.47 ± 0.82	2.47 ± 1.03	15.19	12.79 ± 3.60	0.37 ± 0.01	Undefined
	F[3]	0.17 ± 0.39	0.44 ± 0.10	2.40 ± 0.53	2.42 ± 0.56	16.59	14.91 ± 5.13	0.37 ± 0.01	Undefined
	F[5]	0.21 ± 0.43	0.33 ± 0.06	3.17 ± 0.54	1.70 ± 0.44	20.59	11.51 ± 1.36	0.36 ± 0.01	Undefined
Trifluoromethylbenzene	F[1]	0.10 ± 0.30	1.64 ± 1.99	1.26 ± 0.91	4.66 ± 2.10	9.56	14.84 ± 3.37	0.39 ± 0.02	Undefined
	F[2]	0.10 ± 0.30	0.64 ± 0.37	1.95 ± 0.73	3.10 ± 1.16	9.66	15.37 ± 3.44	0.40 ± 0.02	Undefined
	F[3]	0.10 ± 0.30	2.82 ± 5.74	1.05 ± 0.41	5.00 ± 2.38	9.54	14.94 ± 3.23	0.40 ± 0.02	Undefined
1-chloronaphthalene	Cl	0.37 ± 0.55	0.28 ± 0.02	3.55 ± 0.21	1.39 ± 0.15	33.96	15.53 ± 7.71	0.36 ± 0.00	Undefined
1-phenylethanone	O	0.87 ± 0.66	0.56 ± 0.01	1.79 ± 0.04	3.09 ± 0.05	71.14	1.08 ± 0.01	0.19 ± 0.00	Undefined
Benzaldehyde	O	1.03 ± 0.66	0.78 ± 0.01	1.28 ± 0.02	3.91 ± 0.04	80.79	1.22 ± 0.01	0.18 ± 0.00	Undefined
Nitrobenzene	O[1]	0.14 ± 0.36	0.43 ± 0.13	2.51 ± 0.67	2.34 ± 0.72	13.79	13.60 ± 4.08	0.38 ± 0.01	Undefined
	O[2]	0.14 ± 0.36	0.46 ± 0.15	2.37 ± 0.62	2.48 ± 0.73	13.81	16.48 ± 5.81	0.38 ± 0.01	Undefined
Methylbenzoate	O[1]	0.95 ± 0.67	0.69 ± 0.01	1.45 ± 0.02	3.62 ± 0.04	75.85	1.13 ± 0.01	0.19 ± 0.00	Undefined
	O[2]	0.17 ± 0.38	0.28 ± 0.05	3.63 ± 0.58	1.37 ± 0.43	16.40	25.27 ± 2.00	0.45 ± 0.00	Undefined
2-hydroxy-methylbenzoate	O	0.96 ± 0.58	1.48 ± 0.02	0.67 ± 0.01	5.51 ± 0.03	81.17	1.07 ± 0.00	0.18 ± 0.00	Undefined
	O[1]	0.94 ± 0.64	1.07 ± 0.17	0.96 ± 0.15	4.65 ± 0.39	76.43	1.07 ± 0.13	0.18 ± 0.00	Undefined
	O[2]	0.12 ± 0.33	0.36 ± 0.23	3.43 ± 1.03	1.65 ± 1.10	12.11	23.62 ± 8.28	0.33 ± 0.11	Undefined
	OH	0.05 ± 0.22	0.21 ± 0.04	4.83 ± 0.80	0.66 ± 0.46	5.25	0.40 ± 0.01	0.18 ± 0.01	O-oriented
Methoxybenzene	O	0.36 ± 0.51	0.33 ± 0.02	3.03 ± 0.14	1.78 ± 0.12	34.78	0.42 ± 0.01	0.20 ± 0.00	H-oriented
1,2-dimethoxybenzene	O[1]	0.39 ± 0.54	0.38 ± 0.02	2.62 ± 0.15	2.14 ± 0.14	36.51	20.52 ± 10.11	0.28 ± 0.08	H-oriented
	O[1]	0.39 ± 0.54	0.38 ± 0.05	2.64 ± 0.32	2.14 ± 0.32	36.49	12.48 ± 11.98	0.24 ± 0.00	H-oriented
Phenoxybenzene	O	0.32 ± 0.49	0.29 ± 0.02	3.40 ± 0.18	1.50 ± 0.13	31.12	5.69 ± 10.11	0.23 ± 0.01	Undefined

Colors represent different functional groups: red for oxygen, blue for nitrogen, orange for sulfur and green for halogen containing groups.

(phenylalanine side-chain), our benzene parameters yield a $\Delta G_{hyd} = -3.4$ kJ/mol, a much closer value to the experimental data ($\Delta G_{hyd} = -3.6$ kJ/mol). Nevertheless, the AVED value reveals a underestimation for free energy of hydration in our parameter set. A possible reason is that chemical functions such as nitro, fluorine, chlorine, and aldehydic carbonyls are not commonly found in biomolecules and, therefore, the LJ parameters used in GROMOS53A6 may not be properly extrapolated to synthetic compounds. Moreover, we have tested ether oxygens LJ parameters reported in Horta et al. (2011) in

our pure liquid simulations of [2]furan and [23]methoxybenzene, leading to approximately the same behavior in their respective physical-chemical properties (data not shown).

4.2. Properties in Solution: Influence of Nearby Substitutions in H-Bonds

In order to access quantitative informations regarding how aromatic rings interact with their surroundings, we performed molecular dynamics simulations for 103 aromatic rings most commonly used in drug design, including our 42 molecules

TABLE 5 | Properties of heteroaromatic rings in water. Average H-bonds ($Aver_{HB}$), H-bond residence time (τ_{HB}) is ps, H-bond lifetime ($lifetime_{HB}$) in 1/ps, free-energy of H-bond breakage (ΔG_{HB}) in kJ/mol, percentage of simulation with at least one formed H-bond (*Percent.*), coordination number of water (*CN*), optimal binding distance with water (OBD_{HB}) in nm, and overall water orientation around the heteroatom (*Orientation*).

Molecule	Atom	$Aver_{HB}$	τ_{HB}	$lifetime_{HB}$	ΔG_{HB}	Percent	CN	OBD_{HB}	Orientation
Water	Ow	1.73 ± 0.62	2.11 ± 0.02	0.47 ± 0.00	6.38 ± 0.03	98.58	4.11 ± 2.83	0.18 ± 0.00	Undefined
	OH1	0.87 ± 0.35	1.80 ± 0.03	0.55 ± 0.01	5.98 ± 0.05	86.25	4.11 ± 2.83	0.18 ± 0.00	O-oriented
	OH2	0.86 ± 0.35	1.83 ± 0.03	0.54 ± 0.01	6.03 ± 0.04	86.07	4.11 ± 2.83	0.18 ± 0.00	O-oriented
Imidazole	N^1	0.08 ± 0.27	0.33 ± 0.09	3.27 ± 0.86	1.68 ± 0.69	7.58	26.01 ± 7.18	0.41 ± 0.01	Undefined
	N^1H	0.56 ± 0.52	0.35 ± 0.00	2.89 ± 0.04	1.90 ± 0.03	55.10	34.04 ± 1.08	0.45 ± 0.02	Undefined
	N^3	1.30 ± 0.72	1.01 ± 0.01	0.99 ± 0.00	4.56 ± 0.01	87.72	7.56 ± 12.01	0.20 ± 0.00	Undefined
Thiazole	S^1	0.04 ± 0.20	–	–	–	4.21	16.56 ± 5.11	0.38 ± 0.01	Undefined
	N^3	0.53 ± 0.60	0.37 ± 0.01	2.73 ± 0.08	2.04 ± 0.07	47.16	0.62 ± 0.11	0.22 ± 0.00	Undefined
Benzopyrrole	N^1	0.09 ± 0.29	0.28 ± 0.05	3.68 ± 0.49	1.32 ± 0.37	8.60	15.88 ± 2.99	0.38 ± 0.00	Undefined
	N^1H	0.63 ± 0.51	0.66 ± 0.01	1.50 ± 0.03	3.51 ± 0.04	61.63	21.05 ± 1.45	0.41 ± 0.01	Undefined
Tetrazole	N^4	0.87 ± 0.69	0.54 ± 0.01	1.85 ± 0.03	3.00 ± 0.04	69.85	1.17 ± 0.02	0.21 ± 0.00	Undefined
	N^3	0.89 ± 0.74	0.53 ± 0.02	1.87 ± 0.06	2.97 ± 0.08	68.12	1.09 ± 0.32	0.23 ± 0.00	Undefined
	N^2	0.31 ± 0.51	0.27 ± 0.02	3.75 ± 0.22	1.26 ± 0.15	29.37	26.38 ± 7.22	0.41 ± 0.00	Undefined
	N^1	0.02 ± 0.14	–	–	–	1.95	21.88 ± 2.06	0.41 ± 0.01	Undefined
	N^1H	0.00 ± 0.00	–	–	–	0.00	0.50 ± 0.03	0.24 ± 0.00	O-oriented
Benzeimidazole	N^1	0.06 ± 0.23	0.21 ± 0.03	4.87 ± 0.67	0.62 ± 0.34	5.53	16.49 ± 2.30	0.40 ± 0.01	Undefined
	N^1H	0.78 ± 0.44	1.21 ± 0.02	0.82 ± 0.01	5.01 ± 0.03	77.23	32.26 ± 2.16	0.46 ± 0.01	Undefined
	N^3	1.08 ± 0.71	0.86 ± 0.01	1.16 ± 0.02	4.16 ± 0.04	80.28	1.32 ± 0.01	0.20 ± 0.00	Undefined
7,8-dihydro-1H-purine	N^6H	0.42 ± 0.51	0.34 ± 0.01	2.91 ± 0.09	1.88 ± 0.08	41.30	30.55 ± 3.92	0.46 ± 0.01	Undefined
	N^1	0.04 ± 0.19	0.20 ± 0.02	5.21 ± 0.66	0.46 ± 0.31	3.73	16.89 ± 12.64	0.28 ± 0.00	O-oriented
	N^6	0.04 ± 0.19	–	–	–	3.70	28.25 ± 2.59	0.46 ± 0.01	Undefined
	N^4	0.33 ± 0.51	0.37 ± 0.04	2.76 ± 0.31	2.02 ± 0.29	31.14	24.55 ± 2.24	0.45 ± 0.01	Undefined
	N^1H	0.96 ± 0.21	6.49 ± 0.11	0.15 ± 0.00	9.16 ± 0.04	95.83	0.79 ± 0.65	0.18 ± 0.00	O-oriented
	N^3	1.83 ± 0.70	1.97 ± 0.09	0.51 ± 0.02	6.20 ± 0.11	97.65	3.38 ± 1.14	0.20 ± 0.00	Undefined
1,2,4 - Triazole	N^2	1.50 ± 0.72	1.53 ± 0.04	0.65 ± 0.02	5.59 ± 0.06	92.83	1.70 ± 0.00	0.20 ± 0.00	Undefined
	N^1	0.66 ± 0.66	0.83 ± 0.02	1.20 ± 0.04	4.07 ± 0.07	55.78	2.10 ± 3.51	0.22 ± 0.00	Undefined
	N^1H	0.98 ± 0.15	11.47 ± 0.25	0.09 ± 0.00	10.58 ± 0.05	97.94	3.76 ± 0.00	0.25 ± 0.03	O-oriented
	N^4	0.83 ± 0.68	0.61 ± 0.01	1.63 ± 0.02	3.32 ± 0.04	67.99	0.97 ± 0.01	0.20 ± 0.00	Undefined
Quinazoline	N^1	0.64 ± 0.63	0.49 ± 0.02	2.04 ± 0.07	2.76 ± 0.09	56.17	0.71 ± 0.21	0.21 ± 0.00	Undefined
	N^3	0.43 ± 0.56	0.31 ± 0.01	3.19 ± 0.05	1.65 ± 0.04	39.34	24.86 ± 3.16	0.28 ± 0.08	H-oriented
1H-pyrimidin-2-one	O^2	1.20 ± 0.72	0.79 ± 0.01	1.27 ± 0.02	3.93 ± 0.03	84.99	1.42 ± 0.02	0.20 ± 0.00	Undefined
	N^1H	0.41 ± 0.51	0.33 ± 0.01	3.07 ± 0.13	1.75 ± 0.10	39.74	24.01 ± 4.58	0.44 ± 0.02	Undefined
	N^1	0.01 ± 0.09	–	–	–	0.73	19.00 ± 2.14	0.41 ± 0.00	Undefined
	N^3	0.89 ± 0.62	0.84 ± 0.00	1.19 ± 0.01	4.11 ± 0.01	75.00	1.05 ± 0.00	0.20 ± 0.00	Undefined
4-quinolone	O^4	1.74 ± 0.74	1.39 ± 0.02	0.72 ± 0.01	5.35 ± 0.04	96.17	3.85 ± 1.52	0.19 ± 0.00	Undefined
	N^1	0.01 ± 0.10	–	–	–	1.03	23.69 ± 2.01	0.47 ± 0.01	Undefined
	N^1H	0.66 ± 0.49	0.80 ± 0.02	1.26 ± 0.04	3.96 ± 0.07	65.61	26.90 ± 2.65	0.47 ± 0.01	Undefined
Isoxazole	O^1	0.59 ± 0.62	0.36 ± 0.00	2.82 ± 0.02	1.96 ± 0.02	52.43	7.34 ± 13.27	0.22 ± 0.01	Undefined
	N^2	0.60 ± 0.63	0.35 ± 0.01	2.86 ± 0.05	1.92 ± 0.04	52.00	0.77 ± 0.04	0.24 ± 0.00	H-oriented
Uracil	N^3	0.02 ± 0.16	1.99 ± 1.45	1.04 ± 0.90	5.38 ± 2.21	2.48	17.32 ± 1.01	0.42 ± 0.01	Undefined
	N^3H	0.33 ± 0.49	0.29 ± 0.01	3.47 ± 0.10	1.45 ± 0.07	31.98	25.64 ± 8.27	0.43 ± 0.02	Undefined
	O^2	0.39 ± 0.54	0.28 ± 0.01	3.61 ± 0.13	1.35 ± 0.09	36.17	19.18 ± 8.50	0.37 ± 0.01	Undefined
	O^4	1.24 ± 0.71	0.87 ± 0.01	1.15 ± 0.01	4.19 ± 0.02	86.66	4.08 ± 5.14	0.20 ± 0.00	Undefined
	N^1	0.01 ± 0.07	–	–	–	0.54	29.81 ± 2.46	0.46 ± 0.01	Undefined
	N^1H	0.45 ± 0.52	0.37 ± 0.01	2.67 ± 0.07	2.09 ± 0.06	44.10	30.23 ± 1.97	0.47 ± 0.01	Undefined

(Continued)

TABLE 5 | Continued

Molecule	Atom	$Aver_{HB}$	τ_{HB}	$lifetime_{HB}$	ΔG_{HB}	Percent	CN	OBD_{HB}	Orientation
	N^1H	0.00 ± 0.00	–	–	–	0.00	18.32 ± 2.00	0.40 ± 0.01	Undefined
Pyrazole	N^1	0.00 ± 0.00	–	–	–	0.00	17.76 ± 1.63	0.40 ± 0.00	Undefined
	N^2	0.72 ± 0.66	0.44 ± 0.01	2.29 ± 0.07	2.48 ± 0.08	60.69	0.96 ± 0.03	0.21 ± 0.00	Undefined
Pyrazine	N^1	1.15 ± 0.66	1.15 ± 0.03	0.87 ± 0.02	4.88 ± 0.07	85.83	6.55 ± 10.50	0.19 ± 0.00	Undefined
	N^4	1.15 ± 0.65	1.15 ± 0.02	0.87 ± 0.02	4.86 ± 0.05	85.87	6.66 ± 10.74	0.19 ± 0.00	Undefined
	O^4	1.13 ± 0.73	0.71 ± 0.02	1.41 ± 0.04	3.68 ± 0.07	81.51	1.44 ± 0.02	0.20 ± 0.00	Undefined
1,8-naphthyridin-4(1H)-one	N^8	0.28 ± 0.48	0.28 ± 0.02	3.57 ± 0.28	1.38 ± 0.19	26.76	25.87 ± 2.34	0.45 ± 0.01	Undefined
	N^1	0.05 ± 0.23	0.40 ± 0.14	2.81 ± 0.93	2.10 ± 0.84	5.34	22.03 ± 2.09	0.44 ± 0.01	Undefined
	N^1H	0.40 ± 0.51	0.34 ± 0.02	2.99 ± 0.20	1.82 ± 0.17	39.32	26.16 ± 2.29	0.45 ± 0.01	Undefined
	N^1H	0.40 ± 0.51	0.38 ± 0.01	2.66 ± 0.10	2.10 ± 0.09	39.37	28.47 ± 4.09	0.46 ± 0.02	Undefined
	O^2	0.52 ± 0.60	0.32 ± 0.03	3.13 ± 0.23	1.71 ± 0.19	46.33	17.09 ± 8.14	0.37 ± 0.01	Undefined
	N^7	0.02 ± 0.12	–	–	–	1.51	25.71 ± 2.69	0.45 ± 0.02	Undefined
Xanthine	N^7H	0.47 ± 0.52	0.43 ± 0.01	2.33 ± 0.08	2.43 ± 0.08	46.50	26.50 ± 2.03	0.46 ± 0.01	Undefined
	N^1	0.02 ± 0.15	–	–	–	2.33	21.48 ± 4.05	0.44 ± 0.01	Undefined
	N^3	0.03 ± 0.17	–	–	–	3.09	19.25 ± 5.54	0.41 ± 0.01	Undefined
	O^6	0.46 ± 0.57	0.31 ± 0.01	3.25 ± 0.06	1.61 ± 0.05	42.64	8.82 ± 4.23	0.33 ± 0.06	Undefined
	N^9	0.28 ± 0.47	0.28 ± 0.03	3.61 ± 0.36	1.36 ± 0.25	27.40	26.67 ± 2.40	0.46 ± 0.01	Undefined
	N^1H	0.95 ± 0.24	4.50 ± 0.09	0.22 ± 0.00	8.25 ± 0.05	94.28	1.32 ± 1.05	0.17 ± 0.00	O-oriented
	N^2H	0.48 ± 0.52	0.37 ± 0.01	2.72 ± 0.05	2.04 ± 0.05	46.54	21.76 ± 2.73	0.38 ± 0.01	Undefined
1,2-dihydro-3H-1,2,4-triazol-3-one	N^4	1.21 ± 0.67	1.11 ± 0.01	0.90 ± 0.01	4.80 ± 0.03	87.18	1.39 ± 0.00	0.20 ± 0.00	Undefined
	O^3	1.26 ± 0.76	0.79 ± 0.01	1.27 ± 0.01	3.93 ± 0.02	85.27	1.54 ± 0.02	0.20 ± 0.00	Undefined
	N^1	0.02 ± 0.13	–	–	–	1.75	17.03 ± 9.51	0.28 ± 0.00	O-oriented
	N^2	0.03 ± 0.16	–	–	–	2.52	27.49 ± 5.89	0.38 ± 0.00	Undefined
	S^1	0.02 ± 0.15	–	–	–	2.32	19.74 ± 5.86	0.39 ± 0.01	Undefined
1,3,4 - Thiadiazole	N^3	1.33 ± 0.73	1.17 ± 0.03	0.86 ± 0.02	4.91 ± 0.05	88.26	18.35 ± 13.63	0.21 ± 0.00	Undefined
	N^4	1.34 ± 0.73	1.16 ± 0.01	0.86 ± 0.01	4.89 ± 0.02	88.35	1.70 ± 0.02	0.21 ± 0.00	Undefined
Indoxazine	N^2	0.69 ± 0.65	0.45 ± 0.00	2.20 ± 0.02	2.57 ± 0.02	59.11	0.94 ± 0.02	0.22 ± 0.00	Undefined
	O^1	0.74 ± 0.66	0.48 ± 0.01	2.08 ± 0.05	2.72 ± 0.06	62.08	0.84 ± 0.21	0.21 ± 0.00	Undefined
	N^1H	0.46 ± 0.52	0.40 ± 0.01	2.48 ± 0.09	2.28 ± 0.09	45.20	26.74 ± 2.00	0.45 ± 0.00	Undefined
	N^1	0.02 ± 0.14	–	–	–	1.93	22.39 ± 5.57	0.42 ± 0.01	Undefined
	N^9	0.03 ± 0.17	0.71 ± 0.45	1.99 ± 1.06	3.23 ± 1.48	3.05	20.26 ± 3.47	0.42 ± 0.01	Undefined
3,9-dihydro-6H-purin-6-one	N^9H	0.47 ± 0.52	0.36 ± 0.00	2.80 ± 0.03	1.97 ± 0.03	45.60	26.51 ± 3.63	0.44 ± 0.02	Undefined
	N^3	0.11 ± 0.32	0.47 ± 0.19	2.40 ± 0.71	2.49 ± 0.88	11.22	27.05 ± 1.99	0.46 ± 0.01	Undefined
	O^6	1.35 ± 0.77	0.82 ± 0.03	1.21 ± 0.04	4.05 ± 0.08	87.77	1.68 ± 0.02	0.20 ± 0.00	Undefined
	N^7	0.57 ± 0.61	0.44 ± 0.02	2.28 ± 0.11	2.49 ± 0.12	50.12	0.65 ± 0.15	0.23 ± 0.00	Undefined
Benzofuran	O^1	0.50 ± 0.59	0.35 ± 0.01	2.90 ± 0.10	1.89 ± 0.09	44.67	23.40 ± 11.48	0.32 ± 0.11	Undefined
	N^2	0.40 ± 0.55	0.29 ± 0.02	3.45 ± 0.20	1.46 ± 0.14	36.29	22.45 ± 4.12	0.42 ± 0.01	Undefined
Indazole	N^1	0.17 ± 0.39	0.22 ± 0.02	4.62 ± 0.40	0.75 ± 0.22	16.72	16.16 ± 2.36	0.39 ± 0.01	Undefined
	N^1H	0.55 ± 0.52	0.45 ± 0.00	2.22 ± 0.02	2.55 ± 0.02	53.47	18.47 ± 4.54	0.40 ± 0.01	Undefined
Benzothiophene	S^1	0.14 ± 0.35	0.36 ± 0.09	2.99 ± 0.83	1.91 ± 0.67	13.13	17.61 ± 6.64	0.37 ± 0.00	Undefined
Chromone	O^4	1.17 ± 0.73	0.74 ± 0.01	1.35 ± 0.02	3.78 ± 0.04	83.02	1.46 ± 0.01	0.20 ± 0.00	Undefined
	O^1	0.14 ± 0.35	0.39 ± 0.12	2.81 ± 0.70	2.06 ± 0.71	13.72	25.00 ± 1.49	0.46 ± 0.01	Undefined
1,4-naphthoquinone	O^4	0.64 ± 0.61	0.44 ± 0.01	2.27 ± 0.03	2.49 ± 0.03	56.82	0.83 ± 0.01	0.20 ± 0.00	Undefined
	O^1	0.64 ± 0.61	0.44 ± 0.01	2.25 ± 0.08	2.52 ± 0.08	57.12	0.82 ± 0.02	0.20 ± 0.00	Undefined
	N^1H	0.82 ± 0.41	1.16 ± 0.02	0.86 ± 0.01	4.89 ± 0.04	80.97	14.14 ± 17.25	0.24 ± 0.10	O-oriented
1,2,3 - Triazole	N^3	1.11 ± 0.73	0.78 ± 0.01	1.29 ± 0.02	3.90 ± 0.03	80.38	1.47 ± 0.02	0.21 ± 0.00	Undefined
	N^2	1.09 ± 0.74	0.75 ± 0.01	1.34 ± 0.02	3.81 ± 0.03	78.90	1.47 ± 0.00	0.21 ± 0.00	Undefined

(Continued)

TABLE 5 | Continued

Molecule	Atom	$Aver_{HB}$	τ_{HB}	$lifetime_{HB}$	ΔG_{HB}	Percent	CN	OBD_{HB}	Orientation
	N^1	0.11 ± 0.32	0.21 ± 0.00	4.73 ± 0.09	0.67 ± 0.05	11.02	16.72 ± 8.74	0.39 ± 0.03	Undefined
Pyridazine	N^1	1.42 ± 0.76	1.25 ± 0.01	0.80 ± 0.01	5.09 ± 0.02	89.58	1.83 ± 0.00	0.21 ± 0.00	Undefined
	N^2	1.41 ± 0.76	1.24 ± 0.03	0.81 ± 0.02	5.05 ± 0.07	89.42	1.83 ± 0.00	0.21 ± 0.00	Undefined
Triazine	N^1	0.28 ± 0.48	0.29 ± 0.03	3.46 ± 0.38	1.47 ± 0.27	26.10	29.60 ± 0.96	0.45 ± 0.01	Undefined
	N^3	0.27 ± 0.48	0.29 ± 0.03	3.48 ± 0.35	1.45 ± 0.25	25.94	29.63 ± 1.97	0.46 ± 0.00	Undefined
	N^5	0.27 ± 0.48	0.28 ± 0.02	3.62 ± 0.24	1.34 ± 0.16	25.78	33.15 ± 1.59	0.45 ± 0.01	Undefined
Quinoxaline	N^4	0.34 ± 0.51	0.30 ± 0.02	3.40 ± 0.19	1.50 ± 0.14	32.01	24.66 ± 0.64	0.37 ± 0.10	Undefined
	N^1	0.34 ± 0.51	0.30 ± 0.02	3.34 ± 0.19	1.54 ± 0.14	31.83	25.96 ± 2.58	0.33 ± 0.11	Undefined
Oxazole	O^1	0.34 ± 0.51	0.29 ± 0.01	3.51 ± 0.16	1.42 ± 0.12	31.80	31.43 ± 3.12	0.41 ± 0.10	Undefined
	N^3	0.42 ± 0.56	0.29 ± 0.01	3.48 ± 0.14	1.44 ± 0.10	38.27	33.46 ± 2.32	0.43 ± 0.09	Undefined
Isothiazole	S^1	0.05 ± 0.22	0.70 ± 0.11	1.45 ± 0.20	3.63 ± 0.36	5.11	13.50 ± 1.67	0.37 ± 0.00	Undefined
	N^2	0.30 ± 0.49	0.29 ± 0.02	3.42 ± 0.21	1.48 ± 0.15	28.32	29.65 ± 2.44	0.46 ± 0.01	Undefined
1,3,4 - Oxadiazole	N^3	0.96 ± 0.70	0.65 ± 0.02	1.53 ± 0.04	3.47 ± 0.07	74.33	1.32 ± 0.00	0.22 ± 0.00	Undefined
	N^4	0.96 ± 0.70	0.64 ± 0.01	1.55 ± 0.02	3.44 ± 0.04	73.98	1.31 ± 0.01	0.21 ± 0.00	Undefined
	O^1	0.09 ± 0.29	0.71 ± 0.42	1.88 ± 0.84	3.29 ± 1.36	8.69	29.27 ± 5.26	0.44 ± 0.02	Undefined
1,2,5 - Oxadiazole	O^1	0.64 ± 0.66	0.36 ± 0.01	2.76 ± 0.06	2.01 ± 0.06	53.93	12.92 ± 14.89	0.28 ± 0.09	H-oriented
	N^2	0.35 ± 0.53	0.28 ± 0.02	3.59 ± 0.20	1.37 ± 0.14	32.97	27.66 ± 1.31	0.43 ± 0.01	Undefined
	N^5	0.36 ± 0.53	0.28 ± 0.01	3.54 ± 0.14	1.40 ± 0.10	33.18	29.19 ± 3.89	0.44 ± 0.01	Undefined
1,2,4 - Oxadiazole	N^2	0.57 ± 0.61	0.35 ± 0.01	2.83 ± 0.04	1.95 ± 0.04	50.92	7.40 ± 13.39	0.23 ± 0.01	Undefined
	N^4	0.57 ± 0.57	0.43 ± 0.01	2.30 ± 0.07	2.46 ± 0.07	52.94	0.69 ± 0.01	0.20 ± 0.00	Undefined
	O^1	0.53 ± 0.59	0.34 ± 0.01	2.98 ± 0.05	1.82 ± 0.04	47.71	15.71 ± 18.47	0.33 ± 0.12	Undefined
9H-purine	N^3	0.14 ± 0.35	0.62 ± 0.38	2.12 ± 0.88	2.95 ± 1.29	13.39	22.11 ± 1.98	0.42 ± 0.01	Undefined
	N^9H	0.93 ± 0.28	3.72 ± 0.10	0.27 ± 0.01	7.79 ± 0.07	92.10	0.44 ± 0.00	0.18 ± 0.00	O-oriented
	N^1	0.89 ± 0.64	0.82 ± 0.01	1.22 ± 0.02	4.03 ± 0.04	73.61	1.05 ± 0.01	0.20 ± 0.00	Undefined
	N^9	0.06 ± 0.25	0.23 ± 0.03	4.47 ± 0.62	0.84 ± 0.35	6.42	3.15 ± 3.45	0.29 ± 0.00	O-oriented
	N^7	0.43 ± 0.56	0.34 ± 0.03	2.93 ± 0.23	1.87 ± 0.20	39.57	33.93 ± 0.52	0.29 ± 0.10	H-oriented
1,3-Thiazol-2-amine	N^3	0.33 ± 0.51	0.32 ± 0.03	3.12 ± 0.28	1.72 ± 0.22	30.55	nan ± nan	0.48 ± 0.01	Undefined
	S^1	0.04 ± 0.19	–	–	–	3.62	27.86 ± 3.96	0.45 ± 0.02	Undefined
	N	0.77 ± 0.53	1.33 ± 0.02	0.75 ± 0.01	5.24 ± 0.04	72	0.81 ± 0.00	0.19 ± 0.00	Undefined
	NH^1	0.74 ± 0.46	1.29 ± 0.01	0.78 ± 0.01	5.16 ± 0.03	72.89	1.35 ± 0.38	0.21 ± 0.01	O-oriented
	NH^2	0.73 ± 0.46	1.15 ± 0.01	0.87 ± 0.01	4.88 ± 0.03	72.43	1.20 ± 0.44	0.21 ± 0.01	O-oriented
Cytosine	N^1	0.09 ± 0.29	0.36 ± 0.14	3.07 ± 0.78	1.86 ± 0.81	8.45	25.84 ± 1.36	0.44 ± 0.01	Undefined
	N^1H	0.32 ± 0.48	0.29 ± 0.01	3.41 ± 0.06	1.48 ± 0.04	31.74	29.19 ± 2.52	0.45 ± 0.00	Undefined
	N	0.88 ± 0.53	2.19 ± 0.03	0.46 ± 0.01	6.47 ± 0.04	79.3	8.19 ± 5.54	0.19 ± 0.00	Undefined
	NH^1	0.73 ± 0.46	1.81 ± 0.02	0.55 ± 0.01	6.00 ± 0.02	72.76	1.06 ± 0.48	0.21 ± 0.01	O-oriented
	NH^2	0.70 ± 0.47	1.37 ± 0.02	0.73 ± 0.01	5.30 ± 0.04	69.18	0.87 ± 0.39	0.20 ± 0.00	O-oriented
	O^1	1.20 ± 0.79	0.69 ± 0.02	1.44 ± 0.04	3.62 ± 0.07	81.29	1.40 ± 0.39	0.21 ± 0.00	Undefined
	N^3	0.93 ± 0.73	0.70 ± 0.05	1.44 ± 0.10	3.63 ± 0.18	71.11	1.34 ± 0.32	0.23 ± 0.00	Undefined
Adenine	N^3	1.98 ± 0.68	3.01 ± 0.10	0.33 ± 0.01	7.26 ± 0.08	98.70	3.96 ± 1.48	0.19 ± 0.00	Undefined
	N^9	0.18 ± 0.40	0.31 ± 0.02	3.26 ± 0.27	1.60 ± 0.20	16.99	25.32 ± 2.77	0.35 ± 0.00	Undefined
	N^9H	0.30 ± 0.47	0.35 ± 0.01	2.89 ± 0.11	1.90 ± 0.09	29.54	23.64 ± 1.66	0.34 ± 0.00	Undefined
	N^7	0.17 ± 0.39	0.30 ± 0.02	3.33 ± 0.23	1.55 ± 0.18	16.86	29.43 ± 2.90	0.45 ± 0.01	Undefined
	N^1	0.14 ± 0.36	0.80 ± 0.49	1.96 ± 1.26	3.43 ± 1.72	13.30	21.59 ± 5.25	0.39 ± 0.00	Undefined
	N	0.92 ± 0.48	3.15 ± 0.08	0.32 ± 0.01	7.37 ± 0.06	84.23	4.04 ± 6.16	0.19 ± 0.00	Undefined
	NH^1	0.68 ± 0.48	1.85 ± 0.04	0.54 ± 0.01	6.05 ± 0.05	67.41	0.66 ± 0.06	0.20 ± 0.00	O-oriented

(Continued)

TABLE 5 | Continued

Molecule	Atom	$Aver_{HB}$	τ_{HB}	$lifetime_{HB}$	ΔG_{HB}	Percent	CN	OBD_{HB}	Orientation
5-methylindole	NH^2	0.70 ± 0.47	1.50 ± 0.02	0.67 ± 0.01	5.53 ± 0.04	68.92	0.67 ± 0.03	0.20 ± 0.00	O-oriented
	N^1	0.26 ± 0.47	0.39 ± 0.02	2.56 ± 0.11	2.20 ± 0.11	24.48	12.49 ± 0.43	0.34 ± 0.05	Undefined
	N^1H	0.89 ± 0.33	3.45 ± 0.04	0.29 ± 0.00	7.60 ± 0.03	88.55	0.37 ± 0.00	0.19 ± 0.00	O-oriented
3-methyl-1H-indole	N^1	0.18 ± 0.40	0.35 ± 0.05	2.94 ± 0.40	1.88 ± 0.34	17.01	17.42 ± 2.94	0.38 ± 0.00	Undefined
	N^1H	0.71 ± 0.48	1.07 ± 0.01	0.94 ± 0.01	4.69 ± 0.03	70.01	17.37 ± 2.17	0.39 ± 0.01	Undefined
Paraxanthine	O^6	0.58 ± 0.58	0.48 ± 0.01	2.08 ± 0.05	2.72 ± 0.06	52.88	0.76 ± 0.02	0.21 ± 0.00	Undefined
	N^3	0.01 ± 0.10	–	–	–	1.02	18.20 ± 4.10	0.39 ± 0.01	Undefined
	N^3H	0.54 ± 0.52	0.65 ± 0.02	1.55 ± 0.06	3.45 ± 0.09	52.58	18.43 ± 2.43	0.40 ± 0.01	Undefined
	O^2	0.61 ± 0.61	0.45 ± 0.01	2.22 ± 0.05	2.55 ± 0.06	54.13	0.78 ± 0.02	0.21 ± 0.00	Undefined
	N^9	0.79 ± 0.60	0.86 ± 0.01	1.17 ± 0.02	4.15 ± 0.04	69.54	0.95 ± 0.01	0.20 ± 0.00	Undefined
	N^7	0.00 ± 0.05	–	–	–	0.21	28.11 ± 1.53	0.47 ± 0.00	Undefined
	N^1	0.03 ± 0.16	–	–	–	2.66	24.93 ± 0.00	0.48 ± 0.00	Undefined
Theophylline	N^7H	0.33 ± 0.49	0.33 ± 0.01	3.00 ± 0.11	1.80 ± 0.09	32.06	23.41 ± 1.68	0.44 ± 0.01	Undefined
	O^6	0.30 ± 0.48	0.27 ± 0.01	3.73 ± 0.16	1.27 ± 0.11	28.37	13.20 ± 1.45	0.38 ± 0.01	Undefined
	N^3	0.02 ± 0.15	–	–	–	2.41	20.89 ± 2.00	0.45 ± 0.01	Undefined
	O^2	0.60 ± 0.62	0.40 ± 0.01	2.53 ± 0.09	2.23 ± 0.09	53.03	0.63 ± 0.21	0.22 ± 0.00	Undefined
	N^9	0.16 ± 0.38	0.29 ± 0.03	3.44 ± 0.33	1.48 ± 0.24	15.73	27.76 ± 1.85	0.46 ± 0.01	Undefined
	N^7	0.02 ± 0.13	–	–	–	1.78	23.16 ± 3.82	0.43 ± 0.01	Undefined
	N^1	0.01 ± 0.12	–	–	–	1.48	25.52 ± 2.34	0.48 ± 0.01	Undefined
Theobromine	O^6	0.26 ± 0.46	0.26 ± 0.01	3.89 ± 0.10	1.16 ± 0.06	25.11	12.25 ± 1.29	0.37 ± 0.01	Undefined
	N^3	0.00 ± 0.06	–	–	–	0.33	27.56 ± 1.00	0.48 ± 0.01	Undefined
	O^2	0.97 ± 0.68	0.69 ± 0.01	1.46 ± 0.01	3.59 ± 0.02	76.39	1.22 ± 0.00	0.20 ± 0.00	Undefined
	N^9	0.10 ± 0.30	0.28 ± 0.02	3.54 ± 0.27	1.40 ± 0.19	9.65	17.11 ± 2.33	0.42 ± 0.01	Undefined
	N^7	0.01 ± 0.10	–	–	–	1.01	25.82 ± 1.01	0.47 ± 0.01	Undefined
	N^1H	0.00 ± 0.00	–	–	–	0.00	20.86 ± 1.70	0.41 ± 0.02	Undefined
	N^1	0.03 ± 0.18	2.28 ± 1.56	0.99 ± 0.92	5.67 ± 2.35	3.16	18.46 ± 3.28	0.40 ± 0.00	Undefined
2H-tetrazol-5-thiol	N^1H	0.66 ± 0.50	0.56 ± 0.01	1.79 ± 0.04	3.08 ± 0.06	65.29	24.63 ± 6.12	0.43 ± 0.01	Undefined
	S	0.08 ± 0.28	1.98 ± 2.59	1.55 ± 1.03	4.47 ± 2.73	8.34	24.11 ± 12.41	0.35 ± 0.00	Undefined
	SH	0.65 ± 0.59	0.36 ± 0.01	2.75 ± 0.08	2.02 ± 0.07	59.18	15.22 ± 7.54	0.36 ± 0.00	Undefined
	N^3	1.05 ± 0.75	0.67 ± 0.01	1.50 ± 0.03	3.52 ± 0.06	76.69	1.44 ± 0.02	0.21 ± 0.00	Undefined
	N^2	0.47 ± 0.58	0.34 ± 0.00	2.93 ± 0.03	1.86 ± 0.03	42.55	21.28 ± 4.89	0.40 ± 0.01	Undefined
	N^1	0.01 ± 0.09	–	–	–	0.90	16.82 ± 4.27	0.39 ± 0.02	Undefined
	N^4	0.54 ± 0.61	0.37 ± 0.01	2.68 ± 0.10	2.09 ± 0.09	47.48	31.80 ± 0.00	0.33 ± 0.11	Undefined
3-methylisoxazole	O^1	0.87 ± 0.70	0.59 ± 0.01	1.71 ± 0.02	3.20 ± 0.03	69.34	0.99 ± 0.25	0.21 ± 0.00	Undefined
	N^2	0.94 ± 0.72	0.62 ± 0.01	1.61 ± 0.02	3.35 ± 0.03	72.36	1.32 ± 0.02	0.22 ± 0.00	Undefined
5-methylisoxazole	O^1	1.06 ± 0.71	0.79 ± 0.02	1.27 ± 0.03	3.95 ± 0.06	78.70	1.31 ± 0.02	0.20 ± 0.00	Undefined
	N^2	1.03 ± 0.73	0.73 ± 0.01	1.37 ± 0.02	3.75 ± 0.03	76.61	1.42 ± 0.01	0.22 ± 0.00	Undefined
Methylimidazole	N^3	1.51 ± 0.68	1.51 ± 0.03	0.66 ± 0.01	5.55 ± 0.05	94.20	11.94 ± 12.59	0.19 ± 0.00	Undefined
	N^1	0.03 ± 0.18	0.45 ± 0.28	2.86 ± 1.15	2.20 ± 1.28	3.26	29.76 ± 1.84	0.46 ± 0.01	Undefined
2-Methylimidazole	N^3	1.76 ± 0.68	2.28 ± 0.04	0.44 ± 0.01	6.57 ± 0.05	97.30	3.63 ± 0.94	0.19 ± 0.00	Undefined
	N^1	0.11 ± 0.32	0.23 ± 0.02	4.45 ± 0.34	0.83 ± 0.19	10.86	15.18 ± 1.88	0.40 ± 0.01	Undefined
	N^1H	0.87 ± 0.36	1.86 ± 0.02	0.54 ± 0.01	6.06 ± 0.03	86.05	0.35 ± 0.01	0.19 ± 0.00	O-oriented
Guanine	N^1	0.00 ± 0.06	–	–	–	0.40	6.42 ± 4.70	0.27 ± 0.00	O-oriented
	N^1H	0.98 ± 0.15	11.66 ± 0.29	0.09 ± 0.00	10.62 ± 0.06	97.86	2.00 ± 0.29	0.17 ± 0.00	O-oriented
	N^7	0.98 ± 0.65	0.81 ± 0.01	1.24 ± 0.02	3.99 ± 0.03	78.40	1.19 ± 0.01	0.20 ± 0.00	Undefined
	N^3	1.51 ± 0.64	2.33 ± 0.08	0.43 ± 0.02	6.62 ± 0.09	95.37	2.98 ± 1.13	0.19 ± 0.00	Undefined
	N	0.58 ± 0.57	1.16 ± 0.03	0.86 ± 0.02	4.90 ± 0.06	54.33	0.27 ± 0.02	0.19 ± 0.00	Undefined
	NH^1	0.71 ± 0.47	2.24 ± 0.03	0.45 ± 0.01	6.53 ± 0.03	70.16	29.15 ± 1.28	0.35 ± 0.00	Undefined
	NH^2	0.67 ± 0.48	1.62 ± 0.02	0.62 ± 0.01	5.72 ± 0.03	66.50	24.74 ± 7.45	0.34 ± 0.00	Undefined

(Continued)

TABLE 5 | Continued

Molecule	Atom	$Aver_{HB}$	τ_{HB}	$lifetime_{HB}$	ΔG_{HB}	Percent	CN	OBD_{HB}	Orientation
	O^6	1.91 ± 0.71	2.01 ± 0.02	0.50 ± 0.01	6.26 ± 0.03	98.32	3.73 ± 1.35	0.23 ± 0.05	Undefined
	N^9	0.01 ± 0.09	–	–	–	0.76	3.81 ± 3.08	0.28 ± 0.00	O-oriented
	N^9H	0.97 ± 0.19	11.16 ± 0.09	0.09 ± 0.00	10.51 ± 0.02	96.44	4.90 ± 5.94	0.17 ± 0.00	O-oriented
1-Methylindole	N^1	0.22 ± 0.44	0.65 ± 0.20	1.80 ± 0.84	3.29 ± 0.96	20.67	26.89 ± 0.73	0.47 ± 0.00	Undefined
Chlorobenzene	Cl^1	0.22 ± 0.44	0.34 ± 0.08	3.08 ± 0.70	1.80 ± 0.58	20.83	31.47 ± 1.09	0.36 ± 0.00	Undefined
1,2-dichlorobenzene	Cl^1	0.17 ± 0.39	0.38 ± 0.05	2.70 ± 0.33	2.09 ± 0.32	16.31	19.59 ± 8.61	0.36 ± 0.00	Undefined
	Cl^2	0.17 ± 0.39	0.39 ± 0.05	2.64 ± 0.38	2.14 ± 0.34	16.29	18.60 ± 8.25	0.36 ± 0.00	Undefined
1,3-dichlorobenzene	Cl^1	0.17 ± 0.40	0.38 ± 0.08	2.78 ± 0.63	2.06 ± 0.56	16.74	30.86 ± 3.91	0.36 ± 0.00	Undefined
	Cl^3	0.17 ± 0.39	0.37 ± 0.06	2.79 ± 0.40	2.01 ± 0.37	16.55	26.58 ± 8.67	0.36 ± 0.00	Undefined
1,2,3,4-tetrachlorobenzene	Cl^4	0.13 ± 0.35	0.39 ± 0.12	2.75 ± 0.67	2.11 ± 0.69	12.90	25.88 ± 5.26	0.36 ± 0.00	Undefined
	Cl^1	0.13 ± 0.35	0.43 ± 0.14	2.52 ± 0.58	2.32 ± 0.69	13.06	23.23 ± 6.96	0.37 ± 0.00	Undefined
	Cl^2	0.11 ± 0.32	0.43 ± 0.12	2.47 ± 0.63	2.37 ± 0.66	10.45	22.80 ± 7.24	0.37 ± 0.00	Undefined
	Cl^3	0.11 ± 0.31	0.64 ± 0.32	1.93 ± 0.80	3.14 ± 1.13	10.32	22.24 ± 7.06	0.36 ± 0.00	Undefined
1,2,3,5-tetrachlorobenzene	Cl^5	0.16 ± 0.38	0.29 ± 0.06	3.55 ± 0.69	1.44 ± 0.49	15.90	27.66 ± 8.74	0.36 ± 0.00	Undefined
	Cl^1	0.14 ± 0.36	0.40 ± 0.11	2.68 ± 0.57	2.15 ± 0.60	14.00	23.15 ± 9.67	0.36 ± 0.00	Undefined
	Cl^2	0.11 ± 0.32	0.48 ± 0.25	2.51 ± 0.92	2.46 ± 1.09	10.97	22.95 ± 7.34	0.37 ± 0.00	Undefined
	Cl^3	0.14 ± 0.36	0.79 ± 0.71	1.98 ± 0.84	3.24 ± 1.66	13.90	23.20 ± 8.70	0.36 ± 0.00	Undefined
2-pyridone	O^2	1.55 ± 0.75	1.11 ± 0.02	0.90 ± 0.01	4.79 ± 0.04	93.28	1.82 ± 0.00	0.19 ± 0.00	Undefined
	N^1	0.07 ± 0.27	0.24 ± 0.02	4.21 ± 0.40	0.98 ± 0.24	7.37	19.48 ± 4.86	0.43 ± 0.02	Undefined
	N^1H	0.78 ± 0.43	1.40 ± 0.02	0.71 ± 0.01	5.36 ± 0.03	77.75	26.08 ± 3.66	0.44 ± 0.01	Undefined
1,3,5-triazin-2(1H)-one	N^3	1.09 ± 0.70	1.00 ± 0.03	1.01 ± 0.03	4.52 ± 0.08	80.87	1.35 ± 0.00	0.20 ± 0.00	Undefined
	N^5	0.11 ± 0.32	0.38 ± 0.20	3.10 ± 0.99	1.91 ± 1.04	10.86	26.48 ± 3.24	0.45 ± 0.01	Undefined
	N^1	0.03 ± 0.17	6.76 ± 12.20	1.62 ± 1.41	5.18 ± 4.11	3.06	25.39 ± 7.62	0.43 ± 0.02	Undefined
	N^1H	0.61 ± 0.51	0.55 ± 0.02	1.81 ± 0.06	3.06 ± 0.08	59.92	30.73 ± 1.51	0.46 ± 0.02	Undefined
	O^2	0.61 ± 0.66	0.41 ± 0.02	2.45 ± 0.09	2.31 ± 0.09	51.10	28.96 ± 4.10	0.35 ± 0.00	Undefined
Phenoxazine	O^5	0.68 ± 0.65	0.45 ± 0.01	2.23 ± 0.04	2.54 ± 0.04	58.43	0.83 ± 0.01	0.21 ± 0.00	Undefined
	$N^{10}H$	0.64 ± 0.50	1.10 ± 0.03	0.91 ± 0.02	4.76 ± 0.06	62.98	23.69 ± 5.31	0.45 ± 0.02	Undefined
	N^{10}	0.14 ± 0.36	0.20 ± 0.01	4.98 ± 0.25	0.55 ± 0.13	13.62	14.89 ± 2.51	0.40 ± 0.01	Undefined
7H-purine	N^1	0.40 ± 0.55	0.31 ± 0.01	3.18 ± 0.09	1.66 ± 0.07	37.45	30.48 ± 3.09	0.32 ± 0.10	Undefined
	N^7H	0.48 ± 0.52	0.35 ± 0.01	2.82 ± 0.05	1.96 ± 0.05	47.21	30.09 ± 1.79	0.46 ± 0.01	Undefined
	N^3	0.53 ± 0.61	0.37 ± 0.02	2.68 ± 0.12	2.09 ± 0.11	46.52	28.45 ± 4.00	0.45 ± 0.02	Undefined
	N^9	0.42 ± 0.56	0.32 ± 0.01	3.13 ± 0.08	1.70 ± 0.06	38.40	29.46 ± 1.47	0.41 ± 0.08	Undefined
	N^7	0.02 ± 0.15	1.28 ± 0.78	1.34 ± 1.03	4.52 ± 1.88	2.34	22.55 ± 4.08	0.43 ± 0.01	Undefined
1,4-benzodioxine	O^4	0.49 ± 0.57	0.39 ± 0.01	2.58 ± 0.07	2.18 ± 0.07	45.03	0.50 ± 0.13	0.21 ± 0.00	Undefined
	O^1	0.49 ± 0.57	0.39 ± 0.01	2.58 ± 0.06	2.18 ± 0.06	44.98	0.57 ± 0.02	0.21 ± 0.00	Undefined

Colors represent different functional groups: red for oxygen, blue for nitrogen, orange for sulfur and green for halogen containing groups.

calibration set. These information are condensed in the **Tables 4, 5**. Simulations were carried for 250 ns to properly sample multiple events of H-bond breakages and solvation shell rearrangements.

Our results reveal non-obvious information about the H-bond availability and strength, as in the case of [5]pyridine/[6]pyrimidine/[56]pyrazine/[70]pyridazine/[71]triazine series (**Figure 3**). While exchanging a pyridine by a pyrimidine ring might lead to apparent gain of a H-bond acceptor, nitrogens of pyrimidine present a ΔG_{HB} of nearly 1 kJ/mol lower than

pyridine. Moreover, the *Percent* of time with at least one formed H-bond between water and pyridine nitrogen is higher than the ones in pyrimidine. When comparing pyridine with pyrazine (an addition of another N in *para*), H-bonds are very similar, so as the second and third solvation layers. Also, acceptance capacity in pyrimidine ring is very similar to triazine, where all three nitrogens are located in *meta*. Intriguingly, values for pyridine are very similar to the ones calculated for pyridazine, with a slight increase in OBD_{HB} and a more compact second layer of solvation, as shown in **Figure 3A**. These results suggest that

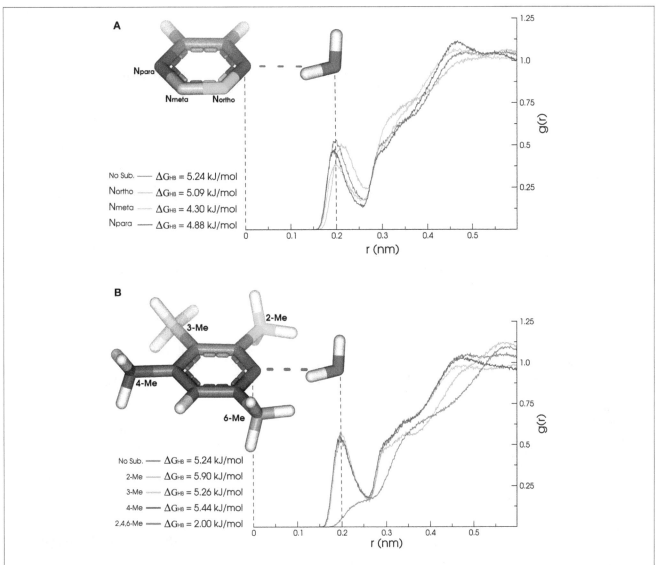

FIGURE 3 | (A) Methyl substituitions: 2-Me (green), 3-Me (yellow), **(B)** Nearby N substitution: N_{ortho} (green), N_{meta} (yellow), 4-Me (purple) and 2,4,6-Me (pink). N_{para} (purple). Solvation properties of aromatic rings in pyridine family. Radial distribution functions (RDFs) and H-bonding strength of N^1 (blue) are affected by substitutions in *ortho*, *meta*, and *para*.

another nitrogen acceptor in *meta* decreases nitrogen acceptance capacity, while another nitrogen acceptor in *ortho* has low effect in H-bond capacity, but a considerable effect in the solvation layers structures. In this sense, these features can impact the binding inside receptors. Pyridazine, for example, has a larger OBD_{HB} than pyridine, suggesting that these molecules can occupy the binding pocket in a different manner, impacting the entropic cost of binding.

Other cases have been equally surprising, like the [39]quinoline/[40]isoquinoline. The main difference between them is the location of the acceptor nitrogen (closer to C^8 in the quinoline fused ring). Counterintuitively, the $Aver_{HB}$ of isoquinoline is slightly lower than for quinoline, such as the τ_{HB}, and the ΔG_{HB} is almost 1.25 kJ/mol lower. The same

properties for pyridine ring are somewhat between these values of quinoline and isoquinoline. In addition, ΔG_{HB} for [51]quinazoline and [72]quinoxaline rings are almost 3 kJ/mol lower than quinoline and isoquinoline. In this sense, quinazoline and quinoxaline would be better candidates in fragment-based drug design due to the lower energetic cost of desolvation, while maintaining the H-bond capacity inside the receptor. Another case in terms of aromatic nitrogen hydrogen bond acceptor is the [37]2,4,6-trimethylpyridine (**Figure 3B**). The presence of methyl groups in both *ortho* positions drastically reduces the availability of H-bonds, as shown in **Figure 3**, and diminish the residence time of the accepted H-bond. But the presence of only one methyl group in *ortho* appears to have a modest effect, slightly favoring the presence of H-bond in nitrogen of [19]2-methylpyridine. Moreover, the second and third solvation layers of 2- and 2,4,6-trimethylpyridine are dismantled, while the same behavior is not observed for [20]3- and [21]4-methylpyridine.

Other non-obvious events can be observed regarding H-bond donation in hydroxyls groups. In case of [12]phenol, the necessary energy to break a donated H-bond (~10 kJ/mol) is almost the double to break an accepted one (~5.70 kJ/mol), in alignment with the QM data reported by Parthasarath et al. (2005) in HF, MP2, and DFT level. And while phenol and [24]phenylmethanol might appear interchangeable during the lead optimization process, the ΔG_{HB} of accepted and donated H-bonds in the hydroxyl group is almost 1 kJ/mol higher for phenylmethanol. While targeting thermodynamics of binding during drug design, these energy costs of desolvation can play a crucial role. As expected, benzenethiol was revealed to be a poor acceptor of hydrogen bonds in our simulations, but a reasonable H-bond donor. In terms of vicinity effects, methylation in *ortho* seems to have little effect on hydroxyl groups, since the properties evaluated for the series [12]phenol/[25]2-methylphenol/[26]3-methylphenol/[27]4-methylphenol have very similar behavior.

It is well– know that halogens are widely used for drug design, and the role of halogen bonds (X-bonds) and H-bonds role have been investigated thoroughly (Rendine et al., 2011; Ford and Ho, 2016; Lin and Mackerell, 2017). In general, the H-bonding strength decreases with the halogen radius (F > Cl > Br > I), while the halogen bond strength increases (Rendine et al., 2011). In this work, we investigated how fluorine and chlorine behave as H-bond acceptors in water. In the case of [7]fluorobenzene, the $\Delta G_{HB} = 1.54 \pm 0.24$ is in accordance with a weak H-bond (Domagała et al., 2017). The other fluorinated rings in the series (1,2-, 1,3-, 1,2,3,4-, and 1,2,3,5-tetrafluorobenzene [8-11]) have similar values, varying from 1.5 to 2.2 kJ/mol. Regarding the chlorinated rings series (chlorobenzene, 1,2-, 1,3-, 1,2,3,4-, and 1,2,3,5-tetrachlorobenzene [94–98]), ΔG_{HB} ranged from 1.80 to 3.24 kJ/mol, contradicting the expected behavior. X-bonding are often poorly described in MM, since it treats atoms as a sphere with isoelectric surface and thus not describing the necessary positive potential required for such interaction. In fact, we have visually evaluated that waters surrounding fluorine and chlorine have their hydrogens oriented toward the halogens, confirming our measure of H-bonds and not X-bonds.

Regarding oxygen atoms within the aromatic ring, $Aver_{HB}$ are generally lower than expected. It is well known that oxygens in heterocycles act as H-bond acceptor (Kaur and Khanna, 2011), but our model does not reproduce this tendency. It is important to notice that GROMOS53A6 does not have specific parameters for oxygens within aromatic rings, and LJ parameters from ethers were employed. Not surprisingly, the calculated properties for the oxygen atom in furan and benzofuran are very similar to methoxybenzene and phenoxybenzene. This result suggests that the description of the properties in aqueous solutions of aromatic rings containing oxygen might be improved by specific LJ parameters. Moreover, we have tested ether LJ parameters reported in Horta et al. (2011) for our simulations of furan and

methoxybenzene in water, yielding lower $Aver_{HB}$ and ΔG_{HB} (data not shown). The new force field parameters developed in this work can be obtained upon request.

4.3. Impacts in Drug Design

Recently, several authors have questioned the LE approach as optimization tool and its actual power to lead to high affinity compounds (Abad-Zapatero, 2007; Morgan et al., 2011; Cavalluzzi et al., 2017). Another recent review (DeGoey et al., 2017) has pointed out the emergence of approved drugs that violate Lipinski's rules of 5 and correlated them to properties such as number of aromatic rings and rotatable bonds. Freire (2009) have proposed an experimental thermodynamic approach to guide the drug design process and these results led to believe that tweaking ligand enthalpy and entropy of binding is not only experimentally possible, but also possible to predict. Therefore, the GROMOS series of force fields present an extra advantage here due to their calibration to reproduce free-energy of solvation and other thermodynamical properties.

In this sense, we have parameterized and validated a calibration set of 42 aromatic rings commonly used in drug design using thermodynamical properties in condensed phase. After, we performed a study with a larger dataset of 103 heteroaromatic rings in order to understand how these molecules interact with water and to prospect and map potential interactions with target-receptors. The water molecules probe the occurrence of hydrogen bonds, and the absence of these interactions, as well as the distance from the first solvation sphere, may probe sites for hydrophobic interactions. With these information at hand, medicinal chemists and pharmacologists may employ quantitative estimations on how each functional group may or may not interact with its target protein, as well as identify the potential influence of close chemical modifications. These properties (and a handful of others) are compiled in **Tables 4, 5**, and can be used as reference during lead optimization process.

The strategy employed here could be used to amplify the spectrum of drug fragments with accurate description of chemical events simulated by molecular dynamics. In addition, it can improve the description of drug-receptor complexation dynamics of other molecules of interest, molecular recognition of drugs and signal transduction mediated by conformational changes of ligands. In fact, by assessing the strength and availability of interactions between aromatic rings and water solvent, the results presented here not only offer detailed quantitative information about potential interactions that each individual aromatic ring can make with its surrounding, but also shed light upon the energetics of biological events, such as dismantling solvation shells — an important step in the ligand binding process.

5. CONCLUSIONS

In this work, we have successfully produced topologies for a calibration set of 42 aromatic rings using as target physicochemical properties of respective organic liquids. Our strategy revealed a very competitive prediction power when compared alongside with other force fields, while presenting a simple approach to describe aromatic rings through molecular dynamics simulations that can be easily extrapolated to other rings. In addition to that, H-bond availability and solvent accessibility are difficult and non-obvious informations to predict from bidimensional data, but still essential for medicinal chemistry purposes. Here, we have simulated in aqueous solvent more than 100 aromatic rings commonly used in drug design in order to assess dynamical chemical properties, such as average H-bonds, their lifetime, residence time and free energy of breakage. Thus, we have described a low cost approach based on molecular dynamics simulations to access valuable information that could be useful both to predict the enthalpic cost of desolvation and for interpretation of pharmacological data by a medicinal chemist or pharmacologist. Our results provide a large database of quantitative information for a total of 103 aromatic rings most commonly used in drug design that can guide medicinal chemists in future drug design efforts.

AUTHOR CONTRIBUTIONS

MP carried out quantum calculations, molecular dynamics simulations, data analyses, and drafted the manuscript. VR contributed in the simulations protocols and manuscript draft. BG wrote in house scripts for dipole-based charge assignment and data analyses. MD contributed to manuscript draft. RL contributed to simulations protocols and manuscript draft. HV contributed to data analyses and manuscript draft.

FUNDING

The authors thank the funding agencies Coordenação de Aperfeiçoamento de Pessoal de Nível Superior (CAPES), Conselho Nacional de Desenvolvimento Científico e Tecnológico (CNPq), and Fundação de Amparo à Pesquisa do Rio Grande do Sul (FAPERGS). This work was partially supported by grants from FAPERGS/PRONUPEQ (16/2551-0000520-6).

ACKNOWLEDGMENTS

Research developed with support of the Centro Nacional de Supercomputação (CESUP), from Universidade Federal do Rio Grande do Sul (UFRGS). We gratefully acknowledge the support of NVIDIA Corporation with the donation of the Titan X Pascal GPU used for this research.

REFERENCES

Abad-Zapatero, C. (2007). Ligand efficiency indices for effective drug discovery. *Expert Opin. Drug Dis.* 2, 469–488. doi: 10.1517/17460441.2.4.469

Abraham, M. J., Murtola, T., Schulz, R., Páll, S., Smith, J. C., Hess, B., et al. (2015). Gromacs: high performance molecular simulations through multi-level parallelism from laptops to supercomputers. *SoftwareX* 1-2, 19–25. doi: 10.1016/j.softx.2015.06.001

Aldeghi, M., Malhotra, S., Selwood, D. L., and Chan, A. W. (2014). Two- and three-dimensional rings in drugs. *Chem. Biol. Drug Des.* 83, 450–461. doi: 10.1111/cbdd.12260

Anderson, A. C. (2003). The process of structure-based drug design. *Chem. Biol.* 10, 787–797. doi: 10.1016/j.chembiol.2003.09.002

Aqvist, J., Medina, C., and Samuelsson, J. E. (1994). A new method for predicting binding affinity in computer-aided drug design. *Protein Eng.* 7, 385–391.

Bajorath, J. (2015). Computer-aided drug discovery. *F1000 Res.* 4:630. doi: 10.12688/f1000research.6653.1

Barker, J. A. and Watts, R. O. (1973). Monte carlo studies of the dielectric properties of water-like models. *Mol. Phys.* 26, 789–792.

Bayly, C. I., Cieplak, P., Cornell, W., and Kollman, P. A. (1993). A well-behaved electrostatic potential based method using charge restraints for deriving atomic charges: the RESP model. *J. Phys. Chem.* 97, 10269–10280.

Bemis, G. W. and Murcko, M. A. (1996). The properties of known drugs. 1. Molecular frameworks. *J. Med. Chem.* 39, 2887–2893.

Berendsen, H. J. C., Postma, J. P. M., van Gunsteren, W. F., DiNola, A., and Haak, J. R. (1984). Molecular dynamics with coupling to an external bath. *J. Chem. Phys.* 81, 3684–3690.

Beutler, T. C., Mark, A. E., van Schaik, R. C., Gerber, P. R., and van Gunsteren, W. F. (1994). Avoiding singularities and numerical instabilities in free energy calculations based on molecular simulations. *Chem. Phys. Lett.* 222, 529–539.

Biela, A., Khayat, M., Tan, H., Kong, J., Heine, A., Hangauer, D., et al. (2012). Impact of ligand and protein desolvation on ligand binding to the S1 pocket of thrombin. *J. Mol. Biol.* 418, 350–366. doi: 10.1016/j.jmb.2012.01.054

Blundell, C. D., Nowak, T., and Watson, M. J. (2016). Measurement, interpretation and use of free ligand solution conformations in drug discovery. *Prog. Med. Chem.* 55, 45–147. doi: 10.1016/bs.pmch.2015.10.003

Blundell, C. D., Packer, M. J., and Almond, A. (2013). Quantification of free ligand conformational preferences by NMR and their relationship to the bioactive conformation. *Bioorg. Med. Chem.* 21, 4976–4987.doi: 10.1016/j.bmc.2013.06.056

Broughton, H. B. and Watson, I. A. (2004). Selection of heterocycles for drug design. *J. Mol. Graph Model.* 23, 51–58.doi: 10.1016/j.jmgm.2004.03.016

Bussi, G., Donadio, D., and Parrinello, M. (2007). Canonical sampling through velocity rescaling. *J. Chem. Phys.* 126:014101. doi: 10.1063/1.2408420

Butler, K. T., Luque, F. J., and Barril, X. (2009). Toward accurate relative energy predictions of the bioactive conformation of drugs. *J. Comput. Chem.* 30, 601–610. doi: 10.1002/jcc.21087

Caleman, C., van Maaren, P. J., Hong, M., Hub, J. S., Costa, L. T., and van der Spoel, D. (2012). Force field benchmark of organic liquids: Density, enthalpy of vaporization, heat capacities, surface tension, isothermal compressibility, volumetric expansion coefficient, and dielectric constant. *J. Chem. Theor. Comput.* 8, 61–74. doi: 10.1021/ct200731v

Cavalluzzi, M. M., Mangiatordi, G. F., Nicolotti, O., and Lentini, G. (2017). Ligand efficiency metrics in drug discovery: the pros and cons from a practical perspective. *Expert Opin. Drug Dis.* 12, 1087–1104. doi: 10.1080/17460441.2017

Csermely, P., Korcsmáros, T., Kiss, H. J., London, G., and Nussinov, R. (2012). Structure and dynamics of molecular networks: A novel paradigm of drug discovery. A comprehensive review. *Pharmacol. Ther.* 138, 333–408. doi: 10.1016/j.pharmthera.2013.01.016

Danishuddin and Khan, A. U. (2016). Descriptors and their selection methods in QSAR analysis: paradigm for drug design. *Drug Discov. Today* 21, 1291–1302. doi: 10.1016/j.drudis.2016.06.013

Daura, X., Mark, A. E., and Van Gunsteren, W. F. (1998). Parametrization of aliphatic CHn united atoms of GROMOS96 force field. *J. Comput. Chem.* 19, 535–547.

DeGoey, D. A., Chen, H. J., Cox, P. B., and Wendt, M. D. (2017). Beyond the rule of 5: lessons learned from AbbVie's drugs and compound collection. *J. Med. Chem.* 61, 2636–2651. doi: 10.1021/acs.jmedchem.7b00717

Dobbs, K. D. and Hehre, W. J. (1986). Molecular orbital theory of the properties of inorganic and organometallic compounds 4. Extended basis sets for third-and fourth-row, main-group elements. *J. Comput. Chem.* 7, 359–378.

Domagała, M., Lutyńska, A., and Palusiak, M. (2017). Halogen bond versus hydrogen bond: The many-body interactions approach. *Int. J. Quantum Chem.* 117:e25348. doi: 10.1002/qua.25348

Feenstra, K. A., Hess, B., and Berendsen, H. J. C. (1999). Improving efficiency of large time-scale molecular dynamics simulations of hydrogen rich systems. *J. Comput. Chem.* 20, 786–798.

Ferenczy, G. G. and Keseru, G. M. (2010). Thermodynamics guided lead discovery and optimization. *Drug Discov. Today* 15, 919–932. doi: 10.1016/j.drudis.2010.08.013

Fock, V. (1930). Näherungsmethode zur Lösung des quantenmechanischen Mehrkörperproblems. *Z. Phys.* 61, 126–148.

Ford, M. C. and Ho, P. S. (2016). Computational tools to model halogen bonds in medicinal chemistry. *J. Med. Chem.* 59, 1655–1670. doi: 10.1021/acs.jmedchem.5b00997

Freire, E. (2009). A thermodynamic approach to the affinity optimization of drug candidates. *Chem. Biol. Drug Des.* 74, 468–472. doi: 10.1111/j.1747-0285.2009.00880.x

Frisch, M. J., Trucks, G. W., Schlegel, H. B., Scuseria, G. E., Robb, M. A., Cheeseman, J. R., et al. (2016). *Gaussian 09, Revision A.02.* Wallingford, CT.

Ganesan, A., Coote, M. L., and Barakat, K. (2017). Molecular dynamics-driven drug discovery: leaping forward with confidence. *Drug Discov. Today* 22, 249–269. doi: 10.1016/j.drudis.2016.11.001

Gao, Q., Yang, L., and Zhu, Y. (2010). Pharmacophore based drug design approach as a practical process in drug discovery. *Curr. Comput. Aid Drug* 6, 37–49. doi: 10.2174/157340910790980151

Gleeson, M. P. (2008). Generation of a set of simple, interpretable ADMET rules of thumb. *J. Med. Chem.* 51, 817–834. doi: 10.1021/jm701122q

Gleeson, M. P., Hersey, A., Montanari, D., and Overington, J. (2011). Probing the links between *in vitro* potency, ADMET and physicochemical parameters. *Nat. Rev. Drug Discov.* 10, 197–208. doi: 10.1038/nrd3367

Gumbart, J. C., Roux, B., and Chipot, C. (2013). Standard binding free energies from computer simulations: what is the best strategy? *J. Chem. Theor. Comput.* 9, 794–802. doi: 10.1021/ct3008099

Halgren, T. A. (1996). Merck molecular force field. II. MMFF94 van der Waals and electrostatic parameters for intermolecular interactions. *J. Comput. Chem.* 17, 520–552.

Hanwell, M. D., Curtis, D. E., Lonie, D. C., Vandermeersch, T., Zurek, E., and Hutchison, G. R. (2012). Avogadro: an advanced semantic chemical editor, visualization, and analysis platform. *J. Cheminformatics* 4:17. doi: 10.1186/1758-2946-4-17

Hartree, D. R. and Hartree, W. (1935). Self-consistent field, with exchange, for beryllium. *Proc. R. Soc. A Math. Phys.* 150, 9–33.

Heinz, T. N., van Gunsteren, W. F., and Hünenberger, P. H. (2001). Comparison of four methods to compute the dielectric permittivity of liquids from molecular dynamics simulations. *J. Chem. Phys.* 115, 1125–1136. doi: 10.1063/1.1379764

Hess, B. (2008). P-LINCS: a parallel linear constraint solver for molecular simulation. *J. Chem. Theor. Comput.* 4, 116–122. doi: 10.1021/ct700200b

Hess, B., Bekker, H., Berendsen, H. J. C., and Fraaije, J. G. E. M. (1997). LINCS: a linear constraint solver for molecular simulations. *J. Comput. Chem.* 18, 1463–1472.

Hopkins, A. L., Keserü, G. M., Leeson, P. D., Rees, D. C., and Reynolds, C. H. (2014). The role of ligand efficiency metrics in drug discovery. *Nat. Rev. Drug Discov.* 13, 105–121. doi: 10.1038/nrd4163

Horta, B. A., Merz, P. T., Fuchs, P. F., Dolenc, J., Riniker, S., and Hünenberger, P. H. (2016). A GROMOS-compatible force field for small organic molecules in the condensed phase: the 2016H66 parameter set. *J. Chem. Theor. Comput.* 12, 3825–3850. doi: 10.1021/acs.jctc.6b00187

Horta, B. A., Fuchs, P. F., van Gunsteren, W. F., and Hünenberger, P. H. (2011). New interaction parameters for oxygen compounds in the GROMOS force field: Improved pure-liquid and solvation properties for alcohols, ethers,

aldehydes, ketones, carboxylic acids, and esters. *J. Chem. Theor. Comput.* 7, 1016–1031. doi: 10.1021/ct1006407

Jordan, A. M. and Roughley, S. D. (2009). Drug discovery chemistry: a primer for the non-specialist. *Drug Discov Today* 14, 731–744. doi: 10.1016/j.drudis.2009.04.005

Jorgensen, W. L., Maxwell, D. S., and Tirado-Rives, J. (1996). Development and testing of the OPLS all-atom force field on conformational energetics and properties of organic liquids. *J. Am. Chem. Soc.* 118, 11225–11236.

Kaur, D. and Khanna, S. (2011). Intermolecular hydrogen bonding interactions of furan, isoxazole and oxazole with water. *Comput. Theor. Chem.* 963, 71–75. doi: 10.1016/j.comptc.2010.09.011

Keserü, G. M. and Makara, G. M. (2009). The influence of lead discovery strategies on the properties of drug candidates. *Nat. Rev. Drug Discov.* 8, 203–212. doi: 10.1038/nrd2796

Kunz, A. P., and van Gunsteren, W. F. (2009). Development of a nonlinear classical polarization model for liquid water and aqueous solutions: COS/D. *J. Phys. Chem. A* 113, 11570–11579. doi: 10.1021/jp903164s

Lee, C. H., Huang, H. C., and Juan, H. F. (2011). Reviewing ligand-based rational drug design: the search for an ATP synthase inhibitor. *Int. J. Mol. Sci.* 12, 5304–5318. doi: 10.3390/ijms12085304

Leeson, P. D. and Springthorpe, B. (2007). The influence of drug-like concepts on decision-making in medicinal chemistry. *Nat. Rev. Drug Discov.* 6, 881–890. doi: 10.1038/nrd2445

Li, S., Smith, D. G., and Patkowski, K. (2015). An accurate benchmark description of the interactions between carbon dioxide and polyheterocyclic aromatic compounds containing nitrogen. *Phys. Chem. Chem. Phys.* 17, 16560–16574. doi: 10.1039/c5cp02365c

Limongelli, V., Bonomi, M., and Parrinello, M. (2013). Funnel metadynamics as accurate binding free-energy method. *Proc. Natl. Acad. Sci. U.S.A.* 110, 6358–6363. doi: 10.1073/pnas.1303186110

Lin, F. Y. and Mackerell, A. D. (2017). Do halogen-hydrogen bond donor interactions dominate the favorable contribution of halogens to ligand-protein binding? *J. Phys. Chem. B* 121, 6813–6821. doi: 10.1021/acs.jpcb.7b04198

Lionta, E., Spyrou, G., Vassilatis, D. K., and Cournia, Z. (2014). Structure-based virtual screening for drug discovery: principles, applications and recent advances. *Curr. Top. Med. Chem.* 14, 1923–1938. doi: 10.2174/1568026614666140929124445

Lounnas, V., Ritschel, T., Kelder, J., McGuire, R., Bywater, R. P., and Foloppe, N. (2013). Current progress in structure-based rational drug design marks a new mindset in drug discovery. *Comput. Struct. Biotechnol. J.* 5:e201302011. doi: 10.5936/csbj.201302011

Matczak, P. and Wojtulewski, S. (2015). Performance of Møller-Plesset second-order perturbation theory and density functional theory in predicting the interaction between stannylenes and aromatic molecules. *J. Mol. Model.* 21, 41. doi: 10.1007/s00894-015-2589-1

Mennucci, B. and Tomasi, J. (1997). Continuum solvation models: a new approach to the problem of solute's charge distribution and cavity boundaries. *J. Chem. Phys.* 106, 5151–5158.

Møller, C. and Plesset, M. S. (1934). Note on an approximation treatment for many-electron systems. *Phys. Rev.* 46, 618–622.

Mondal, J., Friesner, R. A., and Berne, B. J. (2014). Role of desolvation in thermodynamics and kinetics of ligand binding to a kinase. *J. Chem. Theor. Comput.* 10, 5696–5705. doi: 10.1021/ct500584n

Morgan, S., Grootendorst, P., Lexchin, J., Cunningham, C., and Greyson, D. (2011). The cost of drug development: a systematic review. *Health Policy* 100, 4–17. doi: 10.1016/j.healthpol.2010.12.002

Nosé, S. (1984). A molecular dynamics method for simulations in the canonical ensemble. *Mol. Phys.* 52, 255–268.

Oostenbrink, C., Villa, A., Mark, A. E., and van Gunsteren, W. F. (2004). A biomolecular force field based on the free enthalpy of hydration and solvation: the GROMOS force-field parameter sets 53A5 and 53A6. *J. Comput. Chem.* 25, 1656–1676. doi: 10.1002/jcc.20090

Parrinello, M. and Rahman, A. (1981). Polymorphic transitions in single crystals: a new molecular dynamics method. *J. Appl. Phys.* 52, 7182–7190.

Parthasarath, R., Subramanian, V., and Sathyamurthy, N. (2005). Hydrogen bonding in phenol, water, and phenol-water clusters. *J. Phys. Chem. A* 109, 843–850. doi: 10.1021/jp046499r

Paul, S. M., Mytelka, D. S., Dunwiddie, C. T., Persinger, C. C., Munos, B. H., Lindborg, S. R., et al. (2010). How to improve R&D productivity: the pharmaceutical industry's grand challenge. *Nat. Rev. Drug Discov.* 9, 203. doi: 10.1038/nrd3078

Petersson, G. A., Bennett, A., Tensfeldt, T. G., Al-Laham, M. A., Shirley, W. A., and Mantzaris, J. (1988). A complete basis set model chemistry. I. The total energies of closed-shell atoms and hydrides of the first-row elements. *J. Chem. Phys.* 89, 2193–2218.

Rendine, S., Pieraccini, S., Forni, A., and Sironi, M. (2011). Halogen bonding in ligand—receptor systems in the framework of classical force fields. *Phys. Chem. Chem. Phys.* 13:19508. doi: 10.1039/c1cp22436k

Reynolds, C. H. and Holloway, M. K. (2011). Thermodynamics of ligand binding and efficiency. *ACS Med. Chem. Lett.* 2, 433–437. doi: 10.1021/ml2 00010k

Roughley, S. D. and Jordan, A. M. (2011). The medicinal chemist's toolbox: an analysis of reactions used in the pursuit of drug candidates. *J. Med. Chem.* 54, 3451–3479. doi: 10.1021/jm200187y

Rusu, V. H., Baron, R., and Lins, R. D. (2014). PITOMBA: Parameter Interface for Oligosaccharide Molecules Based on Atoms. *J. Chem. Theor. Comput.* 10, 5068–5080. doi: 10.1021/ct500455u

Schuler, L. D., Daura, X., and van Gunsteren, W. F. (2001). An improved FROMOS96 force field for aliphatic hydrocarbons in the condensed phase. *J. Comput. Chem.* 22, 1205–1218. doi: 10.1002/jcc.1078

Shahlaei, M. (2013). Descriptor selection methods in quantitative structure-activity relationship studies: a review study. *Chem. Rev.* 113, 8093–8103. doi: 10.1021/cr3004339

Shirts, M. R. and Pande, V. S. (2005). Comparison of efficiency and bias of free energies computed by exponential averaging, the Bennett acceptance ratio, and thermodynamic integration. *J. Chem. Phys.* 122:144107. doi: 10.1063/1.18 73592

Sliwoski, G., Kothiwale, S., Meiler, J., and Lowe, E. W. (2013). Computational methods in drug discovery. *Pharmacol. Rev.* 66, 334–395. doi: 10.1124/pr.112.007336

Taylor, R. D., MacCoss, M., and Lawson, A. D. (2017). Combining molecular scaffolds from FDA approved drugs: application to drug discovery. *J. Med. Chem.* 60, 1638–1647. doi: 10.1021/acs.jmedchem.6b01367

Taylor, R. D., MacCoss, M., and Lawson, A. D. (2014). Rings in drugs. *J. Med. Chem.* 57, 5845–5859. doi: 10.1021/jm4017625

Tironi, I. G., Sperb, R., Smith, P. E., and van Gunsteren, W. F. (1995). A generalized reaction field method for molecular dynamics simulations. *J. Chem. Phys.* 102, 5451–5459.

Van Gunsteren, W. F. and Berendsen, H. J. C. (1988). A leap-frog algorithm for stochastic dynamics. *Mol. Simulat.* 1, 173–185.

Wang, J., Wolf, R. M., Caldwell, J. W., Kollman, P. A., and Case, D. A. (2004). Development and testing of a general Amber force field. *J. Comput. Chem.* 25, 1157–1174. doi: 10.1002/jcc.20035

Waring, M. J. (2009). Defining optimum lipophilicity and molecular weight ranges for drug candidates-Molecular weight dependent lower log D limits based on permeability. *Bioorg. Med. Chem. Lett.* 19, 2844–2851. doi: 10.1016/j.bmcl.2009.03.109

Waring, M. J. (2010). Lipophilicity in drug discovery. *Expert Opin. Drug Dis.* 5, 235–248. doi: 10.1517/17460441003605098

Welsch, M. E., Snyder, S. A., and Stockwell, B. R. (2010). Privileged scaffolds for library design and drug discovery. *Curr. Opin. Chem. Biol.* 14, 347–361. doi: 10.1016/j.cbpa.2010.02.018

Woo, H. J. and Roux, B. (2005). Calculation of absolute protein-ligand binding free energy from computer simulations. *Proc. Natl. Acad. Sci. U.S.A.* 102, 6825–6830. doi: 10.1073/pnas.0409005102

Zhao, H. and Caflisch, A. (2015). Molecular dynamics in drug design. *Eur. J. Med. Chem.* 91, 4–14. doi: 10.1002/ijch.201400009

Zwanzig, R. W. (1954). High-temperature equation of state by a perturbation method. I. nonpolar gases. *J. Chem. Phys.* 22, 1420–1426.

Identification of a Novel Protein Arginine Methyltransferase 5 Inhibitor in Non-small Cell Lung Cancer by Structure-Based Virtual Screening

Qianqian Wang[1†], Jiahui Xu[1†], Ying Li[1], Jumin Huang[1], Zebo Jiang[1], Yuwei Wang[1], Liang Liu[1*], Elaine Lai Han Leung[1,2,3*] and Xiaojun Yao[1,4*]

[1] State Key Laboratory of Quality Research in Chinese Medicine, Macau Institute for Applied Research in Medicine and Health, Macau University of Science and Technology, Taipa, Macau, [2] State Key Laboratory of Respiratory Diseases, Guangzhou Institute of Respiratory Disease, The First Affiliated Hospital of Guangzhou Medical College, Guangzhou, China, [3] Department of Respiratory Medicine, Taihe Hospital, Hubei University of Medicine, Hubei, China, [4] State Key Laboratory of Applied Organic Chemistry, Department of Chemistry, Lanzhou University, Lanzhou, China

*Correspondence:
Liang Liu
lliu@must.edu.mo
Elaine Lai Han Leung
lhleung@must.edu.mo
Xiaojun Yao
xjyao@must.edu.mo

[†] These authors have contributed equally to this work.

Protein arginine methyltransferase 5 (PRMT5) is able to regulate gene transcription by catalyzing the symmetrical dimethylation of arginine residue of histone, which plays a key role in tumorigenesis. Many efforts have been taken in discovering small-molecular inhibitors against PRMT5, but very few were reported and most of them were SAM-competitive. EPZ015666 is a recently reported PRMT5 inhibitor with a new binding site, which is different from S-adenosylmethionine (SAM)-binding pocket. This new binding site provides a new clue for the design and discovery of potent and specific PRMT5 inhibitors. In this study, the structure-based virtual screening targeting this site was firstly performed to identify potential PRMT5 inhibitors. Then, the bioactivity of the candidate compound was studied. MTT results showed that compound T1551 decreased cell viability of A549 and H460 non-small cell lung cancer cell lines. By inhibiting the methyltransferase activity of PRMT5, T1551 reduced the global level of H4R3 symmetric dimethylation (H4R3me2s). T1551 also downregulated the expression of oncogene FGFR3 and eIF4E, and disturbed the activation of related PI3K/AKT/mTOR and ERK signaling in A549 cell. Finally, we investigated the conformational spaces and identified collective motions important for description of T1551/PRMT5 complex by using molecular dynamics simulation and normal mode analysis methods. This study provides a novel non-SAM-competitive hit compound for developing small molecules targeting PRMT5 in non-small cell lung cancer.

Keywords: protein arginine methyltransferase 5, non-small cell lung cancer, T1551, virtual screening, molecular dynamics simulation

INTRODUCTION

Protein arginine methyltransferases (PRMTs) are a class of enzymes that transfer a methyl group from the cofactor S-adenosylmethionine (SAM) to arginine omega nitrogen of substrate protein. Based on product specificity, PRMTs can be divided into three subclasses: type I, II, and III, which asymmetrically dimethylate, symmetrically dimethylate, and monomethylate their substrates, respectively (Bedford and Clarke, 2009). Protein arginine methyltransferase 5 (PRMT5), as a type II PRMT, is responsible for catalyzing the symmetrical dimethylation of arginine residue of substrate proteins, which has been implicated in diverse cellular and biological processes including transcriptional regulation, RNA metabolism and ribosome biogenesis (Liu et al., 2011; Shilo et al., 2013; Wei et al., 2013; Yang and Bedford, 2013; Deuker and McMahon, 2014; Stopa et al., 2015). An increasing number of studies emphasized that PRMT5 was upregulated in lymphomas, breast cancer, lung cancer, colorectal cancer, and glioblastoma (Ibrahim et al., 2014; Yan et al., 2014; Li et al., 2015; Sheng and Wang, 2016). For instance, Ibrahim et al. (2014) demonstrated that a high cytoplasmic expression of PRMT5 was closely related to high-grade subtypes of primary lung adenocarcinomas and a poor prognosis. Sheng and Wang (2016) pointed out that PRMT5 could regulate multiple signaling pathways to promote lung cancer cell proliferation. All of these suggest that PRMT5 is a promising therapeutic target in lung cancer. However, although many efforts have been made in discovering PRMT5 inhibitors, very few were reported (Alinari et al., 2015; Smil et al., 2015; Mao et al., 2017), and they either occupied SAM-binding site or mimicked SAM. Recently, EPZ015666 has been shown to exhibit remarkably antitumor activity by inhibiting PRMT5, and the pre-clinical studies have also showed that both cell lines and xenograft models of mantle cell lymphoma were sensitive to EPZ015666 (Chan-Penebre et al., 2015). Importantly, the resolved PRMT5-SAM-EPZ015666 crystal complex shows that EPZ015666 does not compete with SAM, but locates in a new pocket (different from SAM-binding site) of PRMT5. This binding site in PRMT5 provides us a new way to discovery and development of more potent and specific PRMT5 inhibitors.

Structure-based virtual screening using molecular docking has become a powerful tool in the drug discovery for rapidly enriching hits from large pools of compound databases. Nowadays, it has been successfully applied to discover novel inhibitors of epigenetic targets, such as SET7, KDM4B, and SIRT2 (Chu et al., 2014; Meng et al., 2015; Huang et al., 2017). The successful use of structure-based virtual screening in the above mentioned epigenetic targets inspires us to identify the novel inhibitor against the non-SAM-binding site of PRMT5. The activity of the identified inhibitors will be further studied on their effects of the biological functions of cancer cells, histone substrate methylation, target gene expression and related signaling pathway. Here, 158 candidate compounds were firstly obtained by the structure-based virtual screening method. MTT assay results showed that among them T1551 had strongest cytotoxicity on A549 non-small cell lung cancer cell line. In addition to inhibiting PRMT5 methyltransferase activity, a series of functional assays showed that T1551 reduced symmetric dimethylation level of H4R3, downregulated the protein expressions of two target genes of PRMT5, FGFR3, and eIF4E, and inhibited the activation of PI3K/AKT/mTOR and ERK signaling. Finally, molecular dynamics simulations and normal mode analysis were performed to study the detailed binding mode and conformational space of T1551/PRMT5 complex. The identification of this novel

PRMT5 inhibitor T1551 and its inhibitory mechanism study will be helpful for the development of PRMT5-targeting cancer treatment.

MATERIALS AND METHODS

Molecular Docking-Based Virtual Screening

Molecular docking-based virtual screening was carried out with Schrödinger software package (Schrödinger, LLC, New York, NY, United States; Schrödinger, 2015). The crystal structure of PRMT5 complexed with cofactor SAM and inhibitor EPZ015666 was derived from Protein Data Bank (PDB ID: 4X61). The protein was first prepared in Protein Preparation Wizard module, including adding hydrogens, refining loop region and minimization. Grid box was generated on the size and center of EPZ015666. Previously, SAM was proved to form crucial cation–π interactions with EPZ015666 and contribute to the binding affinity of PRMT5 inhibitors (Chan-Penebre et al., 2015). Here, to test the role of SAM in docking, enrichment factors (EFs) of virtual screening for PRMT5-EPZ015666 with and without SAM were calculated and compared. Firstly, 16 active derivatives of EPZ015666 were collected from the published paper (Duncan et al., 2015). Eight hundred decoys were then generated at a ratio of 1:50 with DUD-E (Mysinger et al., 2012). All the actives and decoys were docked into EPZ015666 binding site of PRMT5 with and without SAM, respectively. Finally, the 1 and 10% EFs for PRMT5-EPZ015666 and PRMT5-EPZ015666-SAM models were calculated, respectively. For the ligands, prior to virtual screening, a total of 1,671,908 compounds from Chemdiv, Specs and TargetMol databases were filtered by pan-assay interference structures (PAINS) (Baell and Holloway, 2010) and "Lipinski's rule of five" to remove those with false positivity, function group and poor absorption/permeability. Then, the obtained compounds were prepared with Ligand Preparation module. Three-level (HTVS, SP, and XP) molecular docking-based virtual screening was successively performed using Glide module. The top 10% (1,706) compounds ranked by glide score were clustered into 200 groups. By visually inspecting the binding poses of PRMT5-inhibitor, 158 compounds were selected for experimental validation. All compounds were purchased from Topscience company (Shanghai, China).

Cell Culture and Cytotoxicity Assay

A549 and H460 cells (two non-small cell lung cancer cell lines) were purchased from ATCC, cultivated in RPMI 1640 medium supplemented with 10% FBS (Gibco Products, Big Cabin, OK, United States), 1% penicillin-streptomycin solution, and maintained at 37°C in a CO_2 incubator with 5% CO_2. One hundred and fifty-eight compounds from virtual screening were dissolved in DMSO and stored at −40°C. To rapidly identify the compounds with strong inhibitory activity, 20 μM concentration for each compound was firstly used to treat A549 cell line for 72 h. During the MTT assay test, cells were firstly seeded on a 96-well microplate with 3,000 cells/well, cultured overnight for cell adhesion, and treated with DMSO (10.0 μM) or various concentrations (2.5, 5.0, and 10.0 μM) of the studied compound for 24, 48, and 72 h. Then, each well was added 10 μL MTT (5 mg/mL) and incubated for 4 h at 3°C, followed by adding 100 μL acidic isopropanol (10% SDS and 0.01 mol/L HCl). Finally, the absorbance at 570 nm was measured by a Microplate Reader (Tecan US, Inc., Morrisville, NC, United States). Cell viability was calculated relative to untreated controls, and the results were based on at least three independent experiments.

In Vitro Enzymatic Assays

PRMT5 enzymatic assay was carried out by Shanghai ChemPartner Company (998 Halei Road, Pudong New Area, Shanghai, 201203, China), as did previously by Ji et al. (2017). To obtain the specific IC_{50} value, T1551 was diluted into 10 concentrations. PRMT5 protein was purchased from BPS bioscience (Cat. No. 51045), and SAM/SAH were purchased from Sigma. Inc. (Cat. No. A7007-100MG and No. A9384-25MG). T1551 was prepared as 10 mM stock in DMSO and diluted to the final concentration in DMSO. PRMT5 and substrates were incubated with indicated concentrations of T1551 in a 384-well plate for 60 min at room temperature. Then, acceptor and donor solutions were added to label the residual substrates of PRMT5. The labeling process was lasting for 60 min at room temperature, followed by reading endpoint with EnSpire with Alpha mode. In the *in vitro* enzymatic assays, 1% DMSO was used as vehicle control for normalization.

Western Blot Analysis

Cells were washed twice with cold PBS, and lysed in RIPA lysis buffer containing protease and phosphatase inhibitors to extract total protein. Cell lysates were centrifuged for 5 min (12,000 g, 4°C), and the supernatant was collected. Protein concentrations were determined by Bio-Rad protein Assay kit (Bio-Rad, Philadelphia, PA, United States). Equal amounts of protein (50 μg) were separated on a 10% SDS–PAGE gel, and transferred to a nitrocellulose (NC) membrane at 300 mA and 4°C for 1 h. The membrane was incubated with primary antibody (1:1000), and then with a fluorescence-conjugated secondary antibody (1:10000). The primary antibody against PRMT5 was purchased from Merck Millipore Ltd., (Germany); antibodies against H4R3me2s and H4 were purchased from Abcam (Cambridge, MA, United States); antibodies against FGFR3 and eIF4E were purchased from Santa Cruz Biotechnology (Dallas, TX, United States); antibodies against total/phospho-AKT, total/phospho-ERK and total/phospho-mTOR were purchased from Cell Signaling Technology (Danvers, MA, United States). GAPDH was used as the loading control and for normalization. The signal intensity of the membranes was detected with a LI-COR Odyssey Scanner (Belfast, ME, United States).

Molecular Dynamics Simulation

To reveal the interaction features of T1551 and PRMT5, molecular dynamics (MD) simulations were used for sampling the conformational spaces of PRMT5-T1551 complex. Normal mode analysis was used for identifying important collective motions for the complex. All MD simulations were performed with Amber 16 software (Case et al., 2017). The Amber ff14SB force field (Maier et al., 2015) was used for PRMT5, and general amber force field (Wang et al., 2004) was utilized to parameterize inhibitors with their charges assigned by restrained electrostatic potential partial charges. TIP3P water was used to solvate the complex systems, with the solute 12 Å away from water box boundary. Chloride ions were added to neutralize the system. Then, 150 mM NaCl was added to mimic the physiological conditions. After minimization, heating and equilibration, 100 ns production run was carried out without any restraints in NPT ensemble. System temperature and pressure were regulated with Langevin thermostat and Berendsen barostat, respectively. All the bonds involving hydrogen were constrained by SHAKE algorithm allowing an integration time step of 2 fs. Particle mesh Ewald method (Linse and Linse, 2014) was used to calculate long-range electrostatic interactions. The binding free energy of inhibitors and PRMT5 was calculated by molecular mechanics generalized-born surface area (MM-GBSA) method (Hou et al., 2010; Platania et al., 2015; Wang et al., 2017). A single trajectory and three time-frames protocols were adopted here. Specifically, a total of 500 snapshots were extracted from the last 10, 20, and 40 ns trajectory, respectively. The normal mode analysis was performed to identify the collection motions of PRMT5-inhibitor complex during MD simulation, by using cpptraj in Amber 16 and Normal Mode Wizard plugin in VMD 1.9.

Statistical Analysis

Descriptive analytical data were presented as mean ± SEM. Multiple comparisons were evaluated by one-way analysis of variance (ANOVA) using Graph Prim 5.0. $P < 0.05$ was considered statistically significant.

RESULTS

The Selection of Candidate Compounds by Virtual Screening

In this study, we aim to find the non-SAM mimics, so EPZ015666-binding site, not SAM-binding site, was targeted in our virtual screening. Enrichment factor calculations showed that the 1 and 10% EFs for PRMT5-EPZ015666-SAM model were 44.6 and 8.7, higher than that (38.3 and 6.8) for PRMT5-EPZ015666 model. The area under receiver operating characteristic curve (AUC) for the former (0.96) was also higher than that for the latter (0.92). Both of two parameters suggested that SAM was helpful for enriching active compounds in the compound library. Therefore, SAM was remained as a part of the receptor in the screening.

By three-level (HTVS, SP, and XP) screenings, the top-1706 compounds ranked by glide score were remained and then clustered into 200 groups using *k*-means clustering protocol integrated in Canvas 2.4. When selecting the candidate compounds, the following criteria was considered: (1) choosing one compound at most in a group to retain structural diversity; (2) occupying the binding pocket with molecular

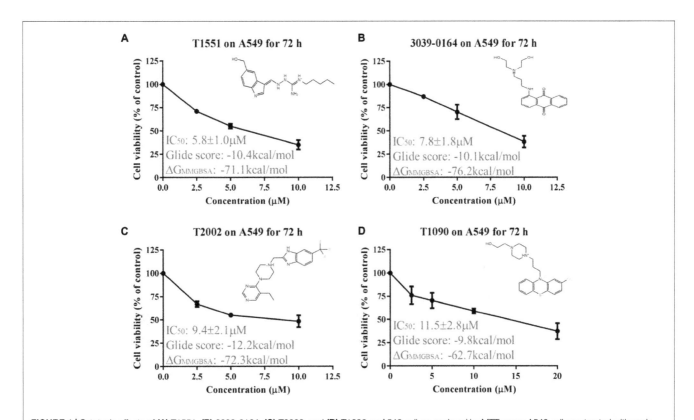

FIGURE 1 | Cytotoxic effects of **(A)** T1551, **(B)** 3039-0164, **(C)** T2002, and **(D)** T1090 on A549 cell, as analyzed by MTT assay. A549 cell was treated with each inhibitor for 72 h, respectively. Results were presented as mean ± SEM (n = 4). Glide score represented the docking score of inhibitor and PRMT5, and ΔG_{MMGBSA} represented the post-docking rescore of inhibitor and PRMT5.

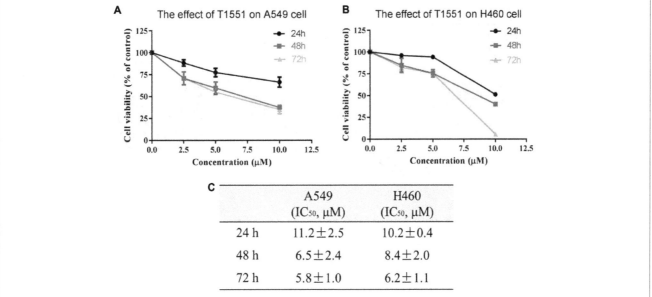

	A549 (IC_{50}, µM)	H460 (IC_{50}, µM)
24 h	11.2±2.5	10.2±0.4
48 h	6.5±2.4	8.4±2.0
72 h	5.8±1.0	6.2±1.1

FIGURE 2 | Cytotoxic effects of T1551 on **(A)** A549 and **(B)** H460 cells by MTT assay. **(C)** IC_{50} values of T1551 on A549 and H460 cell lines. Cells were treated with each inhibitor for 24, 48, and 72 h, respectively. Data was presented as mean ± SEM (n = 4).

size neither too big nor too small; (3) choosing the one with smaller molecular weight or/and lower MM/GBSA score if compounds are similar; (4) forming the reported interactions with the key residues of PRMT5 (Chan-Penebre et al., 2015). For instance, Phe327 forms π–π interactions with THIQ ring of EPZ015666; THIQ forms cation–π interactions

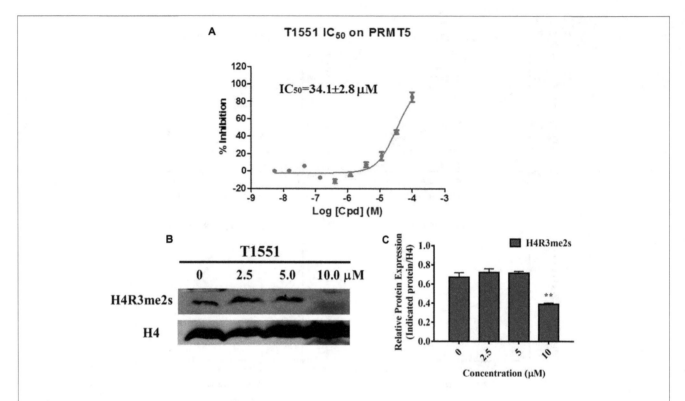

FIGURE 3 | (A) Inhibition of T1551 on PRMT5 methyltransferase activity. **(B)** Protein expression levels of H4R3me2s in A549 cell treated with T1551 at different concentrations (0, 2.5, 5.0, and 10.0 μM). **(C)** Densitometric analysis of band intensities of H4R3me2s. Western blot analysis was performed for 24 h, with at least three independent experiments. Data was presented as mean ± SEM ($n = 3$), with $**p < 0.01$ for comparison between control group (DMSO-treated group) and T1551-treated group.

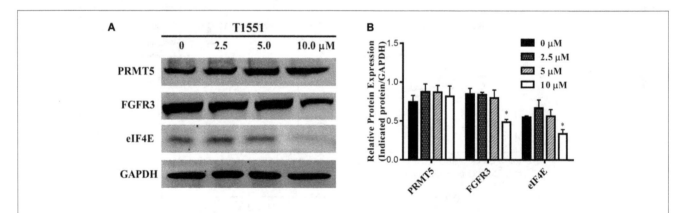

FIGURE 4 | (A) Protein expression levels of oncogene FGFR3 and eIF4E in A549 cell treated with T1551 at different concentrations (0, 2.5, 5.0, and 10.0 μM). **(B)** Densitometric analysis of band intensities of PRMT5, FGFR3, and eIF4E proteins. Western blot analysis was performed for 24 h, with at least three independent experiments. Data was presented as mean ± SEM ($n = 3$), with $*p < 0.05$ for comparison between control group (DMSO-treated group) and T1551-treated group.

with methyl group of SAM; EPZ015666 interacts with the backbone -NH of Phe580 and side chains of Glu444. Based on these, 158 candidates were selected and purchased at last.

T1551 Decreases Cell Viability of A549 Cell

The obtained 158 candidate compounds were then tested for MTT assay to determine their inhibitory activity. Many

recent studies have showed that PRMT5 is upregulated in A549 non-small cell lung cancer cell line (Gu et al., 2012; Wei et al., 2012; Lim et al., 2014). A549 cell line was thus used here. To rapidly identify the compounds with the strong inhibitory activity, 20 μM concentration for each compound was firstly used to treat A549 cell for 72 h. The result showed that among 158 compounds there were four compounds exhibiting the >50% inhibitory percentage on A549 cell at 20 μM. Since T1551 had the strongest inhibitory activity (72 h, 50% inhibition concentration IC_{50} = 5.8 ± 1.0 μM) (**Figure 1**) and was chosen as the hit, a range of T1551 concentrations (0, 2.5, 5.0, and 10.0 μM) for 24, 48, and 72 h were then used to treat A549 to calculate its IC_{50} values. As shown in **Figure 2**, T1551 exhibited significant anti-proliferation on A549 cell at 24 h in a concentration-dependent manner, with the IC_{50} value of 11.2 ± 2.5 μM. The cytotoxic effects of T1551 were also verified using H460 cell, another NSCLC cell line with PRMT5 overexpression (**Figures 2B,C**).

T1551 Inhibits PRMT5 Methyltransferase Activity and Decreases Symmetric Dimethylation Level of Histone 4

AlphaLISA assay was carried out to investigate the influence of T1551 on enzymatic activity of PRMT5. As shown in **Figure 3A**, T1551 inhibited PRMT5 enzyme activity in a dose-dependent manner. The corresponding IC_{50} value was 34.1 ± 2.8 μM, suggesting that T1551 directly inhibited the methyltransferase function of PRMT5. PRMT5-driven methylation of arginine residues can lead to symmetric dimethylation of arginine residue 3 of histone 4 (H4R3me2s), which in turn alters chromatin structure to promote transcriptional repression (Branscombe et al., 2001; Zhao et al., 2009; Chen et al., 2017). To investigate the effect of T1551 on PRMT5 catalytic substrate, we measured the expression level of H4R3me2s protein with and without T1551 in A549 cell. The total H4 was used as loading control. From **Figures 3B,C**, we observed that after the treatment with T1551 for 24 h, the global level of H4R3me2s was notably decreased. Therefore, from the perspective of histone substrate, T1551 indeed inhibited the catalytic ability of PRMT5 methyltransferase.

T1551 Downregulates the Expression of PRMT5 Target Genes

PRMT5 exerts its function by regulating the expression of target genes, such as oncogene FGFR3 and eIF4E (Zhang et al., 2015). FGFR3 and eIF4E were previously reported to frequently overexpress in lung cancer, myeloma, and ovarian cancers (van Rhijn et al., 2001; De Benedetti and Graff, 2004; Culjkovic-Kraljacic et al., 2012), thus playing an important role in tumor occurrence and development. Especially, according to several studies (Desai and Adjei, 2016; Babina and Turner, 2017) recently published, FGFR signaling has been considered as a promising target for lung cancer therapy. As can be seen from **Figure 4**, FGFR3 and eIF4E expressions were significantly decreased in A549 cell treated with 10.0 μM T1551. This reflects that T1551 may reduce FGFR3 and eIF4E expression by inhibiting PRMT5.

T1551 Suppresses the Activation of AKT, ERK, and mTOR

As mentioned above, FGFR3 signaling is an important target for lung cancer treatment. In this FGFR3 pathway, PRMT5 participates in regulating FGFR3 downstream targets such as AKT, ERK, and mTOR (Wei et al., 2012). From the previous study, silencing PRMT5 could reduce FGFR3 expression, leading to the repression of AKT and ERK and subsequent inhibition of mTOR through AKT/mTOR or ERK pathway (Zhang et al., 2015).

To gain further insight into the molecular mechanism underlying PRMT5-dependent regulation of FGFR3, we examined whether T1551 could regulate the activation of AKT, ERK, and mTOR through inhibiting PRMT5. From **Figures 5A,B**, we observed that the protein levels of

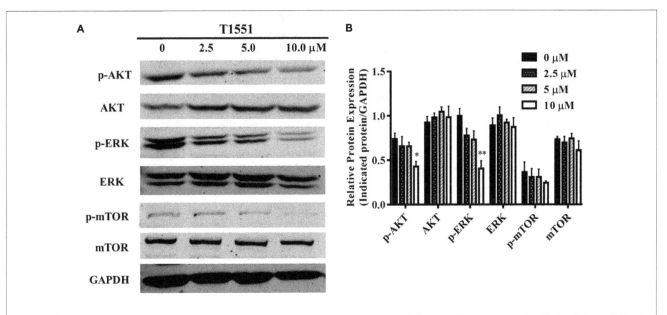

FIGURE 5 | (A) Protein expression levels of p/T-AKT, p/T-ERK, and p/T-mTOR in A549 cell treated with T1551 at different concentrations (0, 2.5, 5.0, and 10.0 μM). **(B)** Densitometric analysis of band intensities of p/T-AKT, p/T-ERK, and p/T-mTOR. Western blot analysis was performed for 24 h, with at least three independent experiments. Data was presented as mean ± SEM (n = 3), with $*p < 0.05$ and $**p < 0.01$ for comparison between control group (DMSO-treated group) and T1551-treated group.

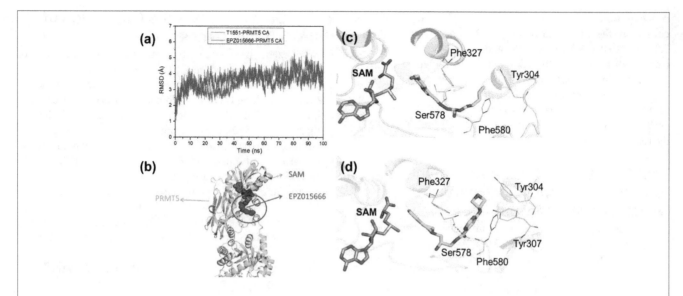

FIGURE 6 | (a) Time series of RMSDs of protein CA atoms during the 100 ns simulation in PRMT5-SAM-T1551 and PRMT5-SAM-EPZ015666 systems. **(b)** Crystal structure of PRMT5-SAM-EPZ015666 (PDBID: 4X61). The binding modes of PRMT5 with **(c)** T1551 and **(d)** EPZ015666. Both two complex structures were extracted from the last equilibrated 20 ns trajectory by clustering analysis.

phosphorylated AKT and ERK were significantly reduced, especially at the 10 μM T1551 concentration, implying that T1551 suppressed the activation of PI3K/AKT/mTOR and ERK signaling mediated by PRMT5.

Inhibition Mechanism of T1551 Inhibitor for PRMT5 Protein

To investigate the detailed binding modes of PRMT5-inhibitors and compare the interaction features of T1551 and EPZ015666 with PRMT5, a single 100 ns MD simulations for PRMT5-SAM-T1551 and PRMT5-SAM-EPZ015666 systems were performed, respectively. Based on the obtained trajectory, with respect to the initial structure, the root-mean-square deviations (RMSDs) of protein CA atoms in PRMT5-SAM-T1551 and PRMT5-SAM-EPZ015666 systems were monitored to assess the overall stability of simulations. From **Figure 6a**, RMSDs of each system almost remained stable from 60 ns, indicating the convergence

of the simulated trajectory. By calculating the binding free energies of PRMT5 with T1551 and EPZ015666, we can identify the energy origin of inhibitors binding to PRMT5. Here, considering the large size of PRMT5 and inhibitor complex (more than 600 residues, **Figure 6b**), entropic contribution was neglected. The predicted ΔG_{GB} for PRMT5-T1551 was higher than that of PRMT5-EPZ015666 (e.g., -32.11 ± 0.14 vs. -40.09 ± 0.18 kcal/mol in last 10 ns) in three replicas, exhibiting a consistent ranking with experimental results (**Table 1**; Chan-Penebre et al., 2015). Among the individual energy parts, van der Waals interaction (ΔE_{vdw}) predominated the total energy in two systems, while non-polar solvation part ($\Delta G_{sol\_np\_GB}$) contributed marginally to inhibitor binding. Therefore, the energetic origin of T1551/EPZ015666 inhibiting PRMT5 is mainly derived from ΔE_{vdw}.

Clustering analysis was used to extract representative structures in simulations. Comparing the binding modes of T1551 and EPZ015666 with PRMT5 (**Figures 6c,d**), we could see

TABLE 1 | The calculated binding free energy and its components (kcal/mol) of PRMT5 with T1551 and EPZ015666 complexes based on the last 10, 20, and 40 ns MD trajectory.

	ΔE_{vdw}	ΔE_{ele}	$\Delta G_{sol\_np\_GB}$	$\Delta G_{sol\_polar\_GB}$	ΔG_{GB}
PRMT5-T1551					
Last 10 ns	-40.98 ± 0.13	-29.73 ± 0.18	-5.49 ± 0.01	44.08 ± 0.13	-32.11 ± 0.14
Last 20 ns	-41.69 ± 0.12	-29.89 ± 0.16	-5.57 ± 0.01	44.64 ± 0.12	-32.50 ± 0.14
Last 40 ns	-41.80 ± 0.12	-30.89 ± 0.19	-5.65 ± 0.01	45.32 ± 0.11	-33.02 ± 0.15
PRMT5-EPZ015666					
Last 10 ns	-49.72 ± 0.15	-43.09 ± 0.50	-6.96 ± 0.01	59.67 ± 0.39	-40.09 ± 0.18
Last 20 ns	-48.98 ± 0.15	-43.72 ± 0.48	-6.94 ± 0.01	58.51 ± 0.38	-41.13 ± 0.17
Last 40 ns	-49.66 ± 0.17	-49.51 ± 0.59	-7.12 ± 0.01	64.17 ± 0.46	-42.12 ± 0.19

ΔG was estimated from gas-phase energy and solvation free energy. The former contains an electrostatic term (ΔE_{ele}) and a van der Waals term (ΔE_{vdw}). The latter is decomposed into polar (ΔG_{sol_polar}) and non-polar solvation energy (ΔG_{sol_np}).

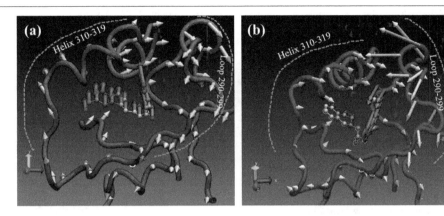

FIGURE 7 | Comparison of effects of **(a)** T1551 and **(b)** EPZ015666 on the collective motion of PRMT5 in the simulation. The mode was obtained by normal mode analysis with Amber16 software and VMD NMWiz plugin. Only the normal modes of T1551 binding domain (10 Å around T1551) were shown here for clarity.

that both inhibitors located in a hydrophobic pocket composed of Tyr304, Phe327, Ser578, and Phe580 when interacting with PRMT5. For EPZ015666, **Figure 6d** showed that its THIQ group formed strong cation–π interactions with partial positively charged methyl group of SAM. Actually, this feature has been reported as a key factor for EPZ015666's efficiency in the previous study (Chan-Penebre et al., 2015). Compared with EPZ015666, although T1551 was lack of THIQ group, its phenyl ring in indole scaffold also formed cation–π interactions with SAM, explaining the inhibitory activity of T1551 against PRMT5 to some extent. Meanwhile, the pyrrole ring of indole group in T1551 formed π–π interactions with Phe327. T1551 also formed a hydrogen bond with the main-chain oxygen atom of Ser578. These together fasten the interactions of T1551 with PRMT5.

Finally, in order to see the effect of inhibitors on conformational space of PRMT5, normal mode analysis was carried out. For clear visualization, only the normal modes of T1551 binding domain (10 Å around T1551) were shown here. From **Figure 7**, it could be observed that the partial collective motion of EPZ015666 was opposite to that of T1551 during the simulation. As for PRMT5, the obvious differences in two complexes were reflected from helix residues 310–319 and loop residues 290–299. In the PRMT5-EPZ015666 system (**Figure 7b**), the helix and loop vibrated in the face–face direction, which seemed like to tighten the binding pocket and thus stabilize EPZ015666 into it. From **Figure 7b**, we also observed that the obviously higher amplitude motion of loop domain made major contributions in it. Nevertheless, in the PRMT5-T1551 system (**Figure 7a**), the helix and loop moved in the back–back direction, which led the pocket not as compact as that in PRMT5-EPZ015666 system. It may be closely associated with that EPZ015666 has better biological activity for PRMT5 than T1551.

DISCUSSION

PRMT5, as currently the only known type II PRMT, is also a member with the few inhibitors reported in PRMT family. As the

relationship of PRMT5 and lung cancer is constantly revealed, it is urgent to search for effective inhibitors targeting PRMT5 for lung cancer therapy. SAM, as the natural substrate of PRMT5, is responsible for providing the methyl group in the process of methyl transfer. To date, most of PRMT5 inhibitors reported were aimed for SAM-binding site and designed to disturb the interaction of SAM and PRMT5 (Alinari et al., 2015; Smil et al., 2015; Mao et al., 2017). However, due to their native binding state, it is difficult to find small molecules with the inhibitory activity stronger than SAM. Fortunately, the discovery of EPZ015666 and its new binding site provides a new clue for developing non-SAM competitive inhibitors.

In this study, we identified T1551 as a non-SAM competitive PRMT5 inhibitor by virtual screening method. Subsequently, the anticancer activity of T1551 against NSCLC was studied from three aspects, namely PRMT5 methyltransferase activity, expression of target genes and signaling pathway mediated by target genes. For the former, the "on-target" and direct inhibitory effect of T1551 was reflected from the low PRMT5 enzymatic activity, and indirect effect was from the low expression level of PRMT5's histone marker (H4R3me2s), which together suggested that T1551 inhibited PRMT5 methyltransferase activity.

For the latter, FGFR3 and eIF4E are two target genes of PRMT5 we focused here. We know that PI3K/AKT/mTOR pathway is a prototypic survival pathway in cancers, whose activation is closely related to cellular proliferation, growth, and mobility. FGFR3 promotes the survival of cancer cells just by stimulating the downstream PI3K/AKT/mTOR pathway (Kang et al., 2007; Hafner et al., 2010). Using RNA interference technology, Zhang et al. (2015) revealed that silencing PRMT5 could significantly downregulate FGFR3 and eIF4E expression. In our study, via inhibiting PRMT5, the identified T1551 was also shown to reduce the protein expressions of oncogene FGFR3 and eIF4E. Despite that the change of phosphorylated mTOR was not significant possibly due to the amplification effect of a signaling cascade, the concurrent reducing of phosphorylated AKT and ERK indicated that T1551 blocked the activation of PI3K/AKT/mTOR and ERK pathways in NSCLC cell line.

Previous studies emphasized that cation–π interaction between the tetrahydroisoquinoline group of EPZ015666 and partial positively charged methyl group of SAM was essential for EPZ015666's higher competitive ability for PRMT5 relative to histone substrate (Chan-Penebre et al., 2015; Duncan et al., 2015). Replacing SAM with SAH, the binding affinity of EPZ015666 and PRMT5 could be decreased more than 100 times. Due to the importance of this feature, in the subsequently structural optimization of EPZ015666, cation–π has always been retained as a crucial interaction (Duncan et al., 2015). By comparing the binding modes of T1551 and EPZ015666 with PRMT5-SAM, we observed that the conformation of T1551 in PRMT5 new pocket was similar to that of EPZ015666. Importantly, the benzene ring of T1551 indole scaffold also formed strong cation–π interactions with the methyl group of SAM. This explains the inhibitory source of T1551 for PRMT5 to some extent.

In summary, a novel PRMT5 inhibitor T1551 with the indole scaffold was identified in this study, whose functional influence on PRMT5 was verified by a series of biological assays and theoretical inhibitory basis on PRMT5 was revealed by molecular dynamic simulation method. These results provide a lead compound for the further design of PRMT5 inhibitors, and contribute to the development of PRMT5-targeting cancer treatment.

AUTHOR CONTRIBUTIONS

XY, EL, and LL conceived the project. XY, EL, and QW designed the experiments. QW, JX, YL, JH, ZJ, and YW carried out the research and data analysis. XY, EL, LL, and QW wrote the paper.

FUNDING

This work was supported by Macao Science and Technology Development Fund (Project Nos: 046/2016/A2, 086/2015/A3, and 005/2014/AMJ).

REFERENCES

Alinari, L., Mahasenan, K. V., Yan, F., Karkhanis, V., Chung, J. H., Smith, E. M., et al. (2015). Selective inhibition of protein arginine methyltransferase 5 blocks initiation and maintenance of B-cell transformation. *Blood* 125, 2530–2543. doi: 10.1182/blood-2014-12-619783

Babina, I. S., and Turner, N. C. (2017). Advances and challenges in targeting FGFR signalling in cancer. *Nat. Rev. Cancer* 17, 318–332. doi: 10.1038/nrc.2017.8

Baell, J. B., and Holloway, G. A. (2010). New substructure filters for removal of pan assay interference compounds (PAINS) from screening libraries and for their exclusion in bioassays. *J. Med. Chem.* 53, 2719–2740. doi: 10.1021/jm901137j

Bedford, M. T., and Clarke, S. G. (2009). Protein arginine methylation in mammals: who, what, and why. *Mol. Cell* 33, 1–13. doi: 10.1016/j.molcel.2008.12.013

Branscombe, T. L., Frankel, A., Lee, J. H., Cook, J. R., Yang, Z. H., Pestka, S., et al. (2001). PRMT5 (Janus kinase-binding protein 1) catalyzes the formation of symmetric dimethylarginine residues in proteins. *J. Biol. Chem.* 276, 32971–32976. doi: 10.1074/jbc.M105412200

Case, D. A., Cerutti, D. S., Cheathamiii, T. E., Darden, T. A., Duke, R. E., Giese, T. J., et al. (2017). *AMBER 16*. San Francisco, CA: University of California.

Chan-Penebre, E., Kuplast, K. G., Majer, C. R., Boriack-Sjodin, P. A., Wigle, T. J., Johnston, L. D., et al. (2015). A selective inhibitor of PRMT5 with *in vivo* and *in vitro* potency in MCL models. *Nat. Chem. Biol.* 11, 432–437. doi: 10.1038/nchembio.1810

Chen, H., Lorton, B., Gupta, V., and Shechter, D. (2017). A TGFβ-PRMT5-MEP50 axis regulates cancer cell invasion through histone H3 and H4 arginine methylation coupled transcriptional activation and repression. *Oncogene* 36, 373–386. doi: 10.1038/onc.2016.205

Chu, C. H., Wang, L. Y., Hsu, K. C., Chen, C. C., Cheng, H. H., Wang, S. M., et al. (2014). KDM4B as a target for prostate cancer: structural analysis and selective inhibition by a novel inhibitor. *J. Med. Chem.* 57, 5975–5985. doi: 10.1021/jm500249n

Culjkovic-Kraljacic, B., Baguet, A., Volpon, L., Amri, A., and Borden, K. L. (2012). The oncogene eIF4E reprograms the nuclear pore complex to promote mRNA export and oncogenic transformation. *Cell Rep.* 2, 207–215. doi: 10.1016/j.celrep.2012.07.007

De Benedetti, A., and Graff, J. R. (2004). eIF-4E expression and its role in malignancies and metastases. *Oncogene* 23, 3189–3199. doi: 10.1038/sj.onc.1207545

Desai, A., and Adjei, A. A. (2016). FGFR signaling as a target for lung cancer therapy. *J. Thorac. Oncol.* 11, 9–20. doi: 10.1016/j.jtho.2015.08.003

Deuker, M. M., and McMahon, M. (2014). Methylation matters in KRAS oncogenesis. *Nature* 510, 225–226. doi: 10.1038/nature13343

Duncan, K. W., Rioux, N., Boriack-Sjodin, P. A., Munchhof, M. J., Reiter, L. A., Majer, C. R., et al. (2015). Structure and property guided design in the identification of PRMT5 tool compound EPZ015666. *ACS Med. Chem. Lett.* 7, 162–166. doi: 10.1021/acsmedchemlett.5b00380

Gu, Z., Gao, S., Zhang, F., Wang, Z., Ma, W., Davis, R. E., et al. (2012). Protein arginine methyltransferase 5 is essential for growth of lung cancer cells. *Biochem. J.* 446, 235–241. doi: 10.1042/BJ20120768

Hafner, C., Di Martino, E., Pitt, E., Stempfl, T., Tomlinson, D., Hartmann, A., et al. (2010). FGFR3 mutation affects cell growth, apoptosis and attachment in keratinocytes. *Exp. Cell Res.* 316, 2008–2016. doi: 10.1016/j.yexcr.2010.04.021

Hou, T., Wang, J., Li, Y., and Wang, W. (2010). Assessing the performance of the MM/PBSA and MM/GBSA methods. 1. The accuracy of binding free energy calculations based on molecular dynamics simulations. *J. Chem. Inf. Model.* 51, 69–82. doi: 10.1021/ci100275a

Huang, S., Song, C., Wang, X., Zhang, G., Wang, Y., Jiang, X., et al. (2017). Discovery of new SIRT2 inhibitors by utilizing a consensus docking/scoring strategy and structure-activity relationship analysis. *J. Chem. Inf. Model.* 57, 669–679. doi: 10.1021/acs.jcim.6b00714

Ibrahim, R., Matsubara, D., Osman, W., Morikawa, T., Goto, A., Morita, S., et al. (2014). Expression of PRMT5 in lung adenocarcinoma and its significance in epithelial-mesenchymal transition. *Hum. Pathol.* 45, 1397–1405. doi: 10.1016/j.humpath.2014.02.013

Ji, S., Ma, S., Wang, W. J., Huang, S. Z., Wang, T. Q., Xiang, R., et al. (2017). Discovery of selective protein arginine methyltransferase 5 inhibitors and biological evaluations. *Chem. Biol. Drug Des.* 89, 585–598. doi: 10.1111/cbdd.12881

Kang, S., Dong, S., Gu, T. L., Guo, A., Cohen, M. S., Lonial, S., et al. (2007). FGFR3 activates RSK2 to mediate hematopoietic transformation through tyrosine phosphorylation of RSK2 and activation of the MEK/ERK pathway. *Cancer Cell* 12, 201–214. doi: 10.1016/j.ccr.2007.08.003

Li, Y., Chitnis, N., Nakagawa, H., Kita, Y., Natsugoe, S., Yang, Y., et al. (2015). PRMT5 is required for lymphomagenesis triggered by multiple oncogenic drivers. *Cancer Discov.* 5, 288–303. doi: 10.1158/2159-8290.CD-14-0625

Lim, J. H., Lee, Y. M., Lee, G., Choi, Y. J., Lim, B. O., Kim, Y. J., et al. (2014). PRMT5 is essential for the eIF4E-mediated 5'-cap dependent translation. *Biochem. Biophys. Res. Commun.* 452, 1016–1021. doi: 10.1016/j.bbrc.2014.09.033

Linse, B., and Linse, P. (2014). Tuning the smooth particle mesh Ewald sum: application to ionic solutions and dipolar fluids. *J. Chem. Phys* 141:184114. doi: 10.1063/1.4901119

Liu, F., Zhao, X., Perna, F., Wang, L., Koppikar, P., and Abdel-Wahab, O. (2011). JAK2V617F-mediated phosphorylation of PRMT5 downregulates its methyltransferase activity and promotes myeloproliferation. *Cancer Cell* 19, 283–294. doi: 10.1016/j.ccr.2010.12.020

Maier, J. A., Martinez, C., Kasavajhala, K., Wickstrom, L., Hauser, K. E., and Simmerling, C. (2015). ff14SB: improving the accuracy of protein side chain and backbone parameters from ff99SB. *J. Chem. Theory Comput.* 11, 3696–3713. doi: 10.1021/acs.jctc.5b00255

Mao, R., Shao, J., Zhu, K., Zhang, Y., Ding, H., Zhang, C., et al. (2017). Potent, selective, and cell active protein arginine methyltransferase 5 (PRMT5) inhibitor developed by structure-based virtual screening and hit optimization. *J. Med. Chem.* 60, 6289–6304. doi: 10.1021/acs.jmedchem.7b00587

Meng, F., Cheng, S., Ding, H., Liu, S., Liu, Y., Zhu, K., et al. (2015). Discovery and optimization of novel, selective histone methyltransferase SET7 inhibitors by pharmacophore-and docking-based virtual screening. *J. Med. Chem.* 58, 8166–8181. doi: 10.1021/acs.jmedchem.5b01154

Mysinger, M. M., Carchia, M., Irwin, J. J., and Shoichet, B. K. (2012). Directory of useful decoys, enhanced (DUD-E): better ligands and decoys for better benchmarking. *J. Med. Chem.* 55, 6582–6594. doi: 10.1021/jm300687e

Platania, C. B., Di Paola, L., Leggio, G. M., Romano, G. L., Drago, F., Salomone, S., et al. (2015). Molecular features of interaction between VEGFA and anti-angiogenic drugs used in retinal diseases: a computational approach. *Front. Pharmacol.* 6:248. doi: 10.3389/fphar.2015.00248

Schrödinger (2015). *Maestro Version 10.2.* New York, NY: Schrödinger.

Sheng, X., and Wang, Z. (2016). Protein arginine methyltransferase 5 regulates multiple signaling pathways to promote lung cancer cell proliferation. *BMC Cancer* 16:567. doi: 10.1186/s12885-016-2632-3

Shilo, K., Wu, X., Sharma, S., Welliver, M., Duan, W., Villalona-Calero, M., et al. (2013). Cellular localization of protein arginine methyltransferase-5 correlates with grade of lung tumors. *Diagn. Pathol.* 8:201. doi: 10.1186/1746-1596-8-201

Smil, D., Eram, M. S., Li, F., Kennedy, S., Szewczyk, M. M., Brown, P. J., et al. (2015). Discovery of a dual PRMT5–PRMT7 inhibitor. *ACS Med. Chem. Lett.* 6, 408–412. doi: 10.1021/ml500467h

Stopa, N., Krebs, J. E., and Shechter, D. (2015). The PRMT5 arginine methyltransferase: many roles in development, cancer and beyond. *Cell. Mol. Life Sci.* 72, 2041–2059. doi: 10.1007/s00018-015-1847-9

van Rhijn, B. W., Lurkin, I., Radvanyi, F., Kirkels, W. J., Van Der Kwast, T. H., and Zwarthoff, E. C. (2001). The fibroblast growth factor receptor 3 (FGFR3) mutation is a strong indicator of superficial bladder cancer with low recurrence rate. *Cancer Res.* 61, 1265–1268.

Wang, J., Wolf, R. M., Caldwell, J. W., Kollman, P. A., and Case, D. A. (2004). Development and testing of a general amber force field. *J. Comput. Chem.* 25, 1157–1174. doi: 10.1002/jcc.20035

Wang, Q., Li, Y., Xu, J., Wang, Y., Leung, E. L. H., Liu, L., et al. (2017). Selective inhibition mechanism of RVX-208 to the second bromodomain of bromo and extraterminal proteins: insight from microsecond molecular dynamics simulations. *Sci. Rep.* 7:8857. doi: 10.1038/s41598-017-08909-8

Wei, H., Wang, B., Miyagi, M., She, Y., Gopalan, B., Huang, D. B., et al. (2013). PRMT5 dimethylates R30 of the p65 subunit to activate NF-κB. *Proc. Natl. Acad. Sci. U.S.A.* 110, 13516–13521. doi: 10.1073/pnas.1311784110

Wei, T. Y. W., Juan, C. C., Hisa, J. Y., Su, L. J., Lee, Y. C. G., Chou, H. Y., et al. (2012). Protein arginine methyltransferase 5 is a potential oncoprotein that upregulates G1 cyclins/cyclin-dependent kinases and the phosphoinositide 3-kinase/AKT signaling cascade. *Cancer Sci.* 103, 1640–1650. doi: 10.1111/j.1349-7006.2012.02367.x

Yan, F., Alinari, L., Lustberg, M. E., Martin, L. K., Cordero-Nieves, H. M., Banasavadi-Siddegowda, Y., et al. (2014). Genetic validation of the protein arginine methyltransferase PRMT5 as a candidate therapeutic target in glioblastoma. *Cancer Res.* 74, 1752–1765. doi: 10.1158/0008-5472.CAN-13-0884

Yang, Y., and Bedford, M. T. (2013). Protein arginine methyltransferases and cancer. *Nat. Rev. Cancer* 13, 37–50. doi: 10.1038/nrc3409

Zhang, B., Dong, S., Zhu, R., Hu, C., Hou, J., Li, Y., et al. (2015). Targeting protein arginine methyltransferase 5 inhibits colorectal cancer growth by decreasing arginine methylation of eIF4E and FGFR3. *Oncotarget* 6, 22799–22811. doi: 10.18632/oncotarget.4332

Zhao, Q., Rank, G., Tan, Y. T., Li, H., Moritz, R. L., Simpson, R. J., et al. (2009). PRMT5-mediated methylation of histone H4R3 recruits DNMT3A, coupling histone and DNA methylation in gene silencing. *Nat. Struct. Mol. Biol.* 16, 304–311. doi: 10.1038/nsmb.1568

Discovery of Potent Disheveled/Dvl Inhibitors Using Virtual Screening Optimized with NMR-Based Docking Performance Index

Kiminori Hori[1], Kasumi Ajioka[2], Natsuko Goda[1], Asako Shindo[3], Maki Takagishi[4], Takeshi Tenno[1,5] and Hidekazu Hiroaki[1,2,5]*

[1] Laboratory of Structural Molecular Pharmacology, Graduate School of Pharmaceutical Sciences, Nagoya University, Nagoya, Japan, [2] Department of Biological Science, School of Science, Nagoya University, Nagoya, Japan, [3] Division of Biological Science, Graduate School of Science, Nagoya University, Nagoya, Japan, [4] Department of Pathology, Graduate School of Medicine, Nagoya University, Nagoya, Japan, [5] BeCellBar LLC, Business Incubation Center, Nagoya University, Nagoya, Japan

Correspondence:
Hidekazu Hiroaki
hiroaki.hidekazu@
f.mbox.nagoya-u.ac.jp

Most solid tumors have their own cancer stem cells (CSCs), which are resistant to standard chemo-therapies. Recent reports have described that Wnt pathway plays a key role in self-renewal and tumorigenesis of CSCs. Regarding the Wnt/β-catenin pathway, Dvl (mammalian Disheveled) is an attractive target of drug discovery. After analyzing the PDZ domain of human Dvl1 (Dvl1-PDZ) using NMR, we subjected it to preliminary NMR titration studies with 17 potential PDZ-binding molecules including CalBioChem-322338, a commercially available Dvl PDZ domain inhibitor. Next, we performed virtual screening (VS) using the program GOLD with nine parameter sets. Results were evaluated using the NMR-derived docking performance index (NMR-DPI). One parameter set of GOLD docking showing the best NMR-DPI was selected and used for the second VS against 5,135 compounds. The second docking trial identified more than 1,700 compounds that exhibited higher scores than CalBioChem-322338. Subsequent NMR titration experiments with five new candidate molecules (NPL-4001, 4004, 4011, 4012, and 4013), Dvl1-PDZ revealed larger chemical shift changes than those of CalBioChem-322338. Finally, these compounds showed partial proliferation inhibition activity against BT-20, a triple negative breast cancer (TNBC) cell. These compounds are promising Wnt pathway inhibitors that are potentially useful for anti-TNBC therapy.

Keywords: Wnt signaling, protein–protein interaction inhibitor, NMR-derived docking performance index, virtual screening, triple negative breast cancer

INTRODUCTION

Poor therapeutic outcomes of chemotherapy against several solid tumors pose a challenge to anti-tumor drug discovery and development. Cancer stem cells (CSCs) are believed to have a pivotal role in malignancy, survival against chemotherapy, and self-renewal of those tumors (Tannishtha et al., 2001). Consequently, CSCs are attractive targets for cancer chemotherapy development (Visvader and Lindeman, 2008). The Wnt/β-catenin pathway, along with Notch and Hedgehog pathways, are important in several CSCs (Reya and Clevers, 2005). In fact, the Wnt pathway has been commonly regarded as the key signaling pathway of self-renewal and anti-differentiation of normal tissue stem cells. Accordingly, proliferation and self-renewal of several CSCs have been demonstrated as dependent on the Wnt pathway. For that reason, Wnt pathway is an attractive target for anti-CSC chemotherapy (Takebe et al., 2011; Holland et al., 2013).

The Wnt/β-catenin pathway is activated by Wnt ligands. Frizzled (Fzd)/LRP co-receptors coordinately bind Wnt, and transduce the signal to cytosolic downstream components including Axin, APC, GSK3β, and CK1. Accordingly, a transcription factor β-catenin is accumulated to induce target gene expression. This signaling system is carried out by a constitutive process of proteasomal degradation of β-catenin at the "Wnt-off" state. Specifically, β-catenin degradation is initiated by phosphorylation by GSK3β. At "Wnt-on" state, then the interaction between Dvl, and Axin inhibits GSK3β, thereby accumulating β-catenin in the cytoplasm and the nucleus. Dvl, a 75 kD multi-domain adaptor protein with Disheveled-aXin (DIX), Post synaptic density-95, Disc large, and Zonular occludens-1 (PDZ), and Disheveled-Egl10-Pleckstrin (DEP) domains (**Figure 2A**), plays a central role in both canonical (β-catenin-dependent) and non-canonical (β-catenin-independent) pathways of Wnt signaling (Gao and Chen, 2010). There are three mammalian Disheveled orthologs, Dvl-1, 2, and 3, in human genome, with functional redundancy. The PDZ domain of Dvl (Dvl-PDZ) specifically interacts to the C-terminus of Fzd (Wong et al., 2003) upon Wnt binding to the extracellular domain of Fzd. Accordingly, Dvl-PDZ is an attractive target for exploring small molecule inhibitors (**Figure 2B**), and has been characterized extensively. For instance, the binding mode of the tripeptides VVV and VWV against Dvl-PDZ has been reported (Lee et al., 2009a). The complex structure of peptide-derived inhibitors and Dvl2-PDZ has also been reported (Zhang et al., 2009). In addition, several reports have described Dvl-PDZ inhibitors, including a peptide-mimic compounds NSC668036 (Shan et al., 2005), 1H-indole-5-carboxylic acid derivative FJ9 (Fujii et al., 2007), sulindac (Lee et al., 2009b), N-benzoyl-2-amino-benzoic acid derivative CalBioChem-322338 (Grandy et al., 2009), and phenoxyacetic acid analogs (Choi et al., 2016). The present study specifically examines N-benzoyl-2-amino-benzoic acid analogs including CalBioChem-322338 because 2-amino-benzoic acid moiety is independently proposed as a key moiety of group-specific inhibitors against several PDZ domains. Therefore, it represents a potential pharmacophore (Tenno et al., 2013). During our research exploring new inhibitors against Zonular Occludens-1 PDZ1 domain (Umetsu et al., 2011), we obtained several N-substituted-2-amino-benzoic acid analogs that are chemically similar to CalBioChem-322338 (**Figure 3** and **Supplementary Figure S1**). The present study evaluates the affinities of those compounds against human Dvl1 PDZ domain (hDvl1-PDZ) using solution NMR experiments (**Figure 2D**).

Virtual screening (VS) of drug candidates, known as high-throughput protein–ligand docking, is a powerful approach. Commercial applications are widely used, such as Glide (Friesner et al., 2004), FRED (McGann, 2011), MOE/ASEDock (Goto et al., 2008), and GOLD (Verdonk et al., 2003), as well as academic applications such as AutoDock

(Goodsell et al., 1996), AutoDock-VINA (Trott and Olson, 2010), and Sievegene (Fukunishi et al., 2005). According their increasing convenience and availability, another practical issue has arisen: VS experiments with different algorithms, different parameter settings, and different target 3D structures might produce disparate results. Consequently, the benchmarking of docking algorithms has come to represent an important issue (McGaughey et al., 2007; Lindh et al., 2015). For the present study, we decided to use GOLD because GOLD is recognized as having acceptably high performance in comprehensive benchmarking throughout several VS programs (Wang et al., 2016). Moreover, results have demonstrated that the experimental tuning of parameter sets and/or the selection of target model structures might greatly improve performance and provide higher accuracy of prediction (Huang and Wong, 2016). Encouraged by that idea proposed by Huang et al., we introduced the idea into our project as a simplified index for evaluating nine docking scoring functions of GOLD. For this study, the index is designated as the NMR-based docking performance index (NMR-DPI).

First, 17 potential PDZ-binding molecules as well as CalBioChem-322338, all of which are N-substituted-2-amino-benzoic acid analogs, were analyzed using NMR chemical shift perturbation (CSP) experiments. We believe that the NMR-CSP experiment is among the easiest and most robust assay methods to compare the affinities of a series of compounds against ^{15}N-labeled small protein (Williamson, 2013). Second, these 17 potential PDZ-binding molecules were docked against hDvl2-PDZ using GOLD with nine different scoring functions. Third, out of the nine scoring functions, we identified the one that is most consistent to the CSP experiments of the 17 compounds. This optimized scoring function was used for a new VS with our in-house focused library, which is a subset of the library LIGANDBOX (Kawabata et al., 2013) containing commercially available 5,135 N-substituted-2-amino-benzoic acid analogs. From the top hit compounds after the new VS experiment, 13 new molecules were purchased: NPL-4001 – NPL-4007, and NPL-4011 – NPL-4016 (**Figure 1**). Our seven original compounds induced markedly larger chemical shift changes upon hDvl1-PDZ than those induced by CalBioChem-322338. The compounds were evaluated further by the cell-based assays as potential Wnt pathway inhibitors. The validity and possible limitations of NMR-DPI were also assessed.

MATERIALS AND METHODS

Preparation of Protein Samples

The expression vector for the recombinant GST-tagged form of prototype hDvl1-PDZ* domain (residues 244–342) was constructed using the PRESAT-vector methodology (Goda et al., 2004). The vector for the GST-tagged hDvl1-PDZ domain (residues 246–340, four amino acids shorter construct) was then produced using the standard PCR cloning technique with pGEX-6P3 plasmid (GE Healthcare, Little Chalfont, United Kingdom). The GST-tagged hDvl2-PDZ domain (residues 262–356) was constructed similarly. Two PDZ domains, residues Cys-Trp near

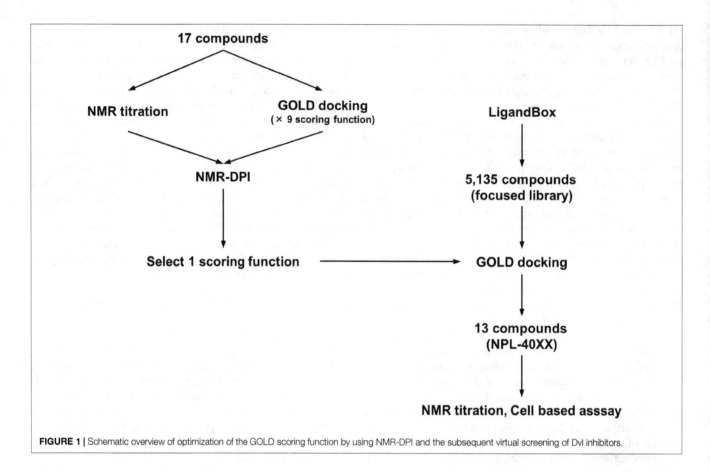

FIGURE 1 | Schematic overview of optimization of the GOLD scoring function by using NMR-DPI and the subsequent virtual screening of Dvl inhibitors.

the C-termini (residues 338–339 and 354–355, respectively, for hDvl1, and hDvl2) were substituted to Ala-Thr to increase protein stability. Since the position of these residues was opposite side to the ligand binding site, we assumed that the mutations affected to neither its affinity nor binding mode to the inhibitors. Isotopically labeled proteins for NMR experiments were generated, respectively, in *E. coli* BL21 (*DE3*) grown in 1 L M9 minimal medium culture at 37°C in the presence of [^{15}N]-NH$_4$Cl and [^{13}C]-glucose (if needed) as the sole nitrogen and carbon sources. The protein expression was induced by addition of final 1 mM of isopropyl-β-D-galactoside, with immediate lowering of the temperature to 20°C. The cells were harvested 20 h after IPTG induction. The harvested cells were then re-suspended in lysis buffer (50 mM Tris–HCl, pH 7.2, and 150 mM NaCl), disrupted by sonication, and clarified by centrifugation. The supernatant was applied to a DEAE–Sepharose^{TM} Fast Flow (GE Healthcare) column. It was then affinity-purified using resin (GST-Accept^{TM}; Nacalai Tesque Inc., Kyoto, Japan). The GST tag was removed by PreScission protease on beads. The protein solution was loaded on a Superdex 75 HR 26/60 column (GE Healthcare) equilibrated with 50 mM Tris–HCl (pH 7.2) and 150 mM NaCl. The purified proteins were concentrated to 0.1 mM (for NMR titration experiment) and were dialyzed against 100 mM potassium phosphate buffer (pH 7.4) containing 0.5 mM EDTA supplemented with 10% D$_2$O and 5% d$_6$-dimethyl sulfoxide. After comparing ^{1}H–^{15}N HSQC spectra of hDvl1 and hDvl2 PDZ domains, we decided to continue further

study of hDvl1-PDZ because of its sharp and well-dispersed HSQC signals. For triple resonance experiments, 0.65 mM of ^{15}N /^{13}C-labeled hDvl1-PDZ was solubilized into 90 mM potassium phosphate buffer (pH 7.4) containing 0.45 mM EDTA supplemented with 10% D$_2$O. ^{15}N-labeled mouse ZO-1 first PDZ domain (residues 18–110, mZO1-PDZ1) was prepared according to an earlier report (Umetsu et al., 2011).

NMR Experiments

For this study, NMR experiments were conducted using NMR spectrometer (600 MHz, Bruker Avance III; Bruker Analytik GmbH, Karlsruhe, Germany) equipped with a cryogenic triple-resonance probe. For assignment of backbone ^{1}H, ^{13}C, and ^{15}N resonances, HNCA, HNCACB, CBCA (CO) NH, HNCO, HN (CA) CO, and 3D ^{15}N-edited-NOESY-HSQC spectra were recorded. For NMR titration experiments, 0.1 mM PDZ domain sample was dissolved in 250 μL of 85 mM potassium phosphate buffer (pH 7.4) containing 0.42 mM EDTA supplemented with 10% D$_2$O and 5% d$_6$-dimethyl sulfoxide (DMSO). Then the ^{1}H–^{15}N HSQC spectra were obtained with and without ligands. In each titration experiment, the final concentration of the compound at 0.2 mM was added to the proteins. All NMR spectra were recorded at 298 K. All spectra were processed using NMRPipe (Delaglio et al., 1995) and were analyzed using the program Sparky 3.114 (Goddard and Kneller, 2004). All chemical shift changes in the ^{1}H–^{15}N HSQC spectra were calculated as $\Delta\delta_{normalized} = \{\Delta\delta(^1H)^2 + [\Delta\delta(^{15}N)/6]^2\}^{1/2}$. The

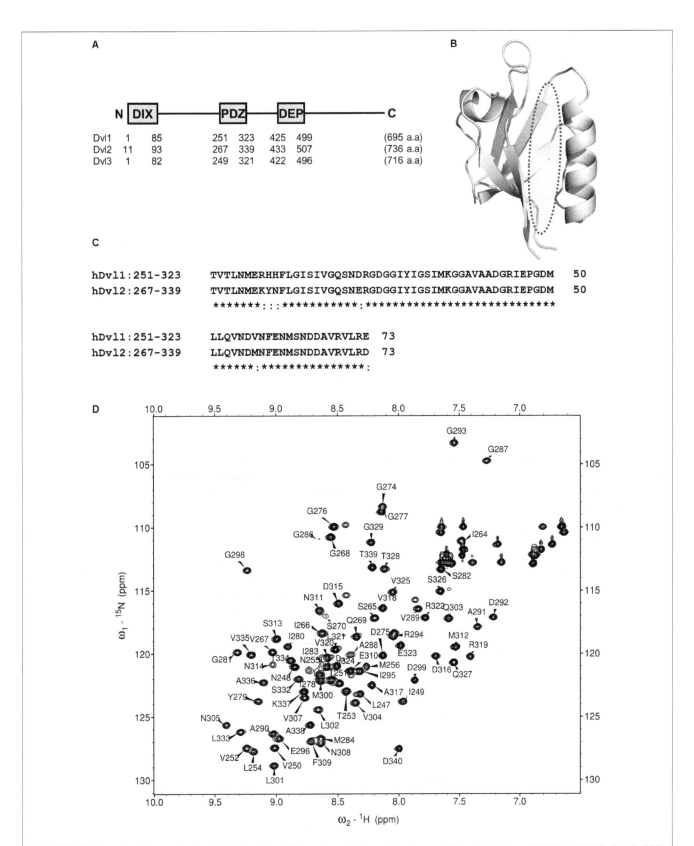

FIGURE 2 | PDZ domain of Dvl as a drug target for Wnt pathway. **(A)** Domain architecture of three human Disheveled orthologs. DIX, DIsheveled-aXin domain, PDZ, Post synaptic density-95, Disc large and Zonular occludens-1domain, DEP, Disheveled-Egl10-Pleckstrin domain. **(B)** Ribbon representation of PDZ domain of Dvl2 (PDB code: 3CBY). A green ellipsoid indicates the position of Fzd binding cleft. **(C)** Multiple sequence alignment of the core region of PDZ domain of human Dvl1 (residues 251–323) and Dvl2 (residues 267–339). Identical amino acids are represented by asterisks. **(D)** A portion of the ^{1}H–^{15}N HSQC spectrum of hDvl1-PDZ illustrating a number of the assigned backbone amide resonances.

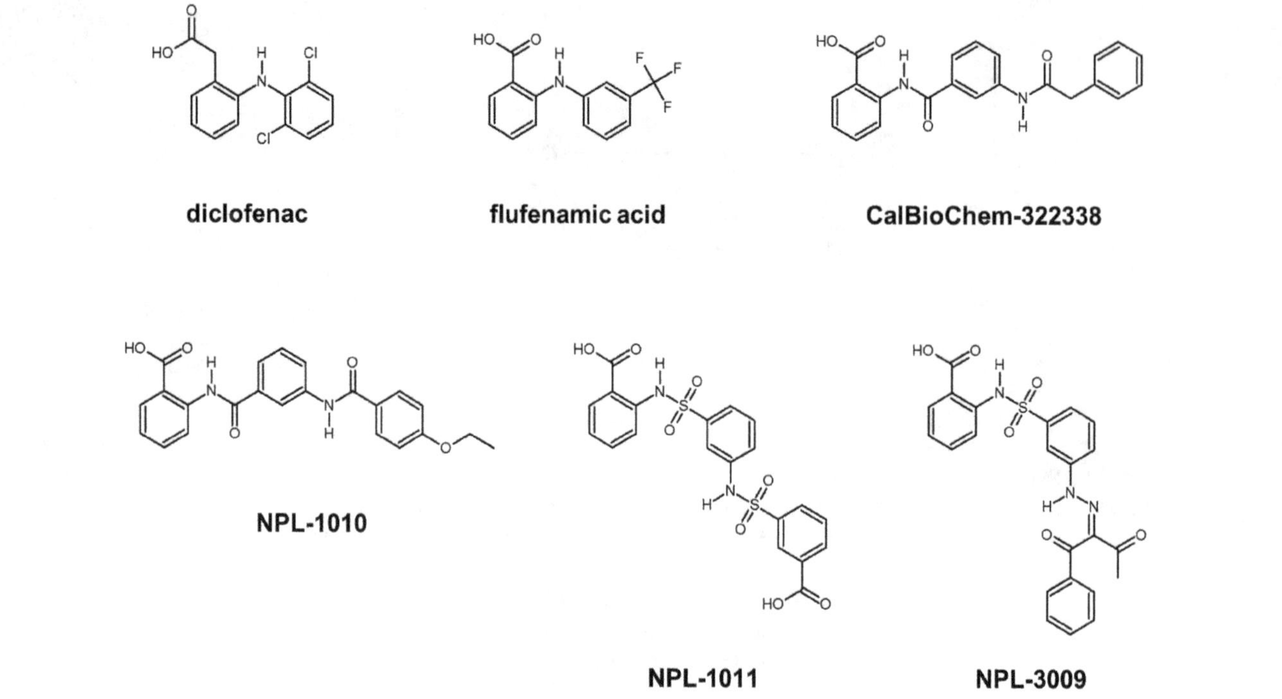

FIGURE 3 | Selected compounds that may bind PDZ domains. Diclofenac and flufenamic acid bind several PDZ domains. CalBioChem-322338 is an example of Dvl-PDZ inhibitors. NPL-1010, 1011, and 3009 are an example of potential hDvl1-PDZ binding compounds.

chemical shift changes were then mapped onto the corresponding residues of the structure of hDvl2-PDZ using PyMol graphic software (Schrödinger, 2015). $\Delta\delta_{ave}$ is the sum of $\Delta\delta_{normalized}$ divided by the total residue number with their residue-specific assignment except the residues with broadened-out signals. After Signals showing marked chemical shift changes were selected, the normalized chemical shift changes were calculated. Non-linear least-squares fitting was applied to estimate the dissociation constant K_D as

$$\Delta\delta_{normalized} = \Delta\delta_{saturated} \times (([R]_{total} + [L]_{total} + K_D) -$$
$$sqrt(([R]_{total} + [L]_{total} + K_D)^2 - 4[R]_{total}$$
$$[L]_{total}))/2[L]_{total} \qquad (1)$$

where $\Delta\delta_{saturated}$ represents the normalized chemical shifts at the saturated point. In addition, $[R]_{total}$ and $[L]_{total}$, respectively, denote the concentrations of PDZ domain and the compound. K_D and $\Delta\delta_{saturated}$ values for the selected residues were optimized simultaneously by using SOLVER function in Microsoft Excel (Microsoft Corp.).

Docking and Virtual Screening Experiments
Prior to the VS experiments, a focused library was constructed by filtering compounds with carboxylic acid moieties, which play a crucially important role in canonical peptide recognition

by many PDZ domains. A focused library was constructed as a subset of the compound database (LIGANDBOX ver. 1306) (Kawabata et al., 2013) based on our earlier observation that diclofenac and flufenamic acid bound several PDZ domains in a group-specific manner (Tenno et al., 2013). We selected and pooled 5,135 compounds of N-substituted 2-amino-benzoic acid and N-substituted 2-amino-benzeneacetic acid. Subsequently, software GOLD suite (ver. 5.32) (Verdonk et al., 2003) was used for molecular docking of the compounds into the structure of hDvl2-PDZ [PDB entry 3CBY (Zhang et al., 2009)]. The GOLD software is based on a genetic algorithm for generating configurations of ligands with the two scoring modes, "simple scoring" and "consensus scoring." Simple scoring uses just a single function out of the four fitness functions. Consensus scoring combines two of four scoring functions, respectively, for initial docking and re-scoring. The present study examined the three scoring functions of ChemScore (CS), GoldScore (GS), and ChemPLP, in the simple scoring mode and the consensus scoring mode, thereby examining nine scoring methods.

Cell-Based Viability Assay
The newly found Dvl-PDZ inhibitors were tested to assess their effectiveness against TNBC cell lines (BT-20) on cell proliferation and viability. For that purpose, luciferase-expressing stable cell lines were chosen, although we did not perform luciferase-based biochemical experiment in this report. The TNBC cell lines BT-20 (BT-20/CMV-Luc, JCRB-1438) were obtained from the JCRB Cell Bank, National Institute of Biomedical Innovation, Health, and Nutrition (Osaka, Japan). The cells were grown in

Minimum Essential Medium Eagle (Earle's salts containing with L-glutamine and sodium bicarbonate; Sigma-Aldrich Corp.), supplemented with 10% fetal bovine serum (FBS) (Biosera, Boussens, France), and 1% Penicillin/Streptomycin antibiotics (Gibco, Grand Island, NY, United States). Cell lines were cultured in a 37°C incubator with a humidified atmosphere of 5% CO_2. Cells were seeded at 15,000 cells/well into 96-well plates. After overnight incubation, cells were treated with d_6-DMSO or 100 μM of each Dvl-PDZ inhibitor (CalBioChem-322338, NPL-4001, 4002, 4007, and 4011–4013) for 96 h. During culture, the media with or without corresponding inhibitors was refreshed every 48 h. After 4 days of culture with the compounds, the cell growth rate was ascertained using WST-8 [2-(2-methoxy-4-nitrophenyl)-3-(4-nitrophenyl)-5-(2,4-disulfophenyl)-2H-tetrazolium] colorimetric assay with a kit (Cell Counting Kit-8®; Dojindo Molecular Technologies Inc., Kumamoto, Japan) according to the manufacturer's instructions. Cell viability was also ascertained after 4 days (Cytotoxicity LDH Assay Kit-WST; Dojindo Molecular Technologies Inc., Japan). The sample absorbance was measured using a microplate reader (EnSpire; PerkinElmer Inc., Waltham, MA, United States). All experiments were performed in triplicate. Each measurement was repeated twice. Statistical tests were performed using Microsoft Office® Excel program.

RESULTS

NMR Analysis of hDvl1-PDZ With Prototype *N*-Substituted 2-Amino-Benzoic Acid Compounds

Before analyzing the interaction between hDvl1-PDZ and the compounds, we completed assignment of the backbone amide signals of hDvl1-PDZ because few signal assignments for hDvl1-PDZ have been published or deposited in the public NMR database (BioMagResBank). The backbone signal assignment was done according to the standard method (Ikura et al., 1990) using software MARS (Jung and Zweckstetter, 2004). The assignment was further confirmed using several inversely ^{14}N-labeled samples (Hiroaki et al., 2011). Out of the 98 residues, 79 residues (81%) were assigned, although seven NH signals at the loop between β1 and β2 strands were missing, probably because of intermediate dynamic motion in the solution. The assignments were labeled on the HSQC spectra (**Figure 2D**).

Subsequently, we performed NMR titration experiments using 17 prototypical *N*-substituted 2-amino-benzoic acid compounds (NPL-1010, 1011, and 3001–3015) (**Figure 3**). In an earlier study, we found from bioinformatics prediction of the eF-seek analysis of all PDZ domains in human genome (Kinoshita et al., 2007; Motono et al., 2011), that flufenamic acid and diclofenac bound several PDZ domains (Tenno et al., 2013). Moreover, we identified the structure of the mouse Zonula ocludens-1 (ZO1)-PDZ1 domain (Umetsu et al., 2011) (PDB: 2RRM) and mouse ligand of numb X1 (LNX1)-PDZ2 domain (PDB: 3VQG, 3VGF, manuscript in preparation). These structures were subjected to VS using GOLD and LIGANDBOX to discover novel PDZ

TABLE 1 | Normalized total CSPs of hDvl1-PDZ induced by 2.0 equations of the prototypical Dvl1-PDZ binding compounds.

Compound ID (NPL-)	$\Delta\delta_{ave}$/ppm	Compound ID (NPL-)	$\Delta\delta_{ave}$/ppm
1010	0.022	3008	0.032
1011	0.022	3009	0.044
3001	0.021	3010	0.027
3002	0.007	3011	0.022
3003	0.003	3012	0.021
3004	0.012	3013	0.022
3005	0.023	3014	0.015
3006	0.019	3015	0.017
3007	0.022	CalBioChem-322338	0.018

domain inhibitors. During that study, we identified the first two prototypical mLNX1-PDZ2 binders (NPL-1010 and 1011), for which direct binding to mLNX1-PDZ2 was confirmed using NMR experiments (manuscript in preparation). Surprisingly, the chemical structure of NPL-1010 closely resembled that of CalBioChem-322338 (**Figure 3**). Accordingly, we proceeded to collect 15 related compounds (NPL-3001–3015) to analyze affinities against both mLNX1-PDZ2 and mZO1-PDZ1 by the combined use of VS and solution NMR. Subsequently, our collected *N*-substituted 2-amino-benzoic acid compounds (NPL-1010, 1011, and 3001–3015) were examined to elucidate whether they bind directly to hDvl1-PDZ, or not. Finally, we found that 12 of 17 compounds tested in this study showed substantial chemical shift changes of amide protons of hDvl1-PDZ larger than that of CalBioChem-322338. All results of chemical shift changes were normalized and were averaged per residue. They are presented in **Table 1** according to descending order of the CSPs. Examples of the chemical shift perturbations are presented in **Figure 4**.

Introduction and Calculation of NMR-Derived Docking Performance Index

Greatly inspired by the idea of fine-tuning of VS parameters and setting them with experimental data to improve VS performance (Huang and Wong, 2016), we modified that original idea to fit the use of our experimental data of NMR titration (CSP) study. For this purpose, we designed a strategy to tune VS parameters with our original NMR-derived docking performance index (NMR-DPI, **Figure 1**). First, NMR titration experiments of hDvl1-PDZ were performed with all 18 compounds as described above. Second, we docked all the 17 *N*-substituted 2-amino-benzoic acid compounds to the hDvl2-PDZ structure (PDB: 3CBY) using the GOLD software. Note that the core region of PDZ domains of human Dvl1 and Dvl2 are 92% identical in amino acid sequences (**Figure 2C**). At that time, the nine docking scoring methods were tested with different combinations of scoring functions, as presented in Table in **Figure 5A**. In our experience, these GOLD scoring functions mutually differ to a great degree. For that reason, it is difficult to determine one of them robustly for any new VS project. Third, the final fitness score of each scoring method was normalized to a value between 0 and 1 as the docking score $D(i, j)$, where i is the index of the scoring methods

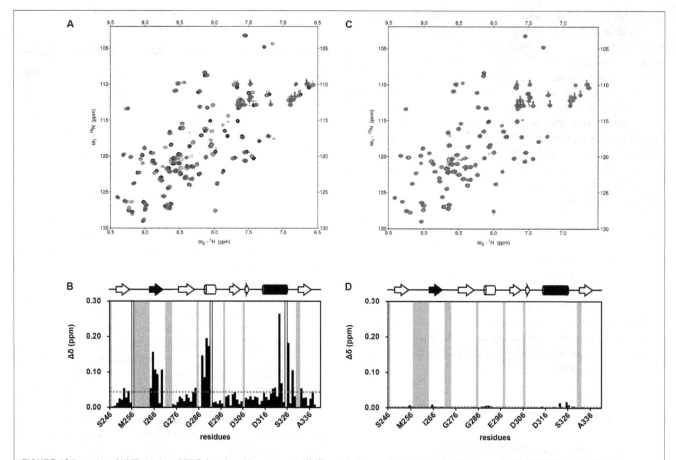

FIGURE 4 | Examples of NMR titration of PDZ domains with compounds **(A,C)** and their normalized chemical shift changes **(B,D)**. **(A,B)** NPL-3009. **(C,D)** NPL-3003. **(A,C)** each overlaid spectrum was derived from 0.1 mM hDvl1-PDZ with (red) and without (black) the 0.2 mM of compound. The signals with markedly large CSPs were boxed and indicated with the residue numbers. **(B,D)** normalized chemical shift changes Δδ is plotted against residue numbers. Gray residues are missing or unassigned residues, and white residues indicate Pro. The secondary structure of hDvl1-PDZ is shown at the top of the figures, whereas α2 and β2 are shown in black.

and j is the name of the compounds. Similarly, the averaged normalized NMR chemical shift change, $N(j)$, was calculated. Finally, NMR-DPI was defined as

$$NMR\_DPI(i) = sqrt\left(\sum^{j}\left(D\left(i,j\right) - N\left(j\right)\right)^2\right) \quad (2)$$

The heat map representation of all docking scores of the 17 compounds with nine scoring functions in GOLD and the normalized averaged NMR chemical shift change for 18 compounds is shown in **Figure 5B**. A bar graph of NMR_DPI is portrayed in **Figure 5C**. The lowest NMR_DPI, which represents the best correlation between the docking score and the NMR CSP experiments, was achieved when the consensus scoring of GS followed by CS was selected.

Advanced Virtual Screening of hDvl1-PDZ Domain Inhibitors

Consensus scoring GS-CS in this order was chosen to perform the advanced VS experiment with GOLD and the specified library, including approximately 5,135 N-substituted-2-amino-benzoic acid compounds. We obtained a list containing 1,770 compounds with scores higher than that of CalBioChem-322338 (score = 59.9). After the selected compounds were purchased (**Figure 6**), they were assessed using NMR-CSP experiments to ascertain whether they were able to bind hDvl1-PDZ. Among them, nine compounds (NPL-4001, 4002, 4004, 4007, and 4011–4016) induced substantial chemical shift changes when added to hDvl1-PDZ: 7 out of 13 (69%) compounds had reasonable affinity against hDvl1-PDZ (**Supplementary Table S1**). Some HSQC spectra are presented in **Supplementary Figure S2** with their chemical structures. The hit rate (69%) is remarkably high, emphasizing the benefit of introducing NMR-DPI combined with VS.

Assessing Physicochemical Properties of the Most Potent hDvl1-PDZ Inhibitor: NPL-4011

Among the 13 newly examined compounds, four (NPL-4007, 4011, 4012, and 4013) possessed a common molecular architecture, with two 2-amino-benzoic acid moieties connected

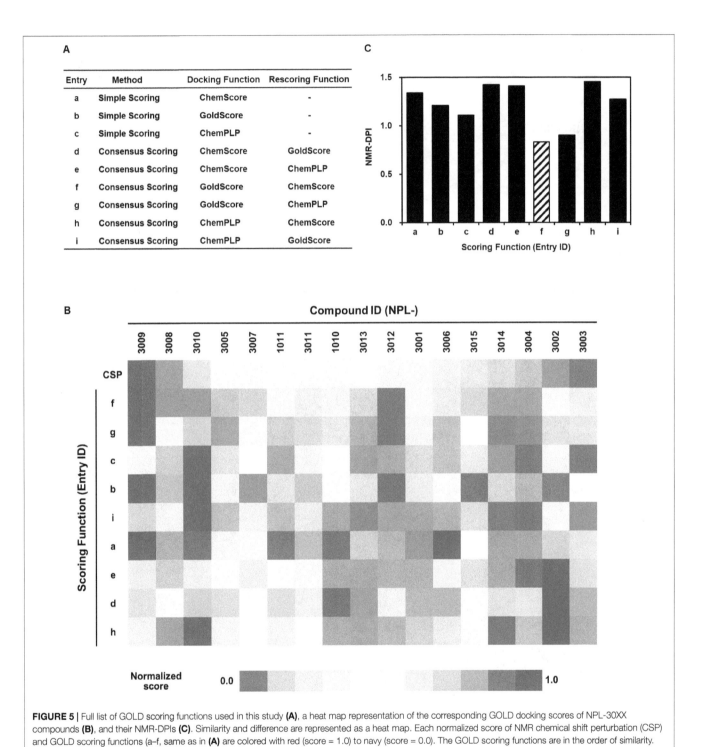

FIGURE 5 | Full list of GOLD scoring functions used in this study **(A)**, a heat map representation of the corresponding GOLD docking scores of NPL-30XX compounds **(B)**, and their NMR-DPIs **(C)**. Similarity and difference are represented as a heat map. Each normalized score of NMR chemical shift perturbation (CSP) and GOLD scoring functions (a–f, same as in **(A)** are colored with red (score = 1.0) to navy (score = 0.0). The GOLD scoring functions are in the order of similarity.

at the 5-position directly or with a single methylene linker (**Figure 6**). NPL-4011 showed a large GOLD VS docking score as well as CSP. Therefore, we determined its K_D further against hDvl1-PDZ using NMR titration experiments (**Figure 7A** and **Supplementary Figure S3A**). First we selected the residues surrounding the ligand binding pocket: D315, V318, L321, R322, and V325. The normalized chemical shift changes of these residues were subjected to non-linear curve fitting to find K_D

(**Figure 7B**), which was 34.5 ± 6.6 μM. Then we compared this value to the commercially available control compound CalBioChem-322338 under the same condition and obtained the value of 954 ± 403 μM (**Supplementary Figures S3C,D**). This K_D value of CalBioChem-322338 is larger than its reported value for mouse Dvl1-PDZ (10.6 ± 1.7 μM) (Grandy et al., 2009) for reasons that remain unknown. Results show that NPL-4011 is a stronger inhibitor than CalBioChem-322338

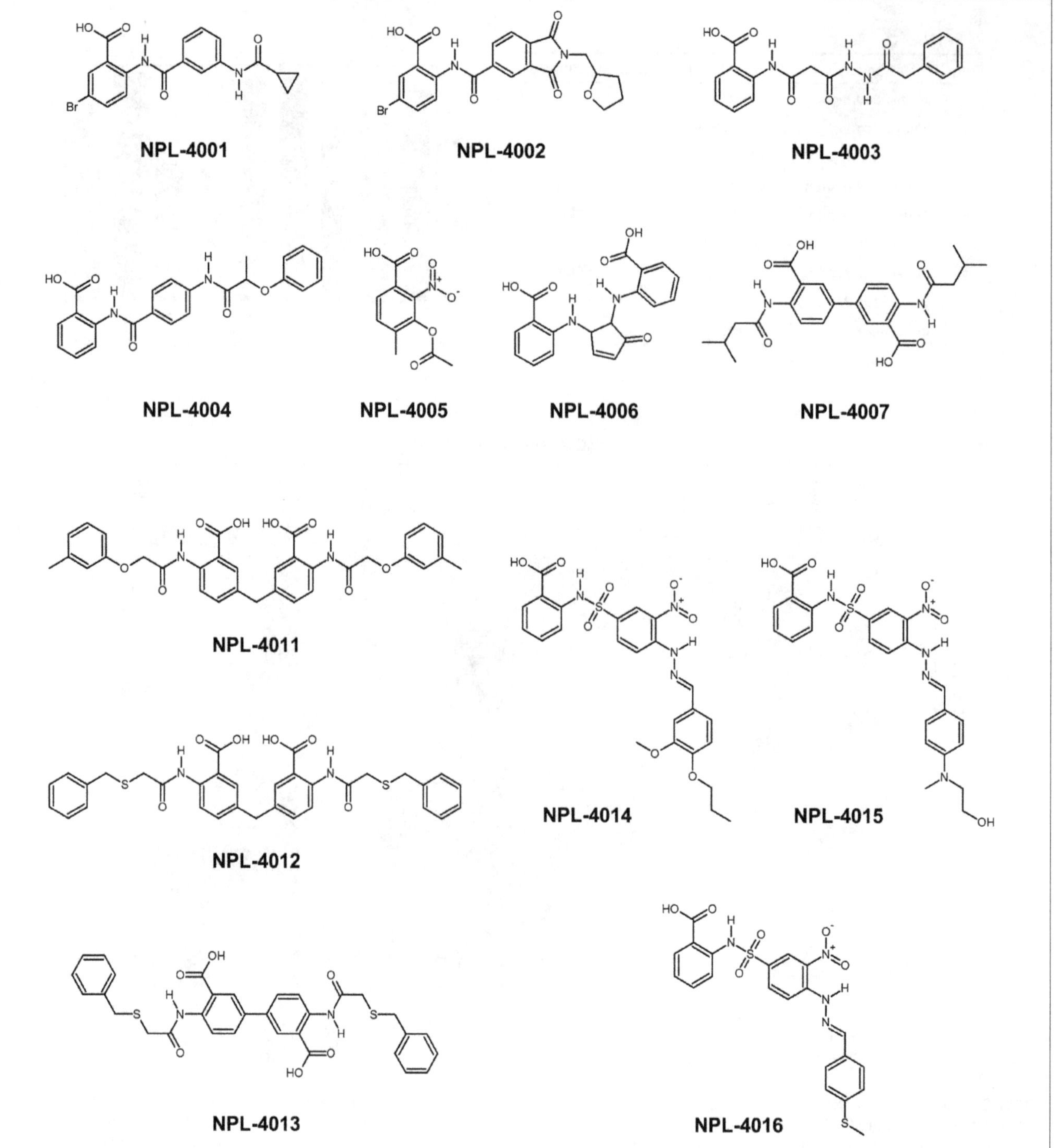

FIGURE 6 | Chemical structure of newly found Dvl-PDZ inhibitor candidates.

when compared under identical conditions using hDvl1-PDZ.

Next, we carefully assessed the docking model of NPL-4011 and Dvl-PDZ generated by GOLD (**Figure 7C**). In the model, the crescent-shaped molecule NPL-4011 is well suited to the long shallow cleft of the ligand binding site of Dvl-PDZ. The residues of hDvl2-PDZ which contact to NPL-4011 are consistent with the residues that showed substantial CSPs at the NMR titration experiments (**Figure 7D**). We examined this binding model further. The lower half part of the symmetrical NPL-4011 molecule fits to the lower half part of the ligand binding cleft of Dvl-PDZ, which corresponds to the "canonical" C-terminal binding pocket common for all other PDZ domains. The upper half part of NPL-4011 also fits to the cleft between two loops:

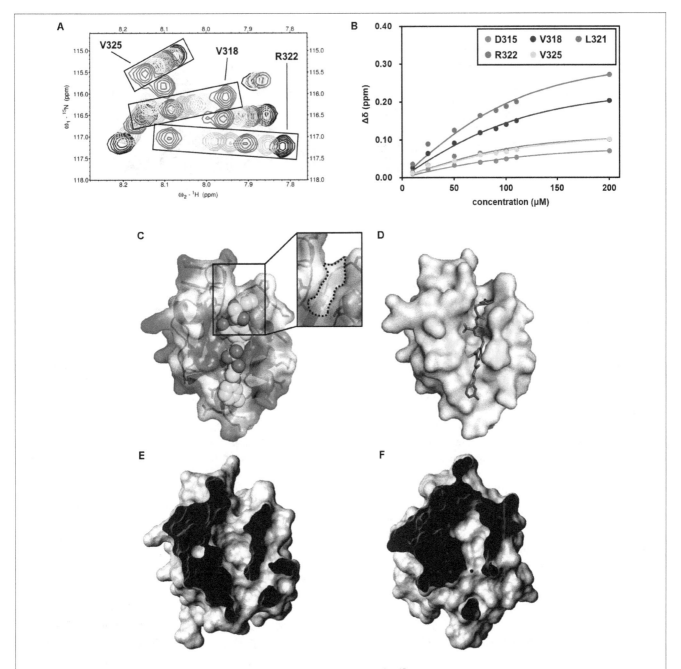

FIGURE 7 | NMR titration experiment of hDvl1-PDZ with NPL-4011. **(A)** Expanded region of ^{1}H–^{15}N HSQC spectra of hDvl1-PDZ with 0 equation. (black), 0.25 equation. (pink), 0.5 equation. (navy), 0.75 equation. (green), 1.0 equation. (orange), 1.2 equation. (yellow), and 2.0 equation. (red) of NPL-4011 were overlaid. The assignments of the signal series are labeled. **(B)** Normalized chemical shift changes of the selected hDvl1-PDZ residues upon titration with NPL-4011. Solid lines indicate the non-linear fitting curves of each signals based on the single-site binding model. **(C)** Example of docking models of hDvl2-PDZ with NPL-4011 predicted by GOLD. The Dvl-PDZ unique cleft is boxed and colored yellow (inset). **(D)** CSPs induced by NPL-4011 binding are mapped on the surface structure of hDvl2-PDZ. **(E,F)** Surface representations of hDvl2-PDZ **(E)** and mouse ZO-1 PDZ1 **(F)** clipped by a front plane. The clipping size is 13.5 Å and the clipped position is 6.5 Å. Many PDZ domains do not possess the groove corresponding to Dvl-PDZ unique cleft which was clearly seen in **(E)**.

β1–β2 loop and α2-β6 loop. This upper cleft is unique to Dvl-PDZ domain (**Figures 7D,E**), which might accommodate binding to "non-canonical" ligands such as the cytosolic regions of Fzd, the physiological partner of Dvl. **Figure 7F** is an example of a close-up view of the representative "canonical" class-III PDZ domain, the first PDZ domain of mouse ZO-1 (mZO1-PDZ1,

PDB:2RRM). The domain does not possess the cleft above the canonical ligand binding pocket because the loop between β1–β2 bends upon and contacts to the end of α2-helix.

This structural difference between Dvl-PDZ and mZO1-PDZ1 invites our speculation that, because of steric crash between the half part of the ligand and the bended β1–β2 loop, NPL-4011

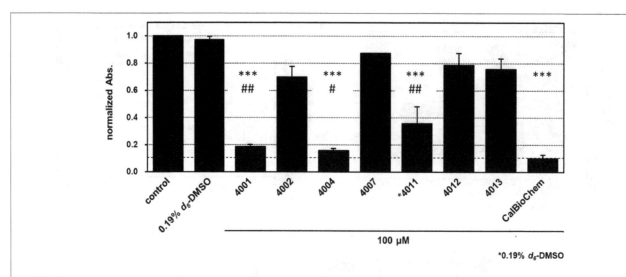

FIGURE 8 | Cell proliferation inhibition of BT-20 triple negative breast cancer cell with indicated compounds, NPL-40XX and CalBioChem-322338. The cells were incubated with 100 μM indicated compounds including final 0.1% d_6-DMSO. Control cells was incubated with the medium containing 0.1% d_6-DMSO. NPL-4011 was examined in the presence of 0.19% d_6-DMSO. The results of normalized absorbance of WST-8 assay with standard deviation were indicated. ***$p < 0.001$ vs. comtrol (0.1 or 0.19% DMSO), ##$p < 0.01$ vs. CalBioCHem-322338, and #$p < 0.05$ vs. CalBioChem-322338, respectively.

(and probably its related molecules, NPL-4007, 4012, and 4013) might not bind mZO1-PDZ1. Instead, the smaller prototype Dvl-PDZ inhibitor CalBioChem-322338 can bind mZO1-PDZ1 because it might only occupy the canonical ligand binding pocket of mZO1-PDZ1 without steric stress. In other words, NPL-4011 is among the more Dvl-specific PDZ domain inhibitors. In order to confirm this speculation, we further performed additional NMR-CSP experiments of mZO1-PDZ1 titrated with NPL-4011 and CalBioChem-322338 (**Supplementary Figure S4**). Assignment of backbone signals were taken from our previous study (Umetsu et al., 2007). In the presence of two equivalent of NPL-4011, mZO1-PDZ1 did not show any chemical shift changes. In contrast, the signals from the residues surrounding the canonical binding site of mZO1-PDZ1 showed substantial CSP upon CalBioChem-322338. Thus, the unique molecular shape of NPL-4011 confined its binding to Dvl-PDZ in more specific manner.

Assessment of Biological Activities of NPL-40XX Compounds

We assessed the inhibitory activity of the selected NPL-40XX compounds toward Wnt signaling pathways in the cultured-cell-based assay. For this purpose, we used BT-20 cell, a triple negative breast cancer (TNBC) cell line. Activation of Wnt signaling pathway is often observed in many cancers. Therefore, Wnt pathway inhibition is a potential therapeutic strategy (Polakis, 2012). Reportedly, activation of Wnt/β-catenin pathway has been observed in TNBC (Geyer et al., 2011; King et al., 2012a,b). For BT-20 cell, overexpression of Fzd 7 (Fzd7) has been reported; shRNA against Fzd7 suppresses the proliferation of BT-20 efficiently (Yang et al., 2011).

We applied cell-based proliferation inhibition assay to concentrations of 100 μM of the compounds, including NPL-4001, 4002, 4004, 4007, 4011–4013, and the control

compounds CalBioChem-322338 (**Figure 8** and **Supplementary Figure S5**). After 4 days of culture with 100 μM of the compounds, NPL-4001 and NPL-4004 showed approximately 80% inhibition of BT-20 cell proliferation, although NPL-4002, 4007, 4012, and 4013 showed no remarkable inhibitory activity. The stronger inhibitor NPL-4011 showed only 60% inhibition, which is less potent to 4001 and 4004. In this condition, the positive control CalBioChem-322338 showed better proliferation inhibitory activity, as 90% inhibition. The results demonstrated that our compound NPL-4011 must provide further improvement in terms of cell-based anticancer activity, although affinity against the target domain was highly optimized.

DISCUSSION

Experimental Aspect of the NMR-Derived Docking Performance Index (NMR-DPI) for Dvl-PDZ Domain Inhibitor Screening

A common tradeoff that arises is that between accurate prediction of binding free energy ΔG in VS and the speed of calculation. Researchers must always confront the dilemmas of "rapidity–inaccuracy" and "sluggishness–accuracy" to process as many compounds as possible during a given period, simplified scoring functions should be chosen rather than the first principle-based force field in simulations between the target protein and ligands. In doing so, although such simplified scoring functions might all be equally inaccurate, eventually some scoring function can be expected to behave better than another for the specified library of the specified compounds. This study demonstrated an experimental strategy to select a better scoring function from the options presented by the GOLD program suite.

For this study, we used the averaged normalized chemical shift changes, $\Delta\delta_{ave}$, instead of K_D for each of 17 training set molecules: 89% (15/17) of them bound to hDvl1-PDZ. According to theory, the maximum value of CSP should be recorded at the saturation point of titration by compounds. At that time, the maximum CSP might vary depending on the chemical structure of ligands. For example, aromatic rings in the ligand might induce larger CSPs upon binding because of the ring current effect. Another important shortcoming of CSP is that it is sensitive to the allosteric conformational changes of the target protein upon ligand binding. Consequently, generally, it is not recommended to use $\Delta\delta_{ave}$ (or other CSP-derived parameters) as an indication of K_D. Irrespective of those shortcomings of CSP, however, we used $\Delta\delta_{ave}$ for this study based on the following two criteria. (1) Only compounds with similar chemical structure were analyzed and compared using $\Delta\delta_{ave}$. (2) Under the experimental conditions we used, the affinity of most ligands was weak. Moreover, they did not saturate to bind against hDvl1-PDZ at 1:2 molecular equivalence. We carefully assessed our experimental system using these two criteria. Finally, we inferred that if the criteria are satisfied, then the use of $\Delta\delta_{ave}$ as an indication of K_D is convenient. Note that it was not feasible to use thermal shift assay to infer the affinity of the compounds in our case because many PDZ domains including hDvl1-PDZ showed no sharp T_m transition curve. In addition, although the CSP experiment requires stable-isotope labeling, the experiment is less troublesome than those of the surface plasmon resonance experiment because it is unnecessary to immobilize the protein to the chip. Accordingly, information of amide NMR signals enables us to discern specific binding from non-specific binding.

Comparison of Biological Activities of NPL-40XX Compounds

Results show that NPL-4011 has stronger affinity against hDvl1-PDZ *in vitro*, but it was a less potent cell growth inhibitor against BT-20 cell than CalBioChem-322338 was. To elucidate this observation in terms of bioavailability, we compared Lipinski's drug-likeness parameters (Lipinski, 2000). The molecular weight of NPL-4011 (580.593) is greater than that of CalBioChem-322338 (373.388). The numbers of H-bond donors are equal (2), although the number of H-bond acceptors of NPL-4011 (8) is double that of CalBioChem-322338 (4). These two parameters violate Lipinski's rule of five. Although the calculated logP-value (1.53 for NPL-4011 and 2.59 for CalBioChem-322338) is the only merit of NPL-4011, it did not contribute to overcoming the other shortcoming. Therefore, we infer that the poor biological activity of NPL-4011 is attributable to its bioavailability. This assumption is partially supported by our other observation. As described above, NPL-4001 and 4004 showed comparable growth inhibition activity to CalBioChem-322338. They are better than NPL-4011. Their Lipinski parameters are, respectively, 402.224 and 403.414 (MW), 1.75, and 2.05 (logP), 2 and 2 (H-bond donors), and 4 and 5 (H-bond acceptors). The numbers of donors and acceptors of H-bond are known to be crucially important to infer biological activity from the cell-based assay.

By contrast, NPL-4011 is expected to be more selective for Dvl-PDZ than the other PDZ domains in human cells because the crescent-shaped molecule fits to the unique cleft of Dvl-PDZ domains. The PDZ domain is the most abundant modular domain in human cell cytosol. Therefore, design of highly specific molecules to one specified PDZ domain might become crucially important. To satisfy both the specificity and the biological activity in terms of bioavailability, a good starting point is our new pharmacophore: bis-benzoic acid moiety. Screening smaller analogs such as NPL-4007 as the seed is better to improve the biological activity of this group of compounds. By contrast, a prodrug strategy starting from NPL-4011 is not recommended because it has already exceeded the drug-likeness parameters.

CONCLUSION

In conclusion, we demonstrated a series of new class of compounds with higher affinity against hDvl1-PDZ. We proposed NMR-DPI as a useful experimental indication to optimize VS in the early stages of drug discovery.

AUTHOR CONTRIBUTIONS

KH and TT performed all the NMR titration experiments and discovered the inhibitors. KH also performed all the cell-based assays assisted by NG and AS. KA initiated the NMR signal assignment of hDvl1 and hDvl2 PDZ domains, whereas KH completed it. NG and TT prepared the plasmid constructs and protein samples of the optimized PDZ domains. The cell and developmental biologists MT and AS designed all the biological assays, set them up, and organized the biological part of the manuscript. HH constructed the focused library, developed the idea of NMR-based DPI, and performed VS. HH wrote the manuscript and organized the project.

FUNDING

This work was supported in part by the Target Protein Research Program from Japan Science and Technology Agency (JST), A-step feasibility study program (AS262Z01275Q and AS242Z00566Q) from JST, Japan Society for the Promotion of Science KAKENHI (15H04337), and the AMED-PDIS from Japan Agency for Medical Research and Development (AMED). This work was also supported by the Princess Takamatsu Cancer Research Fund (15-24726).

ACKNOWLEDGMENTS

The authors would like to thank Fastek Ltd. (Sendai, Miyagi, Japan; http://www.fastekjapan.com/) for the English language review.

REFERENCES

Choi, J., Ma, S., Kim, H.-Y., Yun, J.-H., Heo, J.-N., Lee, W., et al. (2016). Identification of small-molecule compounds targeting the dishevelled PDZ domain by virtual screening and binding studies. *Bioorg. Med. Chem.* 24, 3259–3266. doi: 10.1016/j.bmc.2016.03.026

Delaglio, F., Grzesiek, S., Vuister, G. W., Zhu, G., Pfeifer, J., and Bax, A. (1995). NMRPipe: a multidimensional spectral processing system based on UNIX pipes. *J. Biomol. NMR* 6, 277–293. doi: 10.1007/BF00197809

Friesner, R. A., Banks, J. L., Murphy, R. B., Halgren, T. A., Klicic, J. J., Mainz, D. T., et al. (2004). Glide: a new approach for rapid, accurate docking and scoring. 1. Method and assessment of docking accuracy. *J. Med. Chem.* 47, 1739–1749. doi: 10.1021/jm0306430

Fujii, N., You, L., Xu, Z., Uematsu, K., Shan, J., He, B., et al. (2007). An antagonist of dishevelled protein-protein interaction suppresses -catenin-dependent tumor cell growth. *Cancer Res.* 67, 573–579. doi: 10.1158/0008-5472.CAN-06-2726

Fukunishi, Y., Mikami, Y., and Nakamura, H. (2005). Similarities among receptor pockets and among compounds: analysis and application to in silico ligand screening. *J. Mol. Graph. Model.* 24, 34–45. doi: 10.1016/j.jmgm.2005.04.004

Gao, C., and Chen, Y. G. (2010). Dishevelled: the hub of Wnt signaling. *Cell. Signal.* 22, 717–727. doi: 10.1016/j.cellsig.2009.11.021

Geyer, F. C., Lacroix-Triki, M., Savage, K., Arnedos, M., Lambros, M. B., MacKay, A., et al. (2011). B-Catenin pathway activation in breast cancer is associated with triple-negative phenotype but not with CTNNB1 mutation. *Mod. Pathol.* 24, 209–231. doi: 10.1038/modpathol.2010.205

Goda, N., Tenno, T., Takasu, H., Hiroaki, H., and Shirakawa, M. (2004). The PRESAT-vector: asymmetric T-vector for high-throughput screening of soluble protein domains for structural proteomics. *Protein Sci.* 13, 652–658. doi: 10. 1110/ps.03439004

Goddard, T. D., and Kneller, D. G. (2004). *Sparky 3, 2004, University of California, San Francisco.* Available at: http://www.cgl.ucsf.edu/home/sparky/

Goodsell, D. S., Morris, G. M., and Olson, A. J. (1996). Automated docking of flexible ligands: applications of AutoDock. *J. Mol. Recognit.* 9, 1–5. doi: 10.1002/ (SICI)1099-1352(199601)9:1<1::AID-JMR241>3.0.CO;2-6

Goto, J., Kataoka, R., Muta, H., and Hirayama, N. (2008). ASEDock-docking based on alpha spheres and excluded volumes. *J. Chem. Inf. Model.* 48, 583–590. doi: 10.1021/ci700352q

Grandy, D., Shan, J., Zhang, X., Rao, S., Akunuru, S., Li, H., et al. (2009). Discovery and characterization of a small molecule inhibitor of the PDZ domain of dishevelled. *J. Biol. Chem.* 284, 16256–16263. doi: 10.1074/jbc.M109.00 9647

Hiroaki, H., Umetsu, Y., Nabeshima, Y., Hoshi, M., and Kohda, D. (2011). A simplified recipe for assigning amide NMR signals using combinatorial 14N amino acid inverse-labeling. *J. Struct. Funct. Genomics* 12, 167–174. doi: 10. 1007/s10969-011-9116-0

Holland, J. D., Klaus, A., Garratt, A. N., and Birchmeier, W. (2013). Wnt signaling in stem and cancer stem cells. *Curr. Opin. Cell Biol.* 25, 254–264. doi: 10.1016/j. ceb.2013.01.004

Huang, Z., and Wong, C. F. (2016). Inexpensive method for selecting receptor structures for virtual screening. *J. Chem. Inf. Model.* 56, 21–34. doi: 10.1021/ acs.jcim.5b00299

Ikura, M., Kay, L. E., and Bax, A. (1990). A novel approach for sequential assignment of 1H, 13C, and 15N spectra of larger proteins: heteronuclear triple-resonance three-dimensional NMR spectroscopy. Application to calmodulin. *Biochemistry* 29, 4659–4667. doi: 10.1021/bi00471a022

Jung, Y.-S. S., and Zweckstetter, M. (2004). Mars - Robust automatic backbone assignment of proteins. *J. Biomol. NMR* 30, 11–23. doi: 10.1023/B:JNMR. 0000042954.99056.ad

Kawabata, T., Sugihara, Y., Fukunishi, Y., and Nakamura, H. (2013). LigandBox: a database for 3D structures of chemical compounds. *Biophysics* 9, 113–121. doi: 10.2142/biophysics.9.113

King, T. D., Suto, M. J., and Li, Y. (2012a). The wnt/β-catenin signaling pathway: a potential therapeutic target in the treatment of triple negative breast cancer. *J. Cell. Biochem.* 113, 13–18. doi: 10.1002/jcb.23350

King, T. D., Zhang, W., Suto, M. J., and Li, Y. (2012b). Frizzled7 as an emerging target for cancer therapy. *Cell. Signal.* 24, 846–851. doi: 10.1016/j.cellsig.2011. 12.009

Kinoshita, K., Murakami, Y., and Nakamura, H. (2007). eF-seek: prediction of the functional sites of proteins by searching for similar electrostatic potential and molecular surface shape. *Nucleic Acids Res.* 35, W398–W402. doi: 10.1093/nar/ gkm351

Lee, H.-J., Wang, N. X., Shao, Y., and Zheng, J. J. (2009a). Identification of tripeptides recognized by the PDZ domain of Dishevelled. *Bioorg. Med. Chem.* 17, 1701–1708. doi: 10.1016/j.bmc.2008.12.060

Lee, H.-J., Wang, N. X., Shi, D.-L., and Zheng, J. J. (2009b). Sulindac Inhibits Canonical Wnt Signaling by Blocking the PDZ Domain of the Protein Dishevelled. *Angew. Chem. Int. Ed. Engl.* 48, 6448–6452. doi: 10.1002/anie. 200902981

Lindh, M., Svensson, F., Schaal, W., Zhang, J., Sköld, C., Brandt, P., et al. (2015). Toward a benchmarking data set able to evaluate ligand- and structure-based virtual screening using public HTS data. *J. Chem. Inf. Model.* 55, 343–353. doi: 10.1021/ci5005465

Lipinski, C. A. (2000). Drug-like properties and the causes of poor solubility and poor permeability. *J. Pharmacol. Toxicol. Methods* 44, 235–249. doi: 10.1016/ S1056-8719(00)00107-6

McGann, M. (2011). FRED pose prediction and virtual screening accuracy. *J. Chem. Inf. Model.* 51, 578–596. doi: 10.1021/ci100436p

McGaughey, G. B., Sheridan, R. P., Bayly, C. I., Culberson, J. C., Kreatsoulas, C., Lindsley, S., et al. (2007). Comparison of topological, shape, and docking methods in virtual screening. *J. Chem. Inf. Model.* 47, 1504–1519. doi: 10.1021/ ci700052x

Motono, C., Nakata, J., Koike, R., Shimizu, K., Shirota, M., Amemiya, T., et al. (2011). SAHG, a comprehensive database of predicted structures of all human proteins. *Nucleic Acids Res.* 39, D487–D493. doi: 10.1093/nar/gkq 1057

Polakis, P. (2012). Drugging Wnt signalling in cancer. *EMBO J.* 31, 2737–2746. doi: 10.1038/emboj.2012.126

Reya, T., and Clevers, H. (2005). Wnt signalling in stem cells and cancer. *Nature* 434, 843–850. doi: 10.1038/nature03319

Schrödinger, L. L. C. (2015). *The {PyMOL} Molecular Graphics System, Version~1.8.*

Shan, J., Shi, D.-L., Wang, J., and Zheng, J. (2005). Identification of a Specific Inhibitor of the Dishevelled PDZ Domain †. *Biochemistry* 44, 15495–15503. doi: 10.1021/bi0512602

Takebe, N., Harris, P. J., Warren, R. Q., and Ivy, S. P. (2011). Targeting cancer stem cells by inhibiting Wnt, Notch, and Hedgehog pathways. *Nat. Rev. Clin. Oncol.* 8, 97–106. doi: 10.1038/nrclinonc.2010.196

Tannishtha, R., Morrison, S. J., Clarke, M. F., and Weissman, I. L. (2001). Stem cells, cancer, and cancer stem cells. *Nature* 414, 105–111. doi: 10.1007/978-1-60327-933-8

Tenno, T., Goda, N., Umetsu, Y., Ota, M., Kinoshita, K., and Hiroaki, H. (2013). Accidental interaction between PDZ domains and diclofenac revealed by NMR-assisted virtual screening. *Molecules* 18, 9567–9581. doi: 10.3390/ molecules18089567

Trott, O., and Olson, A. J. (2010). AutoDock Vina. *J. Comput. Chem.* 31, 445–461. doi: 10.1002/jcc.21334

Umetsu, Y., Goda, N., Taniguchi, R., Satomura, K., Ikegami, T., Furuse, M., et al. (2007). Assignment of 1H, 13C and 15N resonances of N-terminal domain of DnaA protein. *Biomol. NMR Assign.* 1, 57–59. doi: 10.1007/s12104-007-9015-2

Umetsu, Y., Goda, N., Taniguchi, R., Satomura, K., Ikegami, T., Furuse, M., et al. (2011). 1H, 13C, and 15N resonance assignment of the first PDZ domain of mouse ZO-1. *Biomol. NMR Assign.* 5, 207–210. doi: 10.1007/s12104-011-9301-x

Verdonk, M. L., Cole, J. C., Hartshorn, M. J., Murray, C. W., and Taylor, R. D. (2003). Improved protein-ligand docking using GOLD. *Proteins* 52, 609–623. doi: 10.1002/prot.10465

Visvader, J. E., and Lindeman, G. J. (2008). Cancer stem cells in solid tumours: accumulating evidence and unresolved questions. *Nat. Rev. Cancer* 8, 755–768. doi: 10.1038/nrc2499

Wang, Z., Sun, H., Yao, X., Li, D., Xu, L., Li, Y., et al. (2016). Comprehensive evaluation of ten docking programs on a diverse set of protein-ligand complexes: the prediction accuracy of sampling power and scoring power. *Phys. Chem. Chem. Phys.* 18, 12964–12975. doi: 10.1039/c6cp01 555g

Discovery of Potent Disheveled/Dvl Inhibitors Using Virtual Screening Optimized with NMR-Based Docking...

95

Williamson, M. P. (2013). Using chemical shift perturbation to characterise ligand binding. *Prog. Nucl. Magn. Reson. Spectrosc.* 73, 1–16. doi: 10.1016/j.pnmrs.2013.02.001

Wong, H.-C., Bourdelas, A., Krauss, A., Lee, H.-J., Shao, Y., Wu, D., et al. (2003). Direct binding of the PDZ domain of Dishevelled to a conserved internal sequence in the C-terminal region of Frizzled. *Mol. Cell* 12, 1251–1260. doi: 10.1016/S1097-2765(03)00427-1

Yang, L., Wu, X., Wang, Y., Zhang, K., Wu, J., Yuan, Y.-C., et al. (2011). FZD7 has a critical role in cell proliferation in triple negative breast cancer. *Oncogene* 30, 4437–4446. doi: 10.1038/onc.2011.145

Zhang, Y., Appleton, B. A., Wiesmann, C., Lau, T., Costa, M., Hannoush, R. N., et al. (2009). Inhibition of Wnt signaling by Dishevelled PDZ peptides. *Nat. Chem. Biol.* 5, 217–219. doi: 10.1038/nchembio.152

Development of an Infrastructure for the Prediction of Biological Endpoints in Industrial Environments: Lessons Learned at the eTOX Project

Manuel Pastor*, Jordi Quintana and Ferran Sanz*

Research Programme on Biomedical Informatics (GRIB), Institut Hospital del Mar d'Investigacions Mèdiques (IMIM), Department of Experimental and Health Sciences, Universitat Pompeu Fabra, Barcelona, Spain

Correspondence:
Manuel Pastor
manuel.pastor@upf.edu
Ferran Sanz
ferran.sanz@upf.edu

In silico methods are increasingly being used for assessing the chemical safety of substances, as a part of integrated approaches involving *in vitro* and *in vivo* experiments. A paradigmatic example of these strategies is the eTOX project http://www.etoxproject.eu, funded by the European Innovative Medicines Initiative (IMI), which aimed at producing high quality predictions of *in vivo* toxicity of drug candidates and resulted in generating about 200 models for diverse endpoints of toxicological interest. In an industry-oriented project like eTOX, apart from the predictive quality, the models need to meet other quality parameters related to the procedures for their generation and their intended use. For example, when the models are used for predicting the properties of drug candidates, the prediction system must guarantee the complete confidentiality of the compound structures. The interface of the system must be designed to provide non-expert users all the information required to choose the models and appropriately interpret the results. Moreover, procedures like installation, maintenance, documentation, validation and versioning, which are common in software development, must be also implemented for the models and for the prediction platform in which they are implemented. In this article we describe our experience in the eTOX project and the lessons learned after 7 years of close collaboration between industrial and academic partners. We believe that some of the solutions found and the tools developed could be useful for supporting similar initiatives in the future.

Keywords: *in silico* toxicology, computational toxicology, predictive models, chemical safety, drug safety, industrial environments, public-private partnership, machine learning

INTRODUCTION

In silico methods are increasingly being used in the assessment of the chemical safety of chemicals as a part of integrated approaches, in which computational tools are used to synergically complement the experimental methods, with the aim of generating better and more efficient predictions of the potential toxicological liabilities of the compounds under study (Luechtefeld et al., 2018). Recent advances in machine learning and deep learning methodologies are demonstrating their effectiveness in this respect (Lenselink et al., 2017; Liu et al., 2017). Moreover, ambitious collaborative initiatives in this field have been set up with the aim of increasing the availability of relevant data frameworks and developing the aforementioned integrative approaches on top of those data. Among these initiatives, EU-ToxRisk (Daneshian et al., 2016), HESS (Sakuratani et al., 2013), TransQST (Maldonado et al., 2017), iPiE (Bravo et al., 2016) and eTOX (Cases et al., 2014; Sanz et al., 2017; Steger-Hartmann and Pognan, 2018) deserve to be highlighted.

In particular, the eTOX project, funded by the Innovative Medicines Initiative, constituted a pioneering exercise of extracting and integrating *in vivo* data from legacy resources at the pharmaceutical industry, and exploiting such data for read-across and the development of predictive models, since one of the aims of the eTOX project was to set up an integrated system for the prediction of toxicological endpoints, with a focus on organ and *in vivo* endpoints. The project faced many challenges, some of which have been described in previous publications (Cases et al., 2014; Sanz et al., 2015, 2017; Steger-Hartmann and Pognan, 2018). Here we wish to share our experiences in an aspect that is often overlooked in this kind of projects, which is how to translate predictive models generated by academia or by Small-Medium Enterprises (SMEs) into a production environment where they can be routinely applied. Irrespectively of the scientific quality of a model, it must meet several requirements to make it amenable for being used by the pharmaceutical industry. This requires building a common understanding between academic and industrial partners, identifying the end-user needs, and making significant efforts to incorporate into the models and the predictive system features that, in spite of their low scientific interest, make the difference between usable and not usable models. In the present article we describe the most significant lessons learned in eTOX, describing some of the problems we identified and describing the solutions applied to solve or mitigate them. Most of these solutions are the result of long hours of discussion, where we learned to understand each other's points of view.

RESULTS

Developing a computational model for predicting a biological endpoint is a complex task. In the case of QSAR-like models, their development involves (at least) the curation of the training series, the selection of appropriate molecular descriptors and machine learning methods, building, validation, and interpretation of the model. However, when the aim is to produce a model that can be used by people outside of the modeler's laboratory, the work has not finished with the generation of the model. There is an additional difficulty if we intend to use the models in industrial environments, particularly if the structures of the compounds should be treated as confidential.

In the following sections we will discuss issues related with the model development and implementation, the need of a standard modeling framework for supporting model development and maintenance, as well as the model documentation and validation.

In the last section we will discuss also the problems related with the confidentiality of the structures for model training and application.

Platform for Model Development and Production

Most of the eTOX models were developed by academic partners and SMEs, located in different European countries. Therefore, the architecture of the system to be developed should support independent and concurrent model development, while model prototypes should be made accessible to the end users (pharmaceutical companies) for early testing. This software platform, designed to increase the model development efficiency, should be compatible with the local deployment of the final system. The final version must be installed physically at the computational resources of the pharmaceutical companies, since the end users considered that only an installation behind the company firewalls guarantees that they could be used on highly confidential compounds corresponding to drug candidates under development.

These requirements made necessary the adoption of technical solutions that facilitate the remote access to the models and the portability of its software implementation, which consisted of two layers of containerization. The outer layer consisted in a self-contained virtual machine (VM), configured to expose a REpresentational State Transfer (REST) web service (Fielding, 2000) to predict the properties of query compounds. VMs were installed at the partners facilities, thus making possible that models developed at remote sites were immediately accessible through a centralized web server which shows all available models through a single graphical interface (see **Figure 1**). The physical location of the server running the computations was completely transparent to the end user.

Figure 2 shows a schematic representation of the setup that was adopted for the development and production of the eTOX models.

The eTOX development setup has the inconvenience that it cannot guarantee an appropriate level of confidentiality on the query structures. These are sent over the Internet, and the computations are carried out in academic servers, some of which do not comply with the strict security requirements necessary to protect confidential structures. For this reason, the testing of the models was carried out using only non-confidential structures and the user interface shows a disclaimer informing of the security risks.

The final version of the system, as mentioned before, was installed locally at the computational facilities of the EFPIA partners (**Figure 2**). The deployment of the system was facilitated by the use of VMs, which can run in heterogeneous computational environments (i.e., diverse operative systems and hardware configurations). The VMs were relatively compact (between 4 and 5 Gb each) and did not have high computational needs (recommended settings were 1 CPU and 2 Gb RAM per VM). The whole system can be accommodated in low-end computational clusters or even in an isolated server with multiple CPUs.

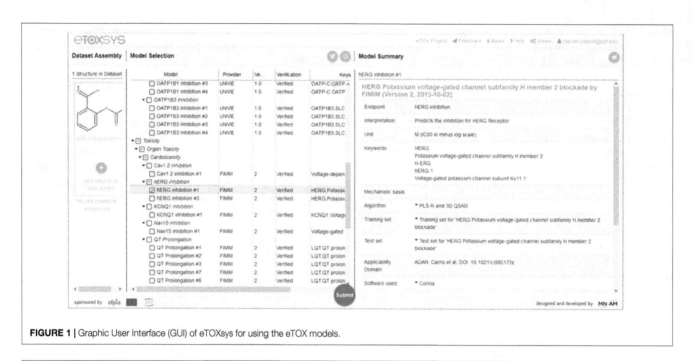

FIGURE 1 | Graphic User Interface (GUI) of eTOXsys for using the eTOX models.

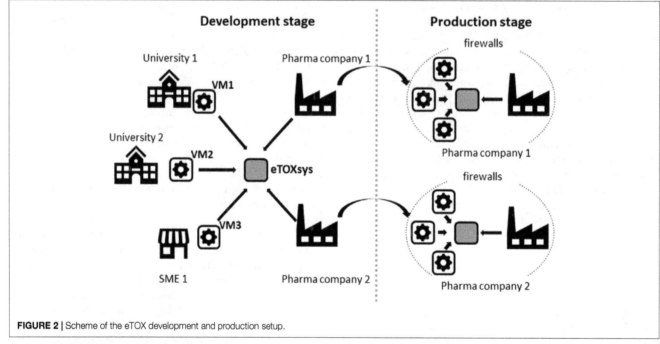

FIGURE 2 | Scheme of the eTOX development and production setup.

In the same way that the VMs provided a layer of standardization for the external access to the models, we had the need of developing an *ad hoc* modeling framework, called eTOXlab (Carrió et al., 2015), which supports modelers in their task of implementing and maintaining the predictive models within the VMs. Essentially, each VM contains an instance of eTOXlab, which can manage multiple models and exposes them as web services using a standard Application Programming Interface (API), as shown in **Figure 3**. All the model inputs and outputs are redirected trough the web services. Therefore, as far as the models are correctly implemented within eTOXlab, they

are perfectly integrated into the project predictive platform and visible in the common interface shown in **Figure 1**.

Model Development and Maintenance

Apart from connecting the individual models to the eTOXsys prediction system, eTOXlab provides additional support for the model development, maintenance, and documentation. Regarding model development by diverse teams of modelers, it is important to make use of common tools providing consistent solutions for tasks that need to be carried out by the different models. An example of this is the structure normalization,

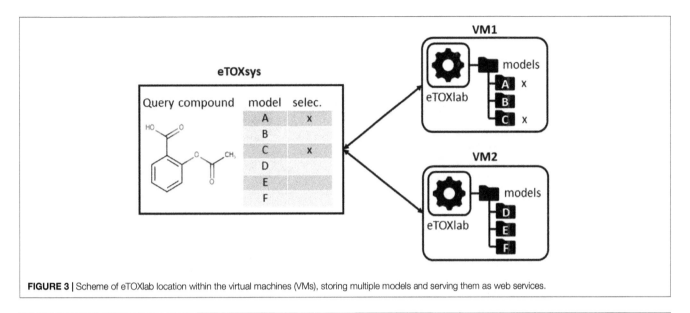

FIGURE 3 | Scheme of eTOXlab location within the virtual machines (VMs), storing multiple models and serving them as web services.

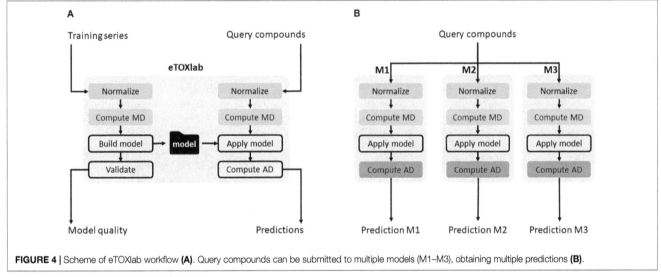

FIGURE 4 | Scheme of eTOXlab workflow **(A)**. Query compounds can be submitted to multiple models (M1–M3), obtaining multiple predictions **(B)**.

since the end user expects that the input structure is internally normalized and processed in the same way by all the models to which it is submitted. The use of a common modeling framework allows employing a common workflow for the building of all the models and for carrying out predictions with them, where the same software tools are used at each step, thus guaranteeing that the results are consistent; an example is structure normalization. Classically, 2D structures of the molecules are entered by the end user using SMILES or SDFiles formats. Before these structures can be processed, they need to be submitted to a normalization protocol that takes care of removing counterions, saturating and ionizing the molecule to a certain pH and, in some cases, generating 3D structures. Ideally, query molecules must be submitted to the same protocol that was applied to the structures of the training series used for developing the models. When the same query molecule is submitted to multiple models at the same time, the protocols must also be consistent. This requirement is easily met by

using the eTOXlab modeling framework. Models implemented in eTOXlab make use of a consistent workflow (**Figure 4**), which processes input molecules in sequential order, submitting them to a normalization tool, an ionization tool and a 3D conversion tool. The tools applied, and the precise parameters used can be customized for each model and are adequately documented, thus guaranteeing a fully consistent treatment in the model training and prediction.

The use of eTOXlab also allowed developing specific components for common tasks. An example of this is ADAN (Carrió et al., 2014), a method specifically developed for assessing the applicability domain of the predictive models developed in eTOX, which is able to generate robust reliability scorings for the predictions. In summary, the ADAN method is based on assessing how far is a query compound from the model applicability domain and, based on this, provide reliability indexes to the predictions. The reliability is translated to pseudo 95% Confidence Interval (CI), thus facilitating the appraisal of

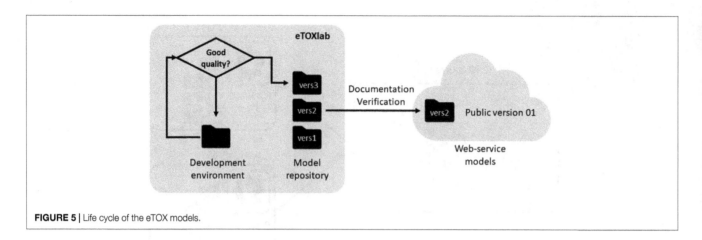

FIGURE 5 | Life cycle of the eTOX models.

the prediction obtained. The ADAN methodology can also be applied to non-QSAR models (Capoferri et al., 2015).

Another task that can be facilitated by the use of a modeling framework like eTOXlab is the maintenance of the models. Given that models are not static entities, once they are developed, they should evolve along the time by incorporating new compounds to the training series, updating of the software used at the different steps or refining the modeling workflow. In any case, every improvement produces a new version of the original model (see **Figure 5**).

In production environments, where important decisions can be based on model results, it is important to maintain a well-ordered inventory of all models and versions developed and use unique identifiers for each of them. As a minimum, the system must allow to reproduce predictions made by any model version.

In eTOX, every model was documented in a central repository, called eTOXvault, where it was assigned a unique public identifier and version number. For models developed within eTOXlab, two circuits of versioning were used. When a model was in development, all the files were stored in a specific development environment (so called "sandbox"). Only models that meet certain quality criteria were copied into a permanent storage space and assigned an internal, sequential version number. Initially these identifiers and version numbers were internal, as they were not exposed to anybody except to the model developer. Once the models were properly documented and verified (as described below), they were assigned an official identifier and version number and they were published as a web service visible to all consortium partners.

Model Documentation and Validation

It is widely accepted that models must be documented. However, we learned that different actors have different expectations and very diverse needs regarding model documentation. Most end users require simple documentation describing, in a concise and non-technical language, what is the precise meaning of the model predictions and how reliable are those. On the other hand, modelers need to document the models at a more detailed level to allow reproducing the models and to facilitate the model maintenance. Potential future uses of the model results for regulatory purposes, recommend following

widely recognized standards, such as the Organization for Economic Co-operation and Development (OECD) guidance document about QSAR modeling (Organisation for Economic Co-operation and Development, 2007), the guidance on the development, evaluation, and application of environmental models published by the US Environmental Protection Agency (EPA) (Environmental Protection Agency, 2009), or the requirements of the European REACH (Benfenati et al., 2011), or the recent efforts from the pharmaceutical industry (Myatt et al., 2018). In eTOX, models were documented following the OECD guidelines, but the sections of the document were reorganized in a way that allow to obtain summary extractions, as we described in a previous paper (Sanz et al., 2015).

To validate a model means to determine if the model is "fit-for-purpose." This task is highly dependent of the use context and cannot be carried out in a general manner for all models. In eTOX the model validation was replaced by a systematic model verification methodology, which guarantees that the model produces the results described in the documentation (Hewitt et al., 2015).

Structure Confidentiality

The eTOX project was a collaborative effort involving several major pharmaceutical companies, which contributed data generated and stored in-house for the training of predictive models. Sharing this information posed a major problem, in particular when it involved the structure of confidential compounds. Predictive models should ideally be built using all available structures and biological annotations available, irrespectively of the partner who contributed this information. Unfortunately, the data protection policies of the different industrial partners imposed obvious limitations, difficult to overcome.

At the beginning of the project we hoped to be able to develop and implement new structure-masking algorithms able to hash the structures into representations usable for building models, but resilient to any effort to reverse-engineer the algorithm and guess the original chemical structure. Our hope was not unfounded, and different similar methods have been published in the past (Tetko et al., 2005; Masek et al., 2008). For this particular purpose, we obtained excellent results using a simple random permutation of the molecular descriptors generated by methods like GRIND or GRIND2 (Pastor et al., 2000; Durán et al., 2008). The permuted vector of descriptors does not allow guessing the original structure, since the permutation destroyed any link between the value of the variables and their physico-chemical interpretation. Moreover, this approach is resistant to brute-force methods (Faulon et al., 2005; Filimonov and Poroikov, 2005), since these methods require the application of the same algorithm to a comprehensive database of structures, and a key element of the hashing algorithm (the random seed of the permutation) is never shared or revealed. The robustness of the algorithm was carefully tested and further demonstrated by code-breaking challenges at the project consortium level, where the hashed representation resisted any effort to identify the original structure. In these exercises, we also demonstrated that the hashed representation preserved all the information existing in the original molecular descriptors, and the models derived from them had equivalent quality.

Unfortunately, in these exercises we found that, beyond the robustness of our masking algorithm, it was impossible to convince the pharmaceutical companies to implement it in the eTOX project since, given the high corporate sensitiveness on the issue, such implementation would require costly external audits that we could not afford. For this reason, we adopted an alternative approach: if the confidential data cannot be taken out of the companies' internal repositories, we can move the whole model building system to the companies, so the models can be built there. Indeed, we took advantage that the eTOXlab-VM containers are already portable model building engines. Without any modification, they can be used to develop fully functional models behind the companies' firewalls. Furthermore, this approach could be even better if the models obtained could be shared without compromising the confidentiality of the training series. In order to make this possible, eTOXlab implements a "safe mode" for building models in a special way, which retains no information at all about the structures or identities of the training series. When configured in this way, the eTOXlab model consists in a small text file, with the values of the coefficients that must be applied to the molecular descriptors computed for future query compounds to estimate their biological activity. This small file can be exported to other partners without any risk since it is easy to audit to guarantee that no sensitive information at all is exported even using an unsecure means (e.g., e-mail, portable USB device).

DISCUSSION

Some of the solutions applied in eTOX for generating a predictive system usable in production environments involve the use of specific software, wrapping the scientific work developed by SMEs and academic partners into a "package" easier to deploy and integrate in corporate settings. The use of this kind of software, which is described in this article as a "modeling framework," adds further advantages, like facilitating the consortium-wide adoption of standard modeling components, and simplifying key steps of the model life cycle, like the model retraining and maintenance. In eTOX, a new modeling framework was developed *ad hoc* for the project (eTOXlab). This software has been released as open source under GNU GPL v3.0 (GNU GPL v3, 2007). The source code of eTOXlab is accessible at https://github.com/phi-grib/eTOXlab. A fully configured VM including eTOXlab is also accessible at http://phi.upf.edu/envoy/. Hence, future projects aiming to develop similar predictive systems have now the option of reusing these resources, either as they are or customizing them to meet specific project needs.

We consider that these resources have value on their own, but they have an additional value as a proof-of-concept, since they demonstrate that they are helpful for making software tools developed by academic and SMEs usable by pharmaceutical companies. **Table 1** lists some of the key features that, in our opinion, such kind of frameworks must incorporate.

Another key element required is the definition and consortium-wide adoption of protocols for labeling, documenting and verifying the models. These are important aspects, which must be negotiated with the end-users for providing fit-for-purpose solutions. In this dialog, the expected use of the predictive system must be identified as soon as possible, since a modeling system aiming to prioritize lead compounds has completely different requirements, in terms of documentation and verification, than a system supporting decisions that could be communicated to regulatory agencies. This consideration should not be interpreted as a justification for considering optional the complete model documentation or the quantification of the prediction uncertainty; however, the standards used in either case are different. For this reason, the requirements derived from all intended model uses must be identified with the help of the end users, clearly defined and translated into system specifications.

One of the most complex aspects in the development of the aforementioned prediction systems is the internal adoption of the

---

TABLE 1 | Features required for the building of a predictive system usable in production environments.

Predictive system component	Feature	Importance
Framework	Support for model development at the academic/SMEs	Must
	Support for model deployment at the end-user site	Must
	Flexible enough to accommodate all modeling methodologies	Must
	Easy model maintenance and retraining	Must
	Pluggable components	Optional
Protocols	Model documentation	Must
	Prediction uncertainty	Must
	Use of international standards (QMRF/QPRF)	Depends on intended use

models by the end-users. The procedures vary from company to company, although they typically involve the validation of the system by comparing the prediction results with other *in silico* or experimental methods. As the structures being used in this comparison are often confidential, in the vast majority of cases the results of such validations are not made public. This is understandable but unfortunate, because this behavior results in a lack of feedback about the final usefulness of the predictive system. A published example of this kind of internal validations was the one carried out by Sanofi on the eTOX QT prolongation model using 434 drug candidates (Amberg et al., 2016).

Another aspect, briefly discussed in this article, is the potential use of portable modeling environments for building and sharing predictive models in which confidential structures are used. In eTOX, this was considered the only acceptable option, while solutions attempting to obfuscate, mask or encrypt the structures (or the molecular descriptors) were considered by the partners too risky to be used in practice. eTOXlab was configured for producing shareable models, which can be safely shared and exported because they contain no trace of the original structures. Similar features can also be easily implemented in other modeling frameworks. Here we want to emphasize the conceptual value of the aforementioned strategy consisting in building the models within the companies and exporting only the model coefficients. The implementation of this strategy only requires the use, across the collaborating partners, of a common modeling framework facilitating the import and export of the model coefficients.

Many of the eTOX partners have continued their collaboration and now participate in a new IMI project (eTRANSAFE)[1], which shares with eTOX the aim to develop predictive systems. The ideas and principles described in this article are being applied, extending and adapting them to meet the objectives of this new project. One part of this effort is the development of a new modeling framework (called Flame), inspired on the same principles of eTOXlab but technologically more advanced. The source code of this software, still in development, is distributed under GNU GPL v3.0 (GNU GPL v3, 2007) and can be accessed at https://github.com/phi-grib/flame.

Finally, a limited version of eTOXsys, including the modeling system described here and a few selected models has been made open to the scientific community and can be accessed at http://etoxsys.eu/.

---

[1] http://etransafe.eu

CONCLUSION

Beyond the concrete database, predictive models and integrated computational system that have been developed, the eTOX project has demonstrated that the successful completion of ambitious industry-oriented collaborative projects requires not only the development and implementation of state-of-the-art scientific approaches, but also the careful implementation of adequate technical and organizational solutions. Among them, the adoption of adequate standards and protocols is a key component. The efforts done in eTOX in this respect are being extended to the new IMI eTRANSAFE project[1], which will jointly exploit preclinical data and clinical safety information for a better prediction of potential human safety liabilities (Sanz et al., 2017).

We hope this paper will contribute to save the readers' time and effort in similar public-private projects, as well as to improve the efficiency in the collaboration between the pharmaceutical industry and external parties in the development and application of computational tools supporting the drug discovery and development pipeline.

AUTHOR CONTRIBUTIONS

FS was the academic coordinator of the eTOX project. MP is a major contributor to the design of the eTOX predictive system described here, even if the credit belongs to the whole eTOX consortium. MP wrote, designed the figures and assembled this manuscript, which was enriched, refined and formatted by FS and JQ.

FUNDING

The eTOX project (Grant Agreement No. 115002), was developed under the Innovative Medicines Initiative Joint Undertaking (IMI), resources of which are composed of a financial contribution from the European Union's Seventh Framework Programme (FP7/2007-2013) and EFPIA companies' in kind contributions. The authors of this article are also involved in other related IMI projects, such as iPiE (no. 115735), TransQST (no. 116030) and eTRANSAFE (no. 777365), as well as the H2020 EU-ToxRisk project (no. 681002).

REFERENCES

Amberg, A., Anger, L., Spirkl, H.-P., Guillon, J.-M., Ballet, V., Schmidt, F., et al. (2016). Cardiosafety in silico prediction - validation results of a multiscale simulation model (eTOX VII). *Toxicol. Suppl. Toxicol. Sci.* 150:2647.

Benfenati, E., Diaza, R. G., Cassano, A., Pardoe, S., Gini, G., Mays, C., et al. (2011). The acceptance of in silico models for reach: requirements, barriers, and perspectives. *Chem. Cent. J.* 5, 1–11. doi: 10.1186/1752-153X-5-58

Bravo, À, Li, T. S., Su, I., Good, B. M., and Furlong, I. (2016). Combining machine learning, crowdsourcing and expert knowledge to detect chemical-induced diseases in text. *Database* 2016:baw094. doi: 10.1093/database/baw094

Capoferri, L., Verkade-Vreeker, M. C. A., Buitenhuis, D., Commandeur, J. N. M., Pastor, M., Vermeulen, N. P. E., et al. (2015). Linear interaction energy based prediction of cytochrome P450 1A2 binding affinities with reliability estimation. *PLoS One* 10:e0142232. doi: 10.1371/journal.pone.0142232

Carrió, P., López, O., Sanz, F., and Pastor, M. (2015). eTOXlab, an open source modeling framework for implementing predictive models in production environments. *J. Cheminform.* 7:8. doi: 10.1186/s13321-015-0058-6

Carrió, P., Pinto, M., Ecker, G., Sanz, F., and Pastor, M. (2014). Applicability domain analysis (ADAN): a robust method for assessing the reliability of drug property predictions. *J. Chem. Inf. Model.* 54, 1500–1511. doi: 10.1021/ci500172z

Cases, M., Briggs, K., Steger-Hartmann, T., Pognan, F., Marc, P., Kleinöder, T., et al. (2014). The eTOX data-sharing project to advance in Silico drug-induced toxicity prediction. *Int. J. Mol. Sci.* 15, 21136–21154. doi: 10.3390/ijms151121136

Daneshian, M., Kamp, H., Hengstler, J., Leist, M., and van de Water, B. (2016). Highlight report: launch of a large integrated European *in vitro* toxicology project: EU-ToxRisk. *Arch. Toxicol.* 90, 1021–1024. doi: 10.1007/s00204-016-1698-7

Durán, Á, Martínez, G. C., and Pastor, M. (2008). Development and validation of AMANDA, a new algorithm for selecting highly relevant regions in molecular interaction fields. *J. Chem. Inf. Model.* 48, 1813–1823. doi: 10.1021/ci800037t

Environmental Protection Agency (2009). *Guidance on the Development, Evaluation, and Application of Environmental Models.* Technical Report EPA/100/K-09/003. Washington, DC: Environmental Protection Agency.

Faulon, J.-L., Brown, W. M., and Martin, S. (2005). Reverse engineering chemical structures from molecular descriptors: how many solutions? *J. Comput. Aided. Mol. Des.* 19, 637–650. doi: 10.1007/s10822-005-9007-1

Fielding, R. T. (2000). *Architectural Styles and the Design of Network-based Software Architectures.* Available at: https://www.ics.uci.edu/~fielding/pubs/dissertation/top.htm

Filimonov, D., and Poroikov, V. (2005). Why relevant chemical information cannot be exchanged without disclosing structures. *J. Comput. Aided. Mol. Des.* 19, 705–713. doi: 10.1007/s10822-005-9014-2

GNU GPL v3 (2007). Available at: http://www.gnu.org/copyleft/gpl.html

Hewitt, M., Ellison, C. M., Cronin, M. T. D., Pastor, M., Steger-Hartmann, T., Munoz-Muriendas, J., et al. (2015). Ensuring confidence in predictions: a scheme to assess the scientific validity of in silico models. *Adv. Drug Deliv. Rev.* 86, 101–111. doi: 10.1016/j.addr.2015.03.005

Lenselink, E. B., Ten Dijke, N., Bongers, B., Papadatos, G., Van Vlijmen, H. W. T., Kowalczyk, W., et al. (2017). Beyond the hype: deep neural networks outperform established methods using a ChEMBL bioactivity benchmark set. *J. Cheminform.* 9:45. doi: 10.1186/s13321-017-0232-0

Liu, J., Patlewicz, G., Williams, A., Thomas, R. S., and Shah, I. (2017). Predicting organ toxicity using in vitro bioactivity data and chemical structure. *Chem. Res. Toxicol.* 30, 2046–2059. doi: 10.1021/acs.chemrestox.7b00084

Luechtefeld, T., Marsh, D., Rowlands, C., and Hartung, T. (2018). Machine learning of toxicological big data enables read-across structure activity relationships (RASAR) outperforming animal test reproducibility. *Toxicol. Sci.* 165, 198–212. doi: 10.1093/toxsci/kfy152

Maldonado, E. M., Leoncikas, V., Fisher, C. P., Moore, J. B., Plant, N. J., and Kierzek, A. M. (2017). Integration of genome scale metabolic networks and gene regulation of metabolic enzymes with physiologically based pharmacokinetics. *CPT Pharmacometrics Syst. Pharmacol.* 6, 732–746. doi: 10.1002/psp4.12230

Masek, B. B., Shen, L., Smith, K. M., and Pearlman, R. S. (2008). Sharing chemical information without sharing chemical structure. *J. Chem. Inf. Model.* 48, 256–261. doi: 10.1021/ci600383v

Myatt, G. J., Ahlberg, E., Akahori, Y., Allen, D., Amberg, A., Anger, L. T., et al. (2018). In silico toxicology protocols. *Regul. Toxicol. Pharmacol.* 96, 1–17. doi: 10.1016/j.yrtph.2018.04.014

Organisation for Economic Co-operation and Development (2007). *Guidance Document on the Validation of (Quantitative) Structure-Activity Relationships (QSAR) Models.* Technical Report ENV/JM/MONO. Paris: Organisation for Economic Co-operation and Development.

Pastor, M., Cruciani, G., McLay, I., Pickett, S., and Clementi, S. (2000). GRid-INdependent descriptors (GRIND): a novel class of alignment-independent three-dimensional molecular descriptors. *J. Med. Chem.* 43, 3233–3243. doi: 10.1021/jm000941m

Sakuratani, Y., Zhang, H. Q., Nishikawa, S., Yamazaki, K., Yamada, T., Yamada, J., et al. (2013). Hazard Evaluation Support System (HESS) for predicting repeated dose toxicity using toxicological categories. *SAR QSAR Environ. Res.* 24, 351–363. doi: 10.1080/1062936X.2013.773375

Sanz, F., Carrió, P., López, O., Capoferri, L., Kooi, D. P., Vermeulen, N. P. E., et al. (2015). Integrative modeling strategies for predicting drug toxicities at the eTox project. *Mol. Inform.* 34, 477–484. doi: 10.1002/minf.201400193

Sanz, F., Pognan, F., Steger-Hartmann, T., and Díaz, C. (2017). Legacy data sharing to improve drug safety assessment: the eTOX project. *Nat. Rev. Drug Discov.* 16, 811–812. doi: 10.1038/nrd.2017.177

Steger-Hartmann, T., and Pognan, F. (2018). Improving the safety assessment of chemicals and drug candidates by the integration of bioinformatics and chemoinformatics data. *Basic Clin. Pharmacol. Toxicol.* doi: 10.1111/bcpt.12956 [Epub ahead of print].

Tetko, I. V., Abagyan, R., and Oprea, T. I. (2005). Surrogate data - a secure way to share corporate data. *J. Comput. Aided. Mol. Des.* 19, 749–764. doi: 10.1007/s10822-005-9013-3

Structural Changes Due to Antagonist Binding in Ligand Binding Pocket of Androgen Receptor Elucidated Through Molecular Dynamics Simulations

Sugunadevi Sakkiah[1], Rebecca Kusko[2], Bohu Pan[1], Wenjing Guo[1], Weigong Ge[1], Weida Tong[1] and Huixiao Hong[1]*

[1] Division of Bioinformatics and Biostatistics, National Center for Toxicological Research, U.S. Food and Drug Administration, Jefferson, AR, United States, [2] Immuneering Corporation, Cambridge, MA, United States

*Correspondence:
Huixiao Hong
huixiao.hong@fda.hhs.gov

When a small molecule binds to the androgen receptor (AR), a conformational change can occur which impacts subsequent binding of co-regulator proteins and DNA. In order to accurately study this mechanism, the scientific community needs a crystal structure of the Wild type AR (WT-AR) ligand binding domain, bound with antagonist. To address this open need, we leveraged molecular docking and molecular dynamics (MD) simulations to construct a structure of the WT-AR ligand binding domain bound with antagonist bicalutamide. The structure of mutant AR (Mut-AR) bound with this same antagonist informed this study. After molecular docking analysis pinpointed the suitable binding orientation of a ligand in AR, the model was further optimized through 1 μs of MD simulations. Using this approach, three molecular systems were studied: (1) WT-AR bound with agonist R1881, (2) WT-AR bound with antagonist bicalutamide, and (3) Mut-AR bound with bicalutamide. Our structures were very similar to the experimentally determined structures of both WT-AR with R1881 and Mut-AR with bicalutamide, demonstrating the trustworthiness of this approach. In our model, when WT-AR is bound with bicalutamide, Val716/Lys720/Gln733, or Met734/Gln738/Glu897 move and thus disturb the positive and negative charge clumps of the AF2 site. This disruption of the AF2 site is key for understanding the impact of antagonist binding on subsequent co-regulator binding. In conclusion, the antagonist induced structural changes in WT-AR detailed in this study will enable further AR research and will facilitate AR targeting drug discovery.

Keywords: androgen receptor, molecular dynamics simulations, induced molecular docking, bicalutamide, agonist, antagonist

INTRODUCTION

The androgen receptor (AR), a member of the nuclear subfamily 3, is a ligand-activated transcriptional factor. AR is expressed in various tissues of different species and regulates many physiological functions including bone density, cognition, muscle hypertrophy, prostate growth and differentiation (Gelmann, 2002). AR and estrogen receptor (ER) are well characterized nuclear receptor target of active endocrine chemicals (Hong et al., 2002; Sakkiah et al., 2016). Copious experimental data and numerous *in silico* predictive models estimate both estrogenic and androgenic activity (Hong et al., 2002, 2003, 2005, 2012, 2015, 2016a,b; Shen et al., 2013; Ng et al., 2014, 2015a,b; Sakkiah et al., 2016; Ye et al., 2016). AR is a well-established drug target for prostate cancer, which is the second most common cancer by occurrence in men in western countries (Damber and Aus, 2008). Both steroid and non-steroid antagonists treat prostate cancer by blocking AR activity. A prolonged treatment course leads to tumor AR mutations, which causes AR antagonists to have a paradoxical effect. A thorough study of WT and mutant AR (Mut-AR) antagonist binding is required to better understand this paradoxical mechanism which limits therapeutic efficacy.

Full-length AR consists of 919 amino acids translated from 8 exons (Kuiper et al., 1989; Lubahn et al., 1989). Like other nuclear receptors, AR consists of three major functional domains: (1) an NH2-terminal domain, (2) a highly conserved DNA binding domain, and (3) a conserved ligand-binding domain (LBD) (Gao et al., 2005; Sakkiah et al., 2016). The hinge region acts as a bridge between the DNA binding domain and the conserved LBD. Both the AR N-terminal activation function 1 (AF1) in the DNA binding domain and the AR C-terminal activation function 2 (AF2) in the LBD control the transcriptional factors in ligand-independent and ligand-dependent manners, respectively. The AR-LBD (hereafter AR-LBD is termed as AR for simplicity) has three different binding or active sites where an agonist or antagonist can bind and alter AR functions: the ligand binding pocket, the AF2 site, and the binding function 3 (BF3) site. An agonist or a competitive antagonist can bind the AR ligand binding pocket to enhance or depress AR function, respectively. The AF2 site plays a major role in co-activator binding, which starts the transcription of AR-regulated genes. A few antagonists were reported to bind to the AF2 site, which directly blocks the binding of a co-activator protein (Axerio-Cilies et al., 2011). The BF3 site is a newly identified AR surface antagonist binding site. An antagonist can bind in any of these described binding sites to suppress AR activity. Antagonist binding causes conformational changes in the AF2 site, rendering it unsuitable for co-activators to bind AR (Estebanez-Perpina et al., 2007; Estébanez-Perpiñá and Fletterick, 2009). The three-dimensional structure of AR consists of 12 bundles of helices forming three layers (**Figure 1**). Among these 12 helices, H12 plays a major role in AR activation and undergoes a considerable conformational change due to the binding of agonist or antagonist in the ligand binding pocket. During agonist or antagonist binding, H12 functions like a "lid" which closes or moves away from the ligand binding pocket, respectively (Bohl et al., 2007; Cantin et al., 2007). When androgen binds the ligand binding pocket of AR, H12 tightly holds co-activator proteins and initiates function. AR antagonists are usually bulkier than agonists and thus require a wider binding pocket than agonists. Due to their larger size, antagonists push the residues in H12 (which is near the ligand binding pocket) outward to expand the active site. These structural changes in the ligand binding pocket cause the AF2 site to undergo conformational changes, preventing co-activator protein binding (Estébanez-Perpiñá and Fletterick, 2009). Some

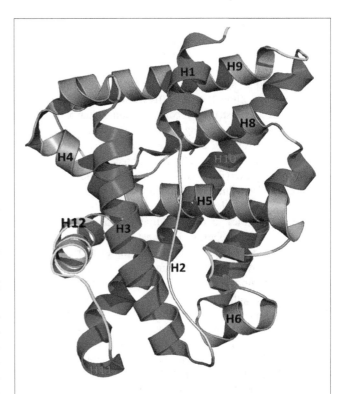

FIGURE 1 | The structure of AR is plotted in a helical bundle composed of 12 helices. These helices are arranged in three layers. Layer 1 has H1, H2, and H3 (magenta), Layer 2 consists of H4, H5, H6, H8, and H9 (gold), and Layer 3 contains H7 and H10 (blue). H12 (in cyan) acts as a lid for the AR ligand binding pocket during binding of agonists and antagonists.

mutations in AR cleverly cause drug resistance by converting AR antagonist properties into agonist properties. Prostate cancer drug resistance is predominantly driven by AR mutations. For example, mutations T877A (Sack et al., 2001; Bohl et al., 2007), W741L/C (Hara et al., 2003), L701A/T877A (Balbas et al., 2013), and F878L (Balbas et al., 2013; Korpal et al., 2013) in the LBD made AR antagonists Flutamide, R-bicalutamide, and Enzalutamide behave as agonists. The mutation T877A significantly increased the activity of AR, as evidenced by the enhanced AR affinity toward progesterone and estrogens (Taplin and Balk, 2004).

There exist 90 crystal structures of AR from different species (rat, mice, chimpanzee, and human) in the Protein Data Bank (PDB[1]) (Berman et al., 2000). Wild type AR (WT-AR) crystal structures exist with either agonists in the ligand binding pocket or antagonists in the AF2 or BF3 sites. Mut-AR crystal structures exist with antagonists in the ligand binding pocket. No 3D structure of WT-AR with an antagonist in the ligand binding pocket has been described, likely because an antagonist binding to the AR-chaperone complex does not disassociate the chaperone from AR (Bohl et al., 2005; Sakkiah et al., 2016). To fill this knowledge gap, the AF2 site structural changes in WT-AR which are induced by antagonist binding could be determined via molecular modeling.

---

[1] www.rcsb.org

Determining the conformation change of a protein induced by a ligand using crystallography is at best time consuming but often infeasible. Several researchers employed molecular dynamics (MD) simulations to characterize H12 structural changes due to antagonists or agonist binding in the AR ligand binding pocket. Zhou J. et al. (2010) utilized replica-exchange MD to characterize structural conformational changes and H12 movement caused by binding of hydroxyflutamide in the ligand binding pocket of WT and mutant (T877A) AR. Using MD simulations, Bisson et al. (2008) proposed that T877A in AR destabilized hydroxyflutamide–Met895 interactions and thus decreased hydroxyflutamide antagonist activity. Additionally, Osguthorpe and Hagler (2011) employed MD simulations and quantum mechanics to discover that an antagonist occupied more space than an agonist, leading to H12 instability. While important contributions to the field, these MD simulations were limited by short time frames and mainly focused on the ligand binding pocket or H12 structural changes (Bisson et al., 2008; Osguthorpe and Hagler, 2011; Liu et al., 2015, 2016, 2017; Wang et al., 2017). Recently, many researchers captured structural changes of various proteins using long time MD simulations (hereafter called "long MD simulations") (Whitten et al., 2005; Dror et al., 2009; Khelashvili et al., 2009; Nury et al., 2010; Gotz et al., 2012; Durrant et al., 2016). For example, Lindorff-Larsen et al. (2011) predicted the folding of 12 proteins using MD simulations ranging from microsecond to a millisecond. Their results unveiled a common principle for the folding of the 12 structurally diverse proteins and more importantly demonstrated that long MD simulations are a power tool to predict and capture protein conformational changes (Lindorff-Larsen et al., 2011). Next, Kumar and Purohit (2014) found that the long MD simulations significantly increased prediction accuracy when studying cancer associated single nucleotide polymorphisms. Thus, long MD simulations overcome many limitations of short-term MD simulations. Duan et al. (2016) conducted 1 μs MD simulations and explored ligand binding pocket changes during agonist and antagonist binding in WT and Mut-AR. Using bias-exchange meta-dynamics to study the free energy profile of agonist and antagonist binding to AR, they observed agonist and antagonist binding driven movement of H12 and structural changes in the ligand binding pocket of WT-AR. They also reported that long MD simulations were required to capture H12 movement, whereas short-term stimulations miscalculated agonist binding induced H12 structural changes (Duan et al., 2016). Hence, in this study, we applied long MD simulations (1 μs) not only to capture H12 movement but also to study AF2 site structural changes due to antagonist binding in the AR ligand binding pocket.

Three AR complex structures were studied to understand the antagonist binding induced structural changes of the AF2 site. R1881 and bicalutamide are, respectively, well-known as an agonist and an antagonist for AR. Structures of AR bound with R1881 and bicalutamide were downloaded from PDB: WT-AR-R1881 (AR with agonist, PDBID: 1E3G) and Mut-AR-bicalutamide (AR with antagonist, PDBID:1Z95). The third AR complex structure, WT-AR-bicalutamide, was absent from PDB and thus was generated using the induced fit molecular

docking (IFD) method (explained in the Section "Materials and Methods"). The IFD method explores both possible binding poses of a ligand in a receptor active site as well as the associated conformational changes of the side chains near the active site. MD simulations are an important tool to study receptor–ligand interactions at an atomic level for a given time frame. MD simulations optimize three-dimensional complex protein structure bound with a ligand obtained from X-ray crystallography or molecular docking. Here, we leveraged the advantages of IFD and MD simulations together to understand the subtle structural changes in WT-AR due to anti-androgen binding and also to elucidate key co-activator binding residues in the WT-AR AF2 site. Each AR complex structure was subjected to 1 μs of MD simulations to resolve important AF2 site residue reformation during the binding of small molecules in WT-AR. Our results will enable design of improved prostate cancer treatments and facilitate endocrine disruption chemical risk assessment through AR-mediated responses.

MATERIALS AND METHODS

Molecular Docking

Rigid docking (only giving flexibility to ligands) might fail to produce a precise ligand pose due to rigidness of the protein. In contrast, IFD gives flexibility to adjust not only the active site but also the side chain orientations of the protein to fit the pose and conformation of the bound ligand (Zhong et al., 2009). Hence, it can generate many protein-ligand complexes by changing the side chains or the backbone of the protein. Glide (docking) and Prime (refinement) modules were used in the IFD to determine the possible binding modes of the ligand and the concomitant binding induced conformational changes.

The IFD (Sherman et al., 2006a,b) module[2] from the Schrodinger-Suite (2016b) was used to dock the AR antagonist, bicalutamide, in WT-AR.

The following steps were involved in the IFD employed here (Wang et al., 2008; Luo et al., 2013):

(i) The protein was refined using the Protein Preparation module.
(ii) Each ligand was docked (Glide module) in a defined region using a softened potential to produce 20 different poses (default setting).
(iii) A sidechain prediction (Prime module) within a given distance of the ligand was conducted for each complex.
(iv) The defined region of the protein-ligand complexes was minimized.
(v) The refined protein-ligand complexes were re-docked using Glide by specifying the lowest energy structure.
(vi) The IFD score (binding energy) was calculated for each complex.

Protein preparation is one of the most important steps in molecular docking and plays a key role in IFD. The three-dimensional atomic coordinates of WT-AR (PDB ID: 1E3G)

---

[2]www.schrodinger.com/induced-fit

(Matias et al., 2000) were retrieved from PDB and used as a receptor for the IFD. The Protein Preparation module[3] was used to add hydrogen atoms and to build the missing side chains, residues, and loops. The OPLS-2001 force field (Jorgensen and Tirado-Rives, 1988; Kaminski et al., 2001; Shivakumar et al., 2010) was used to assign the partial charges. All water molecules were removed and the protein structure was optimized using the OPLS force field. A 10 Å docking grid was generated around the ligand, R1881, in WT-AR. The structure of bicalutamide was obtained from the crystal structure of Mut-AR-bicalutamide (PDB ID: 1Z95) (Bohl et al., 2005) and docked in the generated grid box using Glide XP docking. The Glide XP docking (Halgren et al., 2004; Friesner et al., 2006; Shelley et al., 2007) generated 20 different bicalutamide poses for the WT-AR structural refinements. The Prime module was used to refine the generated WT-AR-bicalutamide complexes. In the Prime refinement, each WT-AR-bicalutamide conformation from the previous step was subjected to side chain and backbone refinements (Jacobson et al., 2004) by selecting the residues within 10 Å from bicalutamide and/or residues from 669 to 918. The Prime energy was calculated and used to rank the refined AR-bicalutamide complexes. The lowest energy conformation (30 kcal/mol) of the refined WT-AR complex was used to re-dock the bicalutamide using Glide XP mode. The most favorable binding pose of bicalutamide in WT-AR was selected based on the IFD score (binding energy). The selected WT-AR-bicalutamide complexes were visualized to check the interactions between bicalutamide and the residues in the ligand binding pocket using Ligand Interactions module in Maestro 11 (Schrodinger-Suite, 2016a).

Molecular Dynamics Simulations

Proteins are dynamic in nature. Thus, understanding atomic level motion is required to capture their profound dynamic mechanisms (Chou and Mao, 1988; Chou et al., 1994; Wang and Chou, 2009). MD simulations have the capacity to analyze the dynamics of an apoprotein or a complex with other molecules in an aqueous environment (Sakkiah et al., 2013a,b). Moreover, MD simulations yield energetically favorable conformations by optimizing a protein-ligand complex, which is needed to understand protein–ligand interactions and ligand binding induced structural changes.

The structures of the WT-AR-bicalutamide complex (obtained from IFD), WT-AR-R1881, (PDBID: 1E3G) (Matias et al., 2000), and the Mut-AR-bicalutamide complex (PDBID: 1Z95) (Bohl et al., 2005) were subjected to MD simulations using the Amber 14 package (Case et al., 2005). Then the topology and coordinate files for the agonist and antagonist were prepared using antechamber. Tleap was used to prepare the topology and coordinate files for the protein as well as to make the AR complex for running MD simulations. Amber03 molecular mechanical force field (Duan et al., 2003) and general AMBER force field (gaff) (Wang et al., 2004) were employed for the protein and ligands (agonist and/or antagonist), respectively. Each of the complex structures were immersed into a rectangular box of TIP3P model water (Jorgensen et al., 1983). The boundaries of

the water box size were 10 Å away from the nearest atoms of the complex. All systems were neutralized by adding Cl^- ions. The Particle Mesh Ewald (PME) (Darden et al., 1993) and SHAKE (Ryckaert et al., 1977) algorithms were used to handle long-range electrostatic interactions for all heavy and hydrogen atoms involved in the covalent bonding. A cutoff of 10 Å was used for the short-range interactions (van der Waals and electrostatic interactions). In the first phase, only the solvents were minimized and equilibrated inside the water box. Then, the whole system was minimized and equilibrated by applying the steepest descent minimization for 1000 cycles, followed by conjugate gradient energy minimization for 4000 cycles. Subsequently the whole system was gradually heated from 0 to 310.15 K over a 100 ps period which was followed by a 250 ps equilibrium simulation for the whole systems. In the second phase, the prepared systems were subjected to 1 μs of MD simulations using Amber14. All MD simulations were performed with a time step of 2 fs. The coordinates were saved for every 1 ps. MD simulations were performed using PyMol (Schrodinger, 2015) and Visual Molecular Dynamics (Humphrey et al., 1996). The Amber package[4] was used to calculate RMSD values for the protein and ligands as well as RMSF values for residues.

RESULTS AND DISCUSSION

IFD Produced a Structure of WT-AR-Bicalutamide for MD Simulations

No crystal structure for WT-AR with an antagonist in the ligand binding pocket has been deposited in PDB (accessed on May 19, 2017). To address this open question, we conducted IFD. Flexibility was given to the active site residues and the

---

[4]http://ambermd.org/doc12/Amber14.pdf

TABLE 1 | Induced fit docking (IFD) score and the key residues involved in hydrogen bond interactions between WT-AR and bicalutamide for the top 5 complexes.

Model #	Glide score	IFD score	Interactions	
			Hydrogen bond	π–Cation
Model-1	−12.75	−600	Leu704, Asn705	Trp741, Phe764
Model-2	−12.11	−600	Leu704, Asn705	Trp741
Model-3	−13.01	−600	Leu704, Asn705, Arg752	Trp741, Phe764
Model-4	−11.78	−598	Leu704, Asn705, Arg752	Trp741, Phe764
Model-5	−11.20	−598	Leu704, Asn705	Phe764

TABLE 2 | Three molecular systems in MD simulations.

#	PDB ID	Ligand	System
1	1E3G	R1881	WT-AR-R1881
2	1Z95	Bicalutamide	WT-AR-bicalutamide
3	1Z95	Bicalutamide	Mut-AR-bicalutamide

---

[3]https://www.schrodinger.com/protein-preparation-wizard

ligand during Glide docking. The whole WT-AR-bicalutamide system was refined using the Prime module to predict the suitable binding orientation of bicalutamide in the ligand binding pocket of WT-AR. Among the 20 models generated for WT-AR-bicalutamide, the top 5 models were selected based on their IFD/Glide scores and checked for residue interactions (**Table 1**). Among these 5 complex structures, Model-1, Model-3, and Model-4 showed a π–cation interaction with Trp741 and Phe764. Trp741 had van der Waals interactions favorable for agonist binding in the ligand binding pocket of WT-AR (Bohl et al., 2005). In contrast, Model-2 and Model-5 failed to form π–cation interactions with Trp741 or Phe874. Model-3, Model-4, and Model-1 had shown three, three, and two hydrogen bond interactions between bicalutamide and WT-AR, respectively. In Model-3 and Model-4, bicalutamide formed hydrogen bond interactions with Leu704, Asn705, and Arg752. Importantly, the hydrogen bond between the agonist/antagonist with Arg752 in WT-AR is crucial for AR activity (Gao et al., 2005; Bohl et al., 2007; Tan et al., 2015). Bicalutamide in Model-1 failed to form hydrogen bond interactions with Arg752. Model-3 had a better binding affinity value than Model-4. Interestingly, bicalutamide in Model-3 showed a bent conformation, which is different from the bicalutamide conformation in the Mut-AR (Gao et al., 2005). Previous evidence proposed that bicalutamide forms a hydrogen bond with residues Arg752, Leu705, Asn705, and Gln711 in Mut-AR (Tan et al., 2015). While Model-3 also formed a hydrogen bond with critical residues (Leu704, Asn705, and

Arg752) it failed to form a hydrogen bond with Gln711 and did not adopt a similar pose with the agonist due to the bulkier tryptophan side chain. Additionally, in Model-3, the 4-fluorophenyl group of bicalutamide moved toward the H12 region to form a suitable position in the WT-AR ligand binding pocket. Hence, Model-3 was selected for subsequent MD simulations of WT-AR-bicalutamide based on IFD score and binding interactions.

System Stability and Fluctuation Analysis Revealed Stability of AR Structures

We used the three molecular systems listed in **Table 2** (WT-AR-R1881, WT-AR-bicalutamide, and Mut-AR-bicalutamide) to analyze the structural changes in WT-AR due to bicalutamide binding in the ligand binding pocket using MD simulations. All trajectory files obtained from the MD simulations were examined for stability and fluctuation of the systems. Metrics of root mean square deviation (RMSD) and root mean square fluctuation (RMSF) were calculated for all systems to measure their energetic stability and the spatial fluctuation of residues, respectively. **Figure 2A** plots the RMSD values of the three systems during the 1 μs simulations. The RMSD values converged in the last 100 ns, indicating that the systems had reached a stable state. The WT-AR-R1881 and Mut-AR-bicalutamide systems were stabilized with an RMSD value of around 2.0 Å, while the WT-AR-bicalutamide system had a higher RMSD value of about 2.5 Å. An average structure was calculated from the last 100 ns for each of the three systems.

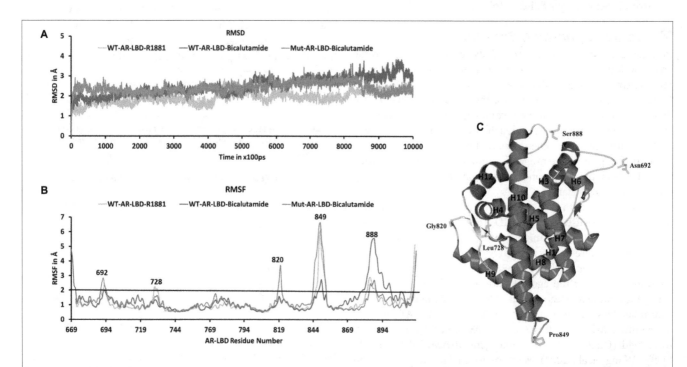

FIGURE 2 | (A) Shows the root mean square deviation (RMSD) plot of the systems during the 1 μs MD simulations. The RMSD values were calculated using AR backbone atoms. The X-axis represents time with a unit of 100 ps and the Y-axis shows RMSD values in Å. **(B)** Shows the root mean square fluctuation (RMSF) of the Cα atoms of AR systems in the 1 μs MD simulations. The X-axis indicates AR residue number and Y-axis represents RMSF in Å. The residues with RMSF > 2 Å are marked. **(C)** Demonstrates the structure of WT-AR-R1881, residues with RMSF > 2 Å in the loop regions are marked. These residues are drawn in a stick model. WT-AR-R1881 is color coded in green, WT-AR-bicalutamide in purple, and Mut-AR-bicalutamide in blue.

The structure with the lowest RMSD value compared with the average structure in last 100 ns was selected as a representative structure for each of the systems to elucidate the structural changes of WT-AR induced by bicalutamide.

Root mean square fluctuation plots were used to analyze flexibility of the residues in AR in the 1 μs MD simulations. Examination of the RMSF plots in **Figure 2B** revealed that WT-AR-bicalutamide had a larger RMSF value compared with WT-AR-R1881 and Mut-AR-bicalutamide near the C-terminal of LBD (mostly near H12). The average RMSF value for WT-AR-bicalutamide, Mut-AR-bicalutamide, and WT-AR-R1881 was 1.29, 1.25, and 1.11 Å, respectively. Five residues (Asn692, Leu728, Gly820, Pro849, and Ser888) in AR had an RMSF of >2.0 Å (**Figure 2B**) and were considered to be flexible residues. These five residues were present in the loop region of AR (**Figure 2C**). The RMSF values of the active site residues were small, demonstrating the stability of the AR active site.

Key Structural Changes in WT-AR Binding Antagonists

The AR ligand binding pocket accommodates both agonists and antagonists. Most antagonists bind in this site and alter the function of AR. The representative structures of WT-AR-R1881 and WT-AR-bicalutamide obtained from the MD simulations were superimposed to examine the difference between the two systems. Several major structural changes were identified in WT-AR due to the bicalutamide binding compared with agonist binding (R1881) (**Figure 3A**). Comparison of WT-AR-bicalutamide with WT-AR-R1881 showed a distortion at the end of H10 due to bicalutamide binding. Several residues in H10 were changed into a loop, which enabled more flexible movement. The structural conversion of H11 into a loop moved H12 away from the AR ligand binding pocket. Moreover, structural changes were observed when comparing WT-AR and Mut-AR bound with bicalutamide (**Figure 3B**). During bicalutamide binding, H11 was retained in the Mut-AR structure but was changed into a loop in the WT-AR structure (marked by the dotted circle in **Figure 3B**). As expected, Mut-AR-bicalutamide had a similar 3D structure to WT-AR-R1881.

The ligand binding pocket area and volume were calculated using the online Computed Atlas of surface Topography of protein server[5]. The area/volume for WT-AR-R1881,

---

[5]http://sts.bioe.uic.edu/castp/calculation.html

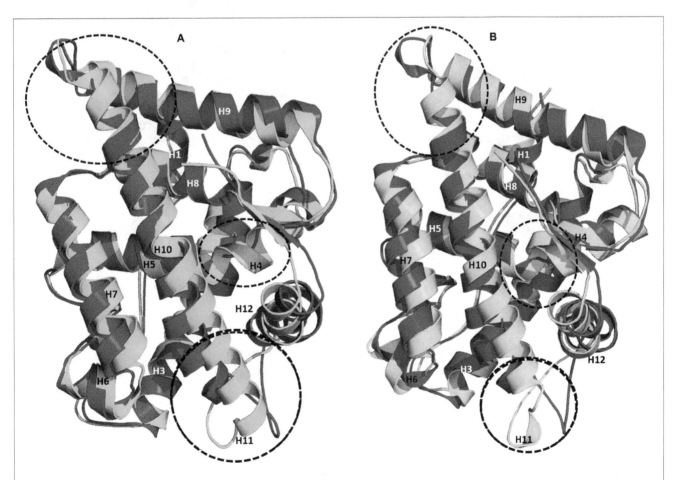

FIGURE 3 | Superimposition of WT-AR-R1881 and WT-AR-bicalutamide **(A)** and superimposition of WT-AR-bicalutamide and Mut-AR-bicalutamide **(B)**. AR-R1881 is drawn in green, WT-AR-bicalutamide in purple, and Mut-AR-bicalutamide in cyan. The black dotted circles mark the structural changes between the two structures.

WT-AR-bicalutamide, and Mut-AR-bicalutamide were 185/90, 528/321, and 366/193, respectively. As expected, area and volume of the ligand binding pocket of WT-AR-bicalutamide were larger than the agonist binding in WT-AR and bicalutamide binding in Mut-AR. Bicalutamide is larger than R1881 and hence moved H12 outward from the ligand binding pocket. The RMSD values comparing the WT-AR-R1881 vs. WT-AR-bicalutamide as well as WT-AR-bicalutamide vs. Mut-AR-bicalutamide were calculated for each residue by superimposing the structures using Visual Molecular Dynamics (Humphrey et al., 1996). The residues were ranked based on the computed RMSD values and are plotted in Supplementary Figure S1. The RMSD values showed a gap between 2.8 and 3 Å in both comparisons

(Supplementary Figures S1A,B). There were 42 and 37 residues with RMSD value greater than 2.8 Å between WT-AR-R1881 and WT-AR-bicalutamide and between WT-AR-bicalutamide and Mut-AR-bicalutamide, respectively. These residues are summarized in Supplementary Tables S1, S2. Twenty-two WT-AR-R1881 vs. WT-AR-bicalutamide residues and 26 WT-AR-bicalutamide vs. Mut-AR-bicalutamide residues were in helices (H3, H7, H9, H10, and H12), while the other residues were in loop regions.

The Trp741 mutation played a major role in the conversion of an AR antagonist into an agonist. The flipped Trp741 side chain moved His874 in H10 away from the ligand binding pocket to accommodate bicalutamide. Leu873, Phe876, Thr877, and

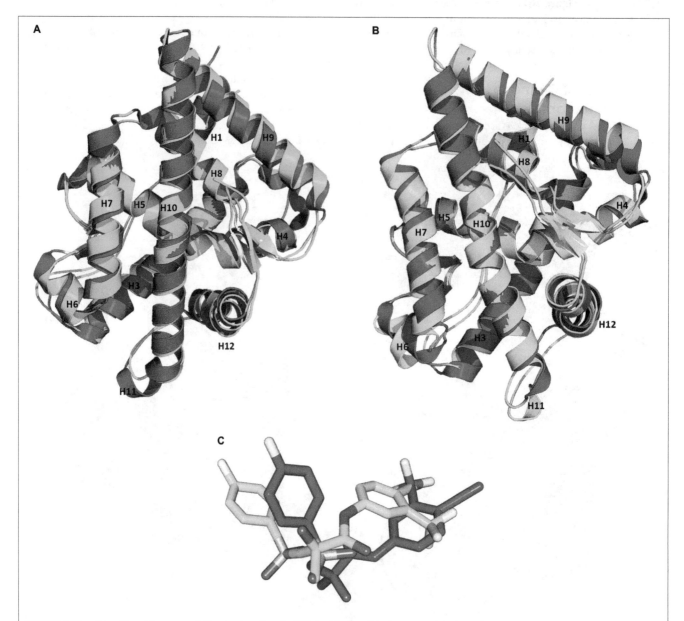

FIGURE 4 | Superimposition of the representative structures from the MD simulations and the X-ray crystal structures from PDB for WT-AR-R1881 (A) vs. Mut-AR-bicalutamide (B). The protein is drawn as a ribbon model. Overlay of bicalutamide structures from PDB are in red and the calculated WT-AR are in cyan (C). The X-ray crystal structure of AR is colored in red, the representative structure of WT-AR-R1881 in green, and Mut-AR-bicalutamide in cyan.

Met895 were the active site residues in the ligand binding pocket showing RMSD values greater than 3 Å between WT-AR-R1881 and WT-AR-bicalutamide. Thr850, Ser851, His874, Phe878, and Leu881 from H10 also had RMSD values greater than 3 Å (Supplementary Table S1). These structural changes drove the ligand binding pocket of WT-AR to expand to accommodate bicalutamide.

The representative structure of WT-AR-R1881 superimposed well with Mut-AR-bicalutamide compared with the superimposition of WT-AR-R1881 and WT-AR-bicalutamide. The H12 residues in Mut-AR-bicalutamide were not very different from the H12 residues in WT-AR-R1881. All residues in Mut-AR had less than 2.5 Å RMSD compared with WT-AR-R1881. Mut-AR-bicalutamide additionally did not experience large structural changes compared to WT-AR-R1881. The mutant residue Trp741Leu in Mut-AR-bicalutamide had a similar conformation to the wild type residue in WT-AR-R1881. The residues showing RMSD greater than 2.8 Å between WT-AR-bicalutamide and WT-AR-R1881 are listed in Supplementary Table S1.

Lastly, Mut-AR-bicalutamide and WT-AR-bicalutamide representative structures were superimposed to identify the crucial residues that played important roles in bicalutamide binding to AR. H11 in WT-AR-bicalutamide changed into a loop. The residues 882–984 in the loop region between H10 and H12 gave more flexibility for H12 to move away from the ligand binding pocket in WT-AR-bicalutamide. All these residues had RMSD values greater than 3.5 Å compared with WT-AR-R1881. Notably, the residues from His885 to Asp890 had RMSD values greater than 6 Å. These residues forming H11 in Mut-AR-bicalutamide reduced the flexibility of the loop and held H12 close to the ligand binding pocket. As expected, these residues showed RMSD values less than 2.8 Å between WT-AR-R1881 and Mut-AR-bicalutamide. Hence, we posit that the structural change of H11 into a loop in WT-AR-bicalutamide plays an essential role in H12 movement and thus makes the AF2 site not suitable for co-activator binding. The residues which are different between Mut-AR-bicalutamide and WT-AR-bicalutamide are listed in Supplementary Table S2.

Superimposition of the X-ray crystal structures and the representative structures from our MD simulations had an RMSD value of 1.10 Å for WT-AR-R1881 (**Figure 4A**) and 1.02 Å for Mut-AR-bicalutamide (**Figure 4B**). This indicates that the selected representative structures do not deviate much from the X-ray crystal structures. Furthermore, the

TABLE 3 | Critical WT-AR AF2 site residues involved in the hydrophobic and hydrogen bond interactions with a co-activator.

PDB ID	Mutation	Hydrophobic interaction	Hydrogen bond interaction
2PKL (Estebanez-Perpina et al., 2007)		Val716, Lys720, Gln733, Met734, Ile 737, Glu893, Met894	
2Q7I (Askew et al., 2007)		Val716, Lys717, Val730, Gln733, Met734, Ile 737, Gln738, Glu893, Met894	Glu897, Lys720
2Q7K (Askew et al., 2007)		Val716, Lys 717, Gln733, Met734, Ile 737, Gln738, Glu893, Met894	Glu897, Lys720
2QPY (Estebanez-Perpina et al., 2007)		Val713, Val716, Lys720, Val730, Gln733, Met734, Gln738, Met894	Glu897, Lys720
4OEY (Hsu et al., 2014)		Val713, Val716, Val730, Gln733, Met734, Ile737, Gln738, Glu893, Met894	Glu897, Lys720
4OEZ (Hsu et al., 2014)		Val716, Phe725, Met734, Ile 737, Gln738, Glu893, Met894	Glu897, Lys720
4OFR (Hsu et al., 2014)		Val716, Phe725, Met734, Ile737, Gln738, Glu893, Met894	Glu897, Lys720, Asp731, Gln733
4OFU (Hsu et al., 2014)		Val713, Val716, Phe725, Met734, Ile737, Gln738, Glu893, Met894	Glu897, Lys720
4OH5 (Hsu et al., 2014)		Val713, Val716, Val730, Gln733, Met734, Ile 737, Gln738, Met894	Glu897, Lys720
4OHA (Hsu et al., 2014)		Val716, Val730, Gln733, Met734, Ile737, Gln738, Glu893, Met894	Glu897, Lys720
4OIL (Hsu et al., 2014)		Val716, Lys 720, Phe725, Met734, Ile737, Gln738, Glu893, Met894	Glu897, Gln733
4OIU (Hsu et al., 2014)		Lys720, Phe725, Met734, Gln738, Glu893	Glu897, Asp731, Gln733
4OJ9 (Hsu et al., 2014)		Val713, Lys720, Phe725, Met734, Ile737, Gln738, Met894	Glu897, Gln733
4OK1 (Hsu et al., 2014)	Trp741Leu, Arg760Ala	Val716, Gln733, Met734, Ile737, Gln738, Met894	Glu897, Lys720
4OKW (Hsu et al., 2014)	Trp741Leu, Arg760Ala	Val716, Phe725, Met734, Ile737, Gln738, Glu893, Met894	Glu897, Lys720, Gln733
4OKX (Hsu et al., 2014)		Val713, Val716, Phe725, Val730, Met734, Ile737, Gln738	Glu897, Lys720, Gln733
4OLM (Hsu et al., 2014)		Val713, Val716, Phe725, Val730, Met734, Ile737, Gln738	Glu897, Gln733

orientations of R1881 and bicalutamide were also similar to the crystal structures. The overlay of bicalutamide from the Mut-AR X-ray crystal structure and the representative WT-AR structure from MD simulations had an RMSD value of 5.2 Å (**Figure 4C**). This comparative analysis confirmed that the representative structures of WT-AR-bicalutamide obtained from the MD simulations are reliable and were not obtained by chance. Therefore, the representative structure of WT-AR-bicalutamide could be reliably used to elucidate the structural changes in WT-AR due to antagonist binding.

Identification of Critical Residues in the AF2 Site

The AR AF2 site is bound by co-activator proteins, which initiates the transcription of target genes. **Table 3** lists the important residues in WT-AR and their interactions with co-activator proteins (Askew et al., 2007; Estebanez-Perpina et al., 2007; Hsu et al., 2014). The interactions between AR and co-activators were identified from 17 WT-AR-agonist and two Mut-AR-agonist complexes in the PDB. Most of the residues (Val713, Val716, Lys717, Lys720, Phe725, Val730, Gln733, Met734, Ile737, Gln738, Glu893, Met894, and Ile898) in the AF2 site formed hydrophobic interactions with co-activator proteins. Five residues (Val716, Met734, Ile737, Gln738, and

Met894) in the AF2 site had hydrophobic interactions with most of the co-activators. Glu897, Lys720, Asp731, and Gln733 formed hydrogen bond interactions with co-activator proteins and Glu897 and Lys720 formed hydrogen bond interactions with most of the co-activators (Askew et al., 2007; Estebanez-Perpina et al., 2007; Hsu et al., 2014). From the structural analysis, it was clear that Val716, Met734, Ile737, Gln738, Met894, Glu897, and Lys720 played a paramount role in tight binding of co-activator proteins.

Comparison of the AF2 site of the three representative structures (WT-AR-R1881, WT-AR-bicalutamide, and Mut-AR-bicalutamide) from the MD simulations shed light on critical residue displacements which prevent co-activator binding. Val713, Val716, Lys717, Lys720, Phe725, Met734, Met894, Glu897, and Ile898 were considerably different between WT-AR-bicalutamide and WT-AR-R1881 (**Figure 5A**). Among these residues, few had a considerable deviation in their side chain. The side chain distances of Glu897 (CD), Gln738 (CD), Met734 (SD), Val716 (O), Lys720 (CG) were 3.8, 4.2, 2.2, 2.0, and 2.2 Å, respectively, between the WT-AR-R1881 and WT-AR-bicalutamide. These residues also had different conformations between WT-AR-bicalutamide and Mut-AR-bicalutamide as depicted in **Figure 5B**, with respective side chain distances of Glu897 (CD), Gln738 (CD), Met734 (SD), Val716 (O), Lys720 (CG) as 3.2, 0.5, 1.8, 1.1, and 3.0 Å.

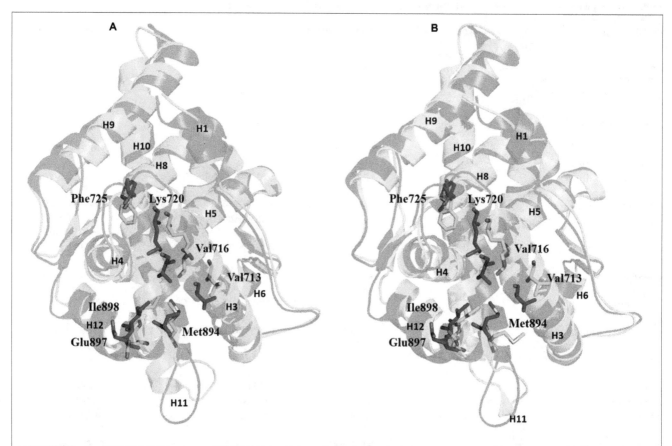

FIGURE 5 | Overlay of WT-AR-R1881 in green and WT-AR-bicalutamide in purple **(A)**. Overlay of WT-AR-bicalutamide in purple and Mut-AR-bicalutamide in cyan **(B)**. The residues with different conformations in the AF2 site are presented as stick models.

Val716, Lys720, and Gln733 were previously experimentally proven to form a charge clump in the AF2 site, which interacts with co-activator proteins (Askew et al., 2007; Estebanez-Perpina et al., 2007; Estébanez-Perpiñá and Fletterick, 2009; Hsu et al., 2014). These residues had a remarkable deviation when comparing between the WT-AR-R1881 and WT-AR-bicalutamide structures in our data. Axerio-Cilies et al. (2011) experimentally proved that Met734 was pushed away from the AF2 site when bicalutamide binds AR. In addition, Zhou X.E. et al. (2010) demonstrated that Glu897 meaningfully interacted with a co-activator protein. Taken together, these previous results support our discovery: when bicalutamide binds WT-AR, Met734, and Glu897 move, which causes structural changes in H12. H12's structural change renders the AF2 site not suitable for co-activator protein binding. Lys720, Glu897, Val716, and Met984 were found to play a major role in the binding of co-activator peptides (He et al., 2004; Hur et al., 2004).

Electrostatic Potential Surface Analysis Revealed That Bicalutamide Binding Disturbed the Positive and Negative Charge Clump in the WT-AR AF2 Site

Electrostatic potential surface analysis is one of the most powerful tools to study intramolecular interactions in a protein and intermolecular interactions between a protein and a small molecule (Sakkiah et al., 2013a). The electrostatic potential surface was calculated only for the critical residues in the AF2 site using PyMol (Baker et al., 2001). PyMol automatically generated the electrostatic potential map and smoothed out the local charge density of the nearby atoms (within 10 Å) without taking solvent

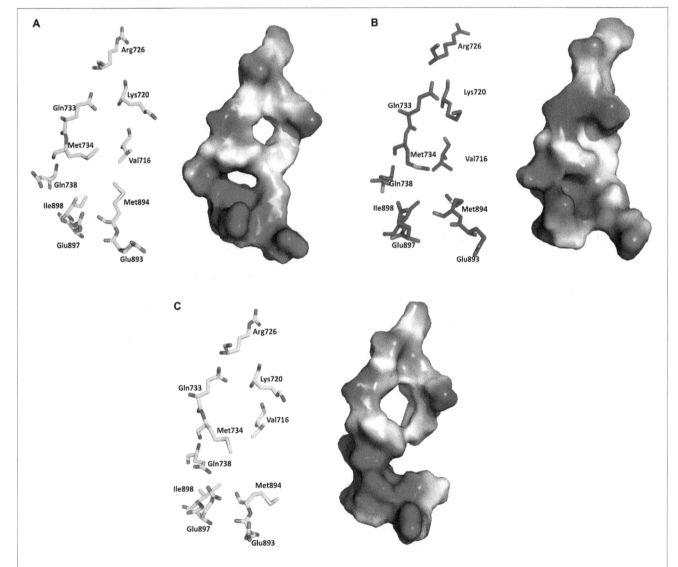

FIGURE 6 | Electrostatic potential surface analysis for the AF2 site in WT-AR-R1881 **(A)**, WT-AR-bicalutamide **(B)**, and Mut-AR-bicalutamide **(C)**. The electrostatic potential surfaces are drawn in the right panels, where red indicates negative and blue indicates positive charges. The corresponding left panels show important residues in stick models.

screening effects into account[6,7]. The electrostatic potential surface of the AF2 site in WT-AR-R1881, WT-AR-bicalutamide, and Mut-AR-bicalutamide is shown in **Figure 6**. WT-AR-R1881 and Mut-AR-bicalutamide had very similar electrostatic potential surfaces in their AF2 site (**Figures 6A,C**), indicating the mutant residues turned the antagonist into an agonist. However, WT-AR-bicalutamide had a very different electrostatic potential surface (**Figure 6B**) compared with the other two structures due to structural changes in the AF2 site caused by the antagonist binding. Five residues (Val716, Lys720, Gln733, Gln738, and Met734) played an important role in bicalutamide binding induced WT-AR AF2 site structural changes. The binding of R1881 in the active site of WT-AR formed a positive (blue) and negative (red) binding region in the AF2 site (**Figure 6A**). Proximal residue contact closed the positive (caused by Gln733, Lys720, and Val716) and negative (caused by Met734, and Gln738) binding sites of the AF2 site in WT-AR-bicalutamide (**Figure 6B**). The critical residues in the Mut-AR-bicalutamide AF2 site (**Figure 6C**) showed a similar type of change compared with Mut-AR-R1881. Previously, it was experimentally proven that the charge clump was formed by residues Lys720 and Glu897 (Estebanez-Perpina et al., 2005; Tan et al., 2015). Co-activators can form hydrogen bond interactions with Lys720 and Glu897, leading to high binding affinity with WT-AR. These hydrogen bonds were distorted due to antagonist binding. Bicalutamide binding in the active site of WT-AR moved Lys720 and Glu897, disturbing the charge clump in the AF2 site and allowing for co-activator binding. Hence, the movement of Lys720, Val716, and Gln733 made the AF2 site unsuitable for co-activator proteins to bind together with bicalutamide. These computational findings give insight into the residues involved in the ligand induced conformational changes of the AF2 site.

CONCLUSION

No structural details of WT-AR when bound by antagonists have been reported to date. Hence, we applied IFD and 1 μs long MD simulations to elucidate the bicalutamide binding induced structural changes of WT-AR's AF2 site. IFD identified a suitable

---

[6] http://www.bccs.uni.no

[7] http://www.bioinfo.no

REFERENCES

Askew, E. B., Gampe, R. T. Jr., Stanley, T. B., Faggart, J. L., and Wilson, E. M. (2007). Modulation of androgen receptor activation function 2 by testosterone and dihydrotestosterone. *J. Biol. Chem.* 282, 25801–25816.

Axerio-Cilies, P., Lack, N. A., Nayana, M. R., Chan, K. H., Yeung, A., Leblanc, E., et al. (2011). Inhibitors of androgen receptor activation function-2 (AF2) site identified through virtual screening. *J. Med. Chem.* 54, 6197–6205. doi: 10.1021/jm200532b

Baker, N. A., Sept, D., Joseph, S., Holst, M. J., and Mccammon, J. A. (2001). Electrostatics of nanosystems: application to microtubules and the ribosome. *Proc. Natl. Acad. Sci. U.S.A.* 98, 10037–10041.

pose of bicalutamide in the ligand binding pocket of WT-AR. The best WT-AR-bicalutamide structure was selected based both on IFD score and on bicalutamide interactions with the critical residues in the ligand binding pocket of WT-AR. The complexes (WT-AR-R1881, WT-AR-bicalutamide, and Mut-AR-bicalutamide) were optimized by MD simulations using Amber 14. Our results clearly pinpointed residues Val716, Lys720, Gln733 and Met734, Gln738, and Glu897 as playing a pivotal role in the formation of the AF2 site in AR. Structural changes or movement of these residues due to bicalutamide binding changed the structure of the AF2 site, making it unsuitable for co-activator protein binding. The electrostatic potential map clearly revealed that the movement of these residues due to bicalutamide binding disturbed the positive and negative charge clump in the AF2 site of WT-AR. The positive clump in the AF2 site was distorted due to the movement of residues Lys720, Val716, and Gln733. Experimental validation is needed to confirm the mechanism by which bicalutamide binding induced WT-AR AF2 structural changes impact recruitment of co-factors.

AUTHOR CONTRIBUTIONS

SS and HH conceived the experiment(s). SS, BP, and WGe conducted the experiments. SS, BP, and WGo analyzed the results. SS, WT, HH, and RK wrote the manuscript. All authors reviewed and approved the manuscript.

FUNDING

This research was supported in part by an appointment to the Research Participation Program at the National Center for Toxicological Research (SS, BP, and WGo) administered by the Oak Ridge Institute for Science and Education through an interagency agreement between the U.S. Department of Energy and the U.S. Food and Drug Administration.

Balbas, M. D., Evans, M. J., Hosfield, D. J., Wongvipat, J., Arora, V. K., Watson, P. A., et al. (2013). Overcoming mutation-based resistance to antiandrogens with rational drug design. *eLife* 2:e00499. doi: 10.7554/eLife.00499

Berman, H. M., Westbrook, J., Feng, Z., Gilliland, G., Bhat, T. N., Weissig, H., et al. (2000). The protein data bank. *Nucleic Acids Res.* 28, 235–242.

Bisson, W. H., Abagyan, R., and Cavasotto, C. N. (2008). Molecular basis of agonicity and antagonicity in the androgen receptor studied by molecular dynamics simulations. *J. Mol. Graph. Model.* 27, 452–458. doi: 10.1016/j.jmgm.2008.08.001

Bohl, C. E., Gao, W., Miller, D. D., Bell, C. E., and Dalton, J. T. (2005). Structural basis for antagonism and resistance of bicalutamide in prostate cancer. *Proc. Natl. Acad. Sci. U.S.A.* 102, 6201–6206.

Bohl, C. E., Wu, Z., Miller, D. D., Bell, C. E., and Dalton, J. T. (2007). Crystal structure of the T877A human androgen receptor ligand-binding domain complexed to cyproterone acetate provides insight for ligand-induced conformational changes and structure-based drug design. *J. Biol. Chem.* 282, 13648–13655.

Cantin, L., Faucher, F., Couture, J.-F., De Jésus-Tran, K. P., Legrand, P., Ciobanu, L. C., et al. (2007). Structural characterization of the human androgen receptor ligand-binding domain complexed with EM5744, a rationally designed steroidal ligand bearing a bulky chain directed toward helix 12. *J. Biol. Chem.* 282, 30910–30919.

Case, D. A., Cheatham, T. E. III, Darden, T., Gohlke, H., Luo, R., Merz, K. M., et al. (2005). The Amber biomolecular simulation programs. *J. Comput. Chem.* 26, 1668–1688.

Chou, K. C., and Mao, B. (1988). Collective motion in DNA and its role in drug intercalation. *Biopolymers* 27, 1795–1815.

Chou, K. C., Zhang, C. T., and Maggiora, G. M. (1994). Solitary wave dynamics as a mechanism for explaining the internal motion during microtubule growth. *Biopolymers* 34, 143–153.

Damber, J.-E., and Aus, G. (2008). Prostate cancer. *Lancet* 371, 1710–1721.

Darden, T., York, D., and Pedersen, L. (1993). Particle mesh Ewald: an N log(N) method for Ewald sums in large systems. *J. Chem. Phys.* 98, 10089–10092.

Dror, R. O., Arlow, D. H., Borhani, D. W., Jensen, M. O., Piana, S., and Shaw, D. E. (2009). Identification of two distinct inactive conformations of the beta2-adrenergic receptor reconciles structural and biochemical observations. *Proc. Natl. Acad. Sci. U.S.A.* 106, 4689–4694. doi: 10.1073/pnas.081106 5106

Duan, M., Liu, N., Zhou, W., Li, D., Yang, M., and Hou, T. (2016). Structural diversity of ligand-binding androgen receptors revealed by microsecond long molecular dynamics simulations and enhanced sampling. *J. Chem. Theory Comput.* 12, 4611–4619. doi: 10.1021/acs.jctc.6b00424

Duan, Y., Wu, C., Chowdhury, S., Lee, M. C., Xiong, G., Zhang, W., et al. (2003). A point-charge force field for molecular mechanics simulations of proteins based on condensed-phase quantum mechanical calculations. *J. Comput. Chem.* 24, 1999–2012.

Durrant, J. D., Bush, R. M., and Amaro, R. E. (2016). Microsecond molecular dynamics simulations of influenza neuraminidase suggest a mechanism for the increased virulence of stalk-deletion mutants. *J. Phys. Chem. B* 120, 8590–8599. doi: 10.1021/acs.jpcb.6b02655

Estebanez-Perpina, E., Arnold, L. A., Nguyen, P., Rodrigues, E. D., Mar, E., Bateman, R., et al. (2007). A surface on the androgen receptor that allosterically regulates coactivator binding. *Proc. Natl. Acad. Sci. U.S.A.* 104, 16074–16079.

Estébanez-Perpiñá, E., and Fletterick, R. J. (2009). "The androgen receptor coactivator-binding interface," in *Androgen Action in Prostate Cancer*, eds J. Mohler and D. Tindall (New York, NY: Springer), 297–311.

Estebanez-Perpina, E., Moore, J. M., Mar, E., Delgado-Rodrigues, E., Nguyen, P., Baxter, J. D., et al. (2005). The molecular mechanisms of coactivator utilization in ligand-dependent transactivation by the androgen receptor. *J. Biol. Chem.* 280, 8060–8068.

Friesner, R. A., Murphy, R. B., Repasky, M. P., Frye, L. L., Greenwood, J. R., Halgren, T. A., et al. (2006). Extra precision glide: docking and scoring incorporating a model of hydrophobic enclosure for protein-ligand complexes. *J. Med. Chem.* 49, 6177–6196.

Gao, W., Bohl, C. E., and Dalton, J. T. (2005). Chemistry and structural biology of androgen receptor. *Chem. Rev.* 105, 3352–3370.

Gelmann, E. P. (2002). Molecular biology of the androgen receptor. *J. Clin. Oncol.* 20, 3001–3015.

Gotz, A. W., Williamson, M. J., Xu, D., Poole, D., Le Grand, S., and Walker, R. C. (2012). Routine microsecond molecular dynamics simulations with AMBER on GPUs. 1. Generalized Born. *J. Chem. Theory Comput.* 8, 1542–1555.

Halgren, T. A., Murphy, R. B., Friesner, R. A., Beard, H. S., Frye, L. L., Pollard, W. T., et al. (2004). Glide: a new approach for rapid, accurate docking and scoring. 2. Enrichment factors in database screening. *J. Med. Chem.* 47, 1750–1759.

Hara, T., Miyazaki, J., Araki, H., Yamaoka, M., Kanzaki, N., Kusaka, M., et al. (2003). Novel mutations of androgen receptor: a possible mechanism of bicalutamide withdrawal syndrome. *Cancer Res.* 63, 149–153.

He, B., Gampe, RT Jr, Kole, A. J., Hnat, A. T., Stanley, T. B., An, G., et al. (2004). Structural basis for androgen receptor interdomain and coactivator interactions

suggests a transition in nuclear receptor activation function dominance. *Mol. Cell* 16, 425–438.

Hong, H., Branham, W. S., Dial, S. L., Moland, C. L., Fang, H., Shen, J., et al. (2012). Rat alpha-Fetoprotein binding affinities of a large set of structurally diverse chemicals elucidated the relationships between structures and binding affinities. *Chem. Res. Toxicol.* 25, 2553–2566. doi: 10.1021/tx3003406

Hong, H., Branham, W. S., Ng, H. W., Moland, C. L., Dial, S. L., Fang, H., et al. (2015). Human sex hormone-binding globulin binding affinities of 125 structurally diverse chemicals and comparison with their binding to androgen receptor, estrogen receptor, and alpha-fetoprotein. *Toxicol. Sci.* 143, 333–348. doi: 10.1093/toxsci/kfu231

Hong, H., Fang, H., Xie, Q., Perkins, R., Sheehan, D. M., and Tong, W. (2003). Comparative molecular field analysis (CoMFA) model using a large diverse set of natural, synthetic and environmental chemicals for binding to the androgen receptor. *SAR QSAR Environ. Res.* 14, 373–388.

Hong, H., Harvey, B. G., Palmese, G. R., Stanzione, J. F., Ng, H. W., Sakkiah, S., et al. (2016a). Experimental data extraction and in silico prediction of the estrogenic activity of renewable replacements for bisphenol A. *Int. J. Environ. Res. Public Health* 13:E705. doi: 10.3390/ijerph13070705

Hong, H., Rua, D., Sakkiah, S., Selvaraj, C., Ge, W., and Tong, W. (2016b). Consensus modeling for prediction of estrogenic activity of ingredients commonly used in sunscreen products. *Int. J. Environ. Res. Public Health* 13, E958.

Hong, H., Tong, W., Fang, H., Shi, L., Xie, Q., Wu, J., et al. (2002). Prediction of estrogen receptor binding for 58,000 chemicals using an integrated system of a tree-based model with structural alerts. *Environ. Health Perspect.* 110, 29–36.

Hong, H., Tong, W., Xie, Q., Fang, H., and Perkins, R. (2005). An in silico ensemble method for lead discovery: decision forest. *SAR QSAR Environ. Res.* 16, 339–347.

Hsu, C. L., Liu, J. S., Wu, P. L., Guan, H. H., Chen, Y. L., Lin, A. C., et al. (2014). Identification of a new androgen receptor (AR) co-regulator BUD31 and related peptides to suppress wild-type and mutated AR-mediated prostate cancer growth via peptide screening and X-ray structure analysis. *Mol. Oncol.* 8, 1575–1587. doi: 10.1016/j.molonc.2014.06.009

Humphrey, W., Dalke, A., and Schulten, K. (1996). VMD: visual molecular dynamics. *J. Mol. Graph.* 14, 33–38.

Hur, E., Pfaff, S. J., Payne, E. S., Grøn, H., Buehrer, B. M., and Fletterick, R. J. (2004). Recognition and accommodation at the androgen receptor coactivator binding interface. *PLoS Biol.* 2:e274. doi: 10.1371/journal.pbio.0020274

Jacobson, M. P., Pincus, D. L., Rapp, C. S., Day, T. J., Honig, B., Shaw, D. E., et al. (2004). A hierarchical approach to all-atom protein loop prediction. *Proteins* 55, 351–367.

Jorgensen, W. L., Chandrasekhar, J., Madura, J. D., Impey, R. W., and Klein, M. L. (1983). Comparison of simple potential functions for simulating liquid water. *J. Chem. Phys.* 79, 926–935.

Jorgensen, W. L., and Tirado-Rives, J. (1988). The OPLS [optimized potentials for liquid simulations] potential functions for proteins, energy minimizations for crystals of cyclic peptides and crambin. *J. Am. Chem. Soc.* 110, 1657–1666.

Kaminski, G. A., Friesner, R. A., Tirado-Rives, J., and Jorgensen, W. L. (2001). Evaluation and Reparametrization of the OPLS-AA force field for proteins via comparison with accurate quantum chemical calculations on peptides. *J. Phys. Chem. B* 105, 6474–6487.

Khelashvili, G., Grossfield, A., Feller, S. E., Pitman, M. C., and Weinstein, H. (2009). Structural and dynamic effects of cholesterol at preferred sites of interaction with rhodopsin identified from microsecond length molecular dynamics simulations. *Proteins* 76, 403–417. doi: 10.1002/prot.22355

Korpal, M., Korn, J. M., Gao, X., Rakiec, D. P., Ruddy, D. A., Doshi, S., et al. (2013). An F876L mutation in androgen receptor confers genetic and phenotypic resistance to MDV3100 (enzalutamide). *Cancer Discov.* 3, 1030–1043. doi: 10.1158/2159-8290.CD-13-0142

Kuiper, G. G., Faber, P. W., Van Rooij, H. C., Van Der Korput, J. A., Ris-Stalpers, C., Klaassen, P., et al. (1989). Structural organization of the human androgen receptor gene. *J. Mol. Endocrinol.* 2, R1–R4.

Kumar, A., and Purohit, R. (2014). Use of long term molecular dynamics simulation in predicting cancer associated SNPs. *PLoS Comput. Biol.* 10:e1003318. doi: 10.1371/journal.pcbi.1003318

Lindorff-Larsen, K., Piana, S., Dror, R. O., and Shaw, D. E. (2011). How fast-folding proteins fold. *Science* 334, 517–520. doi: 10.1126/science.1208351

Liu, H., An, X., Li, S., Wang, Y., Li, J., and Liu, H. (2015). Interaction mechanism exploration of R-bicalutamide/S-1 with WT/W741L AR using molecular dynamics simulations. *Mol. Biosyst.* 11, 3347–3354. doi: 10.1039/c5mb00 499c

Liu, H., Han, R., Li, J., Liu, H., and Zheng, L. (2016). Molecular mechanism of R-bicalutamide switching from androgen receptor antagonist to agonist induced by amino acid mutations using molecular dynamics simulations and free energy calculation. *J. Comput. Aided Mol. Des.* 30, 1189–1200. doi: 10.1007/s10822-016-9992-2

Liu, H., Wang, L., Tian, J., Li, J., and Liu, H. (2017). Molecular dynamics studies on the enzalutamide resistance mechanisms induced by androgen receptor mutations. *J. Cell. Biochem.* 118, 2792–2801. doi: 10.1002/jcb.25928

Lubahn, D. B., Brown, T. R., Simental, J. A., Higgs, H. N., Migeon, C. J., Wilson, E. M., et al. (1989). Sequence of the intron/exon junctions of the coding region of the human androgen receptor gene and identification of a point mutation in a family with complete androgen insensitivity. *Proc. Natl. Acad. Sci. U.S.A.* 86, 9534–9538.

Luo, H.-J., Wang, J.-Z., Deng, W.-Q., and Zou, K. (2013). Induced-fit docking and binding free energy calculation on furostanol saponins from *Tupistra chinensis* as epidermal growth factor receptor inhibitors. *Med. Chem. Res.* 22, 4970–4979.

Matias, P. M., Donner, P., Coelho, R., Thomaz, M., Peixoto, C., Macedo, S., et al. (2000). Structural evidence for ligand specificity in the binding domain of the human androgen receptor. Implications for pathogenic gene mutations. *J. Biol. Chem.* 275, 26164–26171.

Ng, H. W., Doughty, S. W., Luo, H., Ye, H., Ge, W., Tong, W., et al. (2015a). Development and validation of decision forest model for estrogen receptor binding prediction of chemicals using large data sets. *Chem. Res. Toxicol.* 28, 2343–2351. doi: 10.1021/acs.chemrestox.5b00358

Ng, H. W., Shu, M., Luo, H., Ye, H., Ge, W., Perkins, R., et al. (2015b). Estrogenic activity data extraction and in silico prediction show the endocrine disruption potential of bisphenol A replacement compounds. *Chem. Res. Toxicol.* 28, 1784–1795. doi: 10.1021/acs.chemrestox.5b00243

Ng, H. W., Zhang, W., Shu, M., Luo, H., Ge, W., Perkins, R., et al. (2014). Competitive molecular docking approach for predicting estrogen receptor subtype alpha agonists and antagonists. *BMC Bioinformatics* 15(Suppl. 11):S4. doi: 10.1186/1471-2105-15-S11-S4

Nury, H., Poitevin, F., Van Renterghem, C., Changeux, J.-P., Corringer, P.-J., Delarue, M., et al. (2010). One-microsecond molecular dynamics simulation of channel gating in a nicotinic receptor homologue. *Proc. Natl. Acad. Sci. U.S.A.* 107, 6275–6280. doi: 10.1073/pnas.1001832107

Osguthorpe, D. J., and Hagler, A. T. (2011). Mechanism of androgen receptor antagonism by bicalutamide in the treatment of prostate cancer. *Biochemistry* 50, 4105–4113. doi: 10.1021/bi102059z

Ryckaert, J.-P., Ciccotti, G., and Berendsen, H. J. C. (1977). Numerical integration of the cartesian equations of motion of a system with constraints: molecular dynamics of n-alkanes. *J. Comput. Phys.* 23, 327–341.

Sack, J. S., Kish, K. F., Wang, C., Attar, R. M., Kiefer, S. E., An, Y., et al. (2001). Crystallographic structures of the ligand-binding domains of the androgen receptor and its T877A mutant complexed with the natural agonist dihydrotestosterone. *Proc. Natl. Acad. Sci. U.S.A.* 98, 4904–4909.

Sakkiah, S., Arooj, M., Cao, G. P., and Lee, K. W. (2013a). Insight the C-site pocket conformational changes responsible for sirtuin 2 activity using molecular dynamics simulations. *PLoS One* 8:e59278. doi: 10.1371/journal.pone.0059278

Sakkiah, S., Arooj, M., Kumar, M. R., Eom, S. H., and Lee, K. W. (2013b). Identification of inhibitor binding site in human sirtuin 2 using molecular docking and dynamics simulations. *PLoS One* 8:e51429. doi: 10.1371/journal.pone.0051429

Sakkiah, S., Ng, H. W., Tong, W., and Hong, H. (2016). Structures of androgen receptor bound with ligands: advancing understanding of biological functions and drug discovery. *Expert Opin. Ther. Targets* 20, 1267–1282. doi: 10.1080/14728222.2016.1192131

Schrodinger (2015). *The PyMOL Molecular Graphics System, Version 1.8.* New York, NY: Schrodinger.

Schrodinger-Suite (2016a). *Induced Fit Docking Protocol 2016-2; Glide.* New York, NY: Schrodinger.

Schrodinger-Suite (2016b). *2016-2: Maestro, Schrodinger, LLC, New York, NY, 2016). Schrodinger Release 2016-2.* New York, NY: Schrodinger.

Shelley, J. C., Cholleti, A., Frye, L. L., Greenwood, J. R., Timlin, M. R., and Uchimaya, M. (2007). Epik: a software program for pK$_a$ prediction and protonation state generation for drug-like molecules. *J. Comput. Aided Mol. Des.* 21, 681–691.

Shen, J., Xu, L., Fang, H., Richard, A. M., Bray, J. D., Judson, R. S., et al. (2013). EADB: an estrogenic activity database for assessing potential endocrine activity. *Toxicol. Sci.* 135, 277–291. doi: 10.1093/toxsci/kft164

Sherman, W., Beard, H. S., and Farid, R. (2006a). Use of an induced fit receptor structure in virtual screening. *Chem. Biol. Drug Des.* 67, 83–84.

Sherman, W., Day, T., Jacobson, M. P., Friesner, R. A., and Farid, R. (2006b). Novel procedure for modeling ligand/receptor induced fit effects. *J. Med. Chem.* 49, 534–553.

Shivakumar, D., Williams, J., Wu, Y., Damm, W., Shelley, J., and Sherman, W. (2010). Prediction of absolute solvation free energies using molecular dynamics free energy perturbation and the opls force field. *J. Chem. Theory Comput.* 6, 1509–1519. doi: 10.1021/ct900587b

Tan, M. H. E., Li, J., Xu, H. E., Melcher, K., and Yong, E.-L. (2015). Androgen receptor: structure, role in prostate cancer and drug discovery. *Acta Pharmacol. Sin.* 36, 3–23. doi: 10.1038/aps.2014.18

Taplin, M. E., and Balk, S. P. (2004). Androgen receptor: a key molecule in the progression of prostate cancer to hormone independence. *J. Cell. Biochem.* 91, 483–490.

Wang, H., Aslanian, R., and Madison, V. S. (2008). Induced-fit docking of mometasone furoate and further evidence for glucocorticoid receptor 17α pocket flexibility. *J. Mol. Graph. Model.* 27, 512–521.

Wang, J., Wolf, R. M., Caldwell, J. W., Kollman, P. A., and Case, D. A. (2004). Development and testing of a general amber force field. *J. Comput. Chem.* 25, 1157–1174.

Wang, J. F., and Chou, K. C. (2009). Insight into the molecular switch mechanism of human Rab5a from molecular dynamics simulations. *Biochem. Biophys. Res. Commun.* 390, 608–612. doi: 10.1016/j.bbrc.2009.10.014

Wang, Y., Han, R., Zhang, H., Liu, H., Li, J., Liu, H., et al. (2017). Combined ligand/structure-based virtual screening and molecular dynamics simulations of steroidal androgen receptor antagonists. *BioMed Res. Int.* 2017:3572394. doi: 10.1155/2017/3572394

Whitten, S. T., Garcia-Moreno, E. B., and Hilser, V. J. (2005). Local conformational fluctuations can modulate the coupling between proton binding and global structural transitions in proteins. *Proc. Natl. Acad. Sci. U.S.A.* 102, 4282–4287.

Ye, H., Ng, H. W., Sakkiah, S., Ge, W., Perkins, R., Tong, W., et al. (2016). Pathway analysis revealed potential diverse health impacts of flavonoids that bind estrogen receptors. *Int. J. Environ. Res. Public Health* 13:373. doi: 10.3390/ijerph13040373

Zhong, H., Tran, L. M., and Stang, J. L. (2009). Induced-fit docking studies of the active and inactive states of protein tyrosine kinases. *J. Mol. Graph. Model.* 28, 336–346. doi: 10.1016/j.jmgm.2009.08.012

Zhou, J., Liu, B., Geng, G., and Wu, J. H. (2010). Study of the impact of the T877A mutation on ligand-induced helix-12 positioning of the androgen receptor resulted in design and synthesis of novel antiandrogens. *Proteins* 78, 623–637. doi: 10.1002/prot.22592

Zhou, X. E., Suino-Powell, K. M., Li, J., He, Y., Mackeigan, J. P., Melcher, K., et al. (2010). Identification of SRC3/AIB1 as a preferred coactivator for hormone-activated androgen receptor. *J. Biol. Chem.* 285, 9161–9171. doi: 10.1074/jbc.M109.085779

10

Predicting Off-Target Binding Profiles with Confidence Using Conformal Prediction

Samuel Lampa[1], Jonathan Alvarsson[1], Staffan Arvidsson Mc Shane[1], Arvid Berg[1], Ernst Ahlberg[2] and Ola Spjuth[1]*

[1] *Pharmaceutical Bioinformatics Group, Department of Pharmaceutical Biosciences, Uppsala University, Uppsala, Sweden,*
[2] *Predictive Compound ADME and Safety, Drug Safety and Metabolism, AstraZeneca IMED Biotech Unit, Mölndal, Sweden*

*Correspondence:
Ola Spjuth
ola.spjuth@farmbio.uu.se

Ligand-based models can be used in drug discovery to obtain an early indication of potential off-target interactions that could be linked to adverse effects. Another application is to combine such models into a panel, allowing to compare and search for compounds with similar profiles. Most contemporary methods and implementations however lack valid measures of confidence in their predictions, and only provide point predictions. We here describe a methodology that uses Conformal Prediction for predicting off-target interactions, with models trained on data from 31 targets in the ExCAPE-DB dataset selected for their utility in broad early hazard assessment. Chemicals were represented by the signature molecular descriptor and support vector machines were used as the underlying machine learning method. By using conformal prediction, the results from predictions come in the form of confidence *p*-values for each class. The full pre-processing and model training process is openly available as scientific workflows on GitHub, rendering it fully reproducible. We illustrate the usefulness of the developed methodology on a set of compounds extracted from DrugBank. The resulting models are published online and are available via a graphical web interface and an OpenAPI interface for programmatic access.

Keywords: target profiles, predictive modeling, conformal prediction, machine learning, off-target, adverse effects, workflow

1. INTRODUCTION

Drug-target interactions are central to the drug discovery process (Yildirim et al., 2007), and is the subject of study for the field of chemogenomics (Bredel and Jacoby, 2004), which has emerged and grown over the last few decades. Drugs commonly interact with multiple targets (Hopkins, 2008), and off-target pharmacology as well as polypharmacology have important implications for drug efficacy and safety (Peters, 2013; Ravikumar and Aittokallio, 2018). Organizations involved in drug discovery, such as pharmaceutical companies and academic institutions, use many types of experimental techniques and assays to determine target interactions, including *in vitro* pharmacological profiling (Bowes et al., 2012). However, an attractive complementary method is to use computational (*in silico*) profiling of binding profiles for ligands (Cereto-Massagué et al., 2015), which also opens the possibility to predict hypothetical compounds. A common approach to the target prediction problem is to use a panel of structure-activity relationship (QSAR) models, with one model per target (Hansch, 1969), where chemicals in a knowledge base with known interaction values (numerical or categorical) are described numerically by descriptors, and a statistical learning model is trained to predict numerical values (regression) or categorical values (classification) for new compounds. The recent increase in the number of available SAR data points in interaction databases such as ChEMBL (Gaulton et al., 2017) and PubChem (Wang et al., 2017) makes it feasible to use ligand-based models to predict not only targets but also panels of targets. Several methods and tools are available for target prediction and for constructing and using target profiles. Bender et al. use a Bayesian approach to train models for 70 selected targets and use these for target profiling to classify adverse drug reactions (Bender et al., 2007). Chembench is a web-based portal, which founded in 2008 is one of the first publicly available integrated cheminformatics web portals. It integrates a number of commercial as well as open source tools for dataset creation, validation, modeling and validation. It also supports building ensembles of models, for multiple targets (Walker et al., 2010; Capuzzi et al., 2017). The Online chemical modeling environment (OCHEM), is a web-based platform that intends to serve as multi-tool platform where users can select among the many available alternatives in terms of tools and methods, for all of the steps of creating a predictive model, such as data search, selection of descriptors and machine learning model, as well as assessment of the resulting model. OCHEM also encourages tool authors to contribute with their own tools to be integrated in the platform (Sushko et al., 2011). Yu et al. use Random Forest (RF) and Support Vector Machines (SVM) to predict drug-target interactions from heterogeneous biological data (Yu et al., 2012). TargetHunter (Wang et al., 2013) is another online tool that uses chemical similarity to predict targets for ligands, and show how training models on ChEMBL data can enable useful predictions on examples taken from PubChem bioassays. Yao et al. describe TargetNet (Yao et al., 2016), a web service for multi-target QSAR models; an online service that uses Naïve Bayes. The polypharmacology browser (Awale and Reymond, 2017) is a web-based target prediction tool that queries ChEMBL bioactivity data using multiple fingerprints.

We observe three important shortcomings among previous works. Primarily, available methods for ligand-based target profiling often do not offer valid measures of confidence in predictions, leaving the user uncertain about the usefulness of predictions. Secondly, the majority of the web tools lack an open and standardized API, meaning that it is not straightforward (and in most cases not possible at all) to consume the services programmatically, e.g., from a script or a scientific workflow tool such as KNIME (Mazanetz et al., 2012). Thirdly, previous works do not publish the pre-processing and modeling workflows in reproducible formats, rendering it hard to update the models as data changes, and limits the portability of methods. In fact, most implementations are only accessible from a website without the underlying implementations being openly available for

inspection, which limits both the reproducibility (Stodden et al., 2016), and verifiability (Hinsen, 2018) of their implementation.

We here present an approach for ligand-based target profiling using a confidence framework, delivering target profiles with confidence scores for the predictions of whether a query compound interacts with each target. The confidence scores were calculated using the Conformal Prediction methodology (CP) (Vovk et al., 2005), which has been successfully demonstrated in several recent studies (Norinder et al., 2014, 2016; Cortés-Ciriano et al., 2015; Forreryd et al., 2018). For readers new to the CP methodology, we recommend (Gammerman and Vovk, 2007) for a good and gentle general overview, and Norinder et al. (2014) for a good introduction to CP for cheminformatics. The goal of this study was to create an automated and reproducible approach for generating a predicted target profile based on QSAR binding models, with the models making up the profile published online as microservices and the profile accessible from a web page. Although the models give a confidence measure we also set out to evaluate them on a test set to see how well they performed on representative data. We exemplified the process by creating a profile for the targets for broad early hazard assessment as suggested by Bowes et al. (2012).

2. METHODS

2.1. Training Data

We based this study upon data from the ExCAPE-DB dataset (Sun et al., 2017b). The reason for this is that ExCAPE-DB combines data about ligand-target binding from ChEMBL with similar data from PubChem, where importantly, PubChem contains many true non-actives, which has been shown earlier to result in better models than by using random compounds as non-actives (Mervin et al., 2015). The data in ExCAPE-DB has also gone through extensive filtering and pre-processing, specifically to make it more useful as a starting point for QSAR studies. For more details on the data filtering and processing done in the ExCAPE-DB dataset, we refer to Sun et al. (2017b).

A scientific workflow was constructed to automate the full data pre-processing pipeline. The first step comprises extracting data on binding association between ligands and targets from the ExCAPE-DB dataset (Sun et al., 2017b), more specifically the columns Gene symbol, Original entry ID (PubChem CID or CHEMBL ID), SMILES and Activity flag. This was performed early in the workflow to make subsequent data transformation steps less time-consuming, given the relatively large size of the uncompressed ExCAPE-DB data file (18 GB). From the extracted dataset, all rows for which there existed rows with a conflicting activity value for the same target (gene symbol) and SMILES string, were completely removed. Also, all duplicates in terms of the extracted information (Original entry ID, SMILES, and Activity flag) were replaced by a single entry, and thus deduplicated. Note that deduplication on InChI level was already done in for the ExCAPE-DB dataset in Sun et al. (2017b), but since the signatures descriptor is based on SMILES, which is a less specific chemical format than InChI (certain compounds that are unique in InChI might not be unique in SMILES) this turns

---

Abbreviations: A, Active; ACP, Aggregated Conformal Predictor; CAOF, Class-Averaged Observed Fuzziness; CP, Conformal Prediction; JAR, Java Archive (A file format); MC, M Criterion (Fraction of multi-label predictions); N, Non-active; OF, Observed Fuzziness; QSAR, Quantitative Structure-Activity Relationship; RF, Random Forest; SMILES, Simplified molecular-input line-entry system (A text-based representation of chemical structures); SVM, Support Vector Machines.

out to have resulted in some duplicate and conflicting rows in terms of SMILES still appearing in the dataset. Since this is a potential problem in particular if the exact same SMILES end up in both the training and calibration or test set, we performed this additional deduplication, on the SMILES level[1]. For full information about the pre-processing done by the ExCAPE-DB authors, see Sun et al. (2017b). As a help to the reader we note that the activity flag is – in the ExCAPE-DB dataset—set to active (or "A") if the dose-response value in the binding assays was lower than 10 μM and non-active (or "N") otherwise.

A subset of the panel of 44 binding targets as suggested in Bowes et al. (2012) was selected for inclusion in the study. The selection was based on the criteria that targets should have at least 100 active and at least 100 non-active compounds. In addition some targets were excluded for which data was not found in ExCAPE-DB. This is described in detail below. Some of the gene symbols used in Bowes et al. (2012) were not found in their exact form in the ExCAPE-DB dataset. To resolve this, PubMed was consulted to find synonymous gene symbols with the following replacements being done: *KCNE1* was replaced with *MINK1* which is present in ExCAPE-DB. *CHRNA1* (coding for the $\alpha 1$ sub-unit of the Acetylcholine receptor) was excluded, as it is not present in the dataset (*CHRNA4*, coding for the $\alpha 4$ sub-unit of the Acetylcholine receptor, is present in the dataset). We note though, that both *MINK1* and *CHRNA4* were removed in the filtering step mentioned above, since the dataset did not contain more than 100 active and 100 non-active compounds for *MINK1* nor *CHRNA*. However, since one aim of the study is to present and publish an automated and reproducible data processing workflow, these targets could potentially be included in subsequent runs on later versions of the database with additional data available.

The resulting dataset (named Dataset1) consists of 31 targets (marked as "included" in **Table 1**). For 21 of these targets, the dataset contained less than 10,000 non-active compounds, which makes them stand out from the other datasets, and where some of them contain a problematically low amount of non-actives. These 21 targets are referred to as Dataset2, and their respective target datasets were expanded with randomly selected examples from the ExCAPE-DB dataset which were not reported to be active for the target, thus being "assumed non-active." These target datasets are marked with a ✓ in the "Assumed non-actives added" column of **Table 1**. The number of new examples was chosen such that the total number of non-actives and assumed non-actives added up to twice the number of actives, for each target, respectively. The compounds for the remaining 10 targets, which were not extended with assumed non-actives, were named Dataset3.

In order to validate the predictive ability of the trained models, a new dataset was created (Dataset4) by withholding 1,000 compounds from the ExCAPE-DB dataset, to form an external validation dataset. The compounds chosen to be withheld were the following: (i) all small molecules in DrugBank (version 5.0.11) with status "withdrawn," for which we could find either a PubChem ID or a CHEMBL ID, (ii) a randomly selected subset of the remaining compounds in DrugBank 5.0.11, with status

"approved," for which we could also find PubChem or CHEMBL IDs, until a total number of 1,000 compounds was reached. No regard was paid to other drug statuses in DrugBank such as "investigational."

The relation of the mentioned datasets Dataset1-4 are shown in a graphical overview of how they were created in **Figure 1**, and in **Table 2**, which summarizes in words how each dataset was created.

The Conformal Prediction methodology, in particular with the Mondrian approach, can handle differing sizes of the datasets well (Norinder and Boyer, 2017), and so we see no reason to stick to the exact same number of compounds as the actives. Instead we use an active:non-active ratio of 1:2 between the classes. The justification for this is that the assumed non-actives likely have chemistry coming from a larger chemical space compared to the known compounds, thus by adding more of the assumed non-actives we can hopefully increase the number of examples in the regions of chemical space that are of interest for separating the two classes.

All the targets, with details about their respective number of active and non-active compounds, and whether they are included or not, are summarized in **Table 1**.

2.2. Conformal Prediction
Conformal Prediction (CP) (Vovk et al., 2005) provides a layer on top of existing machine learning methods and produces valid prediction regions for test objects. This contrasts to standard machine learning that delivers point estimates. In CP a prediction region contains the true value with probability equal to $1 - \epsilon$, where ϵ is the selected significance level. Such a prediction region can be obtained under the assumption that the observed data is exchangeable. An important consequence is that the size of this region directly relates to the *strangeness* of the test example, and is an alternative to the concept of a model's *applicability domain* (Norinder et al., 2014). For the classification case a prediction is given as set of conformal *p-values*[2], one for each class, which represent a ranking for the test object. The *p*-values together with the user decided ϵ produces the final prediction set. Conformal Predictors are Mondrian, meaning that they handle the classes independently, which has previously been shown to work very well for imbalanced datasets and remove the need for under/oversampling, boosting or similar techniques (Norinder and Boyer, 2017; Sun et al., 2017a).

Conformal Prediction as originally invented, was described for the online transductive setting, meaning that the underlying learning model had to be retrained for every new test object. Later it was adapted for the off-line inductive setting too, where the underlying model is trained only once for a batch of training examples. The Inductive Conformal Predictor (ICP), which is used in this study, require far less computational resources, but has the disadvantage that a part of the training set must be set aside as a *calibration set*. The remaining data, called *proper training set*, is used to train the learning model. As the partitioning of data into a calibration set and proper training set can have a large influence on the performance of the predictor,

---

[1]https://github.com/pharmbio/ptp-project/blob/c529cf/exp/20180426-wo-drugbank/wo_drugbank_wf.go#L239-L246

[2]The term "*p-values*" in Conformal Prediction does not have the same definition as in statistical hypothesis testing.

TABLE 1 | The panel of targets used in this study, identified by gene symbol.

Gene symbol	Actives	Non-actives (before adding assumed non-actives and deduplication)	Non-actives (after adding assumed non-actives and deduplication)	Assumed non-actives added	Remarks
ACHE	3,160	1,152	5,824	✓	
ADORA2A	5,275	593	10,092	✓	
ADRB1	1,306	149	2,544	✓	
ADRB2	1,955	342,282	341,925		
AR	2,593	4,725	4,866	✓	
AVPR1A	1,055	321,406	321,098		
CCKAR	1,249	132	2,458	✓	
CHRM1	2,776	417,549	358,330		
CHRM2	1,817	152	3,440	✓	
CHRM3	1,676	144	3,234	✓	
CNR1	5,336	400	10,220	✓	
CNR2	4,583	402	8,676	✓	
DRD1	1,732	356,201	355,909		
DRD2	8,323	343,206	342,958		
EDNRA	2,129	124	4,050	✓	
HTR1A	6,555	64,578	64,468		
HTR2A	4,160	359,962	359,663		
KCNH2	5,330	350,773	350,452		
LCK	2,662	283	5,246	✓	
MAOA	1,260	1,083	2,452	✓	
NR3C1	2,525	4,382	4,804	✓	
OPRD1	5,350	826	9,580	✓	
OPRK1	3,672	303,335	303,111		
OPRM1	5,837	2,872	11,252	✓	
PDE3A	197	110	392	✓	
PTGS1	849	729	1,634	✓	
PTGS2	2,862	827	5,162	✓	
SCN5A	316	119	624	✓	
SLC6A2	3,879	218	7,498	✓	
SLC6A3	5,017	106,819	106,594		
SLC6A4	7,228	382	13,660	✓	
ADRA1A	1,782	24			
ADRA2A	839	39			
CACNA1C	166	20			
CHRNA1	–	–			Not in ExCAPE-DB
CHRNA4	256	17			
GABRA1	112	5			
GRIN1	555	92			
HRH1	1,218	65			
HRH2	394	56			
HTR1B	1,262	86			
HTR2B	1,159	66			
HTR3A	584	65			
KCNQ1	37	303,466			
MINK1	929	8			Synonym to KCNE1
PDE4D	484	98			

(Left margin labels: "INCLUDED" beside the first row range; "NOT INCLUDED" beside the second row range.)

Actives and non-actives refer to the number of ligand interactions marked as active and non-active in ExCAPE-DB. The labels "included" and "not included" to the left, for the two row ranges, indicate whether targets did pass the filtering criteria of at least 100 actives and 100 non-actives, to be included.

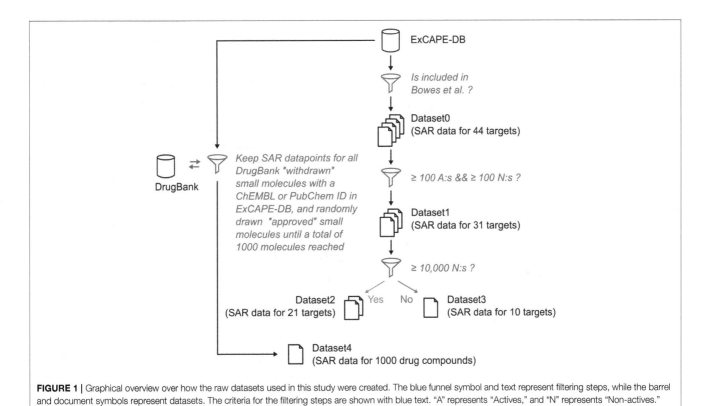

FIGURE 1 | Graphical overview over how the raw datasets used in this study were created. The blue funnel symbol and text represent filtering steps, while the barrel and document symbols represent datasets. The criteria for the filtering steps are shown with blue text. "A" represents "Actives," and "N" represents "Non-actives."

TABLE 2 | Summary of datasets discussed.

Name	Description
Dataset0	SAR data points for all 44 targets in Bowes et al. (2012) which are available in ExCAPE-DB.
Dataset1	SAR data points for the 31 targets in Dataset0 for which there were at least 100 actives and 100 non-actives.
Dataset2	SAR data points for targets with least 10,000 non-actives.
Dataset3	SAR data points for targets which had less than 10,000 non-actives, thus the same as Dataset1 with Dataset2 excluded.
Dataset4	SAR points making up the external test, by extracting rows from ExCAPE-DB for a selected set of 1,000 compounds in DrugBank (All withdrawn, and randomly sampled approved, drugs, until reaching 1,000 drugs).

See also **Figure 1** for a graphical overview of how each dataset was created.

it is common to redo this split multiple times and train an ICP for each such split. This results in a so called Aggregated Conformal Predictor (ACP) that aggregates the predictions for each individual ICP.

In this study we used the Mondrian ACP implementation in the software CPSign (Arvidsson, 2016), leveraging the LIBLINEAR SVM implementation (Fan et al., 2008) together with the signatures molecular descriptor (Faulon et al., 2003). This descriptor is based on the neighboring of atoms in a molecule and has been shown to work well for QSAR studies (Alvarsson et al., 2016; Lapins et al., 2018) and for ligand-based target prediction (Alvarsson et al., 2014). Signatures were

generated with height 1-3, which means that molecular subgraphs including all atoms of distance 1, 2, or 3 from initial atoms, are generated. Support vector machines is a machine learning algorithm which is commonly used in QSAR studies (Norinder, 2003; Zhou et al., 2011) together with molecular signatures and similar molecular descriptors, e.g., the extended connectivity fingerprints (Rogers and Hahn, 2010). As nonconformity measure we used the distance between the classifier's decision surface and the test object, as previously described by Eklund et al. (2015). In order to not use the assumed non-active compounds in Dataset2 in the calibration set of the ICPs, these additional compounds were treated separately, by providing them to the CPSign software with the `--proper-train` parameter, see the CPSign documentation (Arvidsson, 2016). By using this parameter the additional compounds are only added to the proper training set, thus being used for training the underlying SVM model, but not for the calibration of the predictions. This ensures that potentially non-typical chemistry in the additional assumed non-active compounds does not affect the calibration of the predictions in a negative way.

2.3. Hyper-Parameter Tuning

For each of the 31 targets in Dataset1, a parameter sweep was run to find the optimal value of the cost parameter of LIBLINEAR, optimizing modeling efficiency using 10-fold cross validation. The training approach used an Aggregated Conformal Predictor (ACP) with 10 aggregated models. The parameter sweep evaluated three values for the cost parameter for each target; 1, 10, and 100. The efficiency measure used for the evaluation was the observed fuzziness (OF) score described in Vovk et al. (2016) as:

$$OF = \frac{1}{m} \sum_{i=1}^{m} \sum_{y_i \neq y} p_i^y, \qquad (1)$$

where p_i^y is the p-value of the ith test case for class y, and m is the number of test examples, or in our case with only two classes:

$$OF = \frac{\sum\limits_{i,\,y_i=A} p_i^N + \sum\limits_{i,\,y_i=N} p_i^A}{m_A + m_N} \qquad (2)$$

where p_i^N is the ith p-value for class N, p_i^A is the ith p-value for class A and m_A and m_N is the number of test examples in class A and N, respectively. OF is basically an average of the p-values for the wrong class, i.e., lower fuzziness means better prediction.

To study the effect of imbalanced datasets on efficiency, we also implemented a modified version of OF, due to the fact that OF is influenced more by values in the larger class in case of imbalanced datasets, referred to as *class-averaged observed fuzziness* (*CAOF*) as:

$$CAOF = \frac{\sum\limits_{i,\,y_i=A} p_i^N}{m_A} + \frac{\sum\limits_{i,\,y_i=N} p_i^A}{m_N} \qquad (3)$$

with the same variable conventions as above. Where OF is only an average for the p-values in the test set, $CAOF$ averages the contribution from each class separately, meaning that for very imbalanced cases OF is mostly affected by the larger class, while for $CAOF$, both classes contribute equally much, regardless of their respective number of p-values. $CAOF$ was not used for cost selection, but is provided for information in the results from the workflow.

A commonly used efficiency measure in CP is the size of the prediction region or set given by the predictor. In the classification setting, this is expressed as the fraction of *multi-label* predictions. This measure is denoted as the *M criterion* (MC) and described in Vovk et al. (2016):

$$M\ criterion = \frac{1}{m} \sum_{i=1}^{m} \mathbf{1}_{\{|\Gamma_i|>1\}} \qquad (4)$$

where $\mathbf{1}_E$ denotes the indicator function of event E, returning the value 1 if E occurs and 0 otherwise, and Γ_i denotes the prediction set for test example i. A smaller value is preferable.

2.4. Modeling Workflow

Before the training, the CPSign `precompute` command was run, in order to generate a sparse representation of each target's dataset. ACPs consisting of 10 models were then trained for each target using the CPSign `train` command. The cost value used was the one obtained from the hyper-parameter tuning. The observations added as "assumed non-actives" were not included in the calibration set to avoid biasing the evaluation. The computational workflows for orchestrating the extraction of data, model building, and the collection of results for summarizing

and plotting were implemented in the Go programming language using the SciPipe workflow library that is available as open source software at scipipe.org (Lampa et al., 2018b). The cost values for each target are stored in the workflow code, available on GitHub (PTP, 2018). A graphical overview of the modeling workflow is shown in **Figure 2**. More detailed workflow graphs are available in **Supplementary Data Sheet 1**, **Figures S4**, **S5**.

2.5. Model Validation

The models built were validated by predicting the binding activity against each of the 31 targets for all compounds for which there existed known binding data for a particular target in ExCAPE-DB. The validation was done with CPSign's `validate` command, predicting values at confidence levels 0.8 and 0.9.

3. RESULTS

3.1. Published Models

Models for all targets in Dataset1 were produced in the form of portable Java Archive (JAR) files, which were also built into similarly portable Docker containers, for easy publication as microservices. The model JAR files, together with audit log files produced by SciPipe, containing execution traces of the workflow (all the shell commands and parameters) used to produce them, are available for download at Lampa et al. (2018a). The models can be run if obtaining a copy of the CPSign software and a license, from Genetta Soft AB.

3.2. Validity of Models

To check that the Conformal Prediction models are valid (i.e., that they predict with an error rate in accordance to the selected significance level), calibration plots were generated in the cross validation step of the workflow. Three example plots, for three representative targets (the smallest, the median-sized and the largest, in terms of compounds in ExCAPE-DB) can be seen in **Figure 3**, while calibration plots for all targets can be found in the **Supplementary Data Sheet 1** (**Figure S1**). From these calibration plots we conclude that all models produce valid results over all significance levels.

3.3. Efficiency of Models

The efficiency metrics OF, CAOF and MC for Dataset2 (without adding assumed non-actives) are shown in **Figure 4A**. In **Figure 4B**, the same metrics are shown for when all target datasets in Dataset2 have been extended with assumed non-actives, to compensate for these datasets' relative low number of non-actives. We observe that by adding assumed non-actives for datasets with few non-actives, we improve the efficiency of models trained on these datasets. Thus, this strategy of extending the "small" target datasets in Dataset2 was chosen for the subsequent analysis workflows.

3.4. External Validation

In **Figure 5** predicted vs. observed labels for Dataset4 is shown, for confidence levels 0.8 and 0.9, respectively. See the methods section and in particular **Figures 1**, **2**, for information about

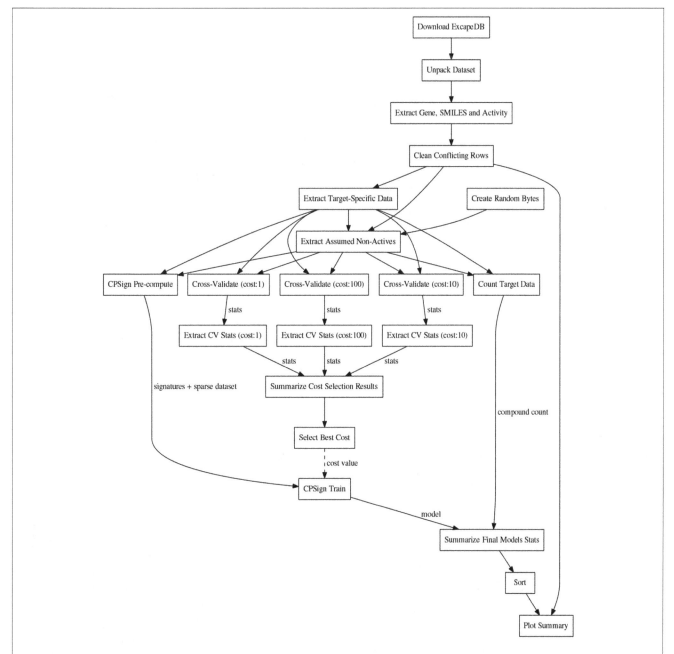

FIGURE 2 | Schematic directed graph of processes and their data dependencies in the modeling workflow used in the experiments in this study. Boxes represent processes, while edges represent data dependencies between processes. The direction of the edges show in which direction data is being passed between processes. The order of execution is here from top to bottom, of the graph. Each experiment contains additions and modifications to the workflow, but the workflow shown here, exemplifies the basic structure, common among most of the workflows. For more detailed workflow plots, see **Supplementary Data Sheet 1**, **Figures S4**, **S5**.

how Dataset4 was created. "A" denotes active compounds and "N" denotes non-active ones. It can be seen how the number of prediction of "Both" labels increase when the confidence level increases from 0.8 to 0.9. This is as expected, as this means that fewer compounds could be predicted to only one label, with the higher confidence level. The number of "Null" predictions decreases at the higher confidence, which is also as expected. The reason is that with a higher confidence, the predictor must consider less probable (in the Conformal Prediction ranking

sense) predictions to be part of the prediction region. This behavior might seem backwards, but at a higher confidence the predictor has to include less likely predictions in order to reach the specified confidence level, which leads to larger prediction sets. For predicted vs. observed labels for each target individually, see **Supplementary Data Sheet 1**, **Figures S2**, **S3**. Because of the fact that CP produces sets of predicted labels, including Null, and Both in this case, the common sensitivity and specificity measures do not have clear definitions in this context. Because

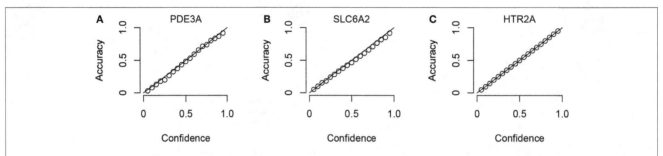

FIGURE 3 | Three representative calibration plots, for models PDE3A **(A)**, SLC6A2 **(B)**, and HTR2A **(C)**, based on the smallest, the median, and the largest target data sets in terms of total number of compounds. The plots show accuracy vs. confidence, for the confidence values between 0.05 and 0.95 with a step size of 0.05.

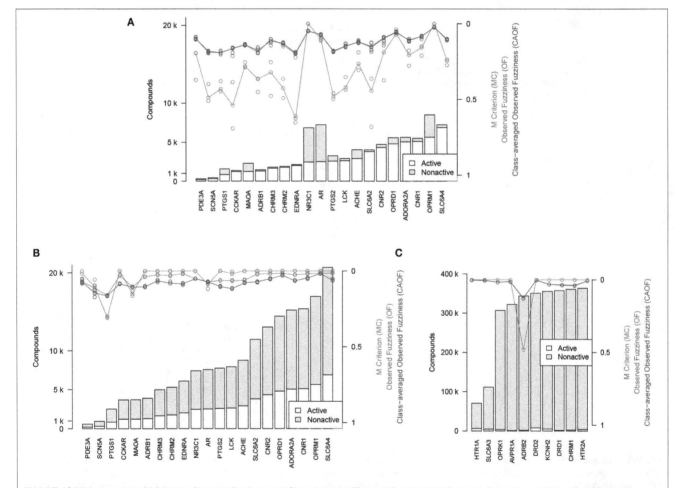

FIGURE 4 | Efficiency metrics (M Criterion, Observed Fuzziness and Class-Averaged Observed Fuzziness) for Dataset1, Dataset2, and Dataset3. **(A)** Dataset2 without extending with assumed non-actives. Circles show individual results from the three replicate runs that were run, while the lines show the median value from the individual replicate results. Targets are here sorted by number of active compounds. **(B)** Dataset2 after extending with assumed non-actives. Circles show individual results from the three replicate runs that were run, while the lines show the median value from the individual replicate results. Targets are here sorted by number of active compounds. **(C)** Dataset3, the 10 largest target datasets, which were not extended with assumed non-actives. Targets are here sorted by total number of compounds.

of this, we have not included calculated values for them but have instead included compound counts for the predicted label sets in **Figure 5** summarized for all targets, and as CSV files in **Supplementary Data Sheet 2** (for 0.8 confidence) and **3** (for 0.9 confidence), for each target specifically.

3.5. Target Profile-as-a-Service

All models based on Dataset2 were published as microservices with REST APIs publicly made available using the OpenAPI specification (Ope, 2018a) on an OpenShift (Ope, 2018b) cluster. A web page aggregating all the models was also created. The

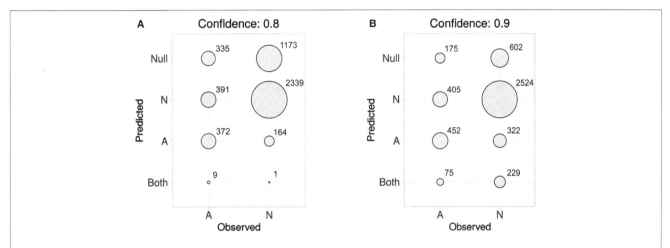

FIGURE 5 | Predicted vs. observed labels, for all targets, for the prediction data, at confidence level 0.8 **(A)** and 0.9 **(B)**. "A" denotes active compounds, and "N" denotes non-active compounds. The x-axis show observed labels (as found in ExCAPE-DB), while the y-axis show the set of predicted labels. The areas of the circles are proportional to the number of SAR data points for each observed label/predicted label combination. For predicted vs. observed labels for each target individually, see **Supplementary Data Sheet 1**, **Figures S2**, **S3**.

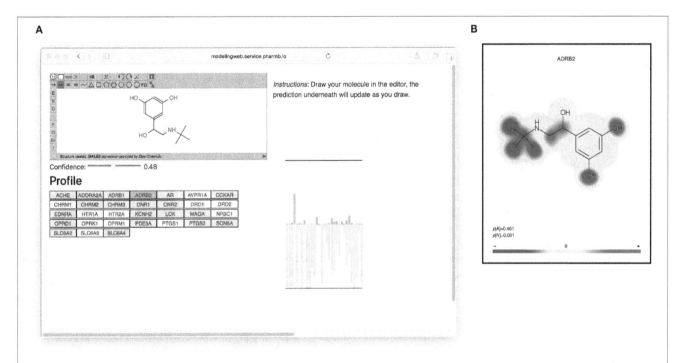

FIGURE 6 | The prediction profile for Terbutaline, a known selective beta-2 adrenergic agonist used as a bronchodilator and tocolytic. **(A)** The profile as seen on the web page (on the right hand in the figure). To show the profile, the user draws a molecule and selects a confidence level, whereafter the profile will update underneath. The profile is shown as a bar plot with two bars for each target: A purple bar, pointing in the upward direction, indicating the size of the p-value of the "Active" label, and a green bar, pointing downwards, indicating the size of the p-value for the "Non-active" label. **(B)** Coloring of which parts of the molecule contributed the most to the prediction for ADBR2. Red color indicates the centers of molecular fragments (of height 1–3) that contributed most to the larger class, while blue color indicates center of fragments contributing most to the smaller class. In this case the larger class is "Active," which can be seen in the size of the p-values in the bottom left of the figure (p[A] = 0.481 >p[N] = 0.001).

OpenAPI specification is a standardization for how REST APIs are described, meaning that there is a common way for looking up how to use the REST API of a web service and that greatly simplifies the process of tying multiple different web services together. It simplifies calling the services from scripts as well as from other web pages, such as the web page (**Figure 6**) that generates a profile image out of the multiple QSAR models. At the top of the web page (see **Figure 6**) is an instance of the JSME editor (Bienfait and Ertl, 2013) in which the user can draw a molecule. As the user draws the molecule, the web page extracts

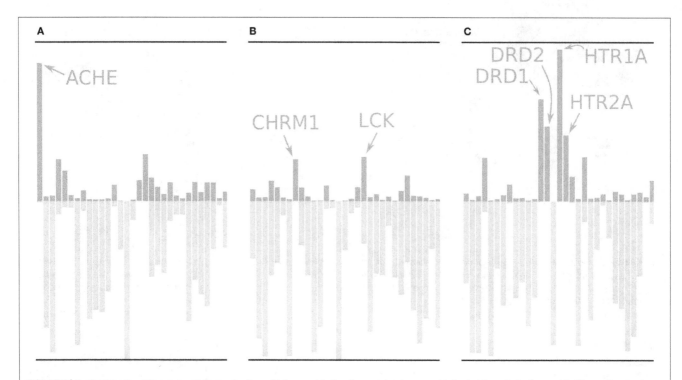

FIGURE 7 | Profiles for a few of the removed drugs using the validation models, i.e., these molecules are not in the training sets for the models. The profiles are shown as bar plots with two bars for each target: A purple bar pointing in the upward direction, indicating the size of the p-value of the "Active" label, and a green bar pointing downwards, indicating the size of the p-value for the "Non-active" label. **(A)** The profile for Tacrine, a centrally acting anticholinesterase, with a distinct peak for the ACHE gene. **(B)** The profile for Pilocarpine, a muscarinic acetylcholine receptor M_1 agonist, with only two moderately higher peaks for active prediction, CHRM1 and LCK. **(C)** The profile for Pergolide, a DRD1, DRD2, HTR1A, and HTR2A agonist, which is reflected by the four highest p-values for an active prediction.

the SMILES from the editor and sends it to the individual model services to get predictions based on all available models. The user can set a threshold for the confidence and get visual feedback on whether the models predict the drawn molecule as active or non-active for each of the targets, at the chosen confidence level. In **Figure 6** on the right side is a graphical profile in the form of a bar plot where confidence of the active label is drawn in the upward direction and the confidence for non-active is drawn in the downward direction. Hovering over a bar in the plot will give information about which model the bar corresponds to. The web page can be accessed at http://ptp.service.pharmb.io/.

3.6. Example Predictions

Using the models built without the external validation dataset (Dataset4), target profiles were predicted for three molecules from the test set (**Figure 7**), i.e., the profiles were made for drugs that the models have not seen before. **Figure 7A** shows the target profile for Tacrine, a centrally acting anticholinesterase, with a distinct peak for the ACHE gene, as expected. Further, we note that most other targets are predicted as non-active with high p-values (green color) or predicted as active with relatively low p-values (purple color). **Figure 7B** shows the target profile for Pilocarpine, a muscarinic acetylcholine receptor M_1 agonist, with a target profile consisting of mostly non-active predictions, and

only two mildly active targets (CHRM1 and LCK). We note that LCK has a similar p-value for active and non-active. For a conformal prediction in the binary classification setting, the *confidence* of a prediction is defined as $1 - p_2$ where p_2 is the lower p-value of the two (Saunders et al., 1999). This means that even if a prediction has one high p-value, its confidence and hence usefulness in a decision setting might still be low. **Figure 7C** shows the target profile for Pergolide, an agonist for DRD1, DRD2, HTR1A, and HTR2A which shows up as the four highest active predictions in the profile.

4. DISCUSSION

We have presented a reproducible workflow for building profiles of predictive models for target-binding. We have exemplified our approach on data from ExCAPE-DB about 31 targets associated with adverse effects and made these models available both via a graphical web interface via an OpenAPI interface for programmatic access and made them available for download. The Conformal Prediction methodology guarantees validity of the models under the exchangeability assumption. We have further showed that our models are indeed valid, with the calibration plots in **Figure 3**.

Based on the efficiency metrics shown in **Figures 4B,C** we see that the efficiency, after adding assumed non-actives to the datasets with very few (under 10,000) non-actives, is clearly improved. Based on the external test set, Dataset4, though, especially based on the plots in **Figure 5**, we see that there is a somewhat higher fraction of observed non-actives ("N") correctly predicted as non-actives, than the fraction of observed actives ("A") correctly predicted as active.

The use of workflows to automate pre-processing and model training and make it completely reproducible has several implications. Primarily, the entire process can be repeated as data change, e.g., when new data is made available or data is curated. In our case, the pre-processing can be re-run when a new version of ExCAPE-DB is released, and new models trained on up-to-date data can be deployed and published without delay. The components of the pre-processing workflow are however general, and can be re-used in other settings as well. Further, a user can select the specific targets that will be pre-processed, and focus the analysis on smaller subsets without having to pre-process and train models on all targets, which could be resource-demanding. With a modular workflow it is also easy to replace specific components, such as evaluating different strategies and modeling methods.

The packaging of models as JAR-files and Docker containers makes them portable and easy to transfer and deploy on different systems, including servers or laptops on public and private networks without cumbersome dependency management. We chose to deploy our services inside the RedHat OpenShift container orchestration system, which has the benefit of providing a resilient and scalable service, but any readily available infrastructure provider is sufficient. The use of OpenAPI for deploying an interoperable service API means that the service is simple to integrate and consume in many different ways, including being called from a web page, (such as our reference page on http://ptp.service.pharmb.io/) but also into third party applications and workflow systems. With the flexibility to consume models on individual level comes the power to put together custom profiles (panels) of targets. In this work we have selected targets based on usefulness in a drug safety setting, but it is easy to envision other types of panels for other purposes. While there has been some previous research on the use of predicted target profiles (Yao et al., 2016; Awale and Reymond, 2017), further research is needed to maximize their usefulness and to integrate with other types of *in vitro* and *in silico* measures. Our methodology and implementation facilitates such large-scale and integrative studies, and paves the way for target predictions that can be integrated in different stages of the drug discovery process.

5. CONCLUSION

We developed a methodology and implementation of target prediction profiles, with fully automated and reproducible data pre-processing and model training workflows to build them. Models are packaged as portable Java Archive (JAR) files, and as Docker containers that can be deployed on any system. We trained data on 31 targets related to drug safety, from the ExCAPE-DB dataset and published these as a predictive profile, using Conformal Prediction to deliver prediction intervals for each target. The example profile is deployed as an online service with an interoperable API.

AUTHOR CONTRIBUTIONS

OS conceived the study. OS, JA, SA, and SL designed the study, interpreted results, and wrote the manuscript. SL implemented the workflow and carried out the analysis. SA extended CPSign with new features. JA, SA, and AB contributed with model deployment and APIs. EA contributed with expertise in target profiles and modeling. All authors read and approved the manuscript.

FUNDING

This study was supported by OpenRiskNet (Grant Agreement 731075), a project funded by the European Commission under the Horizon 2020 Programme.

ACKNOWLEDGMENTS

The computations were performed on resources provided by SNIC through Uppsala Multidisciplinary Center for Advanced Computational Science (UPPMAX) under Project SNIC 2017/7-89.

REFERENCES

Alvarsson, J., Eklund, M., Engkvist, O., Spjuth, O., Carlsson, L., Wikberg, J. E., et al. (2014). Ligand-based target prediction with signature fingerprints. *J. Chem. Inform. Model.* 54, 2647–2653. doi: 10.1021/ci500361u

Alvarsson, J., Lampa, S., Schaal, W., Andersson, C., Wikberg, J. E., and Spjuth, O. (2016). Large-scale ligand-based predictive modelling using support vector machines. *J. Cheminform.* 8:39. doi: 10.1186/s13321-016-0151-5

Arvidsson, S. (2016). *CPSign Documentation*. Available online at: http://cpsign-docs.genettasoft.com (Accessed February 28, 2018).

Awale, M., and Reymond, J. L. (2017). The polypharmacology browser: a web-based multi-fingerprint target prediction tool using ChEMBL bioactivity data. *J. Cheminform.* 9:11. doi: 10.1186/s13321-017-0199-x

Bender, A., Scheiber, J., Glick, M., Davies, J. W., Azzaoui, K., Hamon, J., et al. (2007). Analysis of pharmacology data and the prediction of adverse drug reactions and off-target effects from chemical structure. *ChemMedChem* 2,

861–873. doi: 10.1002/cmdc.200700026

Bienfait, B., and Ertl, P. (2013). JSME: a free molecule editor in JavaScript. *J. Cheminformat.* 5:24. doi: 10.1186/1758-2946-5-24

Bowes, J., Brown, A. J., Hamon, J., Jarolimek, W., Sridhar, A., Waldron, G., et al. (2012). Reducing safety-related drug attrition: the use of *in vitro* pharmacological profiling. *Nat. Rev. Drug Discov.* 11, 909–922. doi: 10.1038/nrd3845

Bredel, M., and Jacoby, E. (2004). Chemogenomics: an emerging strategy for rapid target and drug discovery. *Nat. Rev. Genet.* 5, 262–275. doi: 10.1038/nrg1317

Capuzzi, S. J., Kim, I. S., Lam, W. I., Thornton, T. E., Muratov, E. N., Pozefsky, D., et al. (2017). Chembench: a publicly accessible, integrated cheminformatics portal. *J. Chem. Informat. Model.* 57, 105–108. doi: 10.1021/acs.jcim.6b00462

Cereto-Massagué, A., Ojeda, M. J., Valls, C., Mulero, M., Pujadas, G., and Garcia-Vallve, S. (2015). Tools for *in silico* target fishing. *Methods* 71, 98–103. doi: 10.1016/j.ymeth.2014.09.006

Cortés-Ciriano, I., Bender, A., and Malliavin, T. (2015). Prediction of PARP inhibition with proteochemometric modelling and conformal prediction. *Mol. Inform.* 34, 357–366. doi: 10.1002/minf.201400165

DrugBank (2018). *DrugBank Release Version 5.1.0*. Available online at: https://www.drugbank.ca/releases/latest (Accessed June 20, 2018).

Eklund, M., Norinder, U., Boyer, S., and Carlsson, L. (2015). The application of conformal prediction to the drug discovery process. *Ann. Math. Artif. Intell.* 74, 117–132. doi: 10.1007/s10472-013-9378-2

Fan, R.-E., Chang, K.-W., Hsieh, C.-J., Wang, X.-R., and Lin, C.-J. (2008). LIBLINEAR: a library for large linear classification. *J. Mach. Learn. Res.* 9, 1871–1874.

Faulon, J. L., Visco, D. P., and Pophale, R. S. (2003). The signature molecular descriptor. 1. Using extended valence sequences in QSAR and QSPR studies. *J. Chem. Inform. Comput. Sci.* 43, 707–720. doi: 10.1021/ci020345w

Forreryd, A., Norinder, U., Lindberg, T., and Lindstedt, M. (2018). Predicting skin sensitizers with confidence - Using conformal prediction to determine applicability domain of GARD. *Toxicol. In Vitro* 48, 179–187. doi: 10.1016/j.tiv.2018.01.021

Gammerman, A., and Vovk, V. (2007). Hedging predictions in machine learning. *Comput. J.* 50, 151–163. doi: 10.1093/comjnl/bxl065

Gaulton, A., Hersey, A., Nowotka, M., Bento, A. P., Chambers, J., Mendez, D., et al. (2017). The ChEMBL database in 2017. *Nucleic Acids Res.* 45, D945–D954. doi: 10.1093/nar/gkw1074

Hansch, C. (1969). A quantitative approach to biochemical structure-activity relationships. *Acc. Chem. Res.* 2, 232–239. doi: 10.1021/ar50020a002

Hinsen, K. (2018). Verifiability in computer-aided research: the role of digital scientific notations at the human-computer interface. *PeerJ Comput. Sci.* 4:e158. doi: 10.7717/peerj-cs.158

Hopkins, A. L. (2008). Network pharmacology: the next paradigm in drug discovery. *Nat. Chem. Biol.* 4:682. doi: 10.1038/nchembio.118

Lampa, S., Alvarsson, J., Arvidsson Mc Shane, S., Berg, A., Ahlberg, E., and Spjuth, O. (2018a). Predictive models for off-target binding profiles generation (Version 0.9) [Data set]. *Zenodo*. doi: 10.5281/zenodo.1286304

Lampa, S., Dahlö, M., Alvarsson, J., and Spjuth, O. (2018b). SciPipe - a workflow library for agile development of complex and dynamic bioinformatics pipelines. *bioRxiv*. doi: 10.1101/380808

Lapins, M., Arvidsson, S., Lampa, S., Berg, A., Schaal, W., Alvarsson, J., et al. (2018). A confidence predictor for logD using conformal regression and a support-vector machine. *J. Cheminformat.* 10:17. doi: 10.1186/s13321-018-0271-1

Mazanetz, M. P., Marmon, R. J., Reisser, C. B., and Morao, I. (2012). Drug discovery applications for KNIME: an open source data mining platform. *Curr. Top. Med. Chem.* 12, 1965–1979. doi: 10.2174/156802612804910331

Mervin, L. H., Afzal, A. M., Drakakis, G., Lewis, R., Engkvist, O., and Bender, A. (2015). Target prediction utilising negative bioactivity data covering large chemical space. *J. Cheminformat.* 7, 1–16. doi: 10.1186/s13321-015-0098-y

Norinder, U. (2003). Support vector machine models in drug design: applications to drug transport processes and qsar using simplex optimisations and variable selection. *Neurocomputing* 55, 337–346. doi: 10.1016/S0925-2312(03)00374-6

Norinder, U., and Boyer, S. (2017). Binary classification of imbalanced datasets using conformal prediction. *J. Mol. Graph. Model.* 72, 256–265. doi: 10.1016/j.jmgm.2017.01.008

Norinder, U., Carlsson, L., Boyer, S., and Eklund, M. (2014). Introducing conformal prediction in predictive modeling. a transparent and flexible alternative to applicability domain determination. *J. Chem. Inf. Model.* 54, 1596–603. doi: 10.1021/ci5001168

Norinder, U., Rybacka, A., and Andersson, P. L. (2016). Conformal prediction to define applicability domain - A case study on predicting ER and AR binding. *SAR QSAR Environ. Res.* 27, 303–316. doi: 10.1080/1062936X.2016.1172665

OpenAPI (2018a). *OpenAPI Origin - Open Source Container Application Platform*. Available online at: https://www.openapis.org/ (Accessed June 11, 2018).

OpenShift (2018b). *OpenShift Origin - Open Source Container Application Platform*. Available online at: https://www.openshift.org/ (Accessed June 11, 2018).

Peters, J.-U. (2013). Polypharmacology - foe or friend? *J. Med. Chem.* 56, 8955–8971. doi: 10.1021/jm400856t

PTP (2018). *PTP Project Source Code Repository*. Available online at: https://github.com/pharmbio/ptp-project (Accessed June 20, 2018).

Ravikumar, B., and Aittokallio, T. (2018). Improving the efficacy-safety balance of polypharmacology in multi-target drug discovery. *Exp. Opin. Drug Discov.* 13, 179–192. doi: 10.1080/17460441.2018.1413089

Rogers, D., and Hahn, M. (2010). Extended-connectivity fingerprints. *J. Chem. Inform. Model.* 50, 742–754. doi: 10.1021/ci100050t

Saunders, C., Gammerman, A., and Vovk, V. (1999). "Transduction with confidence and credibility," in *Sixteenth International Joint Conference on Artificial Intelligence (IJCAI '99)* (San Francisco, CA: Morgan Kaufmann Publishers Inc.), 722–726. Available online at: https://eprints.soton.ac.uk/258961/

Stodden, V., McNutt, M., Bailey, D. H., Deelman, E., Gil, Y., Hanson, B., et al. (2016). Enhancing reproducibility for computational methods. *Science* 354, 1240–1241. doi: 10.1126/science.aah6168

Sun, J., Carlsson, L., Ahlberg, E., Norinder, U., Engkvist, O., and Chen, H. (2017a). Applying mondrian cross-conformal prediction to estimate prediction confidence on large imbalanced bioactivity data sets. *J. Chem. Inf. Model.* 57, 1591–1598. doi: 10.1021/acs.jcim.7b00159

Sun, J., Jeliazkova, N., Chupakhin, V., Golib-Dzib, J.-F., Engkvist, O., Carlsson, L., et al. (2017b). ExCAPE-DB: an integrated large scale dataset facilitating big data analysis in chemogenomics. *J. Cheminformat.* 9:17. doi: 10.1186/s13321-017-0203-5

Sushko, I., Novotarskyi, S., Körner, R., Pandey, A. K., Rupp, M., Teetz, W., et al. (2011). Online chemical modeling environment (OCHEM): web platform for data storage, model development and publishing of chemical information. *J. Comput. Aided Mol. Design* 25, 533–554. doi: 10.1007/s10822-011-9440-2

Vovk, V., Fedorova, V., Nouretdinov, I., and Gammerman, A. (2016). "Criteria of efficiency for conformal prediction," in *Conformal and Probabilistic Prediction with Applications*, eds A. Gammerman, Z. Luo, J. Vega, and V. Vovk (Cham: Springer International Publishing), 23–39.

Vovk, V., Gammerman, A., and Shafer, G. (2005). *Algorithmic Learning in a Random World*. New York, NY: Springer Science & Business Media.

Walker, T., Grulke, C. M., Pozefsky, D., and Tropsha, A. (2010). Chembench : a cheminformatics workbench. *Bioinformatics* 26, 3000–3001. doi: 10.1093/bioinformatics/btq556

Wang, L., Ma, C., Wipf, P., Liu, H., Su, W., and Xie, X. Q. (2013). TargetHunter: an *in silico* target identification tool for predicting therapeutic potential of small organic molecules based on chemogenomic database. *AAPS J.* 15, 395–406. doi: 10.1208/s12248-012-9449-z

Wang, Y., Bryant, S. H., Cheng, T., Wang, J., Gindulyte, A., Shoemaker, B. A., et al. (2017). PubChem BioAssay: 2017 update. *Nucleic Acids Res.* 45, D955–D963. doi: 10.1093/nar/gkw1118

Yao, Z. J., Dong, J., Che, Y. J., Zhu, M. F., Wen, M., Wang, N. N., et al. (2016). TargetNet: a web service for predicting potential drug-target interaction profiling via multi-target SAR models. *J. Comput. Aided Mol. Des.* 30, 413–424. doi: 10.1007/s10822-016-9915-2

Yildirim, M. A., Goh, K.-I., Cusick, M. E., Barabási, A.-L., and Vidal, M. (2007). Drug-target network. *Nat. Biotechnol.* 25, 1119–1126. doi: 10.1038/nbt1338

Yu, H., Chen, J., Xu, X., Li, Y., Zhao, H., Fang, Y., et al. (2012). A systematic prediction of multiple drug-target interactions from chemical, genomic, and pharmacological data. *PLoS ONE* 7:e37608. doi: 10.1371/journal.pone.0037608

Zhou, X. B., Han, W. J., Chen, J., and Lu, X. Q. (2011). QSAR study on the interactions between antibiotic compounds and DNA by a hybrid genetic-based support vector machine. *Monatshefte für Chemie-Chemical Monthly* 142, 949–959. doi: 10.1007/s00706-011-0493-7

Genotypic and Phenotypic Factors Influencing Drug Response in Mexican Patients with Type 2 Diabetes Mellitus

Hector E. Sanchez-Ibarra[1], Luisa M. Reyes-Cortes[1], Xian-Li Jiang[2], Claudia M. Luna-Aguirre[1], Dionicio Aguirre-Trevino[1], Ivan A. Morales-Alvarado[1], Rafael B. Leon-Cachon[3], Fernando Lavalle-Gonzalez[4], Faruck Morcos[2,5]* and Hugo A. Barrera-Saldaña[1,6]*

[1] Molecular Genetics Laboratory, Vitagénesis, S.A. de C.V., Monterrey, Mexico, [2] Evolutionary Information Laboratory, Department of Biological Sciences, University of Texas at Dallas, Richardson, TX, United States, [3] Departamento de Ciencias Básicas, Centro de Diagnóstico Molecular y Medicina Personalizada, Vicerrectoría de Ciencias de la Salud, Universidad de Monterrey, Monterrey, Mexico, [4] Servicio de Endocrinología, Hospital Universitario Dr. José E. González, Universidad Autónoma de Nuevo León, Monterrey, Mexico, [5] Center for Systems Biology, University of Texas at Dallas, Richardson, TX, United States, [6] Tecnológico de Monterrey, Monterrey, Mexico

*Correspondence:
Faruck Morcos
faruckm@utdallas.edu
Hugo A. Barrera-Saldaña
habarrera@gmail.com

The treatment of Type 2 Diabetes Mellitus (T2DM) consists primarily of oral antidiabetic drugs (OADs) that stimulate insulin secretion, such as sulfonylureas (SUs) and reduce hepatic glucose production (e.g., biguanides), among others. The marked inter-individual differences among T2DM patients' response to these drugs have become an issue on prescribing and dosing efficiently. In this study, fourteen polymorphisms selected from Genome-wide association studies (GWAS) were screened in 495 T2DM Mexican patients previously treated with OADs to find the relationship between the presence of these polymorphisms and response to the OADs. Then, a novel association screening method, based on global probabilities, was used to globally characterize important relationships between the drug response to OADs and genetic and clinical parameters, including polymorphisms, patient information, and type of treatment. Two polymorphisms, *ABCC8*-Ala1369Ser and *KCNJ11*-Glu23Lys, showed a significant impact on response to SUs. Heterozygous *ABCC8*-Ala1369Ser variant (A/C) carriers exhibited a higher response to SUs compared to homozygous *ABCC8*-Ala1369Ser variant (A/A) carriers (p-value = 0.029) and to homozygous wild-type genotypes (C/C) (p-value = 0.012). The homozygous *KCNJ11*-Glu23Lys variant (C/C) and wild-type (T/T) genotypes had a lower response to SUs compared to heterozygous (C/T) carriers (p-value = 0.039). The screening of OADs response related genetic and clinical factors could help improve the prescribing and dosing of OADs for T2DM patients and thus contribute to the design of personalized treatments.

Keywords: pharmacogenetics, pharmacogenomics, diabetes, sulfonylureas, biguanides, Mexican, direct coupling analysis, direct information

INTRODUCTION

Type 2 Diabetes Mellitus (T2DM) is the most common form of diabetes in adults. T2DM is associated with multiple complications, such as blindness, lower limb amputation, and premature death (Marchetti et al., 2009; Barquera et al., 2013). According to the International Diabetes Federation (IDF), China, India, United States, Brazil, Russia, and Mexico are the countries with the highest incidence. It is estimated that life expectancy is reduced in diabetic individuals by 5–10 years, mainly due to lack of early treatment. In Mexico, the average age for death by diabetes or its complications was 66.7 in 2010, compared with the lifespan of 76 years of non-diabetic individuals (Agudelo-Botero and Davila-Cervantes, 2015). The average annual economic cost from 2006 to 2010 of T2DM patients in Mexico was $941,345,886 USD of direct cost, $177,220,390 USD of indirect cost, and $27,969,427 USD from its complications. This immense cost, coupled with the issues of inequity and access to healthcare in Mexico, where 51% of the cost comes from household income, represents a huge social burden (Arredondo and De Icaza, 2011; Barquera et al., 2013).

Several classes of oral antidiabetic drugs (OADs) are currently available and primarily include agents that stimulate insulin secretion (sulfonylureas), reduce hepatic glucose production (biguanides), delay the digestion and absorption of intestinal carbohydrate (alpha-glucosidase inhibitors), or improve insulin function (thiazolidinediones) (Krentz and Bailey, 2005; Nathan et al., 2009). Additionally, OADs include other classes of drugs such as meglitinides, glucagon-like peptide-1 (GLP-1) agonists, dipeptidylpeptidase-4 (DPP-4) inhibitors, dopamine-2 agonists, and amylin analogs (Inzucchi et al., 2012). There is a wide variability in adverse events and glucose-lowering response to OADs among different patients, which may be attributed to factors like age, sex, and body weight, but also to genetic variation related to pharmacokinetic and pharmacodynamic properties of the OADs (Becker et al., 2013; Emami-Riedmaier et al., 2015).

Biguanide, especially metformin, which is the only one available OAD in some countries, is recommended as the first-choice therapy for T2DM (Inzucchi et al., 2012). Metformin inhibits the activity of mitochondrial respiratory-chain complex I, resulting in decreased ATP synthesis and an accumulation of AMP leading to the activation of AMP-activated protein kinase (AMPK) and the subsequent suppression of hepatic gluconeogenesis (Foretz et al., 2010). Pharmacokinetic studies suggest that metformin is actively absorbed from the gut and is excreted unchanged in the urine (Zhou et al., 2009). The organic cation transporter 1 (OCT1), encoded by *SLC22A1* gene, is expressed in the basolateral membrane of hepatocytes and mediates the metformin uptake, while OCT2 (encoded by *SCL22A2*), expressed in the basolateral membrane of kidney tubular cells, facilitates almost 80% of metformin excretion (Pearson, 2009; Pernicova and Korbonits, 2014). Associations of intronic variants in *SLC22A1* and *SLC22A2* with glucose-lowering response to metformin in T2DM patients have been previously reported (Tkac

et al., 2013). *SLC22A1* gene is highly polymorphic, with common function-reducing polymorphisms such as Arg61Cys (rs12208357), Gly401Ser (rs34130495), and Gly465Arg (rs34059508), which having been associated with decreased transportation and therefore the reduced therapeutic effect of metformin (Distefano and Watanabe, 2010). *In vitro* studies have shown that all three polymorphisms might be associated with reduced metformin uptake (van Dam et al., 2005). However, *in vivo* studies show controversial results (Tzvetkov et al., 2009).

Sulfonylureas (SUs) target an ATP-dependent potassium (K-$_{ATP}$) channel present in pancreatic β-cells. K-$_{ATP}$ channels are hetero-octamers composed of Kir6.2 pore subunit encoded by the gene *KCNJ11*, and the SUR1 receptor subunit encoded by the gene *ABCC8*. SUs lower glycemia by enhancing insulin secretion from pancreatic β-cells by inducing K-$_{ATP}$ channel closure (Tkac, 2015). SUs, such as tolbutamide, glimepiride, and glipizide, are mainly metabolized by the enzyme cytochrome P450 encoded by the *CYP2C9* isoform gene. Several SNPs have been related to their effect on insulin secretion enhancing (Holstein et al., 2005). Reduced drug-metabolizing activity has been reported in individuals carrying two allelic variants namely *CYP2C9*2* (rs1799853) leading to a missense amino acid polymorphism Arg144Cys, and *CYP2C9*3* (rs1057910) leading to the missense amino acid polymorphism Ile359Leu (Huang and Florez, 2011). The Ile359Leu polymorphism has a more profound effect (Ragia et al., 2014). These alleles encode proteins with a diminished enzymatic activity and are correlated with elevated serum levels of SUs (Ragia et al., 2009). However, *CYP2C9*-Arg144Cys polymorphism is not associated with diabetes susceptibility (Semiz et al., 2010).

Regarding SUs target (K-$_{ATP}$ channels), most studies researched two linked non-synonymous common variants in both *ABCC8* and *KCNJ11* genes. *KCNJ11* variants are implicated in glycemic progression to either prediabetes or T2DM. One of the most common *KCNJ11* polymorphisms is Glu23Lys (rs5219). The functional effects of the Glu23Lys variant on insulin secretion and sensitivity yield controversial results, even though recent larger studies demonstrate a significantly reduced insulin secretion, lower insulin levels, and improved insulin sensitivity, consistent with the enhanced K-$_{ATP}$ channels activity in pancreatic β-cells (Villareal et al., 2009). More recently, the associations of the Glu23Lys variant and a different *KCNJ11* variant, Ile1337Val (rs5215), with T2DM have been confirmed in several genome-wide association studies (GWAS), rekindling the interest in its potential role as a genetic marker for T2DM development (Cheung et al., 2011). On the other hand, the *ABCC8*-Ala1369Ser (rs757110) polymorphism has been associated with a reduction of glycated hemoglobin (HbA1c) in the Chinese population with SUs treatment (Feng et al., 2008; Sokolova et al., 2015).

In addition to pharmacogenetic factors, the response to OADs is conditional on different phenotypic or clinical aspects. With the accessibility of cohorts of this T2DM patient information, various statistical approaches can be used to determine the contributing factors affecting response to OADs. Traditional statistical tools are used to measure the co-occurrence of factor variable and treatment response at a time (Turner et al., 2009; Stransky et al., 2015). However, the human trait factors may internally relate or function together to affect the drug response. Although these tests provide real statistical connections among variables in patient data, these relationships tend to be composed with both strong and weak correlations making it difficult to disentangle direct effects that explain the influence of some variables over a factor of interest. Therefore, important efforts have been dedicated to the development of statistical models to better describe relationship networks related to human disease. In the field of pharmacogenomics, a variety of statistical models have been built, such as Bayesian networks and Elastic net regression (Barretina et al., 2012), which have exhibited great performance on finding genes highly connected to drug response. Recently, a global statistical model, direct coupling analysis (DCA), also has been demonstrated to be applicable in pharmacogenetic data (Jiang et al., 2017). DCA efficiently computes estimates of a joint probability distribution of multivariate patient profiles constructed with clinical data. The parameters of such distribution estimated by DCA are used to quantify with high success the degree of connectivity of variables in the model. The ability to disentangle direct couplings from indirect couplings has been successful in the field of structural biology where directly coupled residue pairs have been used to predict co-evolution of amino acids (dos Santos et al., 2015), predict the structure of proteins (Sulkowska et al., 2012) with an accuracy not seen before as well as predict the molecular plasticity and complexes (Morcos et al., 2013; dos Santos et al., 2015). Recently, we have used this framework to study protein expression level–based protein–protein interactions and in a pharmacogenomics approach to infer gene–drug interactions in cancer tissues and cell lines where information on drug sensitivity is available (Jiang et al., 2017). This is the first time that direct information (DI) is used as a metric of correlation in high throughput profiling data. It not only captures the connections between well-known drug response predictors, including some drug targets for certain anti-cancer agents, but also predicts some potential biomarkers and generates gene–drug networks. DCA is used in this study to find highly coupled factors for response to OADs and to construct a network for the patient cohort data. A metric called DI is computed to evaluate the association intensity of two variables, including the connections between two potential factors and between factors and drug response.

In addition to genetic variations traits containing pharmacogenetic data, the phenotypic traits of patients, such as age, sex, health status, have been suggested to have influences on the outcome of OADs treatment for T2DM. Thus, a T2DM patient database including genetic data and patient phenotypic data is advantageous. This study collects 495 T2DM patients with information about age, origin, sex, body index, health status, history of OADs treatment, polymorphisms, and results of glycated hemoglobin (HbA1c) tests. HbA1c is a recognized target for diabetes control used in international guidelines and is the most suitable parameter to be studied in

pharmacogenetic studies (Lo et al., 2012). Here, we propose a new structure-learning approach for Bayesian network construction by using direct information and Chow-Liu trees. Chow-Liu algorithm is commonly used to learn Bayesian network structure (Almudevar, 2010), and mutual information is used by this algorithm to estimate the dependence of two variables (Chen et al., 2008). Due to the better performance of DI on measuring direct associations when compared to mutual information, we integrated DI and the Chow-Liu algorithm to recover global connections between clinical factors for T2DM patients.

Genetic variations or patient phenotypic data affecting the drug responses to T2DM treatments often lead to the necessity of treatment changes and adjustments, resulting in higher expenses for the patients. The aim of this study was to establish an association between patient clinical data, such as habits, treatment history, polymorphisms, and variability in the response to OAD treatments in a Mexican population. Therefore, biomarkers could help prescribe the right drug and its dosage, for better control of the disease and its consequences, including treatment savings and reduced impact in productivity.

MATERIALS AND METHODS

Design

A cross-sectional and retrospective study with convenience sampling was carried out in T2DM patients treated with OADs, in monotherapy or in combination for at least 6 months, to determine possible association between patient data, gene variants, and drug response assessed by HbA1c values. This study was conducted according to Good Clinical Practice standards and guidelines of the Declarations of Helsinki and Tokyo. Furthermore, the protocol was approved by the Ethics and Research Committee from the Medical School of the Universidad Autonoma de Nuevo León (IRB00005579).

Patients

We recruited male and female patients with T2DM from northeastern Mexico who attended the Clinic of Diabetes of the Endocrinology Service at the Dr. José Eleuterio González Hospital in Monterrey, Mexico. The recruitment period lasted 12 months. The inclusion criteria were: patients over 18 years old with T2DM and treated with oral antihyperglycemic agents or OADs, in monotherapy or in combination for at least 6 months. The exclusion criteria were: diabetes type 1, gestational diabetes, other non-T2DM types of diabetes, active cancer, heart failure, co-treatment with corticosteroids or estrogens, conditions that can cause hyperglycemia, addiction to alcohol or illegal drugs, and dementia or severe psychiatric disorders. The co-treatments with corticosteroids and estrogens were excluded. The disease status was confirmed using the American Diabetes Association criteria and a physical examination. Blood pressure, body height, and body weight measurement were done. The body mass index (BMI) was calculated from anthropometric measurements.

All patients were apprised about the aims of the study, and a written informed consent was obtained. In addition, information on the history of diabetes and the presence of arterial hypertension, hyperlipidemia, and chronic-degenerative diseases, smoking status, and other medications was obtained from the medical records and from the interview for inclusion in the study.

Definition of Response

A fasting blood sample was drawn for the determination of HbA1c. HbA1c was measured at least 3 months after drug prescription and determined using Tina-quant® HbA1C Gen. 3 (Cobas-Mira Roche). The approach taken for the treatment of the patients was "treat to target," defined as failure to reach levels of HbA1c $\leq$ 7%. The initial HbA1c of each patient was at least 7%.

DNA Isolation

Peripheral blood from patients was extracted in a tube with EDTA and genomic DNA was isolated with Wizard Genomic DNA Purification Kit (Promega, Madison, WI, United States). Protocol was followed according to manufacturer's instructions. Genomic DNA was quantified by UV absorbance using Nanodrop (Thermo Scientific, Wilmington, DE, United States). The quality of DNA was measured with the A260/280 ratio, a value of 1.8–2 was considered of good quality. Samples were kept at $-20°C$ in small working aliquots until analysis to avoid recurrent cycles of freezing and thawing to minimize degradation.

Pharmacogenetic Tests (Genotyping)

A total of 14 single nucleotide polymorphisms distributed in 5 different genes associated with response to anti-diabetic treatments were genotyped by Real-Time PCR system using validated Genotyping Assays (Applied Biosystems, Foster City, CA, United States) according to the manufacturer's instructions. Two additional polymorphisms in *SLC22A1* gene (Met61Val and Met420Del) were included in the study and analyzed in 50 responders and 50 non-responder patients. These additional polymorphisms were determined by nucleotide sequencing method in a Genetic Analyzer 3100 (Applied Biosystems). As a quality control measure, genotyping for the polymorphisms were required to pass three tests for inclusion in subsequent association studies: the genotype call rate (> 0.90 completeness to obtain 99.8% accuracy), the Hardy-Weinberg equilibrium (HWE) test (p-value > 0.05), and the minor allele frequency (MAF) criterion (> 0.01).

Analysis of Statistical Significance

Standard descriptive and comparative analyses were performed. The responder's phenotypes classification was made using Hb1Ac parameter applied a cut-off $\leq$ 7 for responder's and > 7 for non-responder's [including first-line therapy (FLT), second-line therapy (SLT), third-line therapy (TLT), monotherapy, and combination therapy]. The HWE was determined by comparing the genotype frequencies with the expected values using the maximum likelihood method. To detect significant differences between two groups, Student's t-test or the Mann–Whitney U-test were used for parametric or non-parametric distributions, respectively. Differences between more than two groups were assessed by one-way ANOVA and the Kruskal–Wallis H-test for parametric or non-parametric distributions,

respectively. *Post hoc* tests (LSD and Tamhane's T2) were used for pairwise comparisons. Possible associations between genotypes and phenotypes were assessed using contingency tables X^2 statistics and Fisher's exact tests. The association was evaluated under four different models (dominant, over dominant, recessive, and additive). Odds ratios were estimated with 95% confidence intervals. Aforementioned analyses were performed with SPSS for Windows, V.20 (IBM Corp., Armonk, NY, United States). All p-values were two-tailed. The corrected P (Pc)-values were adjusted by using Bonferroni's correction. A p-value ≤ 0.05 was considered statistically significant.

Computational Modeling: Direct Coupling Analysis

To study the association between diabetes-related SNPs, patient data and antidiabetic drug response, we have developed a metric called DI, which is derived from the inference framework DCA (Morcos et al., 2011). DCA is a statistical method that infers efficiently the parameters of probability distributions with a large set of variables. DCA can be computed efficiently and is able to capture and evaluate direct pairwise correlations among potentially thousands of variable connections. The probability distribution of large sets of data is modeled with the following Boltzmann-like distribution:

$$P(dat) = \frac{1}{Z}\exp\{\sum e_{ij} + \sum h_i\}$$

where *dat* represents a profile with L variables that are indexed by i and j and Z is a normalization constant. The parameters of this distribution are all possible e_{ij} and h_i for $i, j \leq L$ and contain information about pairwise direct connectivity (e_{ij}) of the variables in the dataset. They are typically hard to be calculated exactly, but can be estimated using DCA. Once the parameters have been estimated, we can use them to compute pairwise probabilities. The following expression shows the form of DI based on the probabilities computed using the parameters, e_{ij} and h_i.

$$DI_{ij} = \sum_{x_i, x_j} P_{ij}(x_i, x_j)\log\frac{P_{ij}(x_i, x_j)}{f_i(x_i)f_j(x_j)}$$

Here x_i is the quantized value of the clinical variable in the profile. The values of the DI_{ij} pairs tell us how connected are two variables in the distribution.

Analysis on T2DM Patient Data

The DCA was applied to the complete cohort of data as described in **Figure 1**. The responder's phenotypes classification was made at a cut-off 7 as defined before. Patient's body indexes, such as weight, height, BMI, age, duration of diabetes, systolic pressure, diastolic pressure, are classified based on decade spans. To find the influential factors for response to OADs, a matrix containing all patient phenotypic informatics, 14 polymorphisms, HbA1c test result is generated as the input for DCA algorithm (Morcos et al., 2011). The T2DM database consists of patient profiles from 495 patients, including basic information, first, second, third line therapy information, 14 polymorphisms, health conditions, and

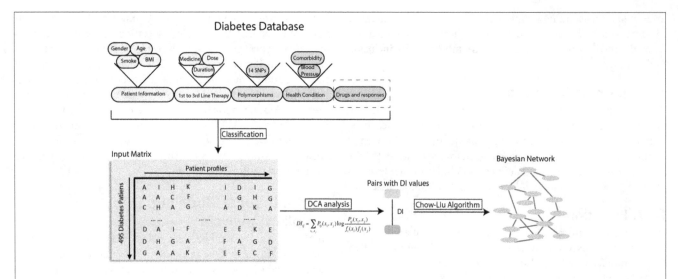

FIGURE 1 | Workflow of global probabilistic modeling on T2DM patient data. Strategy of using T2DM patient datasets to compute the direct information metric between patient genetic or clinical factors and the drug response of OAD treatments. After DI values were calculated, they were used in the Chow-Liu tree for a structural learning for Bayesian network.

the HbA1c test result estimating the glucose-lowering effect of OADs. The patient profile columns also include the 21 OADs separately, representing the usage and doses of a specific OAD for certain patients. All of those profiles data are classified and organized in an input matrix for DCA. DI is computed from DCA as a metric of connectivity strength for pairwise variables. The higher DI values, the stronger the correlation between these two variables. DI has been successfully applied to model molecular interactions in protein folds (Morcos et al., 2011, 2014; dos Santos et al., 2015; Boyd et al., 2016) as well as to identify drug-gene connections in cancer datasets (Jiang et al., 2017). Then, DI values for each variable pair is computed by DCA algorithm and then is used to find a complete network by using a minimum spanning tree approach and then a Bayesian network is built with undirected edges.

Predictive Model for OAD Treatment Response

The direct connectivity (e_{ij}) estimates the strength of couplings between two variables at certain states. The summation of e_{ij} over all of patient profile factors with drug response provides a score to evaluate each patient's glucose lowering response after taking OADs under his specific genetic and clinical profiles.

When summing all the e_{ij} with the j defined as the HbA1c level $\leq$ 7%, the Score represents how likely the patient is responding to the current OAD treatment based on his/her body indexes, treatment strategy, polymorphisms, health condition.

$$Score_{Res} = \sum_i e_{ij}(x_i, Res)$$

where i denotes a genetic or clinical factor of patient, and x_i represents the class of the factor belongs to. Additionally, the score for a patient's inert responses to the OAD is calculated based

on the e_{ij} with j representing HbA1c level > 7%.

$$Score_{NonRes} = \sum_i e_{ij}(x_i, NonRes)$$

The two scores for each patient are compared and the treatment response is predicted based on which score is larger. The leave one out cross-validation is conducted to evaluate the performance of this predictive model.

RESULTS

Descriptive Statistics and Phenotype Classification

A total of 495 patients treated with hypoglycemic drugs were included in this study. The subjects were Mexican, mainly from northeastern of Mexico. The average age of patients was 56.30 ± 12.16 for males and 56.41 ± 11.45 for females. No significant differences were found for the age of diagnosis, diabetes duration, and HbA1c values between males and females. However, the BMI was statistically higher in females (**Table 1**). Regarding to co-morbidities, the most frequent co-morbidity was hypertension with 24.4%, followed by hypertension-dyslipidemia with 13.1%, only dyslipidemia (7.5%), hypothyroidism (6.3%), and hypertension-hypothyroidism (4.6%).

The phenotype classification based on HbA1c values (**Table 1**) was significantly different between the responder's and non-responder's (p = 6.29 × 10^{-68}). More than half of the patients (353) did not respond to any type of therapy (HbA1c > 7%), failing in 71.3% of the cases, and the treatment was effective (HbA1c ≤ 7%) in 142 individuals. The average diagnosis age of non-responders showed significant lower values (p = 4.25 × 10^{-4}) compared to responder's, but showed statistically significant higher values of diabetes duration

TABLE 1 | Demographic and clinical data of patients.

Patients	N	Age	Diagnosis age	Diabetes duration	BMI	HbA1c
Males	156 (31.5%)	56.30 ± 12.16	45.12 ± 12.013	11.45 ± 8.03	28.90 ± 4.46$^{£}$	8.69 ± 2.24
Females	339 (68.5%)	56.41 ± 11.45	45.32 ± 10.705	10.95 ± 8.63	30.66 ± 6.78	8.45 ± 2.10
Non-responders	353 (71.3%)	56.30 ± 11.51	44.14 ± 11.00$^{Δ,¥}$	12.14 ± 8.25¶	29.83 ± 5.95	9.40 ± 1.92$^{£,§}$
MT non-responders	332 (67.1%)	56.47 ± 11.48	44.39 ± 10.95	11.00 ± 8.26	30.00 ± 6.07	9.33 ± 1.94
CT non-responders	30 (6.1%)	55.27 ± 11.51	42.53 ± 11.23	13.07 ± 8.28	28.50 ± 4.80	9.6 ± 1.81
Responders (any type)	142 (28.7%)	56.56 ± 12.09	48.02 ± 10.98	8.54 ± 8.39	30.79 ± 6.72	6.34 ± 0.47
MT responders	127 (25.7%)	55.88 ± 12.08	47.92 ± 11.36	8.06 ± 7.88	30.91 ± 6.72	6.32 ± 0.43
CT responders	7 (1.4%)	65.29 ± 13.16	49.29 ± 6.90	15.43 ± 14.26	25.83 ± 3.78	5.97 ± 0.79
FLT responders	93 (18.8%)	56.61 ± 11.11	49.68 ± 10.83^{j}	6.92 ± 6.89^{C}	31.46 ± 6.85	6.30 ± 0.50
SLT responders	39 (7.9%)	56.77 ± 12.98	46.62 ± 10.33	10.19 ± 8.79	30.13 ± 6.15	6.43 ± 0.41
TLT Responders	10 (2.0%)	55.20 ± 17.69	38.10 ± 9.67	17.10 ± 13.07	27.13 ± 6.88	6.40 ± 0.44

Data presented as mean ± SD. BMI: body mass index; HbA1c: hemoglobin A$_{1c}$; MT: monotherapy; CT: combined therapy; FLT: first-line therapy; SLT: second-line therapy; TLT: third-line therapy. $^{£}p = 0.025$ (male vs. female), $^{Δ}P = 4.25 \times 10^{-4}$ (non-responders vs. responders), $^{¶}p = 2.5 \times 10^{-7}$ (non-responders vs. responders), $^{£}p = 6.29 \times 10^{-68}$ (non-responders vs. responders), $^{¥}p = 1.41 \times 10^{-4}$ (non-responders vs. FLT), $^{P}P = 0.025$ (FLT vs. TLT), $^{C}p \leq 0.049$ (FLT vs. non-responders, SLT, and TLT), and $^{§}p \leq 6.84 \times 10^{-8}$ (non-responders vs. FLT, SLT, TLT).

($p = 2.5 \times 10^{-7}$). A total of 93 patients (18.8%) responded to FLT, and they showed higher values of diagnosis age ($p = 0.025$), although for lower values of diabetes duration ($p \leq 0.049$), compared to responder's to TLT. None other therapies had a significant difference.

The drug most commonly used for the FLT was metformin in monotherapy (46.7%). The second most used drug in FLT was a SU in combination with metformin (34.6%). For SLT and TLT, metformin was also very commonly used (16.7 and 8.0%, respectively). For FLT, SLT, and TLT, the third most common option was SU in monotherapy (9.3, 13.3, and 5.3%, respectively). Insulin was the most common treatment choice in SLT and TLT (55.2 and 69.3%, respectively), although it was the fifth option in FLT (2.2%) (**Table 2**).

Pharmacogenetic Findings by Standard Statistical Methods

The polymorphisms M165I and R400C in *SLC22A2* gene were not in HWE equilibrium. The SNPs G401S and R465G in *SLC22A1* gene, and K432Q in *SLC22A2* gene, had a Minor Allele Frequency (MAF) < 0.01. The polymorphisms were excluded from subsequent analyses. As a result a total of 9 SNPs remained for statistical analysis. Two polymorphisms, Ala1369Ser in gene *ABCC8* and Glu23Lys in gene *KCNJ11*, showed a significant impact on response to SUs.

The effect of *ABCC8*-Ala1369Ser polymorphism on Hb1Ac under SU treatment was statistically significant. Heterozygous variant (C/T) carriers had lower HbA1c values compared to homozygous wild-type (A/A) carriers ($p = 0.029$) and compared to homozygous wild-type and variant (A/A+C/C) carriers ($p = 0.012$). The genotypes resulting from the *KCNJ11*-Glu23Lys polymorphism also had a significant impact on HbA1c under SU treatment. First, the homozygous wild-type and variant (C/C+T/T) carriers had higher HbA1c values ($p = 0.039$) as compared to heterozygous carrier (C/T). None of the other 7 polymorphisms tested had a significant impact on clinical parameters (**Table 3**).

The association was evaluated under genetic models for only nine polymorphisms that had passed a quality control. We found that two of the nine polymorphisms were associated with the responder phenotype. The A/C genotype of *ABCC8*-Ala1369Ser and the C/T genotype of *KCNJ11*-Glu23Lys were significantly associated with responder phenotype using over dominant model. This association remained statistically significant after adjusting using Bonferroni's correction ($p < 0.05$) (**Table 4**).

Pharmacogenetic and Clinical Parametric Findings From T2DM Patient Profiles by Direct Coupling Analysis

The DCA finds factor-drug response connections from a global statistical model computed from an estimate of the joint probability distribution of all clinical variables in the study. **Figure 1** shows the classification process that the patient clinical and genetic data undergoes to form the input discrete matrix for DCA algorithm. The outcome is a set of pairs with DI values. To uncover the minimal set of relevant connections between those factors, a Bayesian network is constructed by using the Chow-Liu algorithm as shown in **Figure 1**. However, this study refines Chow-Liu algorithm by replacing the typical use of mutual information with DI from DCA to calculate the Kullback–Leibler distance. This is a novel approach to generate the Bayesian network. Some factors cluster together and are connected showing previously known relationships, such as the connections between weight, height, BMI, and gender. These known associations of factors can be seen as validation of the links found by the algorithm. The time lengths of treatment (first line and second line), age, age of diagnosis, and diabetes diagnosis span are clustered; however, the treatment history for the third line therapy is more likely to be associated with weight.

In agreement with the pharmacogenomics finding that *KCNJ11* Glu23Lys affects the response to SUs, while *KCNJ11* Glu23Lys is generally connected to response to OADs. However, the *ABCC8* Ala1369Ser variant is not connected to any drug in this network and is linked to *KCNJ11* Ile1337Val variant.

TABLE 2 | Scheme for the treatment of T2DM.

Drug	First-line therapy		Second-line therapy		Third-line therapy	
	N	Percent	N	Percent	N	Percent
Metformin	231	46.7	45	16.7	6	8
Metformin/Sulfonylurea	171	34.6	3	1.1	1	1.3
Sulfonylurea	46	9.3	40	14.8	5	6.8
Other	36	7.2	33	12.2	11	14.6
Insulin	11	2.2	149	55.2	52	69.3
Total	495	100	270	100	75	100

TABLE 3 | Association values between gene polymorphisms and clinical parameters.

Polymorphism	N	BMI	Diagnosis age	HbA1c
		ABCC8-Ala1369Ser		
A/A	180	30.74 ± 6.84	46.23 ± 11.37	$8.69 \pm 2.07^{\Delta}$
A/C	241	29.84 ± 5.93	45.16 ± 11.34	8.34 ± 2.21
C/C	74	29.44 ± 5.26	43.20 ± 9.52	8.74 ± 2.09
A/A+C/C	254	30.36 ± 6.44	45.35 ± 10.93	$8.70 \pm 2.07^{\P}$
		CYP2C9-Arg144Cys		
C/C	423	30.07 ± 6.26	45.41 ± 11.03	8.49 ± 2.17
C/T	67	30.30 ± 6.04	44.69 ± 11.40	8.67 ± 2.00
T/T	5	30.17 ± 2.09	40.00 ± 16.33	9.60 ± 2.13
		CYP2C9-Ile359Leu		
A/A	460	30.06 ± 6.01	45.35 ± 10.96	8.52 ± 2.13
C/A	35	30.67 ± 8.28	44.06 ± 13.24	8.55 ± 2.34
		KCNJ11-Glu23Lys		
C/C	179	30.70 ± 6.87	46.26 ± 11.56	8.64 ± 2.08
C/T	246	29.91 ± 5.96	44.95 ± 11.25	8.37 ± 2.19
T/T	70	29.26 ± 5.01	43.79 ± 9.28	8.75 ± 2.13
C/C+T/T	249	30.29 ± 6.42	45.56 ± 11.00	$8.67 \pm 2.09^{£}$
		KCNJ11-Ile1337Val		
C/C	71	29.36 ± 5.05	43.75 ± 9.22	8.74 ± 2.12
C/T	247	29.97 ± 6.17	44.91 ± 11.34	8.38 ± 2.20
T/T	177	30.59 ± 6.62	46.34 ± 11.46	8.64 ± 2.07
		SLC22A1-Arg61Cys		
C/C	475	30.05 ± 6.21	45.40 ± 11.03	8.53 ± 2.16
C/T	20	31.43 ± 5.83	41.90 ± 13.02	8.51 ± 1.77
		SLC22A1-Met61Val		
G/G	92	30.77 ± 6.22	46.41 ± 9.96	8.18 ± 2.04
A/G	26	29.74 ± 4.45	45.58 ± 14.77	8.14 ± 1.74
A/A	6	28.66 ± 4.03	43.67 ± 10.65	8.15 ± 1.83
		SLC22A2-Ala270Ser		
A/C	58	30.04 ± 6.35	46.03 ± 11.17	8.04 ± 1.56
C/C	437	30.11 ± 6.18	45.15 ± 11.12	8.59 ± 2.20
		SLC22A2-Met420Del		
ATG/ATG	52	30.56 ± 6.30	44.65 ± 9.87	8.35 ± 2.09
ATG/delTGA	49	30.72 ± 5.77	48.10 ± 12.73	8.05 ± 2.00
delGAT/delGAT	23	29.61 ± 4.78	45.13 ± 9.59	8.02 ± 1.56

Data presented as mean ± SD. BMI: body mass index; HbA1c: hemoglobin A1c. $^{\Delta}P = 0.029$ (A/A vs. A/C), $^{\P}p = 0.012$ (A/A+C/C vs. A/C), and $^{£}p = 0.039$ (C/C+T/T vs. C/T).

Polymorphisms in the *SLC22A2* gene have been identified and shown to cause inter-patient variability in the pharmacokinetic and pharmacodynamic profile of metformin. Three gene variants, M165I (rs8177507), Ala270Ser (rs316019), and R400C (rs8177516), of the *SLC22A2* gene were reported with reduced uptake of OCT2 substrate, whereas a fourth one, K432Q (rs8177517), showed an increased uptake activity compared to the wild-type allele. However, attempts to translate those findings

TABLE 4 | Association values between genotypes and response using dominant, over-dominant, and additive models.

Gene	Polymorphism	Model	OR (95% CI)	p-value	Pc-value
ABCC8	Ala1369Ser	Over-dominant (A/A+C/C vs. A/C)	A/A+C/C = 1.33 (1.11–1.59)	0.03	0.04*
			A/C = 0.736 (0.59–0.92)		
KCNJ11	Glu23Lys	Over-dominant (C/C+T/T vs. C/T)	C/C+T/T = 1.27 (1.06–1.51)	0.013	0.018*
			C/T = 0.77 (0.62–0.96)		

*OR: odds ratio; CI: confidence interval; Pc: P-values adjusted by using Bonferroni's correction for multiple comparisons; *p ≤ 0.05.*

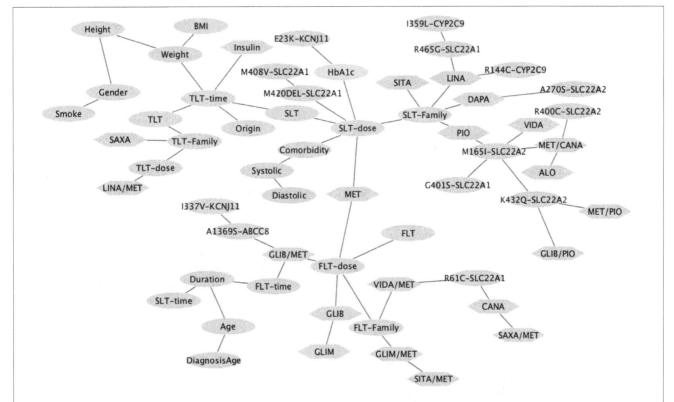

FIGURE 2 | Bayesian network of OADs and factors built from direct information. Hexagonal shapes indicate OADs and ovals denote clinical parameters or polymorphisms.

into altered response to metformin of diabetic patients in several populations have not been successful (Meyer zu Schwabedissen et al., 2010). As shown in **Figure 2**, 3 out of 4 polymorphisms in *SLC22A2* have connections to metformin in combination with other drugs. The genetic variants of *SLC22A2* identified in a Korean population appear to have a significant impact on the disposition of metformin. As expected from the primary distribution of OCT2 in the kidney, the tubular excretion was influenced mainly by the M165I, Ala270Ser, and R400C variants of *SLC22A2*, leading to an increase in plasma metformin concentrations in subjects with these variants (Song et al., 2008). MET is connected to FLT cluster and SLT cluster, being consistent with the fact that MET is the most commonly used drug in FLT and the second common drug in SLT. Two SU drugs, GLIB and GLIM, are connected together.

To systematically investigate the connection between blood glucose lowering outcome and other factors, we studied the couplings between those factors and the drug response HbA1c test results. In the input matrix, the values in columns for each drug identify their presence or absence in the treatment. The overall ranking of each drug response connection is shown in the heatmap of **Figure 3A**. Treatment time and doses are highly associated with HbA1c results. Age and place of origin appear to be strongly influential. The administration of GLIB or MET in monotherapy is also highly connected to HbA1c results, partially corresponding with the fact that Metformin is the most commonly used treatment for T2DM. Among the body indexes parameter, weight and BMI still have high rankings, which suggests that in prediction of treatment outcome those two factors are worthy of consideration. The rankings of

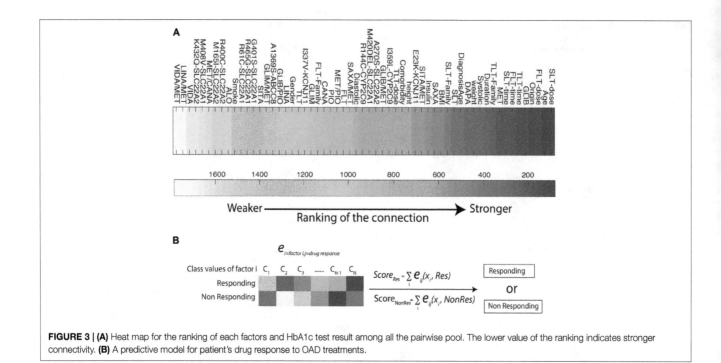

FIGURE 3 | (A) Heat map for the ranking of each factors and HbA1c test result among all the pairwise pool. The lower value of the ranking indicates stronger connectivity. **(B)** A predictive model for patient's drug response to OAD treatments.

polymorphisms have the highest influence at *KCNJ11* Glu23Lys, which is observed to be correlated with drug response to SUs in both the statistical significance study and the DI-based Bayesian network.

In order to predict the glucose-lowering efficacy of each OADs and determine a better therapy strategy based on a given profile of patient, we develop a predictive model on DI (**Figure 3B**). DI is a metric of direct coupling among variables but it does not reveal the directionality of this connection. It is possible to use the parameters of the global joint distribution, to quantify how a large number of factors account for a possible outcome, i.e., responsive or non-responsive treatment. This additive model uses the $e_{ij}(x_i,x_j)$ estimates connecting factors to response with the aims to distinguish between the responder and non-responder group. We conducted a leave one out cross-validation on the 495 T2DM patients dataset, and reached an average of prediction rate at 0.70, with the maximum response vs. non-response prediction rate at 0.76.

DISCUSSION

Association Between Gene Polymorphisms and Clinical Parameters

From the nine analyzed pharamcogentic polymorphisms seeking to explain the relationship between diverse genotypes of diabetic patients and their response to different OADs, only two polymorphisms, *ABCC8*-Ala1369Ser and *KCNJ11*-Glu23Lys, showed a significant impact on response on the reduction of Hb1Ac with SU treatment. None of the other seven polymorphisms tested had a significant impact on clinical parameters. These results confirm the association of *ABCC8*-Ala1369Ser polymorphism and reduction of HbA1c level in

the Chinese population with SU treatment (Feng et al., 2008). Nevertheless, studies in Caucasian populations showed no association of *KCNJ11*-Glu23Lys with Hb1Ac reduction in response to SUs (Ragia et al., 2012).

The *CYP2C9* polymorphisms included in this study, Arg144Cys and I1359L, showed no significant differences in response to SUs in comparison with studies carried on Caucasian population in which they described a higher sensitivity to SUs for Ile359Leu and Arg144Cys variant carriers (Becker et al., 2008; Ragia et al., 2014). The *KCNJ11*-I337 polymorphism showed no evidence of being related in the response to SUs as a study carried on Chinese population suggests (Cheung et al., 2011). The *SLC22A1* polymorphisms, Arg61Cys and Met61Val, showed no significant evidence of being related in the response to metformin in comparison with a study carried in Caucasian population in which they found a significant reduction of Hb1Ac after 6 months of metformin treatment (Tkac et al., 2013). The *SLC22A2* polymorphisms showed no evidence of being related in the response to metformin, contrary of what has been suggested (Avery et al., 2009).

Association Between Genotypes and Phenotypes

Only the A/C nucleotide change from polymorphism Ala1369Ser (gene *ABCC8*) and the C/T nucleotide change from polymorphism Glu23Lys (gene *KCNJ1*) were significantly associated with responder phenotype using an over dominant model. *KCNJ11* and *ABCC8* encode for the subunits KIR6.2 and SUR1, respectively, of the heteroctomer K_{ATP} channel (Emami-Riedmaier et al., 2015). K_{ATP} channels regulate membrane K^+ flux for various cell types including pancreatic β-cells, where increased glucose metabolism results in the closure of the K_{ATP}

channels leading to calcium influx and subsequent insulin secretion (Nathan et al., 2009). Notably, *KCNJ11* and *ABCC8* genes lie close to each other on chromosome 11, with strong linkage disequilibrium. In a Caucasian population study, Ala1369Ser was correlated with Glu23Lys, where for every K allele of *KCNJ11* gene found there was A allele of *ABCC8*, thus constituting a possible haplotype (Florez et al., 2004), whereas several studies and meta-analyses showed the association of *KCNJ11*, but not of *ABCC8* polymorphisms, with susceptibility to type 2 diabetes (van Dam et al., 2005; Gong et al., 2012).

We showed that it is possible to use patient data in this comprehensive study to generate a model of the global distribution of patient profiles. This model includes phenotypic factors, health conditions, treatment information, and polymorphisms with clinical treatment outcome variable. Although we found agreement between the standard statistical tests and the global pairwise DCA model about how *KCNJ11*-Glu23Lys affects the efficacy of SUs drug, we also found novel relationships when modeling the dataset with global techniques. We uncover a network connecting OADs, gene polymorphisms, and patient information. Connections with the HbA1c test and metrics for the association between each pairwise variables can inform better how a large set of factors interact during disease progression.

A predictive model for OAD drug response is proposed based on direct coupling parameters e_{ij} in this study and its predictive performance has been validated by cross validation. The overall prediction rate both for predicting as responding or non-responding can be as high as 0.76. This model has the potential to be used as a guide to modify factors to predict higher response scores. This is a topic of further research that can have applications in personalized therapies. With increasing well-phenotyped cohorts and new methods, such as Next Generation Sequencing and global statistical analyses,

the next few years promise a renewed interest in the use of pharmacogenetics to unravel drug and disease mechanisms, as well as the possibility to individualize T2DM therapy by genotype.

AUTHOR CONTRIBUTIONS

HB-S and LR-C conceived of the idea of analyzing genetic factors altering the oral antidiabetic drugs response in Mexican type II diabetes patients. LR-C, CL-A, HS-I, and IM-A carried out the real-time PCR experiments and Sanger sequencing experiments. FL-G provided the biospecimens and their clinical data. FM, X-LJ, and RL-C analyzed the data and designed the models and the computational framework. X-LJ and FM developed the predictive model. HB-S was in charge of overall direction and planning. HS-I, FM, X-LJ, LR-C, and DA-T wrote the manuscript. HB-S and FM should be considered as co-corresponding authors.

FUNDING

This work was funded by the National Council on Science and Technology (CONACYT) (Grant Nos. 185427, ECO-2015-C01-260826, 294875, and 280114) and funds from the University of Texas at Dallas.

ACKNOWLEDGMENTS

We thank Esteban Lopez for the comments that greatly improved the manuscript. We would also like to show our gratitude to Roxana Rivera, Ph.D., and Ricardo Cerda for their comments on earlier versions of the manuscript.

REFERENCES

Agudelo-Botero, M., and Davila-Cervantes, C. A. (2015). Burden of mortality due to diabetes mellitus in Latin America 2000-2011: the case of Argentina, Chile, Colombia, and Mexico. *Gac. Sanit.* 29, 172–177. doi: 10.1016/j.gaceta.2015.01.015

Almudevar, A. (2010). A hypothesis test for equality of bayesian network models. *EURASIP J. Bioinform. Syst. Biol.* 2010:947564. doi: 10.1155/2010/947564

Arredondo, A., and De Icaza, E. (2011). The cost of diabetes in Latin America: evidence from Mexico. *Value Health* 14(5 Suppl. 1), S85–S88. doi: 10.1016/j.jval.2011.05.022

Avery, P., Mousa, S. S., and Mousa, S. A. (2009). Pharmacogenomics in type II diabetes mellitus management: steps toward personalized medicine. *Pharmgenomics Pers. Med.* 2, 79–91.

Barquera, S., Campos-Nonato, I., Aguilar-Salinas, C., Lopez-Ridaura, R., Arredondo, A., and Rivera-Dommarco, J. (2013). Diabetes in Mexico: cost and management of diabetes and its complications and challenges for health policy. *Glob. Health* 9:3. doi: 10.1186/1744-8603-9-3

Barretina, J., Caponigro, G., Stransky, N., Venkatesan, K., Margolin, A. A., Kim, S., et al. (2012). The cancer cell line Encyclopedia enables predictive modelling of anticancer drug sensitivity. *Nature* 483, 603–607. doi: 10.1038/nature11003

Becker, M. L., Pearson, E. R., and Tkac, I. (2013). Pharmacogenetics of oral antidiabetic drugs. *Int. J. Endocrinol.* 2013:686315. doi: 10.1155/2013/686315

Becker, M. L., Visser, L. E., Trienekens, P. H., Hofman, A., van Schaik, R., and Stricker, B. (2008). Cytochrome P450 2C9*2 and *3 polymorphisms and the

dose and effect of sulfonylurea in type II diabetes mellitus. *Clin. Pharmacol. Ther.* 83, 288–292. doi: 10.1038/sj.clpt.6100273

Boyd, J. S., Cheng, R. R., Paddock, M. L., Sancar, C., Morcos, F., and Golden, S. S. (2016). A combined computational and genetic approach uncovers network interactions of the cyanobacterial circadian clock. *J. Bacteriol.* 198, 2439–2447. doi: 10.1128/JB.00235-16

Chen, X. W., Anantha, G., and Lin, X. T. (2008). Improving Bayesian network structure learning with mutual information-based node ordering in the K2 algorithm. *IEEE Transac. Knowl. Data Eng.* 20, 628–640. doi: 10.1109/Tkde.2007.190732

Cheung, C. Y., Tso, A. W., Cheung, B. M., Xu, A., Fong, C. H., Ong, K. L., et al. (2011). The KCNJ11 E23K polymorphism and progression of glycaemia in Southern Chinese: a long-term prospective study. *PLoS One* 6:e28598. doi: 10.1371/journal.pone.0028598

Distefano, J. K., and Watanabe, R. M. (2010). Pharmacogenetics of anti-diabetes drugs. *Pharmaceuticals* 3, 2610–2646. doi: 10.3390/ph3082610

dos Santos, R. N., Morcos, F., Jana, B., Andricopulo, A. D., and Onuchic, J. N. (2015). Dimeric interactions and complex formation using direct coevolutionary couplings. *Sci. Rep.* 5:13652. doi: 10.1038/srep13652

Emami-Riedmaier, A., Schaeffeler, E., Nies, A. T., Morike, K., and Schwab, M. (2015). Stratified medicine for the use of antidiabetic medication in treatment of type II diabetes and cancer: where do we go from here? *J. Intern. Med.* 277, 235–247. doi: 10.1111/joim.12330

Feng, Y., Mao, G. Y., Ren, X. W., Xing, H. X., Tang, G. F., Li, Q., et al. (2008). Ser1369Ala variant in sulfonylurea receptor gene ABCC8 Is associated with antidiabetic efficacy of gliclazide in Chinese type 2 diabetic patients. *Diabetes Care* 31, 1939–1944. doi: 10.2337/dc07-2248

Florez, J. C., Burtt, N., de Bakker, P. I., Almgren, P., Tuomi, T., Holmkvist, J., et al. (2004). Haplotype structure and genotype-phenotype correlations of the sulfonylurea receptor and the islet ATP-sensitive potassium channel gene region. *Diabetes Metab. Res. Rev.* 53, 1360–1368. doi: 10.2337/diabetes.53.5.1360

Foretz, M., Hébrard, S., Leclerc, J., Zarrinpashneh, E., Soty, M., Mithieux, G., et al. (2010). Metformin inhibits hepatic gluconeogenesis in mice independently of the LKB1/AMPK pathway via a decrease in hepatic energy state. *J. Clin. Invest.* 120, 2355–2369. doi: 10.1172/JCI40671

Gong, B., Yu, J., Li, H., Li, W., and Tong, X. (2012). The effect of KCNJ11 polymorphism on the risk of type 2 diabetes: a global meta-analysis based on 49 case-control studies. *DNA Cell Biol.* 31, 801–810. doi: 10.1089/dna.2011.1445

Holstein, A., Plaschke, A., Ptak, M., Egberts, E. H., El-Din, J., Brockmoller, J., et al. (2005). Association between CYP2C9 slow metabolizer genotypes and severe hypoglycaemia on medication with sulphonylurea hypoglycaemic agents. *Br. J. Clin. Pharmacol.* 60, 103–106. doi: 10.1111/j.1365-2125.2005.02379.x

Huang, C. M., and Florez, J. C. (2011). Pharmacogenetics in type 2 diabetes: potential implications for clinical practice. *Genome Med.* 3:76. doi: 10.1186/gm292

Inzucchi, S. E., Bergenstal, R. M., Buse, J. B., Diamant, M., Ferrannini, E., Nauck, M., et al. (2012). Management of hyperglycaemia in type 2 diabetes: a patient-centered approach. position statement of the American diabetes association (ADA) and the European Association for the Study of Diabetes (EASD). *Diabetologia* 55, 1577–1596. doi: 10.1007/s00125-012-2534-0

Jiang, X. L., Martinez-Ledesma, E., and Morcos, F. (2017). Revealing protein networks and gene-drug connectivity in cancer from direct information. *Sci. Rep.* 7:3739. doi: 10.1038/s41598-017-04001-3

Krentz, A. J., and Bailey, C. J. (2005). Oral antidiabetic agents - Current role in type 2 diabetes mellitus. *Drugs* 65, 385–411. doi: 10.2165/00003495-200565030-00005

Lo, C., Lui, M., Ranasinha, S., Teede, H. J., Kerr, P. G., Polkinghorne, K., et al. (2012). Defining the relationship between HbA(1c) and average plasma glucose in type 2 diabetes and chronic kidney disease. *Diabetologia* 55, S453–S453. doi: 10.1016/j.diabres.2014.01.020

Marchetti, P., Lupi, R., Del Guerra, S., Bugliani, M., D'Aleo, V., Occhipinti, M., et al. (2009). Goals of treatment for Type 2 diabetes beta-Cell preservation for glycemic control. *Diabetes Care* 32, S178–S183. doi: 10.2337/dc09-S306

Meyer zu Schwabedissen, H. E., Verstuyft, C., Kroemer, H. K., Becquemont, L., and Kim, R. B. (2010). Human multidrug and toxin extrusion 1 (MATE1/SLC47A1) transporter: functional characterization, interaction with OCT2 (SLC22A2), and single nucleotide polymorphisms. *Am. J. Physiol. Renal Physiol.* 298, F997–F1005. doi: 10.1152/ajprenal.00431.2009

Morcos, F., Jana, B., Hwa, T., and Onuchic, J. N. (2013). Coevolutionary signals across protein lineages help capture multiple protein conformations. *Proc. Natl. Acad. Sci. U.S.A.* 110, 20533–20538. doi: 10.1073/pnas.1315625110

Morcos, F., Pagnani, A., Lunt, B., Bertolino, A., Marks, D. S., and Sander, C. (2011). Direct-coupling analysis of residue coevolution captures native contacts across many protein families. *Proc. Natl. Acad. Sci. U.S.A.* 108, E1293–E1301. doi: 10.1073/pnas.1111471108

Morcos, F., Schafer, N. P., Cheng, R. R., Onuchic, J. N., and Wolynes, P. G. (2014). Coevolutionary information, protein folding landscapes, and the thermodynamics of natural selection. *Proc. Natl. Acad. Sci. U.S.A.* 111, 12408–12413. doi: 10.1073/pnas.1413575111

Nathan, D. M., Buse, J. B., Davidson, M. B., Ferrannini, E., Holman, R. R., and Sherwin, R. (2009). Medical management of hyperglycemia in type 2 diabetes: a consensus algorithm for the initiation and adjustment of therapy A consensus statement of the American diabetes association and the European association for the study of diabetes. *Diabetes Care* 32, 193–203. doi: 10.2337/dc08-9025

Pearson, E. (2009). Pharmacogenetics in diabetes. *Curr. Diab. Rep.* 9, 172–181. doi: 10.1007/s11892-009-0028-3

Pernicova, I., and Korbonits, M. (2014). Metformin-mode of action and clinical implications for diabetes and cancer. *Nat. Rev. Endocrinol.* 10, 143–156. doi: 10.1038/nrendo.2013.256

Ragia, G., Petridis, I., Tavridou, A., Christakidis, D., and Manolopoulos, V. G. (2009). Presence of CYP2C9*3 allele increases risk for hypoglycemia in Type 2

diabetic patients treated with sulfonylureas. *Pharmacogenomics* 10, 1781–1787. doi: 10.2217/Pgs.09.96

Ragia, G., Tavridou, A., Elens, L., Van Schaik, R. H. N., and Manolopoulos, V. G. (2014). CYP2C9*2 Allele Increases Risk for Hypoglycemia in POR*1/*1 Type 2 Diabetic Patients Treated with Sulfonylureas. *Exp. Clin. Endocrinol. Diabetes* 122, 60–63. doi: 10.1055/s-0033-1361097

Ragia, G., Tavridou, A., Petridis, I., and Manolopoulos, V. G. (2012). Association of KCNJ11 E23K gene polymorphism with hypoglycemia in sulfonylurea-treated Type 2 diabetic patients. *Diabetes Res. Clin. Pract.* 98, 119–124. doi: 10.1016/j.diabres.2012.04.017

Semiz, S., Dujic, T., Ostanek, B., Prnjavorac, B., Bego, T., and Malenica, M. (2010). Analysis of CYP2C9*2, CYP2C19*2, and CYP2D6*4 polymorphisms in patients with type 2 diabetes mellitus. *Bosn. J. Basic Med. Sci.* 10, 287–291. doi: 10.17305/bjbms.2010.2662

Sokolova, E. A., Bondar, I. A., Shabelnikova, O. Y., Pyankova, O. V., and Filipenko, M. L. (2015). Replication of KCNJ11 (p.E23K) and ABCC8 (p.S1369A) Association in Russian diabetes mellitus 2 Type cohort and meta-analysis. *PLoS One* 10:e0124662. doi: 10.1371/journal.pone.0124662

Song, I. S., Shin, H. J., Shim, E. J., Jung, I. S., Kim, W. Y., and Shon, J. H. (2008). Genetic variants of the organic cation transporter 2 influence the disposition of metformin. *Clin. Pharmacol. Ther.* 84, 559–562. doi: 10.1038/clpt.2008.61

Stransky, N., Ghandi, M., Kryukov, G. V., Garraway, L. A., Lehar, J., and Liu, M. (2015). Pharmacogenomic agreement between two cancer cell line data sets. *Nature* 528, 84–87. doi: 10.1038/nature15736

Sulkowska, J. I., Morcos, F., Weigt, M., Hwa, T., and Onuchic, J. N. (2012). Genomics-aided structure prediction. *Proc. Natl. Acad. Sci. U.S.A.* 109, 10340–10345. doi: 10.1073/pnas.1207864109

Tkac, I. (2015). Genetics of Drug Response in Type 2 Diabetes. *Curr. Diab. Rep.* 15:43. doi: 10.1007/s11892-015-0617-2

Tkac, I., Klimcakova, L., Javorsky, M., Fabianova, M., Schroner, Z., and Hermanova, H. (2013). Pharmacogenomic association between a variant in SLC47A1 gene and therapeutic response to metformin in type 2 diabetes. *Diabetes Obes. Metab.* 15, 189–191. doi: 10.1111/j.1463-1326.2012.01691.x

Turner, S. D., Crawford, D. C., and Ritchie, M. D. (2009). Methods for optimizing statistical analyses in pharmacogenomics research. *Expert Rev. Clin. Pharmacol.* 2, 559–570. doi: 10.1586/ecp.09.32

Tzvetkov, M. V., Vormfelde, S. V., Balen, D., Meineke, I., Schmidt, T., and Sehrt, D. (2009). The effects of genetic polymorphisms in the organic cation transporters OCT1, OCT2, and OCT3 on the renal clearance of metformin. *Clin. Pharmacol. Ther.* 86, 299–306. doi: 10.1038/clpt.2009.92

van Dam, R. M., Hoebee, B., Seidell, J. C., Schaap, M. M., de Bruin, T. W., and Feskens, E. J. (2005). Common variants in the ATP-sensitive K+ channel genes KCNJ11 (Kir6.2) and ABCC8 (SUR1) in relation to glucose intolerance: population-based studies and meta-analyses. *Diabetes Med.* 22, 590–598. doi: 10.1111/j.1464-5491.2005.01465.x

Villareal, D. T., Koster, J. C., Robertson, H., Akrouh, A., Miyake, K., and Bell, G. I. (2009). Kir6.2 Variant E23K Increases ATP-Sensitive K(+) channel activity and is associated with impaired insulin release and enhanced insulin sensitivity in adults with normal glucose tolerance. *Diabetes* 58, 1869–1878. doi: 10.2337/db09-0025

Zhou, K. X., Donnelly, L. A., Kimber, C. H., Donnan, P. T., Doney, A. S. F., and Leese, G. (2009). Reduced-Function SLC22A1 polymorphisms encoding organic cation transporter 1 and glycemic response to metformin: a GoDARTS study. *Diabetes Metab. Res. Rev.* 58, 1434–1439. doi: 10.2337/db08-0896

12

Empirical Scoring Functions for Structure-Based Virtual Screening: Applications, Critical Aspects and Challenges

Isabella A. Guedes, Felipe S. S. Pereira and Laurent E. Dardenne*

Grupo de Modelagem Molecular em Sistemas Biológicos, Laboratório Nacional de Computação Científica, Petrópolis, Brazil

Correspondence:
Laurent E. Dardenne
dardenne@lncc.br

Structure-based virtual screening (VS) is a widely used approach that employs the knowledge of the three-dimensional structure of the target of interest in the design of new lead compounds from large-scale molecular docking experiments. Through the prediction of the binding mode and affinity of a small molecule within the binding site of the target of interest, it is possible to understand important properties related to the binding process. Empirical scoring functions are widely used for pose and affinity prediction. Although pose prediction is performed with satisfactory accuracy, the correct prediction of binding affinity is still a challenging task and crucial for the success of structure-based VS experiments. There are several efforts in distinct fronts to develop even more sophisticated and accurate models for filtering and ranking large libraries of compounds. This paper will cover some recent successful applications and methodological advances, including strategies to explore the ligand entropy and solvent effects, training with sophisticated machine-learning techniques, and the use of quantum mechanics. Particular emphasis will be given to the discussion of critical aspects and further directions for the development of more accurate empirical scoring functions.

Keywords: structure-based drug design, molecular docking, virtual screening, scoring function, binding affinity prediction, machine learning

INTRODUCTION

The drug discovery process required to enable a new compound to reach the market as an innovative therapeutic entity is significantly expensive and time-consuming (Mullard, 2014; DiMasi et al., 2016; Mignani et al., 2016). In this context, research groups and pharmaceutical industry have extensively included computer-aided drug design (CADD) approaches in their drug discovery pipeline to increase the potential of finding newer and safer drug candidates (Ban et al., 2017; Barril, 2017; Usha et al., 2017). Structure-based drug design (SBDD) methods, which require the three-dimensional structure of the macromolecular target, have been widely employed in successful campaigns (Bortolato et al., 2012; Danishuddin and Khan, 2015; Rognan, 2017). Although important challenges and some limitations have been addressed, many efforts have been made aiming the improvement of existing methods and the development of innovative approaches. Molecular docking is one of the most used SBDD approaches with several reviews published at the present time (Guedes et al., 2014; Ferreira et al., 2015; Yuriev et al., 2015; Pagadala et al., 2017;

Dos Santos et al., 2018), and has been continuously explored by the scientific community to develop more sophisticated and accurate strategies. Docking aims to predict binding modes and affinity of a small molecule within the binding site of the receptor target of interest, supporting the researcher in the understanding of the main physicochemical features related to the binding process. Docking-based virtual screening (VS) consists of large-scale docking with a growing number of success cases reported (Villoutreix et al., 2009; Matter and Sotriffer, 2011; Rognan, 2017). Examples of docking programs are AutoDockVina (Trott and Olson, 2010), UCSF DOCK (Allen et al., 2015), GOLD (Jones et al., 1997), and Glide (Friesner et al., 2004, 2006a). Beyond the standalone software, web servers such as the DockThor Portal[1] (de Magalhães et al., 2014), MTiOpenScreen[2] (Labbé et al., 2015), HADDOCK[3] (van Zundert et al., 2016), and DOCK Blaster[4] (Irwin et al., 2009) provide to the scientific community friendly user interface and satisfactory time response of docking results.

The fast evaluation of docking poses generated by the search method and the accurate prediction of binding affinity of top-ranked poses is essential in VS protocols. In this context, scoring functions emerge as a straightforward and fast strategy despite limited accuracy, remaining as the main alternative to be applied in VS experiments (Huang et al., 2010). Moreover, the development of more accurate scoring functions is strategic in the field of SBDD and remains a challenging task, especially in the hit-to-lead optimization (Enyedy and Egan, 2008) and *de novo* design (Liu et al., 2017). Although there is no universal scoring function with significant reliability for all molecular systems, some important strategies were explored. Examples of free online resources for predicting protein-ligand binding affinities without the dependency a docking program are BAPPL server[5] (Jain and Jayaram, 2005) CSM-lig[6] (Pires and Ascher, 2016) and K_{DEEP}[7] (Jiménez Luna et al., 2018).

The development of an empirical scoring function requires three components (Pason and Sotriffer, 2016): (i) descriptors that describe the binding event, (ii) a dataset composed of three-dimensional structure of diverse protein–ligand complexes associated with the corresponding experimental affinity data, and (iii) a regression or classification algorithm to calibrate the model establishing a relationship between the descriptors and the experimental affinity. The empirical models differ in the number and type of descriptors; the algorithm adopted for training the model; and the number, the diversity, and the quality data of protein–ligand complexes used during the parameterization process.

According to the algorithm used for training, the scoring function can be linear (i.e., sum of weighted terms) or nonlinear (i.e., nonlinear relationship between the descriptors). It is important to highlight that even the multiple linear regression

(MLR) algorithm, frequently used to calibrate linear scoring functions, is also a machine-learning technique. However, the term "machine-learning-based" scoring function is usually defined in the literature to refer to complex/nonlinear models developed using sophisticated machine-learning techniques to approximate nonlinear problems, such as random forests (RF), support-vector machines (SVM), and deep learning (DL) methods. The linear scoring functions are also referred as "classical" scoring functions. However, we will not adopt the "classical" nomenclature to avoid confusion with scoring functions based on classical force fields. In this work, we will adopt the nomenclature "linear" for the MLR scoring functions and "nonlinear" for models trained with more complex machine-learning techniques.

GOALS OF SCORING FUNCTIONS

During the docking process, the search algorithm investigates a vast amount of conformations for each molecule of the compound library. In this step, the scoring functions evaluate the quality of these docking poses, guiding the search methods toward relevant ligand conformations. The first requirement for a useful scoring function is to be able to distinguish the experimentally observed binding modes – associating them with the lowest binding energies of the energy landscape – from all the other poses found by the search algorithm (*pose prediction*). The second goal is to classify active and inactive compounds (VS), and the third is the prediction of the absolute binding affinity, ranking compounds correctly according to their potency (*binding affinity prediction*) (Jain and Nicholls, 2008; Cheng et al., 2009; Li et al., 2014c). The last one is the most challenging task, mainly in *de novo* design and lead optimization, since small differences in the compound could lead to drastic changes in binding affinity (Schneider and Fechner, 2005). An ideal scoring function would be able to perform the three tasks. However, given several limitations of current scoring functions, they exhibit different accuracies on distinct tasks due to modeling assumptions and simplifications made during their development phase, being intrinsically associated with the main purpose of the evaluated scoring function (Li et al., 2014b). In this context, docking protocols can adopt different scoring functions for each step, e.g., one can use a fast scoring function to predict binding modes and further predict affinities employing a more sophisticated scoring function specific for affinity prediction.

Current docking methods and the associated scoring functions exhibit good pose prediction power if one assumes an adequate preparation of the system and if the target flexibility does not play a significant role (Corbeil et al., 2012; Chaput and Mouawad, 2017). However, the detection of active compounds among a set of decoy compounds and the accurate prediction of binding affinity remain challenging tasks, even when induced fit and entropy effects are not important for binding (Gohlke and Klebe, 2002; Damm-Ganamet et al., 2013; Yuriev and Ramsland, 2013; Grinter and Zou, 2014; Smith et al., 2016). In VS experiments, it is mandatory the use of a scoring function capable of, at least, discriminating active from inactive molecules.

[1] http://www.dockthor.lncc.br
[2] http://bioserv.rpbs.univ-paris-diderot.fr/services/MTiOpenScreen/
[3] http://haddock.science.uu.nl/services/HADDOCK2.2
[4] http://blaster.docking.org/
[5] www.scfbio-iitd.res.in/software/drugdesign/bappl.jsp
[6] structure.bioc.cam.ac.uk/csm_lig
[7] playmolecule.org/Kdeep

Scoring functions are typically divided into three main classes (Wang et al., 2003): *force field-based*, *knowledge-based*, and *empirical*. Liu and Wang (2015) recently proposed a new classification scheme, suggesting classifying current scoring functions as *physics-based*, *regression-based*, *potential of mean force*, and *descriptor-based*. Herein we will follow the traditional classification proposed by Wang et al. (2002) since we believe it is more general and is capable to classify adequately scoring functions according to the main development strategy adopted.

Force field-based functions consist of a sum of energy terms from a classical force field, usually considering the interaction energies of the protein–ligand complex (non-bonded terms) and the internal ligand energy (bonded and non-bonded terms), whereas the solvation energy can be computed by continuum solvation models such as the Poisson–Boltzmann (PB) or the related Generalized Born (GB) (Gilson et al., 1997; Zou and Kuntz, 1999). Examples of force field-based scoring functions include DOCK (Meng et al., 1992) and DockThor (de Magalhães et al., 2014).

Knowledge-based scoring functions are based on the statistical analysis of interacting atom pairs from protein–ligand complexes with available three-dimensional structures. These pairwise-atom data are converted into a pseudopotential, also known as a mean force potential, that describes the preferred geometries of the protein–ligand pairwise atoms. Examples include DrugScore (Velec et al., 2005) and PMF (Muegge, 2006).

Empirical scoring functions are developed to reproduce experimental affinity data (Pason and Sotriffer, 2016) based on the idea that it is possible to correlate the free energy of binding to a set of non-related variables. The coefficients associated with the functional terms are obtained through regression analysis using known binding affinity data of experimentally determined structures. LUDI was the first empirical scoring function developed in the pioneering work of Böhm (1992) for predicting the absolute binding free energy from atomic (3D) structures of protein–ligand complexes. Other examples of empirical scoring functions include ChemScore (Eldridge et al., 1997), ID-Score (Li et al., 2013), and GlideScore (Friesner et al., 2004, 2006a). Some empirical scoring functions (also referred as *hybrid* scoring functions) were developed using a mixture of force field-based, contact-based, and knowledge-based descriptors, such as DockTScore from the DockThor program (empirical and force-field based) (de Magalhães et al., 2014; Guedes et al., 2016), SMoG2016 (empirical and knowledge-based) (Debroise et al., 2017), and GalaxyDock BP2 Score (empirical, knowledge-based, and force-field based) (Baek et al., 2017).

The main focus of this review is the state-of-the-art concerning empirical scoring functions motivated by two main reasons. First, the methodology behind this type of scoring function could be fast enough to be used in large-scale structure-based VS and *de novo* design studies. Secondly, the use of modern sophisticated machine-learning techniques and the increasing availability of protein–ligand structures and measured binding affinity data could increase considerably the accuracy of empirical scoring functions to be useful in computer-aided SBDD experiments. In the following sections, we will discuss crucial aspects concerning their development, successful applications, limitations, and future perspectives.

DESCRIPTORS OF EMPIRICAL SCORING FUNCTIONS

Intermolecular Interactions

Empirical scoring functions have implemented specific terms accounting for intermolecular interactions, such as van der Waals and electrostatic potentials. For example, the Lennard-Jones potential describes the attractive forces (e.g., dispersion forces) and the intrinsic repulsive force between two separated atoms as a function of the interatomic distances (Jones, 1924a,b). Examples of empirical scoring functions using Lennard-Jones potentials are ID-Score (Li et al., 2013) and LISA (Zheng and Merz, 2011). X-Score (Wang et al., 2002) is an example of a scoring function that adopts a softened version of the Lennard-Jones potential instead of the conventional 12-6 potential.

Although all interatomic forces are of electrostatic or electromagnetic origin, the name "electrostatic" is conventionally used to describe forces between polar atoms and is usually represented by the Coulomb potential in both force field-based and empirical scoring functions. Glide (Friesner et al., 2006a) and DockThor (de Magalhães et al., 2014) are examples of scoring functions that implement the Coulomb potential for computing electrostatic interactions.

Some scoring functions include a specific term for hydrogen bonds interactions, commonly through two approaches: (i) by using specific force field-based parameters associated to the van der Waals and electrostatic energy potentials; (ii) by using a directional term, where the hydrogen bond contribution is a function of the deviation of the geometric parameters from those of an ideal hydrogen bond.

GlideScore employs the approach (i) to calculate hydrogen bonds between polar atom pairs, while the Glide XP Score applies the strategy (ii) to account for distinct categories of hydrogen bonds such as neutral–neutral, charged–charged, and neutral–charged interactions (Friesner et al., 2004, 2006b). The DockThor scoring function, which is based on the MMFF94S force field, has also implemented the strategy (i), reducing the size of the polar hydrogen atom when it is involved in hydrogen-bonding interactions (i.e., interacting with a hydrogen bond acceptor) (Halgren, 1996). X-Score adopts the approach (ii) and does not consider explicitly the hydrogen atoms, adopting a concept of "root" atom. In the LUDI implementation of the approach (ii), there are specific parameters for neutral hydrogen bonds and salt bridges (Böhm, 1994). However, some empirical functions do not differentiate hydrogen bonds between charged and neutral atom pairs, e.g., X-Score (Wang et al., 2002) and FlexX (Rarey et al., 1996). ID-Score is an example of a scoring function that uses both approaches: (i) to account for electrostatic interactions between charged groups and (ii) for hydrogen-bonding interactions (Li et al., 2013). The AutoDock4 scoring function employs a directional term based on a 10/12 potential (similar to the Lennard-Jones potential) dependent of the angle deviation from an ideal H-bond interaction with the protein.

Besides the improvement in affinity predictions, the inclusion of a polar desolvation might be crucial to avoid overestimation of hydrogen bonds, since the H-bond formation is directly related with the desolvation of polar atoms.

Despite the importance in considering metal ions, it can be also a source of inaccuracy when using non-specific scoring functions, since the real contribution of interaction metal ions can be underestimated – in the case of simple counting of metal-atom interacting pairs – or overestimated – when using Coulomb potential with formal charges. For example, LUDI (Böhm, 1994), ChemScore (Eldridge et al., 1997), and SFCscore (Sotriffer et al., 2008) implement a contact-based term that attributes 1 to each pair metal–ligand atom within a distance criteria, and lower scores when the distance becomes larger than the specified criteria until an upper limit of distance, attributing the score 0 for larger distances. AutoDock4$_{Zn}$ has implemented a specific force-field-based potential for the zinc ion to consider both geometric and energetic components of the metal–ligand interaction, achieving better performance for pose prediction in redocking experiments (Santos-Martins et al., 2014).

Many studies have highlighted the influence of halogen bonds (X-bonds) on enhancing binding affinity against several targets and the computational methods developed so far (Desiraju et al., 2013; Ford and Ho, 2016). Given the importance of this specific interaction in the hit and lead identification, some scoring functions have incorporated special treatment for X-bonds, such as XBScore (Zimmermann et al., 2015), ScorpionScore (Kuhn et al., 2011), and AutoDockVinaXB (Koebel et al., 2016).

Desolvation

The desolvation contribution to the binding affinity arising from the formation of the protein–ligand complex with the release of water molecules to the bulk solvent can be separated into two distinct effects: the nonpolar and the polar desolvation. The nonpolar desolvation, favorable to binding, is related to the hydrophobic effect when transferring nonpolar molecular surface from the bulk water to a medium that is nonpolar, as is the case of many protein binding cavities (Tanford, 1980; Williams and Bardsley, 1999; Freire, 2008). At the same time, the desolvation of polar or charged groups of the protein or ligand is unfavorable to binding when the formed solute–solvent interactions are not effectively satisfied upon the protein–ligand binding (Blaber et al., 1993; Kar et al., 2013). In this context, many scoring functions have implemented desolvation terms to introduce the hydrophobic effect and/or penalize buried and not interacting polar/charged atoms after protein–ligand binding to improve binding affinity predictions.

The X-Score is a consensus scoring (CS) function based on three distinct strategies to represent the favorable contribution of the desolvation event related to the hydrophobic effect: hydrophobic surface (X-Score^{HS}), hydrophobic matching (X-Score^{HM}), and hydrophobic contact algorithms (X-Score^{HC}) (Wang et al., 2002). The first one is the hydrophobic surface algorithm (X-Score^{HS}), where the hydrophobic effect is proportional to the ligand hydrophobic surface in contact with the solvent accessible surface of the protein. The second is the hydrophobic matching algorithm (X-Score^{HM}), the same

algorithm adopted in the SCORE function (Wang et al., 1998) that calculates the hydrophobic contribution as a function of the logP of each ligand atom and the respective lipophilicity of surrounding protein atoms. The third and simplest method is the hydrophobic contact algorithm (X-Score^{HC}), which approximates the hydrophobic effect through the contact between protein–ligand pairs of lipophilic atoms.

LUDI adopts an approach similar to the X-Score^{HS} (Böhm, 1994), while ChemScore (Eldridge et al., 1997) implements the algorithm similar to the X-Score^{HC}. Fresno scoring function (Rognan et al., 1999) implements a more sophisticated method using the resolution of the linear form of the PB equation using finite difference methods. Cyscore (Cao and Li, 2014) considers the protein shape through a curvature-dependent surface-area term for hydrophobic free energy calculation, leading to a significant improvement on affinity prediction performance on PDBbind benchmarking sets.

The unfavorable desolvation effect from burying polar groups after ligand binding also plays an important role in the binding event, but it is commonly neglected by most scoring functions (Kar et al., 2013; Li et al., 2014c; Cramer et al., 2017). Some efforts have been made to implement specific penalization terms developed with distinct approaches to account for the polar desolvation, such as in the scoring functions ICM (Abagyan et al., 1994; Totrov and Abagyan, 1999; Fernández-Recio et al., 2004), XP GlideScore (Friesner et al., 2006a), LigScore (Krammer et al., 2005), and DockTScore (de Magalhães et al., 2014; Guedes et al., 2016).

The use of more sophisticated methods based on molecular dynamics (MD), such as MM-PBSA and MM-GBSA, have been used in conjunction with empirical scoring functions to predict binding affinities. MM-PBSA and the related MM-GBSA, considered as "end-point" approaches since all calculations are based on the initial and final states of the simulation, rely on MD simulations to compute the polar and nonpolar contributions of the protein–ligand binding event. A classical force field is utilized to compute the potential energy, and the solvation energy is calculated with an implicit solvation model. PB and GB are continuum electrostatic models used to calculate the electrostatic part of the solvation energy that treats the protein and the ligand as low-dielectric regions while considering the aqueous solvent as a high-dielectric medium (Honig et al., 1993). When associated with a surface-area-dependent term (SA), they lead to the implicit solvation models PB (PBSA) (Sitkoff et al., 1994) and Generalized Born (GBSA) (Still et al., 1990; Qiu et al., 1997). Sun et al. (2014) evaluated the performance of MM-PBSA and MM-GBSA methods using several protocols with 1864 protein–ligand complexes from PDBbind v2011 dataset. They concluded that although similar results were observed, MM-GBSA is less sensitive to the investigated systems and is more suitable to be used in general cases (e.g., reverse docking, which is widely used to predict the receptor target(s) of a compound). Inspired by the promising results obtained with GBSA, Zou and Kuntz (1999) implemented a GBSA scheme into the DOCK program as an alternative scoring function and obtained improved binding affinity predictions due to a better description of electrostatic and desolvation effects. More recently,

Zhang X. et al. (2017) also obtained significant improvement on binding affinity prediction of antithrombin ligands when rescoring the top-scored docking poses from VinaLC docking engine with MM-GBSA. Spiliotopoulos et al. (2016) successfully integrated a damped version of MM-PBSA with the HADDOCK scoring function to predict binding poses and affinity of protein–peptide complexes.

Ligand Entropy

Configurational entropy is related to the loss of flexibility of the ligand upon binding. It can be represented as a sum of the conformational (S_{conf}) and the vibrational (S_{vib}^{o}) entropies (Schäfer et al., 2002; Chang et al., 2007). In the energy landscape framework of the protein–ligand binding event, the former reflects the number of occupied energy wells and the last express the average width of the occupied wells. S_{conf} is related to the reduction of the number of ligand accessible conformations upon binding, while S_{vib}^{o} is mainly caused by the restriction of rotational amplitude inside the binding site when compared to the unbounded state (Chang et al., 2007; Gilson and Zhou, 2007).

Given the difficulty in modeling entropic effects for ΔG_{bind}, scoring functions generally neglect their contributions or adopt simplified algorithms to approximate entropies in a straightforward manner (Jain, 2006). Scoring functions such as LUDI (Böhm, 1994) and X-Score (Wang et al., 2002) consider the entropic loss due to the restriction of rotational and translational degrees of freedom implicitly in the regression constant ΔG_0. Surflex approximates such entropic loss as the logarithm of the ligand molecular weight multiplied by a scale factor related to the rough mass dependence of the translational and rotational entropies (Jain, 1996).

The restriction of the rotatable bonds of the ligand after the formation of the protein–ligand complex also promotes an entropic loss (S_{conf}) that is unfavorable to the binding affinity. Some scoring functions have implemented specific terms in a rough approximation to account for entropic contributions of the ligand, as the most used strategies: (i) proportional to the number of rotatable bonds, and (ii) considering the environment of each rotatable bond, i.e., only penalize rotatable bonds that are in contact with the protein. LUDI (Böhm, 1994) and Fresno (Rognan et al., 1999) implement the approach (i) while ChemScore (Eldridge et al., 1997) and ID-Score (Li et al., 2013) use variations of the strategy (ii).

Inspired by the successful application of the energy landscape theory in protein folding and biomolecular binding (Jackson and Fersht, 1991; Miller and Dill, 1997; Baker, 2000), researchers make use of the multiple binding modes predicted by docking programs to describe the binding energy landscape. For example, Wei et al. (2010) developed two new parameters extracted from the multiple binding modes, generated by the AutoDock 3.05 program, and combined them for classification purposes using logistic regression to distinguish true binders among high-scored decoys. The new proposed scheme considered the energy gap (i.e., the difference between the binding energy of the native binding mode and the average binding energy of other binding modes – the *thermodynamic stability* of the native state) and the number of local binding wells (*kinetic accessibility*). This

strategy was successfully applied in the neuraminidase and cyclooxygenase-2 systems from the DUD database, with even improved accuracy when associated with the docking scores. Grigoryan et al. (2012) also successfully applied the energy gap to distinguish true binders from decoys in several protein targets from DUD on single and multiple-receptor VS experiments, achieving superior performance than the ICM scoring function.

Descriptors Based on the Counting of Atom Pairs

With the advance of sophisticated machine-learning algorithms, an increasing number of scoring functions based on a pool of simplistic descriptors have emerged, such as the counting of protein–ligand atom pairs and ligand-based properties. In the literature, such scoring functions are also known as "descriptor-based" or "machine-learning based." It is important to note that this kind of scoring functions are also empirical models, since (i) the algorithms commonly used to derive the models, such as the classical MLR or the robust RF, are machine-learning methods[8], (ii) the attributes used to describe the binding event are, in fact, descriptors, independently of their functional form, physical meaning, and complexity degree.

The success of descriptors based on the simple counting of atom pairs is associated with two important aspects: (i) amount and definition not limited by complex implementations or physical meaning assumptions, and (ii) practically eliminate the necessity of a detailed preparation of the structures, correct assignment of atom types, and physical quantities (e.g., atomic partial charges). Many papers in the recent literature describe outstanding results for binding affinity prediction and active/inactive classification using this more pragmatic approach (Ballester and Mitchell, 2010; Pereira et al., 2016; Wójcikowski et al., 2017). However, the conjunction of nonlinear models and more straightforward atom counting descriptors is subjected to significant criticisms (Gabel et al., 2014). Among the main critics we can highlight: (i) insensitiveness to the protonation state of the ligands and receptor residues; (ii) insensitiveness to the ligand pose; and (iii) facilitate the inclusion of methodological artifacts due to overtraining even when using large training sets.

TRAINING AND TEST SETS

Datasets

The availability of protein–ligand structures with measured binding data has been increased due to efforts on data collection, such as PDBbind-CN (Liu et al., 2015, 2017), DUD-E (Mysinger et al., 2012), and DEKOIS (Bauer et al., 2013) projects.

PDBbind-CN is a source of biomolecular complexes with protein–ligand structure determined experimentally with the associated binding data manually collected from their original reference (Liu et al., 2015). The current release (version 2017)

---

[8]Indeed, according to the IUPAC Recommendations 2015, the term "machine learning" refers to *a computer algorithm that generate empirical models, (...), that is derived from the analysis of a training set for which all the necessary data are available* (Martin et al., 2016).

contains 17,900 structures (14,761 protein–ligand complexes) and is annually updated to keep up with the growth of the Protein Data Bank (Berman et al., 2000). The "refined set" is a subset composed of high-quality datasets constructed according to several criteria concerning the quality of the structures, the affinity data, and the nature of the complex, being considered one of the largest datasets of structures available for the development and validation of docking methodologies and scoring functions. Collected affinities comprise a large interval of values, ranging from 1.2 pM (1.2×10^{-12} M) to 10 mM (1.0×10^{-3} M). Also, PDBbind-CN provides a benchmarking named "core set" widely used for comparative assessment of scoring functions in predicting affinities (Li Y. et al., 2018). The core set is a subset of the refined set constructed using the following protocol: (i) firstly, protein structures with identity of sequence higher than 90% were grouped leading to 65 clusters associated with different protein families; (ii) only the clusters composed of at least five members were considered to construct the core set; and (iii) for each of these clusters, only the complexes with the lowest, the medium, and the highest affinities were selected to the final composition of the core set. A significant drawback of PDBbind-CN datasets is the insufficient information regarding negative data (i.e., experimentally confirmed inactive compounds).

The DUD-E dataset is an enhanced version of the original DUD set and has been widely used to train and validate scoring functions (Huang et al., 2006; Mysinger et al., 2012). It is composed of 102 targets with corresponding active, inactive, marginal, and decoy compounds. Although the number of ligands (i.e., active compounds) significantly varies for each target, a proportion of 50 decoys per ligand is kept for all 102 macromolecules. Decoys are presumed, not experimentally verified, to be inactive compounds since they are chosen to be topologically distinct from ligands but exhibiting similar physicochemical properties. The use of decoys instead of validated inactive compounds remains a major drawback for most datasets since no experimental activity are reported for them, and the number of confirmed inactive molecules is too scarce (Lagarde et al., 2015; Chaput et al., 2016b; Réau et al., 2018).

DEKOIS 2.0 is composed of 81 benchmarking sets for 80 protein targets of therapeutic relevance, including nonconventional targets such as protein–protein interaction complexes (Bauer et al., 2013). Active compounds and the associated binding affinity were retrieved from BindingDB applying several filters to remove pan assay interference (PAINS) compounds, weak binders, reactive groups, and undefined stereocenters. To derive a structurally diverse data set, for each protein target the active compounds were clustered into 40 groups according to the Tanimoto structural similarity and only the most potent compound of each cluster was selected. For each active molecule, 30 structurally diverse decoys molecules from ZINC database were selected according to an improved protocol to that used in the first version of DEKOIS dataset (Vogel et al., 2011), including the detection and removing of latent actives in the decoy set (LADS). Although DUD-E and DEKOIS 2.0 share a common structure of active and decoys compounds, they are complementary since there is a small overlap between them: only

four protein targets present in DEKOIS 2.0 overlaps with the DUD-E dataset.

Scoring functions can be developed based on either experimental structures (i.e., protein–ligand structure experimentally determined) or conformations predicted with docking programs. The structure source (i.e., experimental or docked) is an important point to consider. The use of benchmarking sets such as DUD-E and DEKOIS2.0 is directly dependent on the docking program adopted since the experimental structures of the protein–ligand complexes are not available as in the PDBbind datasets. In fact, the scoring function training or validation in VS experiments using these datasets is performed with no warranty that the ligand poses were correctly predicted.

Training, Validation, and Test Sets

The dataset is commonly separated into three subsets without overlapping structures: (i) the training set, (ii) the validation set, and (iii) the test set (also known as "external validation set").

The *training* set is utilized to calibrate the parameters of the scoring function and to learn the rules that establish a quantitative relationship between the descriptors and the experimental affinity. The *validation* is used to assess the generalization error[9] guiding the model tuning and selection. Once the best model is chosen, it is then applied to the *test* set to evaluate the real predictive capacity of the model.

There is a tradeoff between the size of the training and validation/test sets. Whereas the use of an extensive validation/test set is useful in providing a better estimate of the generalization error, this usually implicates in a smaller dataset to be utilized in the training phase (Abu-Mostafa et al., 2012). Studies evaluating the influence of the training size for the performance of linear and nonlinear scoring functions for affinity prediction demonstrated that MLR becomes insensitive to the growth of the training size whereas larger training sets can lead to an overall better accuracy of nonlinear scoring functions (Ding et al., 2013; Ain et al., 2015; Li et al., 2015a,b; Li H. et al., 2018).

In this context, cross-validation emerges as an alternative strategy to estimate the generalization error without strictly changing the training set size. Cross-validation experiments consist of continuously splitting the original training set of size N into two parts K times (K-fold cross-validation): a smaller set of size V for validation ($V = N/K$) and a larger set of the remaining T instances ($T = N-V$) for training (e.g., leave-one-out cross-validation considers $V = 1$). Different schemes of cross-validation have been adopted and explored to train linear and nonlinear models (Shao, 1993; Golbraikh and Tropsha, 2002; Kramer and Gedeck, 2010; Ballester and Mitchell, 2011; Wójcikowski et al., 2017). For example, in the recent work of Wójcikowski et al. (2017), they performed fivefold cross-validations using the DUD-E dataset. Three distinct splitting strategies were considered: *horizontal*, *vertical*, and *per-target*. In the *horizontal* split, all folds necessarily contain protein–ligand complexes from all protein

---

[9]Generalization error is the expected error when the scoring function is evaluated on a dataset composed of new protein–ligand complexes (i.e., structures not used in the training step).

targets (i.e., each protein target is present in both training and test sets). In the *vertical* split, the protein targets present in the test set do not have representative structures in the training set. This evaluation simulates those cases where the protein target of interest was not present during the training phase. Finally, in the *per-target* split, the training and test are performed for each protein target (i.e., 102 unique machine-learning models relative to the 102 DUD-E targets), simulating the construction and validation of target-specific scoring functions.

It is important to keep in mind that training, validation, and test sets must never have protein–ligand complexes in common at the same time. Furthermore, the test set must be composed of instances not used in the training process at any moment. Thus, the test set must be used only for evaluating the predictive performance of different scoring functions, and no decision should be taken based on the performance for this dataset to avoid useless comparisons due to artificially high correlations.

Benchmarking and Evaluation Metrics

Standard benchmarks are of great importance for an objective assessment of scoring functions providing a reproducible and reliable way to compare different methods. PDBbind (Liu et al., 2015), DUD-E (Mysinger et al., 2012), and DEKOIS 2.0 (Bauer et al., 2013) are examples of widely used benchmarks for evaluating scoring functions.

Many evaluation metrics are used to quantify the performance of scoring functions in pose prediction, active/inactive classification, and affinity prediction. A special issue on *Evaluation of Computational Methods* collects several high-quality papers covering the main aspects of the problem in evaluating and comparing distinct methodologies, highlighting the strengths and weakness of widely used metrics (Stouch, 2008). Recently, Huang and Wong (2016) developed an inexpensive method – the screening performance index (SPI) – to evaluate VS methods that correlate with BEDROC with less computational cost, since it discards the necessity of docking decoy compounds (i.e., only considers the docking of active molecules).

Scoring functions are generally evaluated regarding four aspects related to the three goals of scoring functions aforementioned (Liu et al., 2017):

Docking power: the ability of a scoring function in detecting the native binding mode from decoy poses as the top-ranked solution. The root-mean square deviation (RMSD) is the most commonly used metric to assess the docking power performance.

Screening power: the ability of a scoring function in correctly distinguishing active compounds from inactive molecules. The screening power test does not require that the scoring function correctly predict the absolute binding affinity. The screening power is usually quantified by BEDROC and enrichment factor (EF).

Ranking power: the ability of a scoring function in rank correctly the compounds according to the binding affinities against the *same* target protein. The Spearman correlation coefficient (R_S) and Kendall's tau are metrics widely used for assessing the ranking power of scoring functions.

Scoring power: the ability of a scoring function in rank correctly the compounds according to the binding affinities against *distinct* target proteins. It is important to note that the scoring power test considers the absolute value of the affinity prediction, requiring that the predicted and experimentally observed binding affinities have a linear correlation. This performance is widely assessed by the Pearson correlation coefficient (R_P), and the root-mean squared error (RMSE).

The predictive performance of scoring functions may vary between different benchmarking experiments due to factors such as: (i) composition of the dataset, (ii) structural quality of the complexes, (iii) level of experience of the researches performing the experiments, and (iv) protocol of preparation of the complexes (Yuriev and Ramsland, 2013). Although ranking scoring functions according to their performances for affinity prediction on benchmark sets highlights the more competitive models, it is important to observe that small differences in the calculated performances are generally insufficient to state which scoring function performs better than other when comparing the top-ranked models. Since most benchmarking studies evaluate scoring functions on a few hundred complexes, small differences in Spearman correlation coefficient between 0.05 and 0.15, for example, lack statistical significance (Carlson, 2013, 2016). Thus, larger benchmarking sets composed of high-quality protein–ligand complexes structures are required for a reliable comparison of docking methodologies and scoring functions.

In addition to the well-known benchmarking sets, prospective evaluations are of substantial importance since the blinded predictions simulate real experiments of VS campaigns. Drug Design Data Resource (D3R[10]) periodically provide pharmaceutical-related benchmark datasets and a *Grand Challenge* as a blinded community challenge with unpublished data (Gathiaka et al., 2016). According to the results obtained in the *Grand Challenge 2*, it is clear that the pose prediction task is well performed for many methodologies, but scoring is still a very challenging task, even when the crystal structures are provided (Gaieb et al., 2018). Even with the crystal structures of 36 complexes at *Stage 2*, the maximum Kendall's tau achieved was 0.46, reinforcing the great deal in correctly ranking a set of compounds. Performances and detailed description of the protocols adopted are provided at the D3R *Grand Challenge 2* website[11] and on the scientific reports published on a special issue of Journal of Computer-Aided Molecular Design (Gaieb et al., 2018).

In the last version, D3R *Grand Challenge 3* (GC3), the participants had also to deal with even more challenging tasks, such as the selectivity identification for kinases, assessing the ability of the scoring functions in identifying large changes in affinity due to small structural changes in the ligand (*kinase activity cliff*), and the influence of kinase mutations on protein-ligand affinity (*kinase mutants*).

The broad profile of the D3R *Grand Challenges*, regarding chemical space diversity and affinity data carefully collected, makes their datasets one of the more reliable sources to evaluate docking and scoring methods, providing useful guidelines and

[10]http://www.drugdesigndata.org

[11]https://drugdesigndata.org//about/grand-challenge-2-evaluation-results

best practices for further VS campaigns and methodological improvements.

The Accuracy of Input Structural and Binding Data

Important issues regarding the quality of structural and affinity data must be considered for the development, validation, and application of scoring functions in VS experiments. Reliable protein–ligand structures usually comply these criteria: good resolution (2.5 Å or better), fully resolved electron density for the entire ligand and the surrounding binding-site residues, and without significant influences from crystal packing on the observed binding mode (Cole et al., 2011).

The correct assignment of both protein and ligand protonation/tautomeric states with respect to the experimental pH, Asn/Gln/His flips, and defined stereocenters of the compounds are crucial, requiring a careful inspection of the structures (Kalliokoski et al., 2009; Martin, 2009; Petukh et al., 2013; Sastry et al., 2013). Indeed, the preparation of protein–ligand complexes has a direct influence on training and evaluation of scoring functions, mainly for scoring functions based on force-field descriptors. For example, the initial automatic preparation of the structures performed by PDBbind did not provide an optimized hydrogen bond network and appropriate assignment of protonation/tautomeric states of the α-amylase and MeG2-GHIL complex [**Figure 1**, PDB code 1U33; Numao et al., 2004]. The careful inspection and correction of such complexes comprise a time-consuming and challenging task, but they are particularly important when hydrogen atoms are considered explicitly. In such cases, the wrong orientation of hydrogen atoms can lead to high van der Waals energies, underestimation of hydrogen bond interactions, and incorrect electrostatic repulsions between charged/polar groups. Despite many efforts made for collecting even more extensive and better quality datasets, little attention has been paid to the careful preparation of the protein–ligand structures, usually relying on automatic procedures (Bauer et al., 2013). In this context, scoring functions mainly composed of simple contact-based descriptors (element–element pair counting) emerge to circumvent the complicated preparation required in large datasets for VS.

Especially for affinity prediction purposes, the use of datasets with curated affinity data is essential for reliable predictions and benchmarking. For example, the PDBbind refined set follows several criteria concerning the bioactivity manually collected from the original reference (Liu et al., 2015): (i) only complexes with known dissociation constants (K_d) or inhibition constants (K_i) are allowed, (ii) no complexes with extremely low (K_d or $K_i > 10$ mM) or extremely high (K_d or $K_i < 1$ pM) affinities are accepted, and (iii) estimated values are rejected, e.g., $K_d \sim 1$ nM or $K_i > 10$ μM. Despite the efforts in collecting high-quality affinity data, many factors such as the inherent experimental error can be a source of inaccuracies, limiting the average prediction error achievable on large datasets (Shoichet, 2006; Ferreira et al., 2009; Sotriffer and Matter, 2011; Kramer et al., 2012). Furthermore, the use of decoys instead of confirmed inactive compounds has important impacts in training and measuring

the performance of scoring functions (Chaput et al., 2016b; Réau et al., 2018).

MACHINE LEARNING

Regression and Classification

Scoring functions can be developed using *regression* methods to reproduce continuous (e.g., binding constants) or *classification* methods to reproduce binary affinity data (e.g., active/inactive). It is possible to use scoring functions trained with regression methods to classify active and inactive molecules given a predetermined range of affinity data for defining active and inactive compounds (Ain et al., 2015). It is also possible to use both classification and regression approaches to deal with the same problem of binding affinity prediction. For example, Pason and Sotriffer (2016) used a strategy of classifying the complexes using algorithms such as KNN and further generating linear regression models for each cluster achieving predictive performances comparable to that obtained by the nonlinear scoring function trained with RF. Many sophisticated machine-learning techniques automatically generate local models for similar training points (e.g., locally weighted regression), being able to classify the new instances automatically and use different regression models according to specific properties without explicitly defining classes based on such descriptors.

Linear Versus Nonlinear Scoring Functions

Scoring functions can also be classified as "linear" and "nonlinear" models (Artemenko, 2008).

Linear regression is one of the simplest learning algorithms and is widely used as a starting point in the development of nonlinear regression models (Bishop, 2006). A linear empirical scoring function can be written as a sum of independent terms such as:

$$\Delta G_{binding} = c_0 + c_1 \Delta G_{vdW} + c_2 \Delta G_{hbond} + c_3 \Delta G_{entropy}$$

where c_i is the weighting coefficients of the respective ΔG_i terms, adjusted to reproduce affinity data based on the training set. In the example, ΔG_{vdW} is a van der Waals potential, ΔG_{hbond} is a specific term accounting for hydrogen bonds, and $\Delta G_{entropy}$ is related to the ligand entropic loss upon binding.

The most crucial difference between linear and nonlinear scoring functions is that the former requires a predefined functional form (e.g., the sum of terms in the case of linear scoring functions), whereas the latter implicitly derives the mathematical relationship between the descriptors, allowing the combination of variables and higher order exponents for the terms. This advantage of nonlinear scoring functions partially circumvents the problematic modeling assumptions of linear models (Dill, 1997; Baum et al., 2010; Sotriffer, 2012).

Linear scoring functions developed to date have shown moderate correlations ($R_P \sim 0.6$), whereas nonlinear models achieved significantly better correlations ($R_P > 0.7$) on benchmarking studies (Ashtawy and Mahapatra, 2012;

Empirical Scoring Functions for Structure-Based Virtual Screening: Applications, Critical Aspects...

149

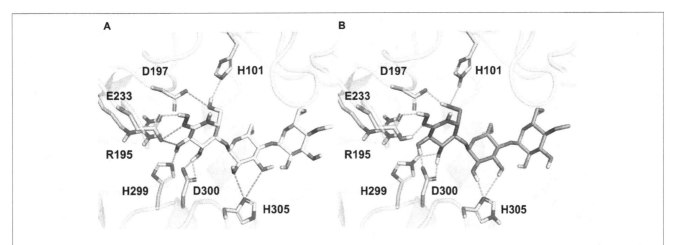

FIGURE 1 | The structure of α-amylase complexed with the inhibitor MeG2-GHIL (PDB code 1U33) as **(A)** provided by PDBbind and **(B)** after manual preparation. Bad and favorable polar contacts are highlighted in orange and green dashes, respectively. D, aspartate; E, glutamate or glutamic acid; H, histidine; R, arginine.

Khamis and Gomaa, 2015; Wang and Zhang, 2017; Wójcikowski et al., 2017). RF, SVM, and more recently, DL, are nonlinear algorithms widely used to develop scoring functions.

The superiority of nonlinear models has also been confirmed through the rebuild of linear scoring functions using nonlinear algorithms, i.e., scoring functions trained with the same original descriptors of the correspondent linear model but with a different regression method. As an example, Zilian and Sotriffer (2013) trained a RF scoring function using the same SFCscore descriptors (named SFCscoreRF) and found a much improved model, with $R = 0.779$ significantly higher than those correlations obtained for the SFScore linear models (Pason and Sotriffer, 2016). Li et al. (2014a) investigated the replacement of MLR by RF for regression using the same Cyscore descriptors and found that the nonlinear model improved the affinity prediction. Furthermore, they also observed that larger training sets and describing the complexes with more descriptors have a positive impact in the predictive performance of the nonlinear models. Pason and Sotriffer (2016) demonstrated that it is possible to achieve similar high performances of nonlinear models through the development of a set of linear scoring functions trained using clustered – smaller and more homogeneous – datasets of protein–ligand complexes. In fact, many machine-learning techniques are based in this approach. For example, locally weighted linear regression automatically generate distinct "local" linear models weighting the training points according to their similarity with the instance to be predicted.

DL is considered as a promising approach to diverse drug discovery projects guided by the successes obtained in image and speech recognition problems (Zhang L. et al., 2017). Such methods take advantage of the recent increase in computational power and the ever-expanding availability of structural and binding data. DL methods are neural networks with many hidden layers, being capable to automatically learn the complicated relationship between the descriptors related to the protein–ligand binding. Recently, DL has been applied for pose/affinity prediction and active/inactive detection, exhibiting

an outstanding performance when compared with several well-performing scoring functions developed with both linear and nonlinear approaches (Wallach et al., 2015; Khamis et al., 2016; Pereira et al., 2016; Ragoza et al., 2017; Jiménez Luna et al., 2018; Nguyen et al., 2018).

Despite nonlinear scoring functions have the main advantage of discarding the necessity of a pre-defined functional form, their main drawback is that they work as "black boxes" since the relationship between the descriptors is often vague, requiring careful use to avoid meaningless interpretations (Gabel et al., 2014). Together with the use of a significant amount of descriptors lacking physical meaning, nonlinear models offer the risk of producing excellent performance indexes due to overfitting and/or bias to the training set construction (e.g., capturing the rules adopted during the selection of active and decoy compounds) (Hawkins, 2004; Abu-Mostafa et al., 2012).

CHALLENGING TOPICS AND PROMISING STRATEGIES

Protein Flexibility

Protein flexibility is still a great challenge for docking programs and scoring functions (Cavasotto and Singh, 2008; Tuffery and Derreumaux, 2012; Buonfiglio et al., 2015; Spyrakis and Cavasotto, 2015; Kurkcuoglu et al., 2018). Most docking methodologies adopt a single, rigid conformation of the receptor, due to the high computational cost and methodological limitations proportional to the increase in the degree of flexibility. However, over the last decades, many strategies have been implemented in docking programs to consider some degree of flexibility in the targeted, such as soft potentials and ensemble docking. In this context, the development of scoring functions adapted for flexible receptor docking is crucial to achieve real improvements in pose and affinity prediction (Totrov and Abagyan, 1997; Wei et al., 2002; Fischer et al., 2014; Ravindranath et al., 2015; Lam et al., 2017; Kong et al., 2018). Ferrari et al. (2004) implemented the fast and methodologically simple soft-docking strategy into the DOCK program, softening the repulsive term of the Lennard-Jones potential, allowing small overlaps between the protein and the ligand atoms. They also validated the methodology in VS studies of potential ligands of the T4 lysozyme and the aldol reductase and obtained better results than using regular docking strategies. Ensemble docking implicitly considers the receptor flexibility by docking the ligand on a set of protein conformations instead of a single conformation, being capable to simulate large-scale receptor flexibility (Korb et al., 2012). Recently, Fischer et al. (2014) successfully identified new ligands targeting specific receptor conformations of cytochrome c peroxidase using a flexible docking method that samples and weights protein conformations guided by experimentally derived conformations, integrating the Boltzmann-weighted energy penalties related with the protein flexibility to the DOCK3.7 scoring function. Despite the many efforts made to include the protein flexibility in VS experiments, the complex and multifactorial framework of flexible protein–ligand binding is still a great challenge (Bottegoni et al., 2011; Nunes-Alves and Arantes, 2014; Antunes et al., 2015; Buonfiglio et al., 2015; Kong et al., 2018). Whereas the high computational cost related with sampling protein conformations and docking large compound libraries can be overcome with the use of high-performance computing platforms, weighing such conformations and integrating them with the scoring functions remains a hindrance for accurate estimation of binding affinities on flexible systems.

Solvation

Water molecules play an essential role in the ligand–protein binding process. Besides the hydrophobic and desolvation effects, individual water molecules can stabilize the ligand binding mode through the formation of water bridges or a water-mediated hydrogen-bond network (Poornima and Dean, 1995; Levy and Onuchic, 2006). The correct prediction of the free energy of binding associated to the ligand displacement of water molecules is a key challenge for the currently available docking scoring functions (Riniker et al., 2012; Spyrakis and Cavasotto, 2015; Bodnarchuk, 2016). An interesting approach is the use of a water-mapping protocol based on the post trajectory analysis of explicit solvent MD. This analysis is based on the inhomogeneous solvation theory and tries to predict the free energy cost of moving a water molecule from a protein hydration site into the bulk solvent (Yang et al., 2013). For instance, in the WScore docking methodology, the location and thermodynamics of explicit waters are predicted using WaterMap and integrated to the scoring function together with a desolvation term to penalize the associated desolvation of polar or uncharged groups of protein or ligand (Murphy et al., 2016). Many solvent mapping methods were evaluated on real drug design studies in a recent paper (Bucher et al., 2018), showing that solvent mapping methods could be important to help ligand optimization and to correctly rank compounds to assist synthetic prioritization. However, these approaches only calculate

the solvent contribution to the free energy and must be combined with other methods to be used for lead optimization or VS.

Recently, Bodnarchuk (2016) published an extensive review of water-placement methods helpful for locating conserved water molecules within the protein binding site to be considered explicitly during the docking simulation. Once the water molecules are identified, some docking engines have implemented strategies to treat water molecules explicitly with adapted scoring functions. The GOLD program considers all-atom and flexible water model able to rotate around its three principal axes, and rewards water displacement in the GoldScore or ChemScore scoring functions according to a balance between the loss of rigid-body entropy and the change in the interaction energies on binding to the protein cavity (Verdonk et al., 2005). In AutoDock4, explicit water molecules of the first hydration shell as represented as uncharged spheres directly attached to the ligand, whereas a hydration force field accounting for the entropic and enthalpic contributions, automatically predicts their potential in mediating protein–ligand interactions (Forli and Olson, 2012).

Covalent Docking

All the discussion made in this review assumes that we are dealing with non-covalent inhibitors. In such cases, the identification and development of computer-aided strategies to identify or improve lead compounds are based on the identification of non-covalent interactions (e.g., electrostatic, van der Waals, hydrophobic interactions) to improve potency or increase selectivity. However, there is a whole class of inhibitors that form a covalent bond with their enzyme/receptor target (De Cesco et al., 2017). Covalent inhibitors can further be divided into two different categories according to whether inhibition is reversible or irreversible (Tuley and Fast, 2018). The development of covalent-docking methodologies capable of dealing with such type of inhibition is very important due to the potential advantages associated with covalent inhibitors (De Cesco et al., 2017), including (i) sustained duration of action leading to less frequent dosing, (ii) increased ligand efficiency, (iii) ability to inhibit targets with shallow binding sites previously categorized as "undruggable," and (iv) increased ability to overcome resistant mutations, among others. The development of non-covalent inhibitors in a drug-design study is usually guided by the optimization of the affinity or dissociation constants (i.e., K_i, K_d, IC$_{50}$). However, dealing with covalent inhibition is even more complex, and in order to address the full potential of a covalent-inhibitor we need not only to measure their affinities but also kinetic binding parameters (e.g., residence time t_r, the average time that a ligand remains bound in the binding site) (De Cesco et al., 2017; Trani et al., 2018). The development of docking methodologies to predict poses and binding affinities of ligands that bind covalently to the receptor is a challenging task. Due to the increasing interest in covalent drugs, many non-covalent docking programs have developed covalent versions and some new docking programs focused on covalent ligands have been developed (Kumalo et al., 2015; Awoonor-Williams et al., 2017; De Cesco et al., 2017). GOLD (Jones et al., 1997), Autodock4 (Bianco et al., 2016), CovalentDock (Ouyang et al., 2013), CovDock (Zhu et al., 2014), DOCKovalent (London et al., 2014), and DOCK-TITE (Scholz et al., 2015) are some examples of docking programs that developed specific methodologies to deal with covalent-docking. These methodologies were discussed in recent reviews addressing covalent-inhibitors and covalent docking (Kumalo et al., 2015; Awoonor-Williams et al., 2017; De Cesco et al., 2017). Some of these methods try to include the complexity of the covalent inhibition introducing modifications into their non-covalent scoring functions. For example, the introduction of a Morse potential to describe the energy associated with the bond formation (CovalentDock). Two critical aspects in the future development of covalent scoring functions are the capacity to predict the kinetics of ligand binding (e.g., residence times) and the intrinsic reactivity of electrophilic and nucleophilic pairs of atoms (De Cesco et al., 2017).

Quantum Mechanics

The use of quantum mechanical methods can improve the description of protein–ligand interactions and, in principle, could provide a more accurate binding affinity (Raha and Merz, 2005; Chaskar et al., 2017; Crespo et al., 2017; Cavasotto et al., 2018). This is particularly true when dealing with systems where the molecular recognition involves bond formation, π-stacking, cation-π, halogen bonding (i.e., σ-hole bonding), and polarization and charge transfer effects (Christensen et al., 2016). These non-classical interactions/effects are beyond the limits of classical methods and represent a significant challenge to the development of scoring functions to be used in computational drug design experiments. In particular, metal ions interactions are essential when dealing with metalloproteins and, due to the large changes in the electronic structure under ligand binding, are also a great challenge. In the last 10 years, important advances were made in computing hardware (e.g., Graphics Processing Units – GPUs), in the development of quantum algorithms to compute molecular wave functions (Dixon and Merz, 1997; Birgin et al., 2013), the development of more reliable semi-empirical quantum methods (Christensen et al., 2016; Yilmazer and Korth, 2016), and development of new hybrid QM/MM methods (Chaskar et al., 2017; Melo et al., 2018). These advances were essential to overcome the bottleneck of the high computational cost and are allowing the increasing use of QM methods in the prediction of protein–ligand binding affinities (Crespo et al., 2017). Recent high-quality reviews cover applications of explicit QM calculations in lead identification and optimization (Adeniyi and Soliman, 2017; Crespo et al., 2017; Cavasotto et al., 2018), development of QM methods for ligand binding affinity calculations (Ryde and Söderhjelm, 2016), and development of semi-empirical QM methods for non-covalent interactions (Christensen et al., 2016; Yilmazer and Korth, 2016).

The results obtained using QM or hybrid QM/MM-based methods are very encouraging when compared to the standard scoring functions, principally when dealing with metalloproteins (Chaskar et al., 2017; Pecina et al., 2018). Wang et al. (2011)

rebuild the AutoDock4 scoring function using ligand partial charges calculated with QM methods and protein charges from the Amber99SB instead of the Gasteiger method, improving both pose and affinity predictions. Moreover, the results from the 2016 D3R Grand Challenge indicate that the use of QM/MM scoring could be a powerful strategy (Gao et al., 2018). Yang et al. (2015) developed and introduced the quantum mechanics-based term XBScore^{QM} as a combination of van der Waals and electrostatic potentials to describe the X-bond interactions into the AutoDock4 scoring function. The new scoring function achieved good performances on both pose and affinity prediction when compared against 12 diverse scoring functions, and increase predictive capacity to deal with protein-ligand complexes with X-bond interactions. Nevertheless, it is important to note that it is not guaranteed that QM-based approaches will always outperform standard scoring functions (Crespo et al., 2017) and they still face the same problems associated with the correct estimation of the solvent and other entropic effects to the protein–ligand binding free energy.

Consensus Scoring

The combination of different scoring functions on a scoring scheme (CS) is considered as a promising data fusion strategy to improve VS enrichment, pose, and affinity prediction (Charifson et al., 1999; Bissantz et al., 2000; Yang et al., 2005; Kaserer et al., 2015; Chaput et al., 2016a; Chaput and Mouawad, 2017; Ericksen et al., 2017). The CS strategy could overcome to some extent the limitations faced by the single-scoring approach, for example, the inconsistent performances across different protein targets and chemical classes (Moitessier et al., 2009). Moreover, CS is frequently used in some extent together with ensemble docking methodology, where different scores are predicted for different conformations of the protein target under investigation (Park et al., 2009, 2010; Paulsen and Anderson, 2009; Kelemen et al., 2016; Baumgartner and Evans, 2018; Li D.-D. et al., 2018).

Since the pioneering work of Charifson et al. (1999), many consensus strategies were developed and assessed on several target proteins, such as cyclooxygenases (Kaserer et al., 2015), and β-secretases (Liu et al., 2012). For instance, Kaserer et al. (2015) applied CS on prospective VS studies against cyclooxygenases 1 and 2 and found that the chance of a compound to be truly active increases when more tools predicted it as active. In the very interesting work of Wang and Wang (2001), they provided a theoretical basis for the effectiveness of CS on affinity prediction. They demonstrated that CS works due to a simple statistical reason related to the law of large numbers: the mean value found by repeated independent predictions tends toward the real and expected value.

Traditional CS approaches combine the predictions of the scoring functions using statistical methods (e.g., arithmetic mean) or voting schemes (i.e., a vote replaces the absolute score predicted by each scoring function) (Terp et al., 2001; Wang and Wang, 2001; Wang et al., 2002; Bar-Haim et al., 2009; Ericksen et al., 2017). Nonlinear CS models were also developed to improve pose prediction and ranking compounds in VS experiments (Betzi et al., 2006; Teramoto and Fukunishi, 2007; Ashtawy and Mahapatra, 2015; Ericksen et al., 2017). For example, Ericksen et al. (2017) developed machine-learning CS using discrete mixture models and gradient boosting to combine the scores from eight docking programs and obtained improved performances than individual scoring functions on 21 targets from DUD-E dataset. In addition, they compared their machine-learning-based CS with individual scoring functions and traditional CS schemed, confirming that CS excel individual scoring functions performances in docking-based VS, being less sensitive to protein target variation.

Tailored Scoring Functions for Protein Targets and Classes

Significant improvements in docking and VS accuracies are reported when employing target-specific scoring functions rather than non-specific models, using as training datasets protein–ligand complexes comprising specific molecular targets instead of a general dataset. Hence, it is expected that they could be more efficient in accounting for specific interactions and particular binding characteristics associated with a target class of interest (Seifert, 2009).

For instance, Logean et al. (2001) adapted the Fresno empirical scoring function to the class I MHC HLA-B*2705 protein with a significant improvement in affinity prediction over six different traditional scoring functions. The GOLD program also implements a modified version of the ChemScore function, with an additional term that accounts for weak hydrogen bonds that claimed to be relevant for some kinase inhibitor binding (Pierce et al., 2002; Verdonk et al., 2004). The HADDOCK$_{PPI}$ is a linear scoring function specifically developed to predict binding affinities of inhibitors of protein–protein interactions (iPPIs), which interact in uncommon binding cavities characterized by higher hydrophobicity, aromaticity, and molecular weight compared to enzyme inhibitors, as usually interacting within flatter, larger, and more hydrophobic binding sites than the enzyme catalytic sites (Morelli et al., 2011; Kuenemann et al., 2014). In a more recent work, a scoring function specific to Heat Shock Protein 90 (HSP90) was successfully designed and applied in VS (Santos-Martins, 2016). In general, nonlinear scoring functions specific for protein classes/targets also achieved superior performance than the generic models (Wang et al., 2015; Ashtawy and Mahapatra, 2018). Still, in the recent work of Wójcikowski et al. (2017), the target-specific scoring functions trained with RF only performed slightly better than generic models, with two-third of them increasing the EF$_{1\%}$ less than 10%. As an intriguing result, they found that tailored scoring functions are more beneficial for the protein targets with less active compounds than the others containing more actives, where the target-specific scoring functions exhibit similar performances to the generic model.

Despite encouraging results obtained for target-specific scoring functions, it is important to highlight that the requirement of a large training set to derive a robust scoring function might become a significant hindrance and source of inaccuracy. To overcome the lack of a sufficient amount of experimental structures, protein–ligand conformations used for training target-specific scoring functions are commonly obtained from docking experiments.

CONCLUSION

The development of accurate empirical scoring functions to predict protein–ligand binding affinities is a key aspect in SBDD. In recent years, the increasing availability of protein–ligand structures with measured binding affinities and data sets containing active, decoy, and true inactive compounds are boosting the use of sophisticated machine-learning techniques to obtain better performing scoring functions. In the coming years, it is expected that the combination of larger training datasets, non-physical/simplified descriptors, and DL techniques will be a very promising research line to improve scoring functions for structure-based VS. Methodological advances will be dependent to the size and quality of the available datasets for training and benchmarking, and great care will be necessary to avoid artificial performances due to the increased capacity of these nonlinear methods to capture bias present in the training data. In this sense, blinded community challenges with unpublished data (e.g., D3R challenge) are essential to address the real performance of scoring functions and docking protocols. Looking to the other side of the methodological spectrum, it is exciting to note that the advance in computing power, the development of new algorithms to introduce protein flexibility and solvation/desolvation effects, and more reliable semi-empirical quantum methods are enabling the development and use of new methodological advances for challenging tasks, such as QM/MM-based methods and entropy estimation.

The full potential of scoring functions will be achieved when models accurate enough to be useful in hit-to-lead optimization and *de novo* design studies are developed. To reach this goal, a scoring function must be sensitive to the docking pose, *right for the right reasons* (Kolb and Irwin, 2009). Reliable predictions of ligand binding affinity remain a big challenge, but we expect that in the next years important advances associated to distinct methodological approaches will be achieved and, probably, will be combined into more effective computer-based drug design protocols.

AUTHOR CONTRIBUTIONS

IG and LD designed, wrote, and edited this review. FP contributed to designing and writing the review.

FUNDING

This work was supported by the Conselho Nacional de Desenvolvimento Científico e Tecnológico (CNPq) (Grant No. 308202/2016-3), Coordenação de Aperfeiçoamento de Pessoal de Nível Superior (CAPES), and Fundação de Amparo à Pesquisa do Estado do Rio de Janeiro (FAPERJ) (Grant No. E-26/010.001229/2015).

REFERENCES

Abagyan, R., Totrov, M., and Kuznetsov, D. (1994). ICM: a new method for protein modeling and design: applications to docking and structure prediction from the distorted native conformation. *J. Comput. Chem.* 15, 488–506. doi: 10.1002/jcc.540150503

Abu-Mostafa, Y. S., Magdon-Ismail, M., and Lin, H.-T. (2012). *Learning From Data.* United States: AMLBook.

Adeniyi, A. A., and Soliman, M. E. S. (2017). Implementing QM in docking calculations: is it a waste of computational time? *Drug Discov. Today* 22, 1216–1223. doi: 10.1016/j.drudis.2017.06.012

Ain, Q. U., Aleksandrova, A., Roessler, F. D., and Ballester, P. J. (2015). Machine-learning scoring functions to improve structure-based binding affinity prediction and virtual screening: machine-learning SFs to improve structure-based binding affinity prediction and virtual screening. *Wiley Interdiscip. Rev. Comput. Mol. Sci.* 5, 405–424. doi: 10.1002/wcms.1225

Allen, W. J., Balius, T. E., Mukherjee, S., Brozell, S. R., Moustakas, D. T., Lang, P. T., et al. (2015). DOCK 6: impact of new features and current docking performance. *J. Comput. Chem.* 36, 1132–1156. doi: 10.1002/jcc.23905

Antunes, D. A., Devaurs, D., and Kavraki, L. E. (2015). Understanding the challenges of protein flexibility in drug design. *Exp. Opin. Drug Discov.* 10, 1301–1313. doi: 10.1517/17460441.2015.1094458

Artemenko, N. (2008). Distance dependent scoring function for describing protein-ligand intermolecular interactions. *J. Chem. Inform. Model.* 48, 569–574. doi: 10.1021/ci700224e

Ashtawy, H. M., and Mahapatra, N. R. (2012). A comparative assessment of ranking accuracies of conventional and machine-learning-based scoring functions for protein-ligand binding affinity prediction. *IEEEACM Trans. Comput. Biol. Bioinforma. IEEE ACM* 9, 1301–1313. doi: 10.1109/TCBB.2012.36

Ashtawy, H. M., and Mahapatra, N. R. (2015). BgN-Score and BsN-Score: bagging and boosting based ensemble neural networks scoring functions for accurate binding affinity prediction of protein-ligand complexes. *BMC Bioinformatics* 16(Suppl. 4):S8. doi: 10.1186/1471-2105-16-S4-S8

Ashtawy, H. M., and Mahapatra, N. R. (2018). Task-specific scoring functions for predicting ligand binding poses and affinity and for screening enrichment. *J. Chem. Inform. Model.* 58, 119–133. doi: 10.1021/acs.jcim.7b00309

Awoonor-Williams, E., Walsh, A. G., and Rowley, C. N. (2017). Modeling covalent-modifier drugs. *Biochim. Biophys. Acta BBA – Proteins Proteom.* 1865, 1664–1675. doi: 10.1016/j.bbapap.2017.05.009

Baek, M., Shin, W.-H., Chung, H. W., and Seok, C. (2017). GalaxyDock BP2 score: a hybrid scoring function for accurate protein–ligand docking. *J. Comput. Aided Mol. Des.* 31, 653–666. doi: 10.1007/s10822-017-0030-9

Baker, D. (2000). A surprising simplicity to protein folding. *Nature* 405, 39–42. doi: 10.1038/35011000

Ballester, P. J., and Mitchell, J. B. O. (2010). A machine learning approach to predicting protein-ligand binding affinity with applications to molecular docking. *Bioinformatics* 26, 1169–1175. doi: 10.1093/bioinformatics/btq112

Ballester, P. J., and Mitchell, J. B. O. (2011). Comments on "leave-cluster-out cross-validation is appropriate for scoring functions derived from diverse protein data sets": significance for the validation of scoring functions. *J. Chem. Inform. Model.* 51, 1739–1741. doi: 10.1021/ci200057e

Ban, F., Dalal, K., Li, H., LeBlanc, E., Rennie, P. S., and Cherkasov, A. (2017). Best practices of computer-aided drug discovery: lessons learned from the development of a preclinical candidate for prostate cancer with a new mechanism of action. *J. Chem. Inform. Model.* 57, 1018–1028. doi: 10.1021/acs.jcim.7b00137

Bar-Haim, S., Aharon, A., Ben-Moshe, T., Marantz, Y., and Senderowitz, H. (2009). SeleX-CS: a new consensus scoring algorithm for hit discovery and lead optimization. *J. Chem. Inform. Model.* 49, 623–633. doi: 10.1021/ci800335j

Barril, X. (2017). Computer-aided drug design: time to play with novel chemical matter. *Expert Opin. Drug Discov.* 12, 977–980. doi: 10.1080/17460441.2017.1362386

Bauer, M. R., Ibrahim, T. M., Vogel, S. M., and Boeckler, F. M. (2013). Evaluation and optimization of virtual screening workflows with DEKOIS 2.0 – A public library of challenging docking benchmark sets. *J. Chem. Inform. Model.* 53, 1447–1462. doi: 10.1021/ci400115b

Baum, B., Muley, L., Smolinski, M., Heine, A., Hangauer, D., and Klebe, G. (2010). Non-additivity of functional group contributions in protein-ligand binding: a comprehensive study by crystallography and isothermal titration calorimetry. *J. Mol. Biol.* 397, 1042–1054. doi: 10.1016/j.jmb.2010.02.007

Baumgartner, M. P., and Evans, D. A. (2018). Lessons learned in induced fit docking and metadynamics in the drug design data resource grand challenge 2. *J. Comput. Aided Mol. Des.* 32, 45–58. doi: 10.1007/s10822-017-0081-y

Berman, H. M., Westbrook, J., Feng, Z., Gilliland, G., Bhat, T. N., Weissig, H., et al. (2000). The protein data bank. *Nucleic Acids Res.* 28, 235–242.

Betzi, S., Suhre, K., Chétrit, B., Guerlesquin, F., and Morelli, X. (2006). GFscore: a general nonlinear consensus scoring function for high-throughput docking. *J. Chem. Inform. Model.* 46, 1704–1712. doi: 10.1021/ci0600758

Bianco, G., Forli, S., Goodsell, D. S., and Olson, A. J. (2016). Covalent docking using autodock: two-point attractor and flexible side chain methods. *Protein Sci. Publ. Protein Soc.* 25, 295–301. doi: 10.1002/pro.2733

Birgin, E. G., Martínez, J. M., Martínez, L., and Rocha, G. B. (2013). Sparse projected-gradient method as a linear-scaling low-memory alternative to diagonalization in self-consistent field electronic structure calculations. *J. Chem. Theory Comput.* 9, 1043–1051. doi: 10.1021/ct3009683

Bishop, C. M. (2006). *Pattern Recognition and Machine Learning.* Switzerland: Springer

Bissantz, C., Folkers, G., and Rognan, D. (2000). Protein-based virtual screening of chemical databases. 1, evaluation of different docking/scoring combinations. *J. Med. Chem.* 43, 4759–4767.

Blaber, M., Lindstrom, J. D., Gassner, N., Xu, J., Heinz, D. W., and Matthews, B. W. (1993). Energetic cost and structural consequences of burying a hydroxyl group within the core of a protein determined from Ala.fwdarw, ser and Val.fwdarw. Thr substitutions in T4 lysozyme. *Biochemistry* (Mosc.) 32, 11363–11373. doi: 10.1021/bi00093a013

Bodnarchuk, M. S. (2016). Water, water, everywhere... It's time to stop and think. *Drug Discov. Today* 21, 1139–1146. doi: 10.1016/j.drudis.2016.05.009

Böhm, H. J. (1992). The computer program LUDI: a new method for the de novo design of enzyme inhibitors. *J. Comput. Aided Mol. Des.* 6, 61–78.

Böhm, H. J. (1994). The development of a simple empirical scoring function to estimate the binding constant for a protein-ligand complex of known three-dimensional structure. *J. Comput. Aided Mol. Des.* 8, 243–256.

Bortolato, A., Perruccio, F., and Moro, S. (2012). "successful applications of in silico approaches for lead/drug discovery," in *In-Silico Lead Discovery*, ed. M. A. Miteva (Emirate of Sharjah: Bentham Science Publishers), 163–175.

Bottegoni, G., Rocchia, W., Rueda, M., Abagyan, R., and Cavalli, A. (2011). Systematic exploitation of multiple receptor conformations for virtual ligand screening. *PLoS One* 6:e18845. doi: 10.1371/journal.pone.0018845

Bucher, D., Stouten, P., and Triballeau, N. (2018). Shedding light on important waters for drug design: simulations versus grid-based methods. *J. Chem. Inform. Model.* 58, 692–699. doi: 10.1021/acs.jcim.7b00642

Buonfiglio, R., Recanatini, M., and Masetti, M. (2015). Protein flexibility in drug discovery: from theory to computation. *ChemMedChem* 10, 1141–1148. doi: 10.1002/cmdc.201500086

Cao, Y., and Li, L. (2014). Improved protein-ligand binding affinity prediction by using a curvature-dependent surface-area model. *Bioinform. Oxf. Engl.* 30, 1674–1680. doi: 10.1093/bioinformatics/btu104

Carlson, H. A. (2013). Check your confidence: size really does matter. *J. Chem. Inform. Model.* 53, 1837–1841. doi: 10.1021/ci4004249

Carlson, H. A. (2016). Lessons learned over four benchmark exercises from the community structure-activity resource. *J. Chem. Inform. Model.* 56, 951–954. doi: 10.1021/acs.jcim.6b00182

Cavasotto, C., and Singh, N. (2008). Docking and high throughput docking: successes and the challenge of protein flexibility. *Curr. Comput. Aided-Drug Des.* 4, 221–234. doi: 10.2174/157340908785747474

Cavasotto, C. N., Adler, N. S., and Aucar, M. G. (2018). Quantum chemical approaches in structure-based virtual screening and lead optimization. *Front. Chem.* 6:188. doi: 10.3389/fchem.2018.00188

Chang, C. A., Chen, W., and Gilson, M. K. (2007). Ligand configurational entropy and protein binding. *Proc. Natl. Acad. Sci. U.S.A.* 104, 1534–1539. doi: 10.1073/pnas.0610494104

Chaput, L., Martinez-Sanz, J., Quiniou, E., Rigolet, P., Saettel, N., and Mouawad, L. (2016a). vSDC: a method to improve early recognition in virtual screening when limited experimental resources are available. *J. Cheminformatics* 8:1. doi: 10.1186/s13321-016-0112-z

Chaput, L., Martinez-Sanz, J., Saettel, N., and Mouawad, L. (2016b). Benchmark of four popular virtual screening programs: construction of the active/decoy dataset remains a major determinant of measured performance. *J. Cheminformatics* 8:56. doi: 10.1186/s13321-016-0167-x

Chaput, L., and Mouawad, L. (2017). Efficient conformational sampling and weak scoring in docking programs? Strategy of the wisdom of crowds. *J. Cheminformatics* 9:37. doi: 10.1186/s13321-017-0227-x

Charifson, P. S., Corkery, J. J., Murcko, M. A., and Walters, W. P. (1999). Consensus scoring: a method for obtaining improved hit rates from docking databases of three-dimensional structures into proteins. *J. Med. Chem.* 42, 5100–5109. doi: 10.1021/jm990352k

Chaskar, P., Zoete, V., and Röhrig, U. F. (2017). On-the-fly QM/MM docking with attracting cavities. *J. Chem. Inform. Model.* 57, 73–84. doi: 10.1021/acs.jcim.6b00406

Cheng, T., Li, X., Li, Y., Liu, Z., and Wang, R. (2009). Comparative assessment of scoring functions on a diverse test set. *J. Chem. Inform. Model.* 49, 1079–1093. doi: 10.1021/ci9000053

Christensen, A. S., Kubaø, T., Cui, Q., and Elstner, M. (2016). Semiempirical quantum mechanical methods for noncovalent interactions for chemical and biochemical applications. *Chem. Rev.* 116, 5301–5337. doi: 10.1021/acs.chemrev.5b00584

Cole, J. C., Korb, O., Olsson, T. S. G., and Liebeschuetz, J. (2011). "The basis for target-based virtual screening: protein structures," in *Methods and Principles in Medicinal Chemistry*, ed. C. Sotriffer (Weinheim: Wiley-VCH Verlag GmbH & Co. KGaA), 87–114. doi: 10.1002/9783527633326.ch4

Corbeil, C. R., Williams, C. I., and Labute, P. (2012). Variability in docking success rates due to dataset preparation. *J. Comput. Aided Mol. Des.* 26, 775–786. doi: 10.1007/s10822-012-9570-1

Cramer, J., Krimmer, S. G., Heine, A., and Klebe, G. (2017). Paying the Price of desolvation in solvent-exposed protein pockets: impact of distal solubilizing groups on affinity and binding thermodynamics in a series of thermolysin inhibitors. *J. Med. Chem.* 60, 5791–5799. doi: 10.1021/acs.jmedchem.7b00490

Crespo, A., Rodriguez-Granillo, A., and Lim, V. T. (2017). Quantum-mechanics methodologies in drug discovery: applications of docking and scoring in lead optimization. *Curr. Top. Med. Chem.* 17, 2663–2680. doi: 10.2174/1568026617666170707120609

Damm-Ganamet, K. L., Smith, R. D., Dunbar, J. B., Stuckey, J. A., and Carlson, H. A. (2013). CSAR benchmark exercise 2011–2012: evaluation of results from docking and relative ranking of blinded congeneric series. *J. Chem. Inform. Model.* 53, 1853–1870. doi: 10.1021/ci400025f

Danishuddin, M., and Khan, A. U. (2015). Structure based virtual screening to discover putative drug candidates: necessary considerations and successful case studies. *Methods* 71, 135–145. doi: 10.1016/j.ymeth.2014.10.019

De Cesco, S., Kurian, J., Dufresne, C., Mittermaier, A. K., and Moitessier, N. (2017). Covalent inhibitors design and discovery. *Eur. J. Med. Chem.* 138, 96–114. doi: 10.1016/j.ejmech.2017.06.019

de Magalhães, C. S., Almeida, D. M., Barbosa, H. J. C., and Dardenne, L. E. (2014). A dynamic niching genetic algorithm strategy for docking highly flexible ligands. *Inform. Sci.* 289, 206–224. doi: 10.1016/j.ins.2014.08.002

Debroise, T., Shakhnovich, E. I., and Chéron, N. (2017). A hybrid knowledge-based and empirical scoring function for protein–ligand interaction: SMoG2016. *J. Chem. Inform. Model.* 57, 584–593. doi: 10.1021/acs.jcim.6b00610

Desiraju, G. R., Ho, P. S., Kloo, L., Legon, A. C., Marquardt, R., Metrangolo, P., et al. (2013). Definition of the halogen bond (IUPAC Recommendations 2013). *Pure Appl. Chem.* 85, 1711–1713. doi: 10.1351/PAC-REC-12-05-10

Dill, K. A. (1997). Additivity principles in biochemistry. *J. Biol. Chem.* 272, 701–704. doi: 10.1074/jbc.272.2.701

DiMasi, J. A., Grabowski, H. G., and Hansen, R. W. (2016). Innovation in the pharmaceutical industry: new estimates of R&D costs. *J. Health Econ.* 47, 20–33. doi: 10.1016/j.jhealeco.2016.01.012

Ding, B., Wang, J., Li, N., and Wang, W. (2013). Characterization of small molecule binding. I. Accurate Identification of Strong Inhibitors in Virtual Screening. *J. Chem. Inform. Model.* 53, 114–122. doi: 10.1021/ci300508m

Dixon, S. L., and Merz, K. M. (1997). Fast, accurate semiempirical molecular orbital calculations for macromolecules. *J. Chem. Phys.* 107, 879–893. doi: 10.1063/1.474386

Dos Santos, R. N., Ferreira, L. G., and Andricopulo, A. D. (2018). Practices in molecular docking and structure-based virtual screening. *Methods Mol. Biol. Clifton NJ* 1762, 31–50. doi: 10.1007/978-1-4939-7756-7_3

Eldridge, M. D., Murray, C. W., Auton, T. R., Paolini, G. V., and Mee, R. P. (1997). Empirical scoring functions: I. The development of a fast empirical scoring function to estimate the binding affinity of ligands in receptor complexes. *J. Comput. Aided Mol. Des.* 11, 425–445.

Enyedy, I. J., and Egan, W. J. (2008). Can we use docking and scoring for hit-to-lead optimization? *J. Comput. Aided Mol. Des.* 22, 161–168. doi: 10.1007/s10822-007-9165-4

Ericksen, S. S., Wu, H., Zhang, H., Michael, L. A., Newton, M. A., Hoffmann, F. M., et al. (2017). Machine learning consensus scoring improves performance across targets in structure-based virtual screening. *J. Chem. Inform. Model.* 57, 1579–1590. doi: 10.1021/acs.jcim.7b00153

Fernández-Recio, J., Totrov, M., and Abagyan, R. (2004). Identification of protein-protein interaction sites from docking energy landscapes. *J. Mol. Biol.* 335, 843–865.

Ferrari, A. M., Wei, B. Q., Costantino, L., and Shoichet, B. K. (2004). Soft docking and multiple receptor conformations in virtual screening. *J. Med. Chem.* 47, 5076–5084. doi: 10.1021/jm049756p

Ferreira, L., dos Santos, R., Oliva, G., and Andricopulo, A. (2015). Molecular docking and structure-based drug design strategies. *Molecules* 20, 13384–13421. doi: 10.3390/molecules200713384

Ferreira, R. S., Bryant, C., Ang, K. K. H., McKerrow, J. H., Shoichet, B. K., and Renslo, A. R. (2009). Divergent modes of enzyme inhibition in a homologous structure-activity series. *J. Med. Chem.* 52, 5005–5008. doi: 10.1021/jm9009229

Fischer, M., Coleman, R. G., Fraser, J. S., and Shoichet, B. K. (2014). Incorporation of protein flexibility and conformational energy penalties in docking screens to improve ligand discovery. *Nat. Chem.* 6, 575–583. doi: 10.1038/nchem.1954

Ford, M. C., and Ho, P. S. (2016). Computational tools to model halogen bonds in medicinal chemistry. *J. Med. Chem.* 59, 1655–1670. doi: 10.1021/acs.jmedchem.5b00997

Forli, S., and Olson, A. J. (2012). A force field with discrete displaceable waters and desolvation entropy for hydrated ligand docking. *J. Med. Chem.* 55, 623–638. doi: 10.1021/jm2005145

Freire, E. (2008). Do enthalpy and entropy distinguish first in class from best in class? *Drug Discov. Today* 13, 869–874. doi: 10.1016/j.drudis.2008.07.005

Friesner, R. A., Banks, J. L., Murphy, R. B., Halgren, T. A., Klicic, J. J., Mainz, D. T., et al. (2004). Glide: a new approach for rapid, accurate docking and scoring. 1. method and assessment of docking accuracy. *J. Med. Chem.* 47, 1739–1749. doi: 10.1021/jm0306430

Friesner, R. A., Murphy, R. B., Repasky, M. P., Frye, L. L., Greenwood, J. R., Halgren, T. A., et al. (2006a). Extra precision glide: docking and scoring incorporating a model of hydrophobic enclosure for protein-ligand complexes. *J. Med. Chem.* 49, 6177–6196. doi: 10.1021/jm051256o

Friesner, R. A., Murphy, R. B., Repasky, M. P., Frye, L. L., Greenwood, J. R., Halgren, T. A., et al. (2006b). Extra precision glide: docking and scoring incorporating a model of hydrophobic enclosure for protein-ligand complexes. *J. Med. Chem.* 49, 6177–6196. doi: 10.1021/jm051256o

Gabel, J., Desaphy, J., and Rognan, D. (2014). Beware of machine learning-based scoring functions-on the danger of developing black boxes. *J. Chem. Inform. Model.* 54, 2807–2815. doi: 10.1021/ci500406k

Gaieb, Z., Liu, S., Gathiaka, S., Chiu, M., Yang, H., Shao, C., et al. (2018). D3R grand challenge 2: blind prediction of protein–ligand poses, affinity rankings, and relative binding free energies. *J. Comput. Aided Mol. Des.* 32, 1–20. doi: 10.1007/s10822-017-0088-4

Gao, Y.-D., Hu, Y., Crespo, A., Wang, D., Armacost, K. A., Fells, J. I., et al. (2018). Workflows and performances in the ranking prediction of 2016 D3R Grand Challenge 2: lessons learned from a collaborative effort. *J. Comput. Aided Mol. Des.* 32, 129–142. doi: 10.1007/s10822-017-0072-z

Gathiaka, S., Liu, S., Chiu, M., Yang, H., Stuckey, J. A., Kang, Y. N., et al. (2016). D3R grand challenge 2015: evaluation of protein-ligand pose and affinity predictions. *J. Comput. Aided Mol. Des.* 30, 651–668. doi: 10.1007/s10822-016-9946-8

Gilson, M. K., Given, J. A., and Head, M. S. (1997). A new class of models for computing receptor-ligand binding affinities. *Chem. Biol.* 4, 87–92.

Gilson, M. K., and Zhou, H.-X. (2007). Calculation of protein-ligand binding affinities. *Annu. Rev. Biophys. Biomol. Struct.* 36, 21–42. doi: 10.1146/annurev.biophys.36.040306.132550

Gohlke, H., and Klebe, G. (2002). Approaches to the description and prediction of the binding affinity of small-molecule ligands to macromolecular receptors. *Angew. Chem. Int. Ed.* 41, 2644–2676.

Golbraikh, A., and Tropsha, A. (2002). Beware of q2! *J. Mol. Graph. Model.* 20, 269–276.

Grigoryan, A. V., Wang, H., and Cardozo, T. J. (2012). Can the Energy gap in the protein-ligand binding energy landscape be used as a descriptor in virtual ligand screening? *PLoS One* 7:e46532. doi: 10.1371/journal.pone.0046532

Grinter, S. Z., and Zou, X. (2014). Challenges, applications, and recent advances of protein-ligand docking in structure-based drug design. *Mol. Basel Switz.* 19, 10150–10176. doi: 10.3390/molecules190710150

Guedes, I. A., Barreto, A. M. S., Miteva, M. A., and Dardenne, L. E. (2016). Development of empirical scoring functions for predicting protein-ligand binding affinity. *Soc. Bras. Bioquim. Biol. Mol.* 1–174.

Guedes, I. A., de Magalhães, C. S., and Dardenne, L. E. (2014). Receptor–ligand molecular docking. *Biophys. Rev.* 6, 75–87. doi: 10.1007/s12551-013-0130-2

Halgren, T. A. (1996). Merck molecular force field. II. MMFF94 van der Waals and electrostatic parameters for intermolecular interactions. *J. Comput. Chem.* 17, 520–552.

Hawkins, D. M. (2004). The problem of overfitting. *J. Chem. Inform. Comput. Sci.* 44, 1–12. doi: 10.1021/ci0342472

Honig, B., Sharp, K., and Yang, A. S. (1993). Macroscopic models of aqueous solutions: biological and chemical applications. *J. Phys. Chem.* 97, 1101–1109. doi: 10.1021/j100108a002

Huang, N., Shoichet, B. K., and Irwin, J. J. (2006). Benchmarking sets for molecular docking. *J. Med. Chem.* 49, 6789–6801. doi: 10.1021/jm0608356

Huang, S.-Y., Grinter, S. Z., and Zou, X. (2010). Scoring functions and their evaluation methods for protein-ligand docking: recent advances and future directions. *Phys. Chem. Chem. Phys.* 12, 12899–12908. doi: 10.1039/c0cp00151a

Huang, Z., and Wong, C. F. (2016). Inexpensive method for selecting receptor structures for virtual screening. *J. Chem. Inform. Model.* 56, 21–34. doi: 10.1021/acs.jcim.5b00299

Irwin, J. J., Shoichet, B. K., Mysinger, M. M., Huang, N., Colizzi, F., Wassam, P., et al. (2009). Automated docking screens: a feasibility study. *J. Med. Chem.* 52, 5712–5720. doi: 10.1021/jm9006966

Jackson, S. E., and Fersht, A. R. (1991). Folding of chymotrypsin inhibitor 2. 1, Evidence for a two-state transition. *Biochemistry (Mosc.)* 30, 10428–10435. doi: 10.1021/bi00107a010

Jain, A. N. (1996). Scoring noncovalent protein-ligand interactions: a continuous differentiable function tuned to compute binding affinities. *J. Comput. Aided Mol. Des.* 10, 427–440.

Jain, A. N. (2006). Scoring functions for protein-ligand docking. *Curr. Protein Pept. Sci.* 7, 407–420.

Jain, A. N., and Nicholls, A. (2008). Recommendations for evaluation of computational methods. *J. Comput. Aided Mol. Des.* 22, 133–139. doi: 10.1007/s10822-008-9196-5

Jain, T., and Jayaram, B. (2005). An all atom energy based computational protocol for predicting binding affinities of protein-ligand complexes. *FEBS Lett.* 579, 6659–6666. doi: 10.1016/j.febslet.2005.10.031

Jiménez Luna, J., Skalic, M., Martinez-Rosell, G., and De Fabritiis, G. (2018). KDEEP: Protein-ligand absolute binding affinity prediction via 3D-convolutional neural networks. *J. Chem. Inform. Model.* 58, 287–296. doi: 10.1021/acs.jcim.7b00650

Jones, G., Willett, P., Glen, R. C., Leach, A. R., and Taylor, R. (1997). Development and validation of a genetic algorithm for flexible docking. *J. Mol. Biol.* 267, 727–748. doi: 10.1006/jmbi.1996.0897

Jones, J. E. (1924a). On the determination of molecular fields, I. From the variation of the viscosity of a gas with temperature. *Proc. R. Soc. Lond. Math. Phys. Eng. Sci.* 106, 441–462. doi: 10.1098/rspa.1924.0081

Jones, J. E. (1924b). On the determination of molecular fields, II. From the equation of state of a gas. *Proc. R. Soc. Lond. Math. Phys. Eng. Sci.* 106, 463–477. doi: 10.1098/rspa.1924.0082

Kalliokoski, T., Salo, H. S., Lahtela-Kakkonen, M., and Poso, A. (2009). The effect of ligand-based tautomer and protomer prediction on structure-based virtual screening. *J. Chem. Inform. Model.* 49, 2742–2748. doi: 10.1021/ci900364w

Kar, P., Lipowsky, R., and Knecht, V. (2013). Importance of polar solvation and configurational entropy for design of antiretroviral drugs targeting HIV-1 protease. *J. Phys. Chem. B* 117, 5793–5805. doi: 10.1021/jp3085292

Kaserer, T., Temml, V., Kutil, Z., Vanek, T., Landa, P., and Schuster, D. (2015). Prospective performance evaluation of selected common virtual screening tools, case study: cyclooxygenase (COX) 1 and 2. *Eur. J. Med. Chem.* 96, 445–457. doi: 10.1016/j.ejmech.2015.04.017

Kelemen, Á. A., Kiss, R., Ferenczy, G. G., Kovács, L., Flachner, B., Lőrincz, Z., et al. (2016). Structure-based consensus scoring scheme for selecting class A aminergic GPCR fragments. *J. Chem. Inform. Model.* 56, 412–422. doi: 10.1021/acs.jcim.5b00598

Khamis, M., Gomaa, W., and Galal, B. (2016). Deep learning is competing random forest in computational docking. arXiv:1608.06665 [Preprint].

Khamis, M. A., and Gomaa, W. (2015). Comparative assessment of machine-learning scoring functions on PDBbind 2013. *Eng. Appl. Artif. Intell.* 45, 136–151. doi: 10.1016/j.engappai.2015.06.021

Koebel, M. R., Schmadeke, G., Posner, R. G., and Sirimulla, S. (2016). AutoDock VinaXB: implementation of XBSF, new empirical halogen bond scoring function, into AutoDock Vina. *J. Cheminform.* 8:27. doi: 10.1186/s13321-016-0139-1

Kolb, P., and Irwin, J. J. (2009). Docking screens: right for the right reasons? *Curr. Top. Med. Chem.* 9, 755–770.

Kong, X., Sun, H., Pan, P., Zhu, F., Chang, S., Xu, L., et al. (2018). Importance of protein flexibility in molecular recognition: a case study on Type-I1/2 inhibitors of ALK. *Phys. Chem. Chem. Phys.* 20, 4851–4863. doi: 10.1039/C7CP08241J

Korb, O., Olsson, T. S. G., Bowden, S. J., Hall, R. J., Verdonk, M. L., Liebeschuetz, J. W., et al. (2012). Potential and limitations of ensemble docking. *J. Chem. Inform. Model.* 52, 1262–1274. doi: 10.1021/ci2005934

Kramer, C., and Gedeck, P. (2010). Leave-cluster-out cross-validation is appropriate for scoring functions derived from diverse protein data sets. *J. Chem. Inform. Model.* 50, 1961–1969. doi: 10.1021/ci100264e

Kramer, C., Kalliokoski, T., Gedeck, P., and Vulpetti, A. (2012). The experimental uncertainty of heterogeneous public ki data. *J. Med. Chem.* 55, 5165–5173. doi: 10.1021/jm300131x

Krammer, A., Kirchhoff, P. D., Jiang, X., Venkatachalam, C. M., and Waldman, M. (2005). LigScore: a novel scoring function for predicting binding affinities. *J. Mol. Graph. Model.* 23, 395–407. doi: 10.1016/j.jmgm.2004.11.007

Kuenemann, M. A., Bourbon, L. M. L., Labbé, C. M., Villoutreix, B. O., and Sperandio, O. (2014). Which three-dimensional characteristics make efficient inhibitors of protein-protein interactions? *J. Chem. Inform. Model.* 54, 3067–3079. doi: 10.1021/ci500487q

Kuhn, B., Fuchs, J. E., Reutlinger, M., Stahl, M., and Taylor, N. R. (2011). Rationalizing tight ligand binding through cooperative interaction networks. *J. Chem. Inform. Model.* 51, 3180–3198. doi: 10.1021/ci200319e

Kumalo, H. M., Bhakat, S., and Soliman, M. E. S. (2015). Theory and applications of covalent docking in drug discovery: merits and pitfalls. *Mol. Basel Switz.* 20, 1984–2000. doi: 10.3390/molecules20021984

Kurkcuoglu, Z., Koukos, P. I., Citro, N., Trellet, M. E., Rodrigues, J. P. G. L. M., Moreira, I. S., et al. (2018). Performance of HADDOCK and a simple contact-based protein-ligand binding affinity predictor in the D3R grand challenge 2. *J. Comput. Aided Mol. Des.* 32, 175–185. doi: 10.1007/s10822-017-0049-y

Labbé, C. M., Rey, J., Lagorce, D., Vavruša, M., Becot, J., Sperandio, O., et al. (2015). MTiOpenScreen: a web server for structure-based virtual screening. *Nucleic Acids Res.* 43, W448–W454. doi: 10.1093/nar/gkv306

Lagarde, N., Zagury, J.-F., and Montes, M. (2015). Benchmarking data sets for the evaluation of virtual ligand screening methods: review and perspectives. *J. Chem. Inform. Model.* 55, 1297–1307. doi: 10.1021/acs.jcim.5b00090

Lam, P. C.-H., Abagyan, R., and Totrov, M. (2017). Ligand-biased ensemble receptor docking (LigBEnD): a hybrid ligand/receptor structure-based approach. *J. Comput. Aided Mol. Des.* 32, 187–198. doi: 10.1007/s10822-017-0058-x

Levy, Y., and Onuchic, J. N. (2006). Water mediation in protein folding and molecular recognition. *Annu. Rev. Biophys. Biomol. Struct.* 35, 389–415. doi: 10.1146/annurev.biophys.35.040405.102134

Li, D.-D., Meng, X.-F., Wang, Q., Yu, P., Zhao, L.-G., Zhang, Z.-P., et al. (2018). Consensus scoring model for the molecular docking study of mTOR kinase inhibitor. *J. Mol. Graph. Model.* 79, 81–87. doi: 10.1016/j.jmgm.2017.11.003

Li, H., Peng, J., Leung, Y., Leung, K.-S., Wong, M.-H., Lu, G., et al. (2018). The impact of protein structure and sequence similarity on the accuracy of machine-learning scoring functions for binding affinity prediction. *Biomolecules* 8:12. doi: 10.3390/biom8010012

Li, Y., Su, M., Liu, Z., Li, J., Liu, J., Han, L., et al. (2018). Assessing protein-ligand interaction scoring functions with the CASF-2013 benchmark. *Nat. Protoc.* 13, 666–680. doi: 10.1038/nprot.2017.114

Li, G.-B., Yang, L.-L., Wang, W.-J., Li, L.-L., and Yang, S.-Y. (2013). ID-score: a new empirical scoring function based on a comprehensive set of descriptors related to protein–ligand interactions. *J. Chem. Inform. Model.* 53, 592–600. doi: 10.1021/ci300493w

Li, H., Leung, K.-S., Wong, M.-H., and Ballester, P. (2015a). Low-quality structural and interaction data improves binding affinity prediction via random forest. *Molecules* 20, 10947–10962. doi: 10.3390/molecules200610947

Li, H., Leung, K.-S., Wong, M.-H., and Ballester, P. J. (2015b). Improving autodock vina using random forest: the growing accuracy of binding affinity prediction by the effective exploitation of larger data sets. *Mol. Inform.* 34, 115–126. doi: 10.1002/minf.201400132

Li, H., Leung, K.-S., Wong, M.-H., and Ballester, P. J. (2014a). Substituting random forest for multiple linear regression improves binding affinity prediction of scoring functions: cyscore as a case study. *BMC Bioinformatics* 15:291. doi: 10.1186/1471-2105-15-291

Li, H., Leung, K.-S., Wong, M.-H., and Ballester, P. J. (2014b). "The impact of docking pose generation error on the prediction of binding affinity," in *Computational Intelligence Methods for Bioinformatics and Biostatistics Lecture Notes in Computer Science*, eds C. D. Serio, P. Liò, A. Nonis, and R. Tagliaferri (Berlin: Springer International Publishing), 231–241. doi: 10.1007/978-3-319-24462-4_20

Li, Y., Han, L., Liu, Z., and Wang, R. (2014c). Comparative assessment of scoring functions on an updated benchmark: 2, evaluation methods and general results. *J. Chem. Inform. Model.* 54, 1717–1736. doi: 10.1021/ci500081m

Liu, J., and Wang, R. (2015). Classification of current scoring functions. *J. Chem. Inform. Model.* 55, 475–482. doi: 10.1021/ci500731a

Liu, S., Fu, R., Zhou, L.-H., and Chen, S.-P. (2012). Application of consensus scoring and principal component analysis for virtual screening against β-secretase (BACE-1). *PLoS One* 7:e38086. doi: 10.1371/journal.pone.0038086

Liu, Z., Li, Y., Han, L., Li, J., Liu, J., Zhao, Z., et al. (2015). PDB-wide collection of binding data: current status of the PDBbind database. *Bioinformatics* 31, 405–412. doi: 10.1093/bioinformatics/btu626

Liu, Z., Su, M., Han, L., Liu, J., Yang, Q., Li, Y., et al. (2017). Forging the basis for developing protein-ligand interaction scoring functions. *Acc. Chem. Res.* 50, 302–309. doi: 10.1021/acs.accounts.6b00491

Logean, A., Sette, A., and Rognan, D. (2001). Customized versus universal scoring functions: application to class I MHC-peptide binding free energy predictions. *Bioorg. Med. Chem. Lett.* 11, 675–679.

London, N., Miller, R. M., Krishnan, S., Uchida, K., Irwin, J. J., Eidam, O., et al. (2014). Covalent docking of large libraries for the discovery of chemical probes. *Nat. Chem. Biol.* 10, 1066–1072. doi: 10.1038/nchembio.1666

Martin, Y. C. (2009). Let's not forget tautomers. *J. Comput. Aided Mol. Des.* 23, 693–704. doi: 10.1007/s10822-009-9303-2

Martin, Y. C., Abagyan, R., Ferenczy, G. G., Gillet, V. J., Oprea, T. I., Ulander, J., et al. (2016). Glossary of terms used in computational drug design, part II (IUPAC Recommendations 2015). *Pure Appl. Chem.* 88, 239–264. doi: 10.1515/pac-2012-1204

Matter, H., and Sotriffer, C. (2011). "Applications and success stories in virtual screening," in *Methods and Principles in Medicinal Chemistry*, ed. C. Sotriffer (Weinheim: Wiley-VCH Verlag GmbH & Co. KGaA), 319–358.

Melo, M. C. R., Bernardi, R. C., Rudack, T., Scheurer, M., Riplinger, C., Phillips, J. C., et al. (2018). NAMD goes quantum: an integrative suite for hybrid simulations. *Nat. Methods* 15, 351–354. doi: 10.1038/nmeth.4638

Meng, E. C., Shoichet, B. K., and Kuntz, I. D. (1992). Automated docking with grid-based energy evaluation. *J. Comput. Chem.* 13, 505–524. doi: 10.1002/jcc.540130412

Mignani, S., Huber, S., Tomás, H., Rodrigues, J., and Majoral, J.-P. (2016). Why and how have drug discovery strategies in pharma changed? What are the new mindsets? *Drug Discov. Today* 21, 239–249. doi: 10.1016/j.drudis.2015.09.007

Miller, D. W., and Dill, K. A. (1997). Ligand binding to proteins: the binding landscape model. *Protein Sci.* 6, 2166–2179. doi: 10.1002/pro.5560061011

Moitessier, N., Englebienne, P., Lee, D., Lawandi, J., and Corbeil, C. R. (2009). Towards the development of universal, fast and highly accurate docking/scoring methods: a long way to go: docking/scoring methods-a review. *Br. J. Pharmacol.* 153, S7–S26. doi: 10.1038/sj.bjp.0707515

Morelli, X., Bourgeas, R., and Roche, P. (2011). Chemical and structural lessons from recent successes in protein-protein interaction inhibition (2P2I). *Curr. Opin. Chem. Biol.* 15, 475–481. doi: 10.1016/j.cbpa.2011.05.024

Muegge, I. (2006). PMF scoring revisited. *J. Med. Chem.* 49, 5895–5902. doi: 10.1021/jm050038s

Mullard, A. (2014). New drugs cost US$2.6 billion to develop. *Nat. Rev. Drug Discov.* 13, 877–877. doi: 10.1038/nrd4507

Murphy, R. B., Repasky, M. P., Greenwood, J. R., Tubert-Brohman, I., Jerome, S., Annabhimoju, R., et al. (2016). WScore: a flexible and accurate treatment of explicit water molecules in ligand-receptor docking. *J. Med. Chem.* 59, 4364–4384. doi: 10.1021/acs.jmedchem.6b00131

Mysinger, M. M., Carchia, M., Irwin, J. J., and Shoichet, B. K. (2012). Directory of useful decoys, enhanced (DUD-E): better ligands and decoys for better benchmarking. *J. Med. Chem.* 55, 6582–6594. doi: 10.1021/jm300687e

Nguyen, D. D., Cang, Z., Wu, K., Wang, M., Cao, Y., and Wei, G.-W. (2018). Mathematical deep learning for pose and binding affinity prediction and ranking in D3R grand challenges. *J. Comput. Aided Mol. Des.* [Epub ahead of print].

Numao, S., Damager, I., Li, C., Wrodnigg, T. M., Begum, A., Overall, C. M., et al. (2004). In situ extension as an approach for identifying novel α-amylase inhibitors. *J. Biol. Chem.* 279, 48282–48291. doi: 10.1074/jbc.M404680 4200

Nunes-Alves, A., and Arantes, G. M. (2014). Ligand-receptor affinities computed by an adapted linear interaction model for continuum electrostatics and by protein conformational averaging. *J. Chem. Inform. Model.* 54, 2309–2319. doi: 10.1021/ci500301s

Ouyang, X., Zhou, S., Su, C. T. T., Ge, Z., Li, R., and Kwoh, C. K. (2013). Covalent dock: automated covalent docking with parameterized covalent linkage energy estimation and molecular geometry constraints. *J. Comput. Chem.* 34, 326–336. doi: 10.1002/jcc.23136

Pagadala, N. S., Syed, K., and Tuszynski, J. (2017). Software for molecular docking: a review. *Biophys. Rev.* 9, 91–102. doi: 10.1007/s12551-016-0247-1

Park, M.-S., Dessal, A. L., Smrcka, A. V., and Stern, H. A. (2009). Evaluating docking methods for prediction of binding affinities of small molecules to the g protein βγ subunits. *J. Chem. Inform. Model.* 49, 437–443. doi: 10.1021/ci800384q

Park, S.-J., Kufareva, I., and Abagyan, R. (2010). Improved docking, screening and selectivity prediction for small molecule nuclear receptor modulators using conformational ensembles. *J. Comput. Aided Mol. Des.* 24, 459–471. doi: 10.1007/s10822-010-9362-4

Pason, L. P., and Sotriffer, C. A. (2016). Empirical scoring functions for affinity prediction of protein-ligand complexes. *Mol. Inform.* 35, 541–548. doi: 10.1002/minf.201600048

Paulsen, J. L., and Anderson, A. C. (2009). Scoring ensembles of docked protein: ligand interactions for virtual lead optimization. *J. Chem. Inform. Model.* 49:2813. doi: 10.1021/ci9003078

Pecina, A., Brynda, J., Vrzal, L., Gnanasekaran, R., Hořejší, M., Eyrilmez, S. M., et al. (2018). Ranking power of the SQM/COSMO scoring function on carbonic anhydrase II-inhibitor complexes. *ChemPhysChem* 19, 873–879. doi: 10.1002/cphc.201701104

Pereira, J. C., Caffarena, E. R., and dos Santos, C. N. (2016). Boosting docking-based virtual screening with deep learning. *J. Chem. Inform. Model.* 56, 2495–2506. doi: 10.1021/acs.jcim.6b00355

Petukh, M., Stefl, S., and Alexov, E. (2013). The role of protonation states in ligand-receptor recognition and binding. *Curr. Pharm. Des.* 19, 4182–4190.

Pierce, A. C., Sandretto, K. L., and Bemis, G. W. (2002). Kinase inhibitors and the case for CH...O hydrogen bonds in protein-ligand binding. *Proteins* 49, 567–576. doi: 10.1002/prot.10259

Pires, D. E. V., and Ascher, D. B. (2016). CSM-lig: a web server for assessing and comparing protein–small molecule affinities. *Nucleic Acids Res.* 44, W557–W561. doi: 10.1093/nar/gkw390

Poornima, C. S., and Dean, P. M. (1995). Hydration in drug design. 1. Multiple hydrogen-bonding features of water molecules in mediating protein-ligand interactions. *J. Comput. Aided Mol. Des.* 9, 500–512.

Qiu, D., Shenkin, P. S., Hollinger, F. P., and Still, W. C. (1997). The GB/SA continuum model for solvation. A fast analytical method for the calculation of approximate born radii. *J. Phys. Chem. A* 101, 3005–3014. doi: 10.1021/jp961992r

Ragoza, M., Hochuli, J., Idrobo, E., Sunseri, J., and Koes, D. R. (2017). Protein-ligand scoring with convolutional neural networks. *J. Chem. Inform. Model.* 57, 942–957. doi: 10.1021/acs.jcim.6b00740

Raha, K., and Merz, K. M. (2005). Large-scale validation of a quantum mechanics based scoring function: predicting the binding affinity and the binding mode of a diverse set of protein-ligand complexes. *J. Med. Chem.* 48, 4558–4575. doi: 10.1021/jm048973n

Rarey, M., Kramer, B., Lengauer, T., and Klebe, G. (1996). A fast flexible docking method using an incremental construction algorithm. *J. Mol. Biol.* 261, 470–489. doi: 10.1006/jmbi.1996.0477

Ravindranath, P. A., Forli, S., Goodsell, D. S., Olson, A. J., and Sanner, M. F. (2015). AutoDockFR: advances in protein-ligand docking with explicitly specified binding site flexibility. *PLoS Comput. Biol.* 11:e1004586. doi: 10.1371/journal.pcbi.1004586

Réau, M., Langenfeld, F., Zagury, J.-F., Lagarde, N., and Montes, M. (2018). Decoys selection in benchmarking datasets: overview and perspectives. *Front. Pharmacol.* 9:11. doi: 10.3389/fphar.2018.00011

Riniker, S., Barandun, L. J., Diederich, F., Krämer, O., Steffen, A., and van Gunsteren, W. F. (2012). Free enthalpies of replacing water molecules in protein binding pockets. *J. Comput. Aided Mol. Des.* 26, 1293–1309. doi: 10.1007/s10822-012-9620-8

Rognan, D. (2017). The impact of in silico screening in the discovery of novel and safer drug candidates. *Pharmacol. Ther.* 175, 47–66. doi: 10.1016/j.pharmthera.2017.02.034

Rognan, D., Lauemoller, S. L., Holm, A., Buus, S., and Tschinke, V. (1999). Predicting binding affinities of protein ligands from three-dimensional models: application to peptide binding to class I major histocompatibility proteins. *J. Med. Chem.* 42, 4650–4658.

Ryde, U., and Söderhjelm, P. (2016). Ligand-binding affinity estimates supported by quantum-mechanical methods. *Chem. Rev.* 116, 5520–5566. doi: 10.1021/acs.chemrev.5b00630

Santos-Martins, D. (2016). Interaction with specific HSP90 residues as a scoring function: validation in the D3R Grand Challenge 2015. *J. Comput. Aided Mol. Des.* 30, 731–742. doi: 10.1007/s10822-016-9943-y

Santos-Martins, D., Forli, S., Ramos, M. J., and Olson, A. J. (2014). AutoDock4Zn: an improved autodock force field for small-molecule docking to zinc metalloproteins. *J. Chem. Inform. Model.* 54, 2371–2379. doi: 10.1021/ci500209e

Sastry, G. M., Adzhigirey, M., Day, T., Annabhimoju, R., and Sherman, W. (2013). Protein and ligand preparation: parameters, protocols, and influence on virtual screening enrichments. *J. Comput. Aided Mol. Des.* 27, 221–234. doi: 10.1007/s10822-013-9644-8

Schäfer, H., Smith, L. J., Mark, A. E., and van Gunsteren, W. F. (2002). Entropy calculations on the molten globule state of a protein: side-chain entropies of α-lactalbumin. *Proteins Struct. Funct. Bioinform.* 46, 215–224. doi: 10.1002/prot.1166

Schneider, G., and Fechner, U. (2005). Computer-based de novo design of drug-like molecules. *Nat. Rev. Drug Discov.* 4, 649–663. doi: 10.1038/nrd1799

Scholz, C., Knorr, S., Hamacher, K., and Schmidt, B. (2015). DOCKTITE-a highly versatile step-by-step workflow for covalent docking and virtual screening in the molecular operating environment. *J. Chem. Inform. Model.* 55, 398–406. doi: 10.1021/ci500681r

Seifert, M. H. J. (2009). Targeted scoring functions for virtual screening. *Drug Discov. Today* 14, 562–569. doi: 10.1016/j.drudis.2009.03.013

Shao, J. (1993). Linear model selection by cross-validation. *J. Am. Stat. Assoc.* 88, 486–494. doi: 10.2307/2290328

Shoichet, B. K. (2006). Interpreting steep dose-response curves in early inhibitor discovery. *J. Med. Chem.* 49, 7274–7277. doi: 10.1021/jm061103g

Sitkoff, D., Sharp, K. A., and Honig, B. (1994). Accurate calculation of hydration free energies using macroscopic solvent models. *J. Phys. Chem.* 98, 1978–1988. doi: 10.1021/j100058a043

Smith, R. D., Damm-Ganamet, K. L., Dunbar, J. B., Ahmed, A., Chinnaswamy, K., Delproposto, J. E., et al. (2016). CSAR benchmark exercise 2013: evaluation of results from a combined computational protein design, docking, and scoring/ranking challenge. *J. Chem. Inform. Model.* 56, 1022–1031. doi: 10.1021/acs.jcim.5b00387

Sotriffer, C. (2012). "Scoring functions for protein-ligand interactions," in *Protein-Ligand Interactions*, ed. H. Gohlke (Weinheim: Wiley-VCH Verlag GmbH & Co. KGaA), 237–263.

Sotriffer, C., and Matter, H. (2011). "The challenge of affinity prediction: scoring functions for structure-based virtual screening," in *Methods and Principles in Medicinal Chemistry*, ed. C. Sotriffer (Weinheim: Wiley-VCH Verlag GmbH & Co. KGaA), 177–221.

Sotriffer, C. A., Sanschagrin, P., Matter, H., and Klebe, G. (2008). SFCscore: scoring functions for affinity prediction of protein-ligand complexes. *Proteins* 73, 395–419. doi: 10.1002/prot.22058

Spiliotopoulos, D., Kastritis, P. L., Melquiond, A. S. J., Bonvin, A. M. J. J., Musco, G., Rocchia, W., et al. (2016). dMM-PBSA: a new HADDOCK scoring function for protein-peptide docking. *Front. Mol. Biosci.* 3:46. doi: 10.3389/fmolb.2016.00046

Spyrakis, F., and Cavasotto, C. N. (2015). Open challenges in structure-based virtual screening: receptor modeling, target flexibility consideration and active site water molecules description. *Arch. Biochem. Biophys.* 583, 105–119. doi: 10.1016/j.abb.2015.08.002

Still, W. C., Tempczyk, A., Hawley, R. C., and Hendrickson, T. (1990). Semianalytical treatment of solvation for molecular mechanics and dynamics. *J. Am. Chem. Soc.* 112, 6127–6129. doi: 10.1021/ja00172a038

Stouch, T. (2008). Editorial: special issue on "evaluation of computational methods." *J. Comput. Aided Mol. Des.* 22:131. doi: 10.1007/s10822-008-9197-4

Sun, H., Li, Y., Tian, S., Xu, L., and Hou, T. (2014). Assessing the performance of MM/PBSA and MM/GBSA methods. 4. Accuracies of MM/PBSA and MM/GBSA methodologies evaluated by various simulation protocols using PDBbind data set. *Phys. Chem. Chem. Phys.* 16, 16719–16729. doi: 10.1039/c4cp01388c

Tanford, C. (1980). *The Hydrophobic Effect: Formation of Micelles and Biological Membranes*, 2nd Edn. New York, NY: Wiley.

Teramoto, R., and Fukunishi, H. (2007). Supervised consensus scoring for docking and virtual screening. *J. Chem. Inform. Model.* 47, 526–534. doi: 10.1021/ci6004993

Terp, G. E., Johansen, B. N., Christensen, I. T., and Jørgensen, F. S. (2001). A new concept for multidimensional selection of ligand conformations (multiselect) and multidimensional scoring (multiscore) of protein-ligand binding affinities. *J. Med. Chem.* 44, 2333–2343. doi: 10.1021/jm001090l

Totrov, M., and Abagyan, R. (1997). Flexible protein-ligand docking by global energy optimization in internal coordinates. *Proteins Suppl.* 1, 215–220.

Totrov, M., and Abagyan, R. (1999). *Derivation of Sensitive Discrimination Potential for Virtual Ligand Screening*. New York, NY: ACM Press, 312–320. doi: 10.1145/299432.299509

Trani, J. M. D., Cesco, S. D., O'Leary, R., Plescia, J., Nascimento, C. J. do, Moitessier, N., et al. (2018). Rapid measurement of inhibitor binding kinetics by isothermal titration calorimetry. *Nat. Commun.* 9:893. doi: 10.1038/s41467-018-03263-3

Trott, O., and Olson, A. J. (2010). AutoDock vina: improving the speed and accuracy of docking with a new scoring function, efficient optimization and multithreading. *J. Comput. Chem.* 31, 455–461. doi: 10.1002/jcc.21334

Tuffery, P., and Derreumaux, P. (2012). Flexibility and binding affinity in protein-ligand, protein-protein and multi-component protein interactions: limitations of current computational approaches. *J. R. Soc. Interface* 9, 20–33. doi: 10.1098/rsif.2011.0584

Tuley, A., and Fast, W. (2018). The taxonomy of covalent inhibitors. *Biochemistry (Mosc.)* 57, 3326–3337. doi: 10.1021/acs.biochem.8b00315

Usha, T., Shanmugarajan, D., Goyal, A. K., Kumar, C. S., and Middha, S. K. (2017). Recent updates on computer-aided drug discovery: time for a paradigm shift. *Curr. Top. Med. Chem.* 17, 3296–3307. doi: 10.2174/1568026618666180101163651

van Zundert, G. C. P., Rodrigues, J. P. G. L. M., Trellet, M., Schmitz, C., Kastritis, P. L., Karaca, E., et al. (2016). The HADDOCK2.2 web server: user-friendly integrative modeling of biomolecular complexes. *J. Mol. Biol.* 428, 720–725. doi: 10.1016/j.jmb.2015.09.014

Velec, H. F. G., Gohlke, H., and Klebe, G. (2005). DrugScore(CSD)-knowledge-based scoring function derived from small molecule crystal data with superior recognition rate of near-native ligand poses and better affinity prediction. *J. Med. Chem.* 48, 6296–6303. doi: 10.1021/jm050436v

Verdonk, M. L., Berdini, V., Hartshorn, M. J., Mooij, W. T. M., Murray, C. W., Taylor, R. D., et al. (2004). Virtual screening using protein-ligand docking: avoiding artificial enrichment. *J. Chem. Inform. Model.* 44, 793–806. doi: 10.1021/ci034289q

Verdonk, M. L., Chessari, G., Cole, J. C., Hartshorn, M. J., Murray, C. W., Nissink, J. W. M., et al. (2005). Modeling water molecules in protein-ligand docking using GOLD. *J. Med. Chem.* 48, 6504–6515. doi: 10.1021/jm050543p

Villoutreix, B., Eudes, R., and Miteva, M. (2009). Structure-based virtual ligand screening: recent success stories. *Comb. Chem. High Throughput Screen.* 12, 1000–1016. doi: 10.2174/138620709789824682

Vogel, S. M., Bauer, M. R., and Boeckler, F. M. (2011). DEKOIS: demanding evaluation kits for objective in silico screening – A versatile tool for benchmarking docking programs and scoring functions. *J. Chem. Inf. Model.* 51, 2650–2665. doi: 10.1021/ci2001549

Wallach, I., Dzamba, M., and Heifets, A. (2015). AtomNet: a deep convolutional neural network for bioactivity prediction in structure-based drug discovery. arXiv:1510.02855 [Preprint].

Wang, C., and Zhang, Y. (2017). Improving scoring-docking-screening powers of protein–ligand scoring functions using random forest. *J. Comput. Chem.* 38, 169–177. doi: 10.1002/jcc.24667

Wang, J.-C., Lin, J.-H., Chen, C.-M., Perryman, A. L., and Olson, A. J. (2011). Robust scoring functions for protein-ligand interactions with quantum chemical charge models. *J. Chem. Inform. Model.* 51, 2528–2537. doi: 10.1021/ci200220v

Wang, R., Lai, L., and Wang, S. (2002). Further development and validation of empirical scoring functions for structure-based binding affinity prediction. *J. Comput. Aided Mol. Des.* 16, 11–26.

Wang, R., Liu, L., Lai, L., and Tang, Y. (1998). SCORE: a new empirical method for estimating the binding affinity of a protein-ligand complex. *J. Mol. Model.* 4, 379–394. doi: 10.1007/s008940050096

Wang, R., Lu, Y., and Wang, S. (2003). Comparative evaluation of 11 scoring functions for molecular docking. *J. Med. Chem.* 46, 2287–2303. doi: 10.1021/jm0203783

Wang, R., and Wang, S. (2001). How does consensus scoring work for virtual library screening? An idealized computer experiment. *J. Chem. Inform. Comput. Sci.* 41, 1422–1426.

Wang, Y., Guo, Y., Kuang, Q., Pu, X., Ji, Y., Zhang, Z., et al. (2015). A comparative study of family-specific protein–ligand complex affinity prediction based on random forest approach. *J. Comput. Aided Mol. Des.* 29, 349–360. doi: 10.1007/s10822-014-9827-y

Wei, B. Q., Baase, W. A., Weaver, L. H., Matthews, B. W., and Shoichet, B. K. (2002). A model binding site for testing scoring functions in molecular docking. *J. Mol. Biol.* 322, 339–355.

Wei, D., Zheng, H., Su, N., Deng, M., and Lai, L. (2010). Binding energy landscape analysis helps to discriminate true hits from high-scoring decoys in virtual screening. *J. Chem. Inform. Model.* 50, 1855–1864. doi: 10.1021/ci900463u

Williams, D. H., and Bardsley, B. (1999). Estimating binding constants – The hydrophobic effect and cooperativity. *Perspect. Drug Discov. Des.* 17, 43–59. doi: 10.1023/A:1008770523049

Wójcikowski, M., Ballester, P. J., and Siedlecki, P. (2017). Performance of machine-learning scoring functions in structure-based virtual screening. *Sci. Rep.* 7:46710. doi: 10.1038/srep46710

Yang, J.-M., Chen, Y.-F., Shen, T.-W., Kristal, B. S., and Hsu, D. F. (2005). Consensus scoring criteria for improving enrichment in virtual screening. *J. Chem. Inform. Model.* 45, 1134–1146. doi: 10.1021/ci050034w

Yang, Y., Lightstone, F. C., and Wong, S. E. (2013). Approaches to efficiently estimate solvation and explicit water energetics in ligand binding: the use of WaterMap. *Exp. Opin. Drug Discov.* 8, 277–287. doi: 10.1517/17460441.2013.749853

Yang, Z., Liu, Y., Chen, Z., Xu, Z., Shi, J., Chen, K., et al. (2015). A quantum mechanics-based halogen bonding scoring function for protein-ligand interactions. *J. Mol. Model.* 21:138. doi: 10.1007/s00894-015-2681-6

Yilmazer, N. D., and Korth, M. (2016). Prospects of applying enhanced semi-empirical QM methods for 2101 virtual drug design. *Curr. Med. Chem.* 23, 2101–2111.

Yuriev, E., Holien, J., and Ramsland, P. A. (2015). Improvements, trends, and new ideas in molecular docking: 2012-2013 in review: improvements, trends, and new ideas in molecular docking. *J. Mol. Recognit.* 28, 581–604. doi: 10.1002/jmr.2471

Yuriev, E., and Ramsland, P. A. (2013). Latest developments in molecular docking: 2010-2011 in review. *J. Mol. Recognit. JMR* 26, 215–239. doi: 10.1002/jmr.2266

Zhang, L., Tan, J., Han, D., and Zhu, H. (2017). From machine learning to deep learning: progress in machine intelligence for rational drug discovery. *Drug Discov. Today* 22, 1680–1685. doi: 10.1016/j.drudis.2017.08.010

Zhang, X., Perez-Sanchez, H., and Lightstone, F. C. (2017). A comprehensive docking and MM/GBSA rescoring study of ligand recognition upon binding antithrombin. *Curr. Top. Med. Chem.* 17, 1631–1639. doi: 10.2174/1568026616666161117112604

Zheng, Z., and Merz, K. M. (2011). Ligand identification scoring algorithm (LISA). *J. Chem. Inform. Model.* 51, 1296–1306. doi: 10.1021/ci2000665

Zhu, K., Borrelli, K. W., Greenwood, J. R., Day, T., Abel, R., Farid, R. S., et al. (2014). Docking covalent inhibitors: a parameter free approach to pose prediction and scoring. *J. Chem. Inform. Model.* 54, 1932–1940. doi: 10.1021/ci500118s

Zilian, D., and Sotriffer, C. A. (2013). SFCscore RF: a random forest-based scoring function for improved affinity prediction of proteinŰligand complexes. *J. Chem. Inf. Model.* 53, 1923–1933. doi: 10.1021/ci400120b

Zimmermann, M. O., Lange, A., and Boeckler, F. M. (2015). Evaluating the potential of halogen bonding in molecular design: automated scaffold decoration using the new scoring function XBScore. *J. Chem. Inform. Model.* 55, 687–699. doi: 10.1021/ci5007118

Zou, X., and Kuntz, I. D. (1999). Inclusion of solvation in ligand binding free energy calculations using the generalized-born model. *J. Am. Chem. Soc.* 121, 8033–8043. doi: 10.1021/ja984102p

Using Machine Learning to Predict Synergistic Antimalarial Compound Combinations with Novel Structures

Daniel J. Mason [1,2], Richard T. Eastman [3], Richard P. I. Lewis [1], Ian P. Stott [4], Rajarshi Guha [3*†] and Andreas Bender [1*]

[1] Department of Chemistry, Centre for Molecular Informatics, University of Cambridge, Cambridge, United Kingdom, [2] Healx Ltd., Cambridge, United Kingdom, [3] Division of Preclinical Innovation, National Center for Advancing Translational Sciences, National Institutes of Health, Rockville, MD, United States, [4] Unilever Research and Development, Wirral, United Kingdom

*Correspondence:
Rajarshi Guha
rajarshi.guha@gmail.com
Andreas Bender
ab454@cam.ac.uk

The parasite *Plasmodium falciparum* is the most lethal species of Plasmodium to cause serious malaria infection in humans, and with resistance developing rapidly novel treatment modalities are currently being sought, one of which being combinations of existing compounds. The discovery of combinations of antimalarial drugs that act synergistically with one another is hence of great importance; however an exhaustive experimental screen of large drug space in a pairwise manner is not an option. In this study we apply our machine learning approach, Combination Synergy Estimation (CoSynE), which can predict novel synergistic drug interactions using only prior experimental combination screening data and knowledge of compound molecular structures, to a dataset of 1,540 antimalarial drug combinations in which 22.2% were synergistic. Cross validation of our model showed that synergistic CoSynE predictions are enriched $2.74\times$ compared to random selection when both compounds in a predicted combination are known from other combinations among the training data, $2.36\times$ when only one compound is known from the training data, and $1.5\times$ for entirely novel combinations. We prospectively validated our model by making predictions for 185 combinations of 23 entirely novel compounds. CoSynE predicted 20 combinations to be synergistic, which was experimentally validated for nine of them (45%), corresponding to an enrichment of $1.70\times$ compared to random selection from this prospective data set. Such enrichment corresponds to a 41% reduction in experimental effort. Interestingly, we found that pairwise screening of the compounds CoSynE individually predicted to be synergistic would result in an enrichment of $1.36\times$ compared to random selection, indicating that synergy among compound combinations is not a random event. The nine novel and correctly predicted synergistic compound combinations mainly (where sufficient bioactivity information is available) consist of efflux or transporter inhibitors (such as hydroxyzine), combined with compounds exhibiting antimalarial activity alone (such as sorafenib, apicidin, or dihydroergotamine). However, not all compound synergies could be rationalized easily in this way. Overall, this study highlights the potential for predictive modeling to expedite the discovery of novel drug combinations in fight against antimalarial resistance, while the underlying approach is also generally applicable.

Keywords: synergy, combinations, malaria, plasmodium falciparum, artificial intelligence, modeling

INTRODUCTION

Malaria is a deadly and worldwide disease, with an estimated 445,000 deaths globally in 2016, of which 91% are estimated to have occurred in Africa (World Health Organisation, 2017). Despite global mortality rates declining by 62% between 2000 and 2015, this disease remains a major killer for children under 5 years, with a young life being taken every 2 min (World Health Organisation, 2017).

When exposed to antimalarial compounds, the malaria-causing parasite *Plasmodium falciparum* can over time develop resistance to different therapies and *via* a number of distinct mechanisms (Mita and Tanabe, 2012). This tendency has rendered many antimalarial therapies ineffective in the past, and continues to threaten the current standards of care. In order to combat resistance, options include the design or discovery of new antimalarial compound classes or analogs that offer increased efficacy over those with prior use. However, in the present time, and in absence of these novel discoveries, the current World Health Organization (WHO) guidelines state that combinations of at least two effective antimalarial medicines with different modes of action need to be administered in order to help protect against resistance (World Health Organisation, 2015). At present, the standard of care listed by WHO includes artemisinin-based combination therapies (ACT), such as artemether with lumefantrine, artesunate with amodiaquine, and dihydroartemisinin with piperaquine (**Figure 1**). Resistance to artemisinins has arisen more recently in South East Asia (World Health Organisation, 2017), raising concern on the future effectiveness of ACTs since resistance to the ACT partner drug significantly decreases the clinical efficacy of the combination therapy (Bacon et al., 2007). Alarmingly, this concern has recently been confirmed in Cambodia, in the form of resistance to the first line treatment dihydroartemisinin-piperaquine by *P. falciparum* strain *PfPailin* (Imwong et al., 2017). The evolution and spread of multidrug resistant organisms renders the selection of novel drug combinations only a viable medium-term option, and there is continued effort to map ACT partner drugs by the World Wide Antimalarial Resistance Network (World Wide Antimalarial Resistance Network, 2014).

The combined properties resulting from a mixture of drugs is not always equivalent to the sum of their parts. Drug combinations are well-known to result in an increase or decrease in measured therapeutic efficacy (synergy or antagonism, respectively), result in no difference in effectiveness (additivity), or present an increase or decrease in the number of side effects experienced (drug-drug interactions, which would then also possibly represent synergy, albeit of undesired effects; Lehár et al., 2009; Tatonetti et al., 2012). In the case of malaria (and probably many other diseases one wants to treat), the desired effect sought after is usually synergy, i.e., a drug combination for which the antimalarial effect is greater than that observed by each compound alone, and greater than what would be expected by assuming solely additivity of compound effect (Sucher, 2014). In this case lower doses of each individual compound would be required, thereby potentially achieving the desired efficacy with in many cases reduced side-effects (Csermely et al., 2005).

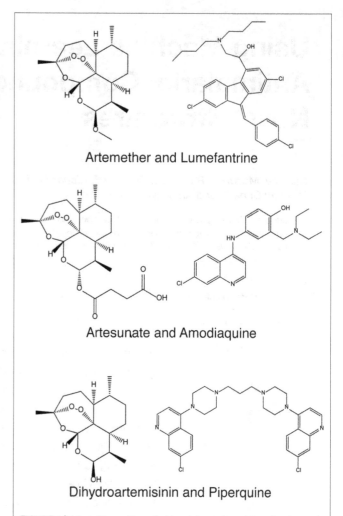

FIGURE 1 | Artemether and Lumefantrine, Artesunate and Amodiaquine, and Dihydroartemisinin and Piperaquine are antimalarial combinations recommended by the WHO as the current standard of care to help protect against drug resistance in *P. falciparum*.

Antimalarial drug combinations can be either novel, or represent the repurposing of drugs used previously for other purposes, such as in the use of tricyclic antidepressants in chloroquine-resistant strains of *P. falciparum* (Bitonti et al., 1988). High throughput screening for antimalarial compound combinations is one mechanism by which discovery of novel combinations may be found faster (Mott et al., 2015). However, the discovery of synergistic combinations is experimentally challenging: As the number of compounds increases, very quickly too does the number of potential combinations, in particular when considering multiple replicates, the requirement of screening concentration matrices, and possibly against different strains of the pathogen. For example, 100 compounds screened pairwise results in 4,950 compound combinations, and testing for synergy in a 6 × 6 dose-response matrix altogether requires 178,200 data points (with numbers increasing further when taking into account replicates, different strains, etc.; Cokol et al., 2014). Increasing the search space by the addition of just 25 more compounds would require over 100,000 further data points, due to combinatorial explosion.

Computational approaches have been investigated as a means to predict the synergistic interaction of compounds previously, with methods that utilize networks of pathways and simulation (Lehár et al., 2007; Nelander et al., 2008; Miller et al., 2013; Huang et al., 2014; Patel et al., 2014; Zhang et al., 2014), relationships between physicochemical properties (Yilancioglu et al., 2014), chemogenomics approaches (Bansal et al., 2014; Wildenhain et al., 2015; KalantarMotamedi et al., 2018), and single agent efficacies (Gayvert et al., 2017) and/or combinations (Menden et al., 2018) measured across multiple cell lines (for recent reviews of compound combination modeling and perspectives, see Bulusu et al., 2016; Weinstein et al., 2017; Tsigelny, 2018). A disadvantage to many of these approaches is that they often require experimental knowledge of underlying biological interactions between drugs and disease, or chemogenomic or phenotypic readouts (Jansen et al., 2009; Bansal et al., 2014; Wildenhain et al., 2015; Menden et al., 2018). This data may be difficult to obtain, non-existent, or expensive to collect enough to create a predictive model from. In addition, the prediction of novel combinations themselves will rely on the same experimental descriptors being available for each new compound.

In order to address these problems, we have developed CoSynE (Combination Synergy Estimation; Mason et al., 2017). CoSynE constructs predictive models from existing combination screening data, and utilizes only the known structures of compounds that have been part of these screens. As such, CoSynE requires only two pieces of information, namely a list of compounds together with their structural representations, and a list of compound combinations together with a label whether the action of each combination was found to be synergistic, antagonistic, or additive (depending on the criteria for those categories one finds appropriate in a particular case). The compounds are transformed into two classes of representation by CoSynE: Firstly, a compound structure fingerprint (SFP; a 2048-bit Morgan Fingerprint), and secondly a predicted target fingerprint representing bioactivity spectra [TFP; 1,080 predicted protein target binding probabilities above a training cut-off, using PIDGIN (Mervin et al., 2015)]. This hence yields three classes of models: SFP, TFP, and STFP (a concatenation of the SFP and TFP fingerprints). These fingerprints are used as input to machine learning models that make inferences between a particular representation and the experimentally observed synergy. A number of models are optimized for the prediction of synergistic combinations, and the best-performing final model is selected following a rigorous cross-validation procedure, where either both compounds are known to the model, one compound is unknown, or both are unknown, such that the ability of CoSynE to extrapolate to novel chemical space may be inferred (**Figure 2**).

We have previously applied CoSynE to the prediction of novel antibiotic combinations effective against *E. coli* (Mason et al., 2017). In this initial study, CoSynE was trained upon 156 pairs of 18 compounds using the SFP representation of combinations (since in preliminary studies other types of descriptors were found to lead to inferior performance), which was then used to pre-screen a set of 123 combinations, comprising compounds that were known and/or unknown to the model. After prospective validation, 10 novel synergistic combinations were confirmed from a list of 12 that were highlighted by CoSynE. The results from our previous study correspond to a 2.8-fold enrichment in the discovery of synergistic combinations vs. that expected by random selection from the same set of compounds.

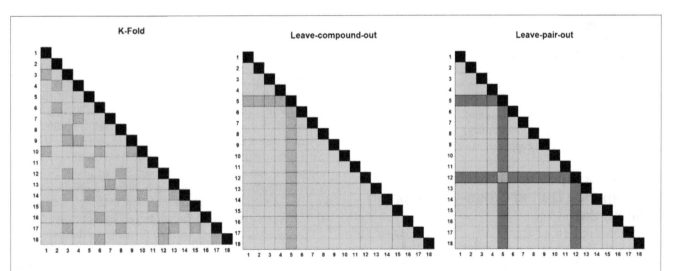

FIGURE 2 | Three different rounds of cross-validation (CV) were employed to test model performance prior to making final predictions. Numbers on axes represent compound IDs in a compound combination training dataset. K-fold randomly selects a 1/K fraction of combinations to remove from the training data and predict in each round; Leave One Compound Out (LOCO) chooses pairs to remove based upon one compound in each round, and Leave One Pair Out chooses pairs to remove based upon a choice of two compounds in each round. Green; training combinations; blue; test combinations, red; held-out combinations, black; self-self crosses (not included in training data).

In the present study, we were starting with a much larger training dataset consisting of 1,540 combinations of 56 compounds tested against *P. falciparum* (Mott et al., 2015). Next, CoSynE was used to pre-screen a library of 23 compounds *unknown to the model* (see Methods section for compound selection process) by predicting which combinations of those compounds are likely to exhibit novel antimalarial synergy.

These predictions were prospectively validated by carrying out a full pairwise experimental screen of all 23 compounds the model could have chosen from (in order to also provide a negative control, i.e., testing of compound combinations not predicted to be synergistic by the model). This validation represents making predictions in entirely novel compound space, where both compounds have not been seen by the model before, which is a very tough challenge, compared to our previous study (and many other studies) which mostly included compounds that were previously known to the model. However, prospective validation in the present study showed CoSynE predictions to be enriched with 1.70 times more synergistic combinations than expected by random selection (over an already rather high baseline synergy level, see details below), and hence also predictions in novel chemical space are enriched over random.

RESULTS AND DISCUSSION

Similarity of Training and Validation Sets

Clustered hierarchical similarities are shown for whole and scaffold structures in **Supplementary Figure 1**. In general, there is little structural similarity between compounds in the training data compared to the prospectively tested data. Compounds which formed the top five most synergistic combinations in both the training and validation datasets are shown in dimensionally-reduced chemical space in **Figure 3**. The lack of a clear clustering between the top synergistic compound structures in either datasets demonstrates the difficulty in selection of compounds to screen simply *via* structural similarity alone. In addition to the observation that synergy is more commonly observed for drugs targeting the same processes (Brochado et al., 2018), the relationship between compound structure-related properties and synergistic interaction has been shown previously [such as lipophilicity and synergy in the case of anti-fungals (Yilancioglu et al., 2014)]. Overall, the inference of complex relationships, such as these on a scale that may quickly explode to intractable proportions is a task highly applicable to machine learning.

Dataset Composition and Model Performance During Cross-Validation on Training Set

The number of high quality (HQ) training combinations per dataset (see Methods section for definition) and synergy type is shown in **Table 1**. The Dd2 dataset contains the greatest number of HQ combinations (1,245), followed by 3d7 (1,194), and then Hb3 (1,159). This was reflected in the results of the 5-fold leave-one-compound-out (LOCO) and leave-one-pair-out (LOPO) cross-validation routines (**Supplementary Table 1**), which showed the Dd2 model to outperform 3d7 and Hb3.

The mean average Matthews Correlation Coefficient (MCC) score for each strain (i.e., across all fingerprint type and all CV routines) were 0.19 (Dd2), 0.18 (3d7), and 0.11 (Hb3). Although these MCC scores are not particularly high in absolute terms (particularly since the more difficult CV routines bring the scores down, while considering that a score of 0 is equivalent to random selection), the Dd2 dataset was chosen for use in the remainder of the study due to the expectation of relatively greater performance in a prospective validation, in addition to the greater number of high quality data points upon which the model is trained upon.

The Dd2 dataset model was further examined in terms of the performance for each of the descriptor types, the results of which are displayed in **Table 2**. During 5-fold CV (where a random subset of 20% of the training data is held out to test upon), each descriptor type for Dd2 showed similar performance, with a cross-descriptor average MCC of 0.46 and a cross-descriptor average 2.78-fold enrichment (compared to random selection) of synergistic combinations correctly predicted by the model. However, for the more challenging leave-one-compound-out (LOCO) CV, the SFP model significantly outperformed the others, with MCC scores of 0.27 (SFP), 0.03 (TFP), and 0.03 (STFP). Moving on to the most difficult leave-one-pair-out (LOPO) CV routine, the performance was still greatest for the SFP model with a precision of 0.33 and recall of 0.01 (corresponding to an MCC of 0.02). Although recall (number of synergistic compounds in the test data that were identified correctly) is very low, the precision (number of synergistic combinations correctly identified in all that were predicted to be synergistic) is greater at 0.33. This is still useful in practice since it suggests *we are only likely to find the minority of all synergistic combinations in a dataset, but 33% of those combinations predicted to be synergistic will indeed turn out to be synergistic combinations.* Compared to our previous study where CoSynE was applied to antibiotic combinations (Mason et al., 2017), the LOPO CV performance was qualitatively similar with a high precision and low recall (1.0 and 0.2, respectively) for a SFP fingerprint on the training data. Since the coverage of chemical space in this dataset overall is quite low it is likely that the model has not been exposed to enough diversity to make confident predictions about many of the compounds, and so the recall score is low as a result.

A possible reason behind the low performance of the TFP descriptor models is that the protein targets from PIDGIN are of human origin, and are unlikely to provide a useful representation of target interactions in *P. falciparum*. However, it is the case that orthologous proteins exist between *Homo sapiens* and *P. falciparum*, and it has previously been shown that the number of conflicting bioactivities between human and ortholog targets in public databases is comparatively low (Mervin et al., 2018), which supports the use of human targets as bioactivity spectra in this indirect manner. It has also been shown that bioactivity spectra can be used more generally as a descriptor that captures biologically relevant information, and can outperform chemical descriptors in the identification of compounds with similar bioactivities [see Petrone et al. (Petrone et al., 2012) Bender et al. (Bender et al., 2006), Kauvar et al. (Kauvar et al., 1995), Riniker et al. (Riniker et al., 2014), and Paricharak et al. (Paricharak et al., 2016)]. These, together with the lack of predictive modeling tools

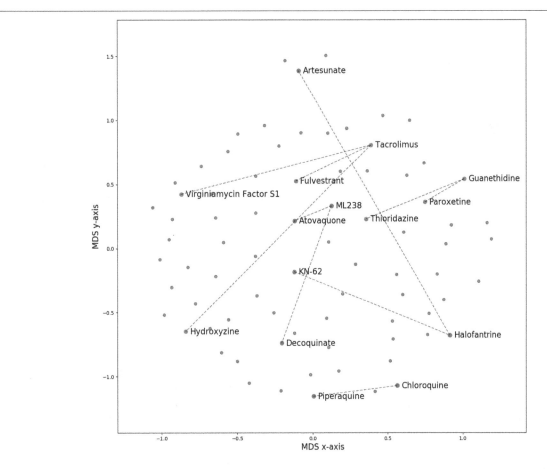

FIGURE 3 | Multi-Dimensional Scaling (MDS) plot of chemical space for all compounds used in this study, based upon pairwise similarity of radius 2, 2,048-bit Morgan fingerprints. Compounds that comprise the top five synergistic combinations in the training (red dots) and prospective validation (green dots) datasets are highlighted, together with their synergistic connection. The lack of a clear clustering suggests that pairs of synergistic compounds do not always arise from those in distinct or well-defined chemical space. Out of these predictions in green, none were predicted by CoSynE, but paroxetine + guanethidine would be discovered following the indirect route described in the Results section, and is the second-most synergistic combination in the validation dataset. Structures for validation and training compounds are included in **Supplementary Tables 5, 7**, respectively.

available to predict potential *P. falciparum* targets from a given compound structure, provided the reasoning behind our choice of entire bioactivity spectra against proteins as a descriptor type.

Since we are carrying out the toughest validation possible for our model by exploring novel areas of chemical space (i.e., the compounds to be prospectively validated in this study are not present in the training data), the most-challenging LOPO scenario represents the predictions we wish to make. The CV performance results suggest that by using the SFP descriptor model, we may expect an approximate 1.5-fold enrichment of synergistic combinations in those predicted from our novel compounds compared to random selection (although this enrichment appears low, note that there is already a high baseline of synergy within the dataset which this suggests could be increased further and that the prediction of synergy for entirely unseen data is the most difficult test of a predictive model possible). The SFP descriptor model was therefore selected as the most suitable candidate for this study, which is the same class of descriptor used in our previous study which successfully identified antibacterial combinations (Mason et al., 2017).

Prospective Validation of CoSynE Predictions

The library of 23 compounds that were selected for prospective validation resulted from predictions generated by a developmental version of CoSynE that had previously virtually screened 21 million DrugBank combinations using the same training data, alongside a different approach that was developed in parallel to CoSynE (KalantarMotamedi et al., 2018; see Experimental section for details). From this library of 23 compounds (and a possible 253 combinations), a total of 20 combinations comprising 12 distinct individual compounds were predicted to be synergistic, and these were submitted for prospective experimental validation. The prospective validation found that 9 of these 20 combinations (i.e., 45%) exhibited antimalarial synergy (defined in this study as $\gamma \leq 0.96$). These predicted synergistic combinations are shown in **Table 3** where the range of γ is 0.917–0.958 (compared to the full prospective screen shown in **Supplementary Table 2**, where the range of γ is 0.88–0.959). The nine synergistic combinations that were correctly predicted comprise only seven compounds of the 23

TABLE 1 | Dataset statistics.

Strain	Synergistic combinations	Additive combinations	Antagonistic combinations	Total
TRAINING COMBINATIONS (HQ)				
3d7	264 (22.1%)	762 (63.8%)	168 (14.1%)	1,194
Dd2	277 (22.2%)	817 (65.6%)	151 (12.1%)	1,245
Hb3	242 (20.9%)	767 (66.2%)	150 (12.9%)	1,159
PROSPECTIVELY VALIDATED COMBINATIONS (HQ)				
3d7	18 (15.1%)	100 (84%)	1 (0.8%)	119
Dd2	49 (26.5%)	134 (72.4%)	2 (1.1%)	185
Hb3	29 (35.8%)	52 (64.2%)	0	81

Counts for the number of synergistic, additive, and antagonistic compounds in each of the datasets available for the current study, after filtering for high quality (HQ) data. The Dd2 training dataset had the highest number of HQ datapoints, which was reflected during cross validation (CV). The Dd2 dataset also contained the highest number of HQ datapoints in the prospectively validated dataset.

TABLE 2 | Dd2 training performance.

CV	Descriptor	MCC	F1	AUC	Pr	Re	Ac	Ef	Rank
5-Fold	SFP	0.45	0.56	0.84	0.61	0.53	0.82	2.74	2
	TFP	0.44	0.55	0.83	0.60	0.51	0.81	2.69	3
	STFP	0.47	0.57	0.84	0.64	0.52	0.83	2.89	1
	Cross-descriptor average	**0.46**	**0.56**	**0.84**	**0.62**	**0.52**	**0.82**	**2.78**	
LOCO	SFP	0.27	0.31	0.81	0.52	0.33	0.77	2.36	1
	TFP	0.03	0.08	0.58	0.07	0.11	0.76	0.31	3
	STFP	0.03	0.32	0.55	0.23	0.89	0.31	1.04	2
	Cross-descriptor average	**0.11**	**0.23**	**0.64**	**0.28**	**0.44**	**0.61**	**1.24**	
LOPO	SFP	0.02	0.01	0.44	0.33	0.01	0.78	1.50	1
	TFP	−0.02	0.10	0.49	0.20	0.07	0.73	0.89	3
	STFP	0.02	0.36	0.47	0.23	0.82	0.34	1.02	2
	Cross-descriptor average	**0.01**	**0.16**	**0.47**	**0.25**	**0.30**	**0.62**	**1.14**	

The results from three increasingly difficult rounds of cross validation (CV); shuffled and stratified 5-fold CV, leave one compound out (LOCO), and leave one pair out (LOPO), for each model type (SFP, structural fingerprint; TFP, target fingerprint; and STFP, combined structure-target fingerprint). Since the current study concerns the prediction of novel compound combinations, our chosen model followed the expected performance of the SFP model during LOPO CV, since this is the most challenging test of the model. AUC, area under receiver operating curve; Pr, precision; Re, recall; Ac, accuracy; Ef, enrichment factor. The "cross descriptor average" is the average score for each metric across each cross validation routine.

that were provided to CoSynE. These seven compounds were further investigated using the literature, in order to identify a biological rationale for their selection, and are depicted in **Table 4**. It should be noted that five out of these seven compounds were found to also have self-self ꭣvalues that would be classed as synergistic by the threshold that was trained upon, instead of additive (as one would expect). Inclusion of this observation in a predictive model would additionally include the experimental data for self-self crosses for all compounds, which may not be feasible. Instead, this highlights a current limitation of synergy quantification based upon experimental dose-response matrices, whereby the underlying metric should include these crosses as an additional parameter (see Experimental for details). In the present study however, the model has successfully predicted combinations of drugs that produced ꭣvalues below a cutoff at a rate of 45%, demonstrating the ability to reduce search space significantly.

The following seven compounds were part of the nine combinations that were prospectively validated as

being synergistic; dihydroergotamine (in four of the combinations), apicidin (three combinations), hydroxyzine (three combinations), trifluoperazine (three combinations), sorafenib (two combinations), virginiamycin factor S1 (two combinations), and guanethidine (one combination). The Tanimoto similarity of each compound vs. the training compounds is shown in **Supplementary Figure 2**, which shows apicidin has the greatest similarity among validation compounds to the training compounds at 39.1% (to gramicidin). Virginiamycin factor S1 is the next-closest compound to the training data, with a 30.7% similarity to gramicidin, followed by hydroxyzine (26.2% to piperaquine), trifluoperazine (24.6% to piperaquine), dihydroergotamine (23.5% to gramicidin), sorafenib (19.8% to nilotinib), and guanethidine (15.9% to pyronaridine). Overall, these greatest similarities to the training compounds are on the more-similar end of the distribution curve, but the overall similarity is still quite low. Compounds that form both the validation and training compounds are listed in **Supplementary Tables 5, 7**.

TABLE 3 | Dd2 SFP predictions.

Combination ID	Drug1 name (PubChem ID)	Drug2 name (PubChem ID)	Predicted probability of being synergistic	Prospectively derived γ (synergy ≤0.96)
NCGC00167488 NCGC00021152	Sorafenib (216239)	Hydroxyzine (3658)	0.4	0.917
NCGC00263624 NCGC00017400	Apicidin (6918328)	Dihydroergotamine (10531)	0.42	0.924
NCGC00016272 NCGC00013226	Guanethidine (3518)	Trifluoperazine (5566)	0.36	0.926
NCGC00021152 NCGC00017400	Hydroxyzine (3658)	Dihydroergotamine (10531)	0.4	0.932
NCGC00167488 NCGC00013226	Sorafenib (216239)	Trifluoperazine (5566)	0.43	0.937
NCGC00181117 NCGC00017400	Virginiamycin s1 (46937022)	Dihydroergotamine (10531)	0.49	0.941
NCGC00263624 NCGC00021152	Apicidin (6918328)	Hydroxyzine (3658)	0.47	0.952
NCGC00263624 NCGC00181117	Apicidin (6918328)	Virginiamycin s1 (46937022)	0.62	0.957
NCGC00017400 NCGC00013226	Dihydroergotamine (10531)	Trifluoperazine (5566)	0.43	0.958

The 9 combinations out of 20 predicted by CoSynE, which were prospectively validated to be synergistic, which cover a total of 7 unique compounds. The probability of being synergistic that was assigned by CoSynE is shown, which does not correlate with the experimentally quantified degree of synergy.

Out of the nine true positive synergistic predictions, four combinations involved one compound (namely, either hydroxyzine or guanethidine) known as a drug efflux pump inhibitor in other species (further details given below), which may also facilitate accumulation of a respective antimalarial partner drug in *P. falciparum*. Drug efflux pump inhibition has previously been suggested as attractive in combating resistance, whereby the intracellular concentration of an active compound is otherwise strongly restricted by the microorganism (Alibert-Franco et al., 2009). Firstly, hydroxyzine is a compound with antihistamine and central nervous system (CNS) properties that has been shown to act as an efflux pump inhibitor in bacteria, and also affects Quorum Sensing (QS) (Aybey et al., 2014). QS is a system of stimulus and coordination among microorganisms, which *P. falciparum* may use to detect conditions of the external environment (Wu et al., 2016), such as overcrowding, in order to keep the parasite population under control in the host (Mutai and Waitumbi, 2010). Hydroxyzine was correctly predicted to be synergistic in combination with sorafenib, apicidin, or dihydroergotamine. Sorafenib is a tyrosine kinase inhibitor used in the treatment of cancer that inhibits parasite egress from the host cell (Gaji et al., 2014), and is annotated with activity against both 3D7 and Dd2 strains of *P. falciparum* in PubChem (Pathak et al., 2015; Kim et al., 2016). Apicidin is a potent inhibitor of histone deacetylase [HDA; of which the *P. falciparum* ortholog PfHDA2 exists (Coleman et al., 2014)] and this mechanism of inhibition is responsible for the antiprotozoal properties of the drug (Darkin-Rattray et al., 1996; Engel et al., 2015). Dihydroergotamine is a known inhibitor of *P. falciparum* (Weisman et al., 2006), which may target a serotonin 5-HT1a-like receptor in the parasite thought to be a nutrient channel critical for parasite development (Hanoun

et al., 2003; Locher et al., 2003). Ergotamine, the structural analog of dihydroergotamine was one compound involved in a docking study looking for competitive inhibitors for the enzyme *P. falciparum* lactate dehydrogenase (*Pf*LDH), upon which the parasite is dependent for energy production where it achieved a reasonably good docking score (Penna-Coutinho et al., 2011). The combination of these active compounds with the hydroxyzine efflux pump inhibition and QS action may be responsible for the observed synergy in these cases. Secondly, guanethidine is annotated as active against human multidrug resistance protein 1 (MDR-1) in a screen for compounds that compete for this transporter as a means to increase accumulation of active compounds in cells (AID:377). A plasmodium ortholog of MDR-1, PfMDR1 exists (Hyde, 2007), and if guanethidine competes for PfMDR1, this may explain a potential mechanism for synergy, since PfMDR1 is important for transporting substrates from the cytoplasm into the lysosomal-like parasite digestive vacuole (Reiling and Rohrbach, 2015). Guanethidine alone does not show activity against *P. falciparum* (Chong et al., 2006), but was correctly predicted to show synergy in combination with trifluoperazine. Trifluoperazine is an antipsychotic drug and a potent inhibitor of *P. falciparum* calcium-dependent protein kinase 4 (PfCDPK4) (Cavagnino et al., 2011), and so would represent the anti-malarial compound in this combination. To the authors' knowledge, these may be novel modes of action for the use of hydroxyzine and guanethidine in context of *P. falciparum*. Since the training dataset did not include compounds explicitly annotated as targeting *P. falciparum* efflux pumps [with the exception of primaquine, which exhibits synergy with chloroquine through inhibiting the *P. falciparum* Chloroquine Resistance Transporter; PfCRT (Bray et al., 2005)]. Further experimental validation

TABLE 4 | Synergistic drugs correctly predicted by CoSynE.

Drug name	Depiction	Notes
Apicidin		Known to target histone deacetylase and has previously shown activity against P. falciparum via inhibition of apicomplexan histone deacetylase (HDA) (Darkin-Rattray et al., 1996).
Dihydroergotamine		An inhibitor of P. falciparum (Weisman et al., 2006), and is annotated in PubChem as being active in several assays. May target a serotonin 5-HT1a-like receptor in the parasite thought to be a nutrient channel (Hanoun et al., 2003; Locher et al., 2003). Structural analog ergotamine achieved reasonably good docking score in a study searching for competitive inhibitors for *Pf*LDH (Penna-Coutinho et al., 2011).
Guanethidine		Annotated in PubChem as having an inconclusive potency against P. falciparum of 5.72 uM (AID:504834). Also annotated as active against MDR-1 (AID:377); the P. falciparum analog of which (pfmdr1) is involved in resistance and guanethidine may therefore play a role in preventing drug efflux (Hyde, 2007)
Hydroxyzine		Shown to act as an efflux pump inhibitor in bacteria (Aybey et al., 2014). Also affects Quorum Sensing in microorganisms (Aybey et al., 2014).

(Continued)

TABLE 4 | Continued

Drug name	Depiction	Notes
Sorafenib tosylate		Tyrosine kinase inhibitor that exhibits antimalarial properties, and has been shown to inhibit the function of calcium-dependent protein kinase 3 in P. falciparum (PfCDPK1), which affects parasite egress from the host cell (Gaji et al., 2014). Sorafenib is an antitumor drug annotated in PubChem with activity against both 3D7 and DD2 strains, as well as RKL9, MRC2, and 7G8 with IC50s of 1.66–2.64 uM (Pathak et al., 2015). This compound was also tested in combination with artesunate in the study, however the mode of action was found to be antagonistic, while for another tyrosine kinase inhibitor, imatinib, combination with artesunate demonstrated synergy.
Trifluoperazine		Calmodulin inhibitor, and a potent antiplasmodial inhibitor of calcium-dependent protein kinase 4 (PfCDPK4) (Cavagnino et al., 2011).
Virginiamycin s1		An antibiotic that is annotated as targeting 60S Ribosomal Protein L37 in PubChem. Similar in structure to azithromycin (which is known to target apicoplast 50S ribosomal subunit and inhibit P. falciparum).

Depiction and description of the seven compounds that were part of combinations predicted to be synergistic by CoSynE.

would be required to confirm this mechanistic hypothesis of the synergies observed experimentally.

Three of the remaining five combinations that were correctly predicted involve a combination of the previously detailed compounds that were the "active" partner drugs to those with expected efflux pump inhibitors (apicidin-dihydroergotamine, trifluoperazine-sorafenib, and trifluoperazine-dihydroergotamine). The observed synergy in these may exert their synergistic effect through their differing mechanisms.

The final two correctly predicted combinations involve virginiamycin factor S1, a macrolide antibiotic annotated as active against P. falciparum proliferation (AID:504749), with either apicidin or dihydroergotamine. Antibiotics may exhibit antimalarial properties, albeit slow-acting, by targeting the apicoplast during development (Dahl et al., 2006; Barthel et al., 2008; Chakraborty, 2016). Macrolides are known for their effectiveness in treatment of uncomplicated malaria in combination with quinine, where the main mechanism of action involves binding to ribosomal proteins, but suffer due to poor pharmacological properties (Gaillard et al., 2016). The combination of virginiamycin S1 targeting the apicoplast, and apicidin targeting plasmodium orthologs of histone deacetylase, such as PfHDA2 (Darkin-Rattray et al., 1996; Coleman et al., 2014; Engel et al., 2015) suggests that this combination puts pressure on the developmental and growth stages of the parasite. The combination of potential nutrient channel and energy inhibition properties of dihydroergotamine (Hanoun et al., 2003; Locher et al., 2003; Penna-Coutinho et al., 2011) with the apicoplast-targeting mechanism of virginiamycin S1 also suggests pressure being put on the developmental and growth stages. However, since this work used asynchrous parasite cultures to assess compound efficacy, and given that apicoplast-targeting molecules don't typically affect the first replication cycle upon drug pressure [where they are instead exhibiting a "delayed death" phenotype (Dahl and Rosenthal, 2007)], this apicoplast-targeting mechanism is unlikely to have been observed. Unfortunately, the combination of macrolides and dihydroergotamine has been reported to produce clinically significant adverse drug reactions (Horowitz et al., 1996), which means this particular combination would not be suitable as a potential treatment.

Full Pairwise Synergy Screen of 23 Compounds

A subsequent full pairwise experimental screen of all 23 compounds was also carried out (**Supplementary Table 3**), in order to assess the performance of CoSynE for the prediction of completely novel combinations of compounds acting synergistically. Comparison of the overall number of synergistic combinations that were found (49 out of 185, or 26%, see **Table 1**), compared to the number that was present among those predicted by CoSynE (9 out of 20, or 45%) showed that we achieved a 1.70-fold enrichment (0.45/0.265); approximately that which was expected from our LOPO CV performance. This level of enrichment is significant in the search for antimalarial compound combinations in practical terms, where a 41% reduction [1 − (1/1.70)] in the total number of measurements required is a very attractive prospect in terms of both time and cost. Although this performance is attractive, the model is still far from ideal and requires further refinement to increase both the precision (0.45) and recall (0.18) seen in **Table 5**. On the other hand it should be noted that the baseline of obtaining synergy in 26.5% of cases is a rather high baseline, which the model was able to increase further to nearly half of all synergistic predictions being true positives (more precisely, to 45% of all combinations).

Potential for Indirect Discovery of Synergistic Combinations

We next investigated the hypothetical scenario where all compounds that are part of combinations predicted to be synergistic by CoSynE were screened in a fully pairwise manner, to see whether CoSynE could indirectly expand the discovery of novel combinations. Interpreted differently, we investigated whether synergy between compounds is "clustered"—and whether the knowledge that a compound has shown synergy before increases the chances that it will show synergy also in combination with other compounds (with the limitation of our validation being the limited sampling of chemical space, which may or may not generalize to "all" chemical space). Each combination in the prospective validation dataset for Dd2 involving any of the 12 compounds that were part of a combination predicted to be synergistic was extracted, yielding a total of 61 combinations, out of which 36% were found to be synergistic (22 combinations in **Supplementary Table 4**). This proportion of synergistic combinations is hence higher (by 9.5% in absolute terms, and 36% in relative terms) than the 26.5% found in all of the 185 HQ validation combinations, which corresponds to an enrichment of 1.36× compared to random selection. However, to some extent this enrichment may be slightly inflated due to CoSynE having identified drug efflux pump inhibitors in the model. Among the synergistic combinations in this subset indirectly found through CoSynE is guanethidine (antiplasmodial and active against MDR1) and paroxetine (annotated in DrugBank as targeting MDR1, antibacterial activity via efflux pump and QS inhibition Aybey et al., 2014, and antiplasmodial activity Chong et al., 2006 including AID:524790–524796), with a γscore of 0.889. This combination is more synergistic than all those directly predicted by CoSynE, and is the second-most synergistic combination among all HQ combinations in the validation dataset. This suggests that by not only screening compound combinations predicted to be synergistic by CoSynE, but *all combinations* of the compounds predicted to be part of *any* combination predicted to be synergistic will still increase the likelihood of identifying further synergistic combinations. This also is in line with previous studies, which have found that while synergy to an extent depends on the properties of both compounds in a combination, there is still a significant bias in chemical space, with some parts of it being significantly more frequently part of synergistic compounds combinations than others (Weinstein et al., 2017).

Along these lines, we believe that an iterative screening procedure could be followed in an industrial setting, whereby predictions are made, screened, and then fed back into CoSynE for training before further predictions are made. Such iterative approaches have been investigated in the literature (Paricharak et al., 2016), and could enable gradual expansion of chemical and/or biological space, in particular with current improvements in cherry picking compounds in such iterative screening settings.

CONCLUSION

In this work, we describe the application of our compound combination prediction method, CoSynE, to a recently published compound combination screening dataset for *P. falciparum*, and the results to a prospective validation of our predictions. When we used our final CoSynE model to predict synergistic combinations ($\gamma \leq 0.96$) from a library of compounds previously

TABLE 5 | Dd2 SFP Performance.

Descriptor	Predicted synergistic combinations	Experimentally validated as synergistic	MCC	F1	AUC	Pr	Re	Ac	Ef
SFP	20	9	0.15	0.26	0.63	0.45	0.18	0.72	1.70

Overall performance of the Dd2 SFP model, after the full pairwise screen of prospective compounds was carried out. Overall, the precision and recall for the prediction of novel synergistic combinations, however this still provides greater enrichment of synergistic combinations than expected by random selection (1.70-fold) from the prospectively validated dataset. AUC, area under receiver operating curve; Pr, precision; Re, recall; Ac, accuracy; Ef, enrichment factor.

unknown to the model for *P. falciparum* Dd2, 45% of the predicted combinations (9 out of 20) were experimentally confirmed as being synergistic, corresponding to a 1.70-fold enrichment of synergistic combinations than that expected by randomly selection from the validation dataset. This is of practical significance when combinatorial explosion and experimental cost for combination screening is taken into account. Furthermore, a 2.36-fold enrichment was observed during cross validation when one compound is unknown, and 2.74-fold when both compounds are known to the model (but only in different combinations). In addition, it was found that screening only compounds part of combinations CoSynE predicted to be synergistic would yield 9.5% more synergistic combinations in absolute terms (and 36% in relative terms) than expected by random selection alone.

The combinations that were prospectively validated from our predictions mainly involve one compound with antimalarial activity coupled to another targeting potential drug efflux or substrate transport mechanisms in *P. falciparum*. These results in particular suggest that the approach we describe can capture meaningful information that enables the prediction of synergy, which is corroborated by our previous study involving antibiotic combinations.

CoSynE offers an advantage over similar methods that require data, such as differential gene expression analysis, or single agent efficacies across multiple cell lines related to the target, in that the only information required to make new predictions is the provision of chemical structure information. The use of CoSynE to make predictions for other therapeutic areas requires only a dataset of combination screening results together with compound structural information, and may also predict for higher orders of combinations (e.g., combinations of 3, 4, and above), should training data with a meaningful measure of synergy be made available. Our approach may be employed to prioritize screening of new combinations, thus reducing the potential burden and cost of combinatorial explosion in the search for future antimalarial compound combinations that exhibit synergy.

EXPERIMENTAL

Experimental Screening of Compound Combinations

Training data was obtained from a publicly available dataset of antimalarial compound combinations from a high-throughput screen against 3D7, Dd2, and HB3 strains of *P. falciparum* (assay IDs 1463, 1464 and 1465, which can be

found at https://tripod.nih.gov/matrix-client/?p=183; Mott et al., 2015). Compounds were acoustically dispensed and read at 72 h as previously described (Mott et al., 2015). Matrix combination response was calculated based upon relative SYBRGreen intensity values, compared to controls (Mott et al., 2015). The prospective validation data was screened using the same method as the training data. This validation dataset includes both single-agent and combination responses, and can be found at https://tripod.nih.gov/matrix-client/?p=1261. The 23 compounds that comprised the validation dataset are listed in **Supplementary Table 5**, the experimental data used to validate the Dd2 model is listed in **Supplementary Table 3**, and reproducibility of assay results is detailed in **Supplementary Table 6**.

Compound Combination Datasets and Synergy

The training data used in this study consisted of 1,540 combinations of 56 antimalarial compounds that exhibit different modes of action, which were screened against the 3D7, Dd2, and HB3 strains of *P. falciparum*. The 56 compounds that formed this screen are listed in **Supplementary Table 7**. Synergy metrics and data quality (QC) were pre-determined from a 6 × 6 dose-response matrix of each combination, where inhibition of the parasite in infected red blood cells was measured. The QC score for a combination was precomputed from a set of heuristics described in Mott et al. (2015), that takes in to account the quality of the single agent dose response, DMSO activity and the smoothness of the dose combination response matrix. This yields a value between 0 and 18, where lower values indicate higher quality. Only high quality (HQ) experimental readouts were kept that have a QC score ≤3, which provided 1,194 HQ combinations for 3D7, 1,245 for Dd2, and 1,159 for HB3 (**Table 1**; training dataset). For the validation dataset, the same filtering rules applied to 209 combinations of 23 compounds provided 119 for 3D7, 185 for Dd2, and 81 for HB3 (**Table 1**; validation dataset).

The metric used to interpret synergy in our modeling approach was gamma (γ), which is a combination of the Highest Single Agent (HSA; also known as Gaddum's non-interaction model) and Bliss independence. Based upon a 6 × 6 dose-response matrix of compound A and compound B at concentration x and y vs. inhibition of *P. falciparum*, the variable γ is computed to minimize the following function (Cokol et al., 2014).

$$\Sigma \left[f\left(A_{[x]} + B_{[y]}\right) - \gamma \times max\left\{f\left(A_{[x]}\right), f\left(B_{[y]}\right)\right\}\right]^2 \quad (1)$$

This yields a positive value, where synergy is characterized as <1, additivity as $=1$, and antagonism as >1. In order to classify each of the combination readouts, we set a maximum γ cutoff for synergy of 0.96, and minimum cutoff for antagonism of 1.04, with the remainder assigned as additive. This cutoff value was empirically chosen to provide a degree of separation between antagonism and synergy in the training data, while aiming to keep the balance of each class similar across strains. Although not explicitly investigated during the study, we expect that making the γ cutoff larger may lead to an increased enrichment of synergistic combinations being predicted, while making it smaller may affect the model robustness by decreasing the number of synergistic training datapoints further.

One limitation with regard to the pre-processing of experimental combination responses during our study is that measurement of self-crosses using the Bliss model component of γ may in fact produce values which are classed as synergistic. For example, apicidin in combination with itself in the validation dataset shows a γ value of 0.895, whereas our cut-off for the training data was 0.96. In other words, this self-cross should be labeled as "synergistic" according to our criteria, whereas self-interaction should be additive; this is a well-known phenomenon among synergy measures, where a generalizable and robust model is yet to be identified (Bulusu et al., 2016). We chose to apply the cut-off of 0.96 that was used for the training data to enable our assessment of validation predictions "in the eyes of the model" with respect to training criteria, yielding 49 synergistic combinations in the Dd2 validation dataset. Compounds with self-cross γ values lower than our training data cut-off include trifluoperazine, raloxifene, guanethidine, hydroxyzine, megestrol acetate, FK-506, fulvestrant, sorafenib, apicidin, and ingenol mebutate. Since these cover five out of the seven compounds in **Table 3**, any future investigation into combinations involving these compounds based solely upon γ values should bear this in mind (i.e., eight out of our nine predictions in **Table 3**). Although it is not clear precisely how to overcome this limitation, future models that additionally train upon the validation dataset might take these self-crosses into account more explicitly by lowering synergistic cut-offs on a per-combination basis, or seek to find a way of incorporating this into the synergy metric itself. All self-crosses for the validation data may be found at https://tripod.nih.gov/matrix-client/?p=1261, and minimum significance ratios for the validation compounds that were screened are detailed in **Supplementary Table 6**.

Prior Selection of Validation Compounds

The selection of compound combinations for screening and validation of our models were based upon a version of CoSynE much earlier in development. Several CoSynE models were trained upon the same dataset as described in this report, except the range of additivity for γ was narrower at 0.975–1.025 (opposed to 0.96–1.04). The resulting models were used to predict enumerated combinations of approved, investigational, and experimental compounds in DrugBank (Wishart et al., 2006), which amounted to around 21 million combinations for prediction. Of these, approximately 1.2 million combinations were predicted to be synergistic, and 10 combinations needed to be selected for the prospective validation. This selection was achieved by manually reviewing the top-ranked combinations (sorted by the probability of being synergistic that was assigned to each combination by CoSynE), and taking into consideration the prevalence of each compound throughout the list of combination predictions, followed by examining the literature co-occurrence of each predicted combination's compounds together with mention of *P. falciparum* in PubMed. These 10 chosen combinations comprised 18 compounds, and were submitted for testing together with an additional 10 selected from a different approach developed in parallel by KalantarMotamedi et al. (2018).

Out of the total number of compounds among the 20 combinations primarily suggested for testing, only the 23 compounds shown in **Supplementary Table 5** were available for purchase at the time, which meant few original predictions could be prospectively validated. The decision was made to instead use a more recent version of CoSynE to predict which combinations of these 23 compounds were synergistic, finally yielding the dataset in this study. Interestingly, **Table 1** shows that the number of antagonistic combinations observed in the validation dataset is significantly lower compared to the training dataset, while at the same time the number classed as additive or synergistic has increased. This reduction in the number of antagonistic combinations as a result of virtually screening a library of intractable size suggests that the approach taken by CoSynE, together with the process of manually reviewing the top predictions, aids the discovery of synergistic combinations.

Comparison to a Similar Study Conducted in Parallel

The approach by KalantarMotamedi et al. (2018) differs from that described in this work primarily by the usage of gene expression data. Firstly, differential gene expression profiles of mild vs. severe malaria patient peripheral blood samples were used to predict potentially active single antimalarial agents by comparison of drug gene perturbations through a modified Gene Set Enrichment Analysis (GSEA) approach (Subramanian et al., 2005) applied to the Library of INtegrated Cellular Signatures (LINCS) Phase I database (Subramanian et al., 2017). Secondly, a Random Forest model was trained on the same dataset of 1,540 combinations from NCATS as in the present study, and human target predictions and pathway annotations were used to infer which drug combinations may interact synergistically. Finally, the single agents identified by the GSEA approach to human blood samples were enumerated as pairs and predicted by the Random Forest model as synergistic/non-synergistic. These predicted combinations were ranked based upon the predicted probability of being synergistic, and the top 17 compound combinations were selected for prospective experimental testing (covering a total of 14 single agents). This approach reported an overall average precision of 0.488 and recall of 0.755 (F1 = 0.593) for experiments across the three strains of *P. falciparum* where drug combinations were predicted to be synergistic at a cutoff for synergy of $\gamma \leq 0.975$. Among the 14 single agents in 17 combinations

Kalantar-Motamedi et al. selected for prospective validation were seven that overlapped with the 12 drugs in 20 combinations CoSynE predicted for prospective validation; ciprofloxacin, wortmannin, paroxetine, raloxifene, apicidin, trifluoperazine, and hydroxyzine. The only combination of these overlapping compounds that was correctly predicted to be synergistic in both CoSynE and the method described by Kalantar-Motamedi et al. was apicidin-hydroxyzine. Since CoSynE is not constrained to compounds that are only present in the Connectivity-Map (Lamb et al., 2006) or LINCS databases (instead needing only knowledge of compound structure) it is difficult to draw a direct and fair comparison of overall performance. However, for the same experimental γ cutoff applied to the total pool of 185 prospective combinations in the current study that denotes a synergistic combination, CoSynE achieved precision of 0.45 and recall of 0.18 (F1 = 0.26). While the precision of CoSynE for the prospectively validated combinations is close to that reported by Kalantar-Motamedi et al. recall in this instance is much lower. However, it should be noted this overall performance still represents greater enrichment of synergistic combinations being discovered than by random selection (see **Table 5**), and CoSynE is not limited by the requirement for gene expression data to be made available for the compounds that are to be predicted.

Combination Descriptors

We represented each compound combination as an array of features in three ways. A Structural Fingerprint (SFP) descriptor based upon the molecular structure of each compound in a combination, a Target Fingerprint (TFP) descriptor based upon probabilistic combination of predicted target affinity probabilities per compound, and a concatenation of these two previous descriptors (Structure-Target; STFP). This provided three descriptor sets for which models were trained.

Structural fingerprints were generated by first obtaining SMILES representation PubChem (Kim et al., 2016) for each compound that was screened in the training data, before standardizing this representation with ChemAxon JChem Standardizer (ChemAxon, 2014) according to the protocol defined by PIDGIN (Mervin et al., 2015). Standardized SMILES were then loaded into RDKit v2015[1] and 2,048-bit Morgan fingerprints with radius 2 were generated, yielding arrays of 2,048 integer features. A given combination of two compounds was represented as the bitwise average of these features, yielding possible values of 0, 0.5, and 1 per feature, which formed the SFP descriptor. A Morgan fingerprint was chosen for this study due to generally outperforming the MACCS fingerprint in this dataset [however the MACCS fingerprint was found to outperform Morgan when CoSynE was used to predict antibiotic combinations (Mason et al., 2017)]. The SMILES representation was also used as input for PIDGIN (Mervin et al., 2015), where the probability of binding below the training cut-off of 10 μM for each compound vs. 1,080 human protein targets was predicted, yielding arrays of 1,080 floating point value features between 0 and 1. A given combination considered the probability of binding to each protein target by each compound from the following function, such that the maximum affinity a combination of

compounds may have is 100% [i.e., a value of 1.0; Equation (2)], which formed the TFP descriptor. The rationale behind the use of this function for TFP was that the probability of a protein being inhibited cannot be more than 100%, but the more compounds in a single combination that are predicted to target the protein, the more this is likely to be the case.

$$p\left(Combination,\ TargetN\right) = 1 - \left(1 - p\left(Compound1,\ TargetN\right)\right) \times \left(1 - p\left(Compound2,\ TargetN\right)\right) \quad (2)$$

Model Construction and Performance Testing

Model settings were optimized prior to construction of the final models, and all machine learning capabilities were carried out using SciKit-Learn v0.17 (Pedregosa et al., 2011).

The 1,245 Dd2 compound combinations that formed our training data each has either between 1,080, 2,048, or 3,128 features per combination (depending on the descriptor used), meaning that the feature space is larger than the number of combinations. It is therefore necessary to remove any features that are not useful for training prior to constructing the final models. Training data was scaled to unit variance with a zero-centered mean, and starting from $N = 1$, the top N percentile of features within the training data [as determined by ANOVA F-classifier score in SciKit-Learn v0.17 (Pedregosa et al., 2011)] was selected to train upon using a Support Vector Machine Classifier (SVC, optimization parameters detailed in **Supplementary Methods**), together with the synergy type labels per combination, to construct a classifier. This classifier then predicted the synergy label for test data that has had the same features selected, and the outcome of this test was scored using the Matthews Correlation Coefficient [MCC, Equation (3)] with respect to the ability for correctly predicting a synergistic combination. Due to the consideration of all possible outcomes of a classification problem (true positive; TP, false positive; FP, true negative; TN, false negative; FN), the MCC score offers benefit over performance metrics, such as the Area Under Receiver Operating Curve (AU-ROC) and Accuracy, which ignore TN and TN, and FP and FN predictions, respectively.

$$MCC = \frac{TP \times TN - FP \times FN}{\sqrt{(TP + FP)(TP + FN)(TN + FP)(TN + FN)}} \quad (3)$$

This process was repeated 10 times per N, by stratified and shuffled 5-fold cross validation, to finally yield 99 averaged MCC scores. These top N selected features that resulted in the highest MCC score overall were subsequently used by CoSynE in the final model training round, in order to test model performance in different scenarios. The top N selected features per model are detailed in **Supplementary Methods**. While CoSynE will label predicted combinations as synergistic, additive, or antagonistic, during model optimization only the prediction of synergistic combinations is carried out.

The second round that results in selection of the final model involved construction of a number of different classifiers [Bernoulli Naïve Bayes, Support Vector Machine, Random Forest, Extra Trees, and Decision Tree, SciKit-Learn v0.17

---

[1]Landrum, G. *RDKit: Open-Source Cheminformatics*. Available online at: http://www.rdkit.org

(Pedregosa et al., 2011)], which were subject to grid search parameter optimization (optimization parameters detailed in **Supplementary Methods**). The selection of the best model parameters was based upon 10 repeats of stratified and shuffled 5-fold cross validation, which represents a scenario where the training data has prior knowledge of both compounds per combination (**Figure 3**). Each model with a new set of parameters was then subjected to two further rounds of validation of increasing difficulty; Leave One Compound Out (LOCO; in which one compound in a combination is made unknown to the model), and Leave One Pair Out (LOPO; in which both compounds are made unknown to the model). This provided a view on model performance when looking to extend the compounds used in combination with those already known (LOCO) or, in the toughest case, searching for novel combinations of unknown compounds (LOPO). The choice of final model settings was based upon performance in terms of the MCC score for the prediction of synergistic combinations in each of these scenarios.

In each test and train split of the data, feature selection and scaling were based solely upon the training data to ensure that no information from the test set was used in the model generation step. Final model settings are detailed in **Supplementary Table 7**.

AUTHOR CONTRIBUTIONS

DM created the tool and wrote the majority of the manuscript. RL provided advice with respect to the training dataset. RG and RE carried out the experimental work. IS and AB obtained funding, supervised and provided advice.

FUNDING

This work was supported by a grant from Unilever Research and Development to DM (MA-2013-00588), and an ERC Starting Grant (MIXTURE) to AB.

REFERENCES

Alibert-Franco, S., Pradines, B., Mahamoud, A., Davin-Regli, A., and Pagès, J.-M. (2009). Efflux mechanism, an attractive target to combat multidrug resistant *Plasmodium falciparum* and *Pseudomonas aeruginosa*. *Curr. Med. Chem.* 16, 301–317. doi: 10.2174/092986709787002619

Aybey, A., Usta, A., and Demirkan, E. (2014). Effects of psychotropic drugs as bacterial efflux pump inhibitors on quorom sensing regulated behaviors. *J. Microbiol. Biotechnol. Food Sci.* 4, 128–131. doi: 10.15414/jmbfs.2014.4.2.128-131

Bacon, D. J., Jambou, R., Fandeur, T., Le Bras, J., Wongsrichanalai, C., Fukuda, M. M., et al. (2007). World Antimalarial Resistance Network (WARN) II: *in vitro* antimalarial drug susceptibility. *Malar. J.* 6:120. doi: 10.1186/1475-2875-6-120

Bansal, M., Yang, J., Karan, C., Menden, M. P., Costello, J. C., Tang, H., et al. (2014). A community computational challenge to predict the activity of pairs of compounds. *Nat. Biotechnol.* 32, 1213–1222. doi: 10.1038/nbt.3052

Barthel, D., Schlitzer, M., and Pradel, G. (2008). Telithromycin and quinupristin-dalfopristin induce delayed death in *Plasmodium falciparum*. *Antimicrob. Agents Chemother.* 52, 774–777. doi: 10.1128/AAC.00892-07

Bender, A., Jenkins, J. L., Glick, M., Deng, Z., Nettles, J. H., and Davies, J. W. (2006). "Bayes affinity fingerprints" improve retrieval rates in virtual screening and define orthogonal bioactivity space: when are multitarget drugs a feasible concept? *J. Chem. Inf. Model.* 46, 2445–2456. doi: 10.1021/ci600197y

Bitonti, A. J., Sjoerdsma, A., McCann, P. P., Kyle, D. E., Oduola, A. M., Rossan, R. N., et al. (1988). Reversal of chloroquine resistance in malaria parasite *Plasmodium falciparum* by desipramine. *Science* 242, 1301–1303. doi: 10.1126/science.3057629

Bray, P. G., Deed, S., Fox, E., Kalkanidis, M., Mungthin, M., Deady, L. W., et al. (2005). Primaquine synergises the activity of chloroquine against chloroquine-resistant *P. falciparum*. *Biochem. Pharmacol.* 70, 1158–1166. doi: 10.1016/j.bcp.2005.07.021

Brochado, A. R., Telzerow, A., Bobonis, J., Banzhaf, M., Mateus, A., Selkrig, J., et al. (2018). Species-specific activity of antibacterial drug combinations. *Nature* 559, 259–263. doi: 10.1038/s41586-018-0278-9

Bulusu, K. C., Guha, R., Mason, D. J., Lewis, R. P. I., Muratov, E., Kalantar Motamedi, Y., et al. (2016). Modelling of compound combination effects and applications to efficacy and toxicity: state-of-the-art, challenges and perspectives. *Drug Discov. Today* 21, 225–238. doi: 10.1016/j.drudis.2015.09.003

Cavagnino, A., Rossi, F., and Rizzi, M. (2011). The potent antiplasmodial calmodulin-antagonist trifluoperazine inhibits *Plasmodium falciparum*

calcium-dependent protein kinase 4. *Protein Pept. Lett.* 18, 1273–1279. doi: 10.2174/092986611797642742

Chakraborty, A. (2016). Understanding the biology of the *Plasmodium falciparum* apicoplast, an excellent target for antimalarial drug development. *Life Sci.* 158, 104–110. doi: 10.1016/j.lfs.2016.06.030

ChemAxon. (2014). *J. Chem. Standardizer*. Available online at: https://chemaxon.com/products/chemical-structure-representation-toolkit

Chong, C. R., Chen, X., Shi, L., Liu, J. O., and Sullivan, D. J. (2006). A clinical drug library screen identifies astemizole as an antimalarial agent. *Nat. Chem. Biol.* 2, 415–416. doi: 10.1038/nchembio806

Cokol, M., Chua, H. N., Tasan, M., Mutlu, B., Weinstein, Z. B., Suzuki, Y., et al. (2014). Systematic exploration of synergistic drug Pairs. *Mol. Syst. Biol.* 7, 544–544. doi: 10.1038/msb.2011.71

Coleman, B. I., Skillman, K. M., Jiang, R. H. Y., Childs, L. M., Altenhofen, L. M., Ganter, M., et al. (2014). A *Plasmodium falciparum* histone deacetylase regulates antigenic variation and gametocyte conversion. *Cell Host Microbe* 16, 177–186. doi: 10.1016/j.chom.2014.06.014

Csermely, P., Agoston, V., and Pongor, S. (2005). The efficiency of multi-target drugs: the network approach might help drug design. *Trends Pharmacol. Sci.* 26, 178–182. doi: 10.1016/j.tips.2005.02.007

Dahl, E. L., and Rosenthal, P. J. (2007). Multiple antibiotics exert delayed effects against the *Plasmodium falciparum* apicoplast. *Antimicrob. Agents Chemother.* 51, 3485–3490. doi: 10.1128/AAC.00527-07

Dahl, E. L., Shock, J. L., Shenai, B. R., Gut, J., DeRisi, J. L., and Rosenthal, P. J. (2006). Tetracyclines specifically target the apicoplast of the malaria parasite *Plasmodium falciparum*. *Antimicrob. Agents Chemother.* 50, 3124–3131. doi: 10.1128/AAC.00394-06

Darkin-Rattray, S. J., Gurnett, A. M., Myers, R. W., Dulski, P. M., Crumley, T. M., Allocco, J. J., et al. (1996). Apicidin: a novel antiprotozoal agent that inhibits parasite histone deacetylase. *Proc. Natl. Acad. Sci. U.S.A.* 93, 13143–13147. doi: 10.1073/pnas.93.23.13143

Engel, J. A., Jones, A. J., Avery, V. M., Sumanadasa, S. D. M., Ng, S. S., Fairlie, D. P., et al. (2015). Profiling the anti-protozoal activity of anti-cancer HDAC inhibitors against plasmodium and trypanosoma parasites. *Int. J. Parasitol. Drugs Drug Resist.* 5, 117–126. doi: 10.1016/j.ijpddr.2015.05.004

Gaillard, T., Dormoi, J., Madamet, M., and Pradines, B. (2016). Macrolides and associated antibiotics based on similar mechanism of action like lincosamides in malaria. *Malar. J.* 15:85. doi: 10.1186/s12936-016-1114-z

Gaji, R. Y., Checkley, L., Reese, M. L., Ferdig, M. T., and Arrizabalaga, G. (2014).

Expression of the essential kinase PFCDPK1 from *Plasmodium falciparum* in *Toxoplasma gondii* facilitates the discovery of novel antimalarial drugs. *Antimicrob. Agents Chemother.* 58, 2598–2607. doi: 10.1128/AAC.02261-13

Gayvert, K. M., Aly, O., Platt, J., Bosenberg, M. W., Stern, D. F., and Elemento, O. (2017). A computational approach for identifying synergistic drug combinations. *PLOS Comput. Biol.* 13:e1005308. doi: 10.1371/journal.pcbi.1005308

Hanoun, N., Saurini, F., Lanfumey, L., Hamon, M., and Bourgoin, S. (2003). Dihydroergotamine and its metabolite, 8'-hydroxy-dihydroergo-tamine, as 5-HT 1A receptor agonists in the rat brain. *Br. J. Pharmacol.* 139, 424–434. doi: 10.1038/sj.bjp.0705258

Horowitz, R. S., Dart, R. C., and Gomez, H. F. (1996). Clinical ergotism with lingual ischemia induced by clarithromycin-ergotamine interaction. *Arch. Intern. Med.* 156, 456–458. doi: 10.1001/archinte.1996.00440040134015

Huang, L., Li, F., Sheng, J., Xia, X., Ma, J., Zhan, M., et al. (2014). DrugComboRanker: drug combination discovery based on target network analysis. *Bioinformatics* 30, i228–i236. doi: 10.1093/bioinformatics/btu278

Hyde, J. E. (2007). Drug-resistant malaria–an insight. *FEBS J.* 274, 4688–4698. doi: 10.1111/j.1742-4658.2007.05999.x

Imwong, M., Hien, T. T., Thuy-Nhien, N. T., Dondorp, A. M., and White, N. J. (2017). Spread of a single multidrug resistant malaria parasite lineage (PfPailin) to Vietnam. *Lancet Infect. Dis.* 17, 1022–1023. doi: 10.1016/S1473-3099(17)30524-8

Jansen, G., Lee, A. Y., Epp, E., Fredette, A., Surprenant, J., Harcus, D., et al. (2009). Chemogenomic profiling predicts antifungal synergies. *Mol. Syst. Biol.* 5, 338. doi: 10.1038/msb.2009.95

KalantarMotamedi, Y., Eastman, R. T., Guha, R., and Bender, A. (2018). A systematic and prospectively validated approach for identifying synergistic drug combinations against malaria. *Malar. J.* 17, 160. doi: 10.1186/s12936-018-2294-5

Kauvar, L. M., Higgins, D. L., Villar, H. O., Sportsman, J. R., Engqvist-Goldstein, A., Bukar, R., et al. (1995). Predicting ligand binding to proteins by affinity fingerprinting. *Chem. Biol.* 2, 107–118. doi: 10.1016/1074-5521(95)90283-X

Kim, S., Thiessen, P. A., Bolton, E. E., Chen, J., Fu, G., Gindulyte, A., et al. (2016). PubChem substance and compound databases. *Nucleic Acids Res.* 44, D1202–D1213. doi: 10.1093/nar/gkv951

Lamb, J., Crawford, E. D., Peck, D., Modell, J. W., Blat, I. C., Wrobel, M. J., et al. (2006). The connectivity map: using gene-expression signatures to connect small molecules, genes, and disease. *Science* 313, 1929–1935. doi: 10.1126/science.1132939

Lehár, J., Krueger, A. S., Avery, W., Heilbut, A. M., Johansen, L. M., Price, E. R., et al. (2009). Synergistic drug combinations tend to improve therapeutically relevant selectivity. *Nat. Biotechnol.* 27, 659–666. doi: 10.1038/nbt.1549

Lehár, J., Zimmermann, G. R., Krueger, A. S., Molnar, R. A., Ledell, J. T., Heilbut, A. M., et al. (2007). Chemical combination effects predict connectivity in biological systems. *Mol. Syst. Biol.* 3:80. doi: 10.1038/msb4100116

Locher, C. P., Ruben, P. C., Gut, J., and Rosenthal, P. J. (2003). 5HT1A serotonin receptor agonists inhibit *Plasmodium falciparum* by blocking a membrane channel. *Antimicrob. Agents Chemother.* 47, 3806–3809. doi: 10.1128/AAC.47.12.3806-3809.2003

Mason, D. J., Stott, I., Ashenden, S., Weinstein, Z. B., Karakoc, I., Meral, S., et al. (2017). Prediction of antibiotic interactions using descriptors derived from molecular structure. *J. Med. Chem.* 60, 3902–3912. doi: 10.1021/acs.jmedchem.7b00204

Menden, M. P., Wang, D., Guan, Y., Mason, M., Szalai, B., Bulusu, K. C., et al. [Preprint] (2018). A Cancer Pharmacogenomic Screen Powering Crowd-Sourced Advancement of Drug Combination Prediction. *bioRxiv.* doi: 10.1101/200451.

Mervin, L. H., Afzal, A. M., Drakakis, G., Lewis, R., Engkvist, O., and Bender, A. (2015). Target prediction utilising negative bioactivity data covering large chemical space. *J. Cheminform.* 7:51. doi: 10.1186/s13321-015-0098-y

Mervin, L. H., Bulusu, K. C., Kalash, L., Afzal, A. M., Svensson, F., Firth, M. A., et al. (2018). Orthologue chemical space and its influence on target prediction. *Bioinformatics* 34, 72–79. doi: 10.1093/bioinformatics/btx525

Miller, M. L., Molinelli, E. J., Nair, J. S., Sheikh, T., Samy, R., Jing, X., et al. (2013). Drug synergy screen and network modeling in dedifferentiated liposarcoma

identifies CDK4 and IGF1R as synergistic drug targets. *Sci. Signal.* 6:ra85. doi: 10.1126/scisignal.2004014

Mita, T., and Tanabe, K. (2012). Evolution of *Plasmodium falciparum* drug resistance: implications for the development and containment of artemisinin resistance. *Jpn. J. Infect. Dis.* 65, 465–475. doi: 10.7883/yoken.65.465

Mott, B. T., Eastman, R. T., Guha, R., Sherlach, K. S., Siriwardana, A., Shinn, P., et al. (2015). High-throughput matrix screening identifies synergistic and antagonistic antimalarial drug combinations. *Sci. Rep.* 5:13891. doi: 10.1038/srep13891

Mutai, B. K., and Waitumbi, J. N. (2010). Apoptosis stalks *Plasmodium falciparum* maintained in continuous culture condition. *Malar. J.* 9 , S6. doi: 10.1186/1475-2875-9-S3-S6

Nelander, S., Wang, W., Nilsson, B., She, Q.-B., Pratilas, C., Rosen, N., et al. (2008). Models from experiments: combinatorial drug perturbations of cancer cells. *Mol. Syst. Biol.* 4, 216. doi: 10.1038/msb.2008.53

Paricharak, S., IJzerman, A. P., Bender, A., and Nigsch, F. (2016). Analysis of iterative screening with stepwise compound selection based on novartis in-house HTS data. *ACS Chem. Biol.* 11, 1255–1264. doi: 10.1021/acschembio.6b00029

Patel, K., Batty, K. T., Moore, B. R., Gibbons, P. L., and Kirkpatrick, C. M. (2014). Predicting the parasite killing effect of artemisinin combination therapy in a murine malaria model. *J. Antimicrob. Chemother.* 69, 2155–2163. doi: 10.1093/jac/dku120

Pathak, V., Colah, R., and Ghosh, K. (2015). Tyrosine kinase inhibitors: new class of antimalarials on the horizon? *Blood Cells. Mol. Dis.* 55, 119–126. doi: 10.1016/j.bcmd.2015.05.007

Pedregosa, F., Varoquaux, G., Gramfort, A., Michel, V., Thirion, B., Grisel, O., et al. (2011). Scikit-learn: machine learning in python. *J. Mach. Learn. Res.* 12, 2825–2830. Available online at: http://scikit-learn.org

Penna-Coutinho, J., Cortopassi, W. A., Oliveira, A. A., França, T. C. C., and Krettli, A. U. (2011). Antimalarial activity of potential inhibitors of *Plasmodium falciparum* lactate dehydrogenase enzyme selected by docking studies. *PLoS ONE* 6:e21237. doi: 10.1371/journal.pone.0021237

Petrone, P. M., Simms, B., Nigsch, F., Lounkine, E., Kutchukian, P., Cornett, A., et al. (2012). Rethinking molecular similarity: comparing compounds on the basis of biological activity. *ACS Chem. Biol.* 7, 1399–1409. doi: 10.1021/cb3001028

Reiling, S. J., and Rohrbach, P. (2015). Monitoring PfMDR1 transport in *Plasmodium falciparum*. *Malar. J.* 14:270. doi: 10.1186/s12936-015-0791-3

Riniker, S., Wang, Y., Jenkins, J. L., and Landrum, G. A. (2014). Using information from historical high-throughput screens to predict active compounds. *J. Chem. Inf. Model.* 54, 1880–1891. doi: 10.1021/ci500190p

Subramanian, A., Narayan, R., Corsello, S. M., Peck, D. D., Natoli, T. E., Lu, X., et al. (2017). A next generation connectivity map: L1000 platform and the first 1,000,000 profiles. *Cell* 171, 1437–1452.e17. doi: 10.1016/j.cell.2017.10.049

Subramanian, A., Tamayo, P., Mootha, V. K., Mukherjee, S., Ebert, B. L., Gillette, M. A., et al. (2005). Gene set enrichment analysis: a knowledge-based approach for interpreting genome-wide expression profiles. *Proc. Natl. Acad. Sci. U.S.A.* 102, 15545–15550. doi: 10.1073/pnas.0506580102

Sucher, N. J. (2014). Searching for synergy *in silico, in vitro* and *in vivo. Synergy* 1, 30–43. doi: 10.1016/j.synres.2014.07.004

Tatonetti, N. P., Ye, P. P., Daneshjou, R., and Altman, R. B. (2012). Data-driven prediction of drug effects and interactions. *Sci. Transl. Med.* 4, 125ra31. doi: 10.1126/scitranslmed.3003377

Tsigelny, I. F. (2018). Artificial intelligence in drug combination therapy. *Brief. Bioinform.* doi: 10.1093/bib/bby004. [Epub ahead of print].

Weinstein, Z. B., Bender, A., and Cokol, M. (2017). Prediction of synergistic drug combinations. *Curr. Opin. Syst. Biol.* 4, 24–28. doi: 10.1016/j.coisb.2017. 05.005

Weisman, J. L., Liou, A. P., Shelat, A. A., Cohen, F. E., Guy, R. K., and DeRisi, J. L. (2006). Searching for new antimalarial therapeutics amongst known drugs. *Chem. Biol. Drug Des.* 67, 409–416. doi: 10.1111/j.1747-0285.2006. 00391.x

Wildenhain, J., Spitzer, M., Dolma, S., Jarvik, N., White, R., Roy, M., et al. (2015). Prediction of synergism from chemical-genetic interactions by machine learning. *Cell Syst.* 1, 383–395. doi: 10.1016/j.cels.2015.12.003

Wishart, D. S., Knox, C., Guo, A. C., Shrivastava, S., Hassanali, M., Stothard, P., et al. (2006). DrugBank: a comprehensive resource for *in silico* drug discovery and exploration. *Nucleic Acids Res.* 34, D668–D672. doi: 10.1093/nar/gkj067

World Health Organisation (2015). *WHO-Guidelines for the Treatment of Malaria. 3rd Edn.* Geneva: World Health Organization.

World Health Organisation. (2017). *WHO-World Malaria Report 2017.* Geneva: World Health Organisation.

World Wide Antimalarial Resistance Network (2014). *ACT Partner Drug Molecular Surveyor: Mapping Resistance Marker Data.* Available online at: http://www.wwarn.org/molecular/surveyor/#0 (Accessed September 17, 2017).

Wu, Y., Cruz, L. N., Szestak, T., Laing, G., Molyneux, G. R., Garcia, C. R. S., et al. (2016). An external sensing system in plasmodium falciparum-infected erythrocytes. *Malar. J.* 15:103. doi: 10.1186/s12936-016-1144-6

Yilancioglu, K., Weinstein, Z. B., Meydan, C., Akhmetov, A., Toprak, I., Durmaz, A., et al. (2014). Target-independent prediction of drug synergies using only drug lipophilicity. *J. Chem. Inf. Model.* 54, 2286–2293. doi: 10.1021/ci500276x

Zhang, Y., Smolen, P., Baxter, D. A., and Byrne, J. H. (2014). Computational analyses of synergism in small molecular network motifs. *PLoS Comput. Biol.* 10:e1003524. doi: 10.1371/journal.pcbi.1003524

Molecular Connectivity Predefines Polypharmacology: Aliphatic Rings, Chirality and sp^3 Centers Enhance Target Selectivity

Stefania Monteleone, Julian E. Fuchs† and Klaus R. Liedl**

Institute of General, Inorganic and Theoretical Chemistry, Center of Molecular Biosciences, University of Innsbruck, Innsbruck, Austria

Correspondence:
Klaus R. Liedl
klaus.liedl@uibk.ac.at
Julian E. Fuchs
julian.fuchs@uibk.ac.at

Dark chemical matter compounds are small molecules that have been recently identified as highly potent and selective hits. For this reason, they constitute a promising class of possible candidates in the process of drug discovery and raise the interest of the scientific community. To this purpose, Wassermann et al. (2015) have described the application of 2D descriptors to characterize dark chemical matter. However, their definition was based on the number of reported positive assays rather than the number of known targets. As there might be multiple assays for one single target, the number of assays does not fully describe target selectivity. Here, we propose an alternative classification of active molecules that is based on the number of known targets. We cluster molecules in four classes: black, gray, and white compounds are active on one, two to four, and more than four targets respectively, whilst inactive compounds are found to be inactive in the considered assays. In this study, black and inactive compounds are found to have not only higher solubility, but also a higher number of chiral centers, sp^3 carbon atoms and aliphatic rings. On the contrary, white compounds contain a higher number of double bonds and fused aromatic rings. Therefore, the design of a screening compound library should consider these molecular properties in order to achieve target selectivity or polypharmacology. Furthermore, analysis of four main target classes (GPCRs, kinases, proteases, and ion channels) shows that GPCR ligands are more selective than the other classes, as the number of black compounds is higher in this target superfamily. On the other side, ligands that hit kinases, proteases, and ion channels bind to GPCRs more likely than to other target classes. Consequently, depending on the target protein family, appropriate screening libraries can be designed in order to minimize the likelihood of unwanted side effects early in the drug discovery process. Additionally, synergistic effects may be obtained by library design toward polypharmacology.

Keywords: dark chemical matter, drug discovery, molecular descriptors, stereochemistry, chemical properties, screening library design, off-targets, drug repurposing

INTRODUCTION

Drug discovery for a specific target is a long process that starts from hit finding: in the past high throughput screening (HTS) of huge compound libraries was the most common process in pharmaceutical companies. However, the chemical space that the HTS can reach is restricted to the molecules that were previously synthesized and included in the screened library. This certainly precludes the discovery of new compounds, as the chemical space is much wider and the use of limited knowledge makes the hit discovery challenging (Dobson, 2004; Reymond, 2015).

To overcome these disadvantages, computational techniques can be applied in order to speed up the process of drug design and to perform *de novo* drug design. One of the most popular methods is virtual screening, that is the identification of possible candidates for assays by considering their molecular properties (ligand-based) and/or their interactions with the macromolecular binding partner (typically a protein) when its structure is available (structure-based) (Kirchmair et al., 2009; von Grafenstein et al., 2014; Kaserer et al., 2015; Vuorinen and Schuster, 2015). Different virtual compound libraries can be designed, depending on the target properties and on the desired pharmacokinetics (Lionta et al., 2014). Therefore, fragment-based and relatively small focused libraries have found great success: a wider chemical space is covered by virtually assembling many different building blocks as in combinatorial synthesis (Chevillard and Kolb, 2015; Reymond, 2015) or by building compounds directly starting from the structure complex with the first fragment (Srinivas Reddy et al., 2013).

Furthermore, virtual libraries can be properly designed in order to identify active compounds, which also exhibit suitable ADMET (absorption, distribution, metabolism, excretion, and toxicity) properties (Gleeson, 2008). The Lipinski's rule of five (Lipinski, 2004) helps in identifying orally active compounds, but does not fully describe all facets of druggability. For instance, today the *in silico* assessment of molecular toxicity is still challenging (Roncaglioni et al., 2013; Raies and Bajic, 2016), but at the same time necessary to establish early and *in silico* if a molecule could cause toxic side effects, rather than in the later preclinical phase by experimental assays, which are expensive and time consuming (Peters et al., 2012). On one side, it is undoubted that side effects take place when a molecule is active on multiple targets and, hence, by definition promiscuous (Wang and Greene, 2012). On the other side, promiscuity can represent also an advantage, where the goal of the drug development is to obtain a polypharmacological effect, especially in the treatment of diseases that involve multiple targets (Anighoro et al., 2014; Rastelli and Pinzi, 2015).

To this purpose, the computation of molecular properties has been established not only to discriminate between inactive and active, weak and potent compounds, but also between promiscuous and selective ligands. For instance, Lovering et al. (2009) showed that target selectivity increases with the number of chiral centers and with higher molecular complexity, described as fraction of carbon sp^3 atoms. Moreover, the presence of amines and high clogP values negatively affect target selectivity (Lovering, 2013). Indeed, many promiscuous compounds are positively charged at physiological pH, as emerged also from the analysis of a Roche dataset (Peters et al., 2009).

With the recent identification of "dark chemical matter" (DCM) as promising starting point for drug discovery (Macarron, 2015; Wassermann et al., 2015), chemical properties of this potentially highly selective compound species are in the focus of interest. Wassermann et al. (2015) use descriptors based on the two-dimensional (2D) compound structures and describe subtle shifts in their distributions toward higher solubility (logS), lower hydrophobicity (logP), smaller molecular weight (MW) and lower amount of rings for DCM versus compounds that are frequently active in HTS assays (Wassermann et al., 2015). They define DCM as molecules that are inactive in at least 100 assays, presuming that these compounds would hit only few possible targets. However, there are compounds, which are listed as DCM, but they are active on many different targets. For example, CID1048281 (Supplementary Figure 1) is considered DCM because it is inactive in more than 650 assays, but it is also active in other six assays in PubChem, which test the activity on unrelated targets (RAR-related orphan receptor gamma, aldehyde dehydrogenase, tyrosyl-DNA phosphodiesterase, ATPase, bromodomain adjacent to zinc finger domain and shiga toxin).

On the other side, many assays may be available for the same target and the number of negative test outcomes does not necessarily correctly depict target selectivity. For example, there are 245 small-molecule bioassays reported on PubChem for the adrenoreceptor beta 1 and more than 350 for the beta 2 subtype. Moreover, most of these bioassays are not specific for a receptor subtype or are simply confirmatory. In order to overcome this pitfall, Wassermann et al. (2015) filtered the set of bioassays by removing redundant readouts for the same target.

As shown, it is extremely hard to determine the target selectivity of a molecule solely on the base of its assay positive or negative outcomes. For this reason, we propose an alternative classification of active molecules, on the base of the number of targets they hit, in order to investigate target selectivity and/or polypharmacology in the early phase of the drug discovery process. In detail, we distinguish between molecules that are selective toward one single protein and other compounds that are active on multiple targets. In this way, it is possible to identify which molecular properties enhance target selectivity and which protein families are likely to constitute off-targets.

MATERIALS AND METHODS

Ligand Dataset Retrieval

We extracted the set of 139,352 DCM compounds from Novartis and PubChem (Kim et al., 2015) as InChi (IUPAC International Chemical Identifier) from the Supporting Information of Wassermann et al. (2015) and downloaded the 3D coordinates of 139,328 molecules from the PubChem Compound database (Kim et al., 2016).

The set of active compounds was extracted from PubChem BioAssay (Wang et al., 2017) using the list of 459 bioassays provided by Wassermann et al. (2015). Active compounds (256,448) were extracted via their compound identifiers (CIDs), downloaded as 3D coordinates (237,510) and pooled to a single set of 376,838 compounds.

Furthermore, we performed a filtering step to remove duplicates within the dataset. To this purpose we used the RDKit (RDKit, 2015) chemoinformatics toolkit. Moreover, we removed the compounds that were active but without any specified targets (14,464). Our final dataset included 341,599 molecules.

Computation of Molecular Descriptors

The PubChem coordinate files contained already precomputed 2D descriptors, including MW, number of heavy atoms, defined and undefined stereocenters, H-bond donors and acceptors, which were considered for our analysis as provided.

Additionally, we calculated logS (Hou et al., 2004) and $logP_{(o/w)}$ using the MOE (Molecular Operating Environment, version 2015.1001) (MOE, 2016) molecular descriptor tools and the atomic geometries with MOE's Scientific Vector Language (SVL) function "aGeometry" together with the SMARTS matching function "sm_MatchAll." In detail, aGeometry returns the hybridization of an atom and sm_MatchAll searches for specific SMARTS patterns, which we used to count non-ring and non-terminal carbon atoms. For instance, sp^3 carbon atoms are counted by matching "CH_2" SMARTS codes. In order to restrict the count to non-ring and non-terminal atoms, we specified "!r" and "!H3" respectively.

Furthermore, we used RDKit (RDKit, 2015) to count the number of single and fused aromatic and aliphatic rings as well as the number of carbon–carbon and carbon–nitrogen double bonds based on SMILES codes.

Statistical analysis, including the two-sided Wilcoxon rank-sum test and Kolmogorov–Smirnov test, was performed using R (R Development Core Team, 2010) (Supplementary Tables 2–4).

Target Retrieval and Analysis

Assay and target information for all compounds have been retrieved from the PubChem database by querying the compounds identifiers (CID) against the assay summary webpage. Active targets with specified gene id were considered for Uniprot (Bateman et al., 2015; The UniProt Consortium, 2017) retrieval, in order to convert the gene id to the associated protein's Uniprot accession number.

We assigned the protein superfamily for every target, by searching Uniprot accession numbers into lists of GPCRs, kinases, proteases, and ion channels. We obtained the lists of 3,092 GPCRs, 1,365 kinases and 11,606 proteases from Uniprot, and the list of 899 ion channels from ChEMBL (Bento et al., 2014) and IUPHAR/BPS Guide to Pharmacology (Southan et al., 2016).

We counted the number of targets on which a molecule is found to be active and clustered active ligands in three classes: black compounds are active only on one single target, gray compounds are active on two to four targets and white compounds are active on more than four targets. We defined these cut-off values in order to obtain a comparable number of molecules in every subset: 73,383 black, 103,025 gray, 87,303 white, 77,888 inactive compounds (compound set provided via SI).

Figures are generated by using MATLAB (MATLAB, 2012), R (R Development Core Team, 2010) and ChemDraw (PerkinElmer Informatics, 1998–2015).

RESULTS

Molecular Descriptors

We analyzed the distributions of 2D molecular descriptors within the compound sets (inactive, black, gray, and white). We find that chirality enhances target selectivity. For instance, molecules become more selective if they present at least one chiral center: inactive and black compounds contain a higher number of defined R/S stereocenters with respect to white molecules (**Figure 1A**). On the contrary, the absence of a chiral center enhances promiscuity, as described by the percentage of white molecules (~79% versus ~62% in black ones) (Supplementary Table 1).

On the opposite, if at least a carbon–carbon or carbon–nitrogen double bond is present, molecules tend to be white and, hence, more promiscuous (**Figure 1B**). Otherwise, if they do not have any double bonds, they tend to be inactive or black (~85% versus ~69% in white ones) (Supplementary Table 1).

These findings are also confirmed by the analysis of atomic geometries: non-ring and non-terminal sp^3 carbon atoms enhance selectivity (**Figure 1C**); about 42% of white compounds do not include any sp^3 carbon atoms, with respect to ~27% of inactive and black ones (Supplementary Table 1).

We also computed the molecular descriptors that were reported by Wassermann et al. (2015). However, our results show that the MW is not able to properly describe target selectivity: indeed, black compounds do not follow the expected trend, as they show MWs which are comparable to those of white molecules (**Figure 1D**). This finding disagrees with Wassermann et al. (2015), because our dataset does not include all molecules that were considered in the Novartis analysis, but only those that were reported in the publication. As this descriptor appears dataset dependent, we discarded it.

Additionally, the number of rings differs between these classes: black compounds exhibit higher numbers of aliphatic rings (~36% of black molecules have one aliphatic ring, with respect to 30% of white ones) (**Figure 1E**). By contrast, white compounds show higher numbers of fused aromatic rings (~35% with respect to 26% of inactive molecules) (**Figure 1F**). Indeed, more than half of the selective molecules has at least one aliphatic ring (~53% of inactive and ~51% of black compounds) and no fused aromatic rings (~71 of inactive and 62% of black compounds).

Furthermore, inactive and black compounds exhibit higher values of logS compared to gray and white compounds, especially for logS in the range between −2 and −4 (**Figure 2A**). By contrast, the opposite trend is observed for lower solubility: half of white molecules shows a logS value lower than −5, whereas only 20% of inactive and ~30% of black compounds have similar solubility (Supplementary Table 1).

Consequently, lipophilicity increases with the number of targets: gray and white molecules show higher SlogP values than inactive and black ones (**Figure 2B**). For instance, ~36% of white compounds show SlogP values that are higher than 4, whereas selective molecules (~33% of inactive and ~29% of black compounds) exhibit SlogP values which are in the range between 2 and 3.

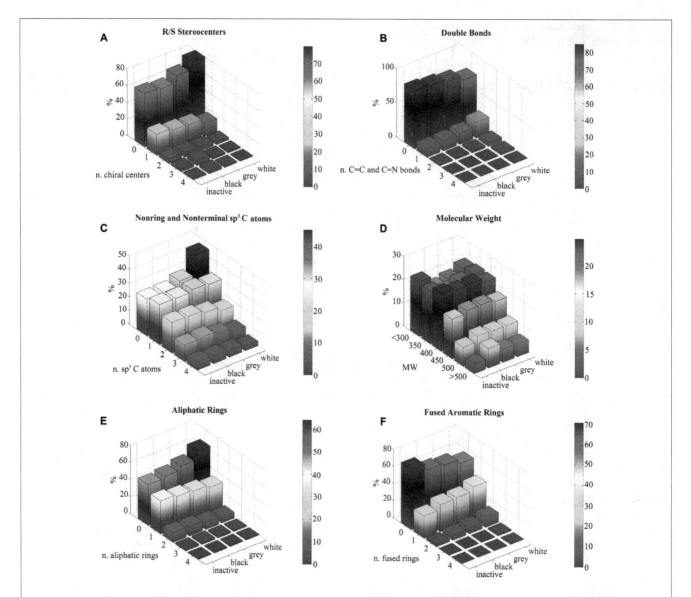

FIGURE 1 | Statistical analysis of molecular descriptors per ligand class (inactive, black, gray, and white). Data are represented as 3D bar plots, colored according to the percentage values for each subset (see color bar). **(A)** The number of R/S stereocenters per molecule shows that most of white compounds have no chiral centers, whereas inactive molecules show the highest percentage of compounds with one stereocenter. **(B)** The number of carbon–carbon or carbon–nitrogen double bonds is higher for white ligands compared to the other classes, which normally have none. **(C)** Inactive and black sets exhibit higher content of non-ring and non-terminal sp^3 carbon atoms with respect to white compounds, which tend to be sp^2 hybridized. **(D)** The molecular weight (MW) is similar for all subsets in the range 300–500 Da, but shows different results for smaller and higher values. Indeed, inactive and white compounds exhibit higher percentages for values lower than 300 Da, with respect to black and gray sets. On the contrary, black compounds can be rather complex structures as their MW can be higher than 500 Da. The MW axis is divided into different ranges and its labels represent the highest boundary. For instance, "350" indicates compounds with MW values between 300 and 350. **(E)** Most of white molecules have no aliphatic rings, which characterize instead inactive and black datasets. **(F)** In contrast, a higher number of fused aromatic rings is a chemical feature of white molecules.

Calculating these molecular descriptors, it is possible to predict which building blocks characterize black compounds and, therefore, can be used for synthesis of new selective drug candidates.

Target Analysis

Our dataset includes ligands that bind to a variety of targets, 2,715 in total. For instance, 10.98% of the targets are represented by G-protein coupled receptors (GPCRs), 13.41% by kinases, 10.68%

by ion channels and 5.78% by proteases (**Figure 3**). About 60% of the targets comprise other enzymes, receptors or transcription factors that do not fall into these four major target classes.

G-protein coupled receptor ligands are more selective than other classes, as the number of black compounds is higher (14.30%) with respect to other targets (5.80% ion channels, 6.25% ion channels, 9.21% kinases) (**Figure 4**). For example, CID 2983576 is a ligand that binds to the human cholinergic muscarinic receptor 4 and is inactive toward other muscarinic

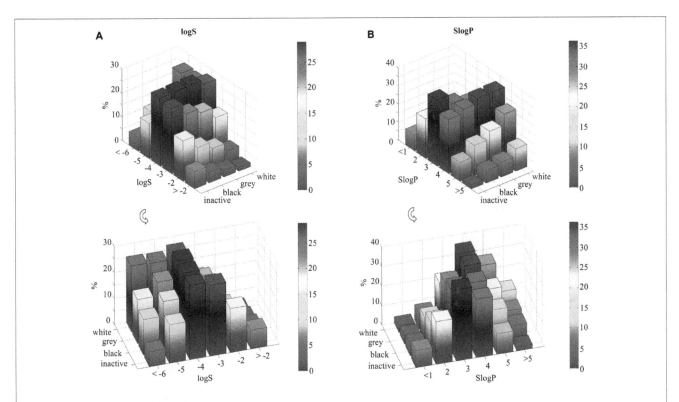

FIGURE 2 | Statistical analysis of molecular solubility (logS) and hydrophobicity (SlogP) per ligand class (inactive, black, gray, and white). Data are represented as 3D bar plots, colored according to the percentage values for each subset (see color bar). The logS and SlogP axes are divided into different ranges and labels represent the highest boundary of each range. (A) Molecular solubility, reported as logS, is higher for inactive and black compounds for values higher than −4. Whereas white compounds have logS values lower than −4. (B) White compounds show SlogP values higher than 4. In contrast, inactive and black molecules have values lower than 4.

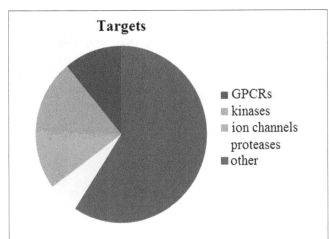

FIGURE 3 | Statistical analysis of targets that are present in the entire dataset. In total, we identified 2,715 different targets. GPCRs represent 10.98%, kinases 13.41%, ion channels 10.68%, and proteases 5.78%. Other targets include further enzymes, nuclear receptors, and transcription factors.

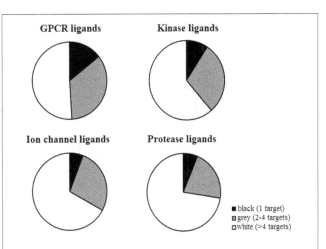

FIGURE 4 | Distribution of black, gray, and white compounds in every target class. The number of black compounds is higher for GPCR ligands (14.30%) compared to other targets (5.80% ion channels, 6.25% ion channels, 9.21% kinases). In contrast, ion channels and proteases have higher percentages of white molecules.

receptor subtypes (**Figure 5**). As many other black compounds, it contains a chiral center, an aliphatic ring, several non-ring and non-terminal sp^3 carbon atoms (5) and has a low logP value (2.2).

Ligands that bind to ion channels and proteases tend to be more promiscuous (**Figure 4**). This is particularly pronounced for proteases, where 62% of ligands can bind to more than four non-protease targets (**Figure 6**). For example, CID 646260 is active on caspase 3 and other non-protease targets, such as GPCRs and other enzymes.

In contrast, only 37% of GPCR ligands binds to other proteins beyond GPCRs. For instance, only 13% of GPCR ligands bind to kinases, 16% to proteases and 24% to ion channels.[1]

Instead, kinase ligands are able to bind to many non-kinase targets. For example, compound CID 1005278 binds not only to kinases (such as RIPK), but also to potassium channels (such as KCNQ1), dopamine receptors (D1 and D3), proteases and other non-kinase targets. However, analysis of intra-class activity shows that kinase ligands in general bind only to one kinase (for example, CID 2283311 is a black molecule that is active only on MAP3K3). This evidence is surprising, as kinases are known to be promiscuous, especially toward other kinases (Davis et al., 2011). However, the number of kinase ligands in our dataset is relatively small (27,935) and we might miss information from unselective ligands that were not included in the analysis.

Furthermore, ion channel, protease and kinase ligands exhibit higher chances to bind to GPCRs: almost half of ion channel (49%), 36.6% of protease and 35% of kinase ligands bind to GPCRs as well. However, this trend cannot be observed for proteases, kinases or ion channels, as they exhibit lower probabilities to bind to these target classes (Supplementary Figure 2).

DISCUSSION

The escape from flatland has already been described as a valuable approach to improve clinical success (Lovering et al., 2009) and the unique activity profiles of highly potent and selective molecules might be the underlying principle. It is chemically intuitive that more complex molecular shapes restrict the diversity of binding partners and provide selectivity gains (Mendez-Lucio and Medina-Franco, 2017). A criterion favoring complex 3D shapes, with chiral centers and high sp^3 carbon contents, low number of double bonds and fused aromatic rings, in candidate molecules might complement widely accepted criteria for drug-likeness solely based on 2D molecular properties, like solubility and MW (Lipinski, 2004; Leeson and Springthorpe, 2007).

We also believe that these molecular properties highly affect the target selectivity. Indeed, already Lovering et al. (2009) stated that the degree of saturation is able to distinguish marketed drugs from drug-like molecules. In detail, compounds that have success through clinical trials are characterized by increased saturation and the presence of chiral centers. For instance, our findings confirm that the sp^3 conformation is a key feature to obtain target selectivity and in turn to improve clinical success in the process of drug development.

These molecular descriptors, together with solubility and lipophilicity, may be readily applied as an additional selection criterion for promising starting points in early stage drug discovery. Wassermann et al. (2015) have shown DCM is more soluble than active molecules. Our results are in agreement with their findings, as selective compounds are more soluble than promiscuous ones.

In contrast, MW does not properly distinguish between inactive and white molecules as shown in other datasets. For

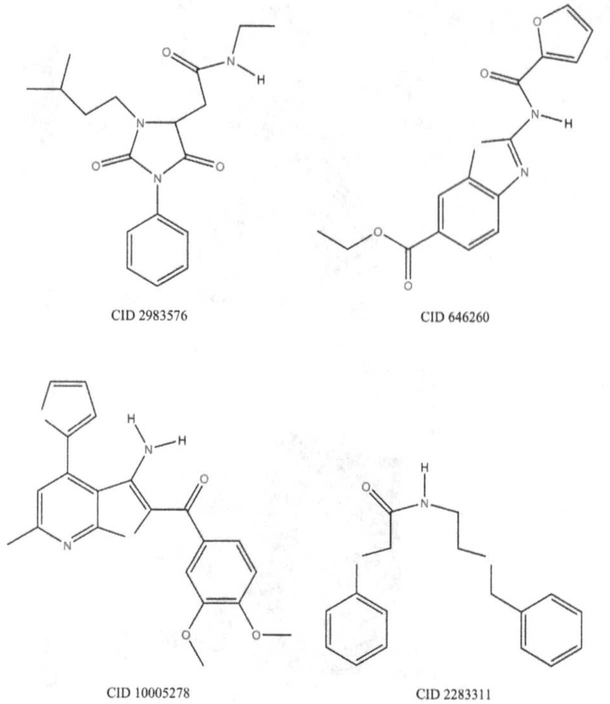

FIGURE 5 | Ligands that represent the dataset. Compounds are labeled according to the compound identifier (CID) from PubChem. CID 2983576 is a selective GPCR ligand: its absolute stereochemistry is undefined in PubChem and, hence, not shown here. CID 646260 is a protease ligand, which binds also to other non-protease targets. CID 1005278 is a kinase ligand that binds also to other non-kinase targets. CID 2283311 is a selective kinase ligand that is active only on one target.

instance, promiscuity is enhanced by lower values of MW in a dataset from Pfizer (Hopkins et al., 2006), but higher values in datasets from Novartis (Azzaoui et al., 2007), Roche (Peters et al., 2009) and Boehringer Ingelheim (Muegge and Mukherjee, 2016).

We also considered further molecular descriptors, such as the number of hydrogen bond donors and acceptors, but they do not allow to distinguish between selective and promiscuous compounds (Supplementary Table 1), as also shown by Novartis (Azzaoui et al., 2007) and Roche (Peters et al., 2009).

In our dataset many ligands are promiscuous and, hence, can effectively hit off-targets, which are represented by all other targets that a molecule can bind besides the intended target (Rudmann, 2013).

However, in our dataset GPCR ligands are highly selective. This evidence appears to be in contrast to previous knowledge, as GPCRs are known to be promiscuous targets, especially if their ligands are not peptidic or small molecules (Paolini et al., 2006). For instance, our results may change by considering specialized datasets, such as PDSP Ki database (Roth et al., 2000).

Additionally, our analysis shows that ligands from other target protein families can easily bind GPCRs. Indeed, there are great overlaps between all four target classes that we considered (Supplementary Figure 2) and we do not know if these molecules were developed firstly as GPCR ligands or not.

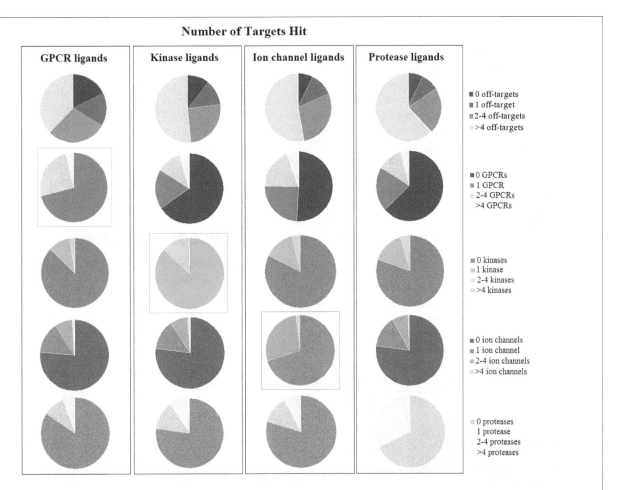

FIGURE 6 | Number of targets hit by every ligand class (GPCRs, kinases, ion channels, and proteases). The first row shows if ligands can hit other targets that are not included in their own target class: for instance, GPCR ligands might hit only GPCRs (indicated as "0 off-targets") or also other non-GPCR targets (larger number of off-targets). The following rows of pie charts show the number of ligands that hit a specific target class: for instance, GPCR ligands hit at least one GPCR, whereas kinase or ion channel or protease ligands can hit GPCRs or not (indicated as "0 GPCRs"). The same is shown for all four target classes. Intra-class selectivity is highlighted by colored boxes around the pie charts.

The identification of a GPCR as off-target is extremely important, as the activity on specific GPCRs is also related to severe side effects, e.g., cardiovascular diseases. Indeed, 5-HT2B has been identified as cause of valvulopathy and led to the withdrawal of drugs from the market (Huang et al., 2009).

Our results show that protease ligands can bind to many off-targets: indeed, it can be difficult to achieve target selectivity within related proteases (Drag and Salvesen, 2010) but strategies to rationally improve the selectivity profiles of protease inhibitors based on substrate peptide data and experimental 3D structures have been described (Fuchs et al., 2013).

In our dataset, kinase ligands seem to be selective toward only one kinase member rather than to more targets in the same protein family. However, this unexpected outcome can be explained by the relatively low amount of kinases ligands that is present in the dataset. Kinase ligands are indeed generally known to be promiscuous, but some of them exhibit higher selectivity, especially if they bind to the pocket close to the ATP site and prefer a specific conformation of the activation loop (Davis

et al., 2011). Moreover, in our dataset we identify even more pronounced polypharmacology within and between other target classes. For instance, ion channel ligands overlap with GPCR ligands, as they frequently exhibit a common ligand scaffold, which includes an amine linked to an aromatic ring by an alkylic chain that is present in benzodiazepines or dihydropyridines. In addition, ion channels constitute a common off-target, causing cardiac adverse effects. Indeed, hERG potassium channels are responsible of arrhythmias, in particular torsades de pointes, and many antipsychotics and other drugs bind to these channels as off-targets, increasing the risk of cardiovascular diseases (Silvestre and Prous, 2007). As example, the antihistaminic terfenadine was withdrawn from the market for its toxic adverse effect, that was caused by this off-target activity (Monahan et al., 1990).

This analysis bring us to ask if we can identify likely off-targets in the early discovery process. Normally, in the

early steps, target selectivity is considered only among related targets, which are proteins that belong to the same protein early steps, target selectivity is considered only among related targets, which are proteins that belong to the same protein family, since high structure and ligand similarity is expected. In this case, target selectivity can be rationalized, e.g., via X-ray structures of targets and off-targets. However, several adverse side effects are caused by distant or nearly unrelated targets. For this reason, the prediction of ligand binding is still challenging and the use of cheminformatics tools can guide the medicinal chemists in identifying the chemical features that typically cause promiscuity (Besnard et al., 2012). Nevertheless, the training of virtual screening models is limited by the use of biased ligand sets. Indeed, our analysis show that results highly depend on the selected dataset, which affected the distribution of the physico-chemical properties and target classes. Therefore we expect that based on the desired target, specialized datasets can be used to further improve the performance of *in silico* models.

In particular, screening libraries can be properly designed by taking into account molecular properties, such as stereochemistry, atomic geometries and rings, besides solubility and lipophilicity. Many predesigned compound libraries are already freely available online and could be easily filtered or prioritized by using these 2D descriptors, without the need of applying a time consuming and computationally demanding generation of 3D conformers.

CONCLUSION

A good starting point for the design of a selective drug should favor aliphatic over aromatic rings, alkylic chains containing sp^3 carbon atoms over double bonds, and stereocenters over achiral atoms. Even though the introduction of chiral centers can make the synthesis more challenging, the gain in target selectivity may be considerable.

On the other hand, polypharmacology could be achieved by introducing flat chemical moieties, such as fused aromatic rings and double bonds. However, this could bring not only additional desired, but also undesired side effects.

AUTHOR CONTRIBUTIONS

SM and JF performed the research. SM, JF, and KL designed the study and contributed to the preparation of the manuscript.

FUNDING

The research of the manuscript was supported by funding of the Austrian Science Fund FWF with respect to the project "Targeting Influenza Neuraminidase" (P23051).

REFERENCES

Anighoro, A., Bajorath, J., and Rastelli, G. (2014). Polypharmacology: challenges and opportunities in drug discovery. *J. Med. Chem.* 57, 7874–7887. doi: 10.1021/jm5006463

Azzaoui, K., Hamon, J., Faller, B., Whitebread, S., Jacoby, E., Bender, A., et al. (2007). Modeling promiscuity based on in vitro safety pharmacology profiling data. *Chemmedchem* 2, 874–880. doi: 10.1002/cmdc.200700036

Bateman, A., Martin, M. J., O'donovan, C., Magrane, M., Apweiler, R., Alpi, E., et al. (2015). UniProt: a hub for protein information. *Nucleic Acids Res.* 43, D204–D212. doi: 10.1093/nar/gku989

Bento, A. P., Gaulton, A., Hersey, A., Bellis, L. J., Chambers, J., Davies, M., et al. (2014). The ChEMBL bioactivity database: an update. *Nucleic Acids Res.* 42, D1083–D1090. doi: 10.1093/nar/gkt1031

Besnard, J., Ruda, G. F., Setola, V., Abecassis, K., Rodriguiz, R. M., Huang, X. P., et al. (2012). Automated design of ligands to polypharmacological profiles. *Nature* 492, 215–220. doi: 10.1038/nature11691

Chevillard, F., and Kolb, P. (2015). SCUBIDOO: a large yet screenable and easily searchable database of computationally created chemical compounds optimized toward high likelihood of synthetic tractability. *J. Chem. Inform. Model.* 55, 1824–1835. doi: 10.1021/acs.jcim.5b00203

Davis, M. I., Hunt, J. P., Herrgard, S., Ciceri, P., Wodicka, L. M., Pallares, G., et al. (2011). Comprehensive analysis of kinase inhibitor selectivity. *Nat. Biotechnol.* 29, 1046–U1124. doi: 10.1038/nbt.1990

Dobson, C. M. (2004). Chemical space and biology. *Nature* 432, 824–828. doi: 10.1038/nature03192

Drag, M., and Salvesen, G. S. (2010). Emerging principles in protease-based drug discovery. *Nat. Rev. Drug Discov.* 9, 690–701. doi: 10.1038/nrd3053

Fuchs, J. E., Von Grafenstein, S., Huber, R. G., Kramer, C., and Liedl, K. R. (2013). Substrate-driven mapping of the degradome by comparison of sequence logos. *PLoS Comput. Biol.* 9:e1003353. doi: 10.1371/journal.pcbi.1003353

Gleeson, M. P. (2008). Generation of a set of simple, interpretable ADMET rules of thumb. *J. Med. Chem.* 51, 817–834. doi: 10.1021/jm701122q

Hopkins, A. L., Mason, J. S., and Overington, J. P. (2006). Can we rationally design promiscuous drugs? *Curr. Opin. Struct. Biol.* 16, 127–136. doi: 10.1016/j.sbi.2006.01.013

Hou, T. J., Xia, K., Zhang, W., and Xu, X. J. (2004). ADME evaluation in drug discovery. 4. Prediction of aqueous solubility based on atom contribution approach. *J. Chem. Inf. Comput. Sci.* 44, 266–275. doi: 10.1021/ci034184n

Huang, X. P., Setola, V., Yadav, P. N., Allen, J. A., Rogan, S. C., Hanson, B. J., et al. (2009). Parallel functional activity profiling reveals valvulopathogens are potent 5-hydroxytryptamine(2B) receptor agonists: implications for drug safety assessment. *Mol. Pharmacol.* 76, 710–722. doi: 10.1124/mol.109.058057

Kaserer, T., Beck, K. R., Akram, M., Odermatt, A., and Schuster, D. (2015). Pharmacophore models and pharmacophore-based virtual screening: concepts and applications exemplified on hydroxysteroid dehydrogenases. *Molecules* 20, 22799–22832. doi: 10.3390/molecules201219880

Kim, S., Thiessen, P. A., Bolton, E. E., and Bryant, S. H. (2015). PUG-SOAP and PUG-REST: web services for programmatic access to chemical information in PubChem. *Nucleic Acids Res.* 43, W605–W611. doi: 10.1093/nar/gkv396

Kim, S., Thiessen, P. A., Bolton, E. E., Chen, J., Fu, G., Gindulyte, A., et al. (2016). PubChem substance and compound databases. *Nucleic Acids Res.* 44, D1202–D1213. doi: 10.1093/nar/gkv951

Kirchmair, J., Distinto, S., Markt, P., Schuster, D., Spitzer, G. M., Liedl, K. R., et al. (2009). How to optimize shape-based virtual screening: choosing the right query and including chemical information. *J. Chem. Inform. Model.* 49, 678–692. doi: 10.1021/ci8004226

Leeson, P. D., and Springthorpe, B. (2007). The influence of drug-like concepts on decision-making in medicinal chemistry. *Nat. Rev. Drug Discov.* 6, 881–890. doi: 10.1038/nrd2445

Lionta, E., Spyrou, G., Vassilatis, D. K., and Cournia, Z. (2014). Structure-based virtual screening for drug discovery: principles, applications and recent advances. *Curr. Top. Med. Chem.* 14, 1923–1938. doi: 10.2174/1568026614666140929124445

Lipinski, C. A. (2004). Lead- and drug-like compounds: the rule-of-five revolution. *Drug Discov. Today Technol.* 1, 337–341. doi: 10.1016/j.ddtec.2004.11.007

Lovering, F. (2013). Escape from Flatland 2: complexity and promiscuity. *Medchemcomm* 4, 515–519. doi: 10.1039/c2md20347b

Lovering, F., Bikker, J., and Humblet, C. (2009). Escape from Flatland: increasing saturation as an approach to improving clinical success. *J. Med. Chem.* 52, 6752–6756. doi: 10.1021/jm901241e

Macarron, R. (2015). Chemical libraries: how dark is HTS dark matter? *Nat. Chem. Biol.* 11, 904–905. doi: 10.1038/nchembio.1937

MATLAB (2012). *Matlab R2012a*. Natick, MA: The MathWorks Inc.

Mendez-Lucio, O., and Medina-Franco, J. L. (2017). The many roles of molecular complexity in drug discovery. *Drug Discov. Today* 22, 120–126. doi: 10.1016/j.drudis.2016.08.009

MOE (2016). *Molecular Operating Environment, 2015.1001*. Montreal, QC: Chemical Computing Group Inc.

Monahan, B. P., Ferguson, C. L., Killeavy, E. S., Lloyd, B. K., Troy, J., and Cantilena, L. R. (1990). Torsades-de-pointes occurring in association with terfenadine use. *JAMA* 264, 2788–2790. doi: 10.1001/jama.1990.03450210088038

Muegge, I., and Mukherjee, P. (2016). Performance of dark chemical matter in high throughput screening. *J. Med. Chem.* 59, 9806–9813. doi: 10.1021/acs.jmedchem.6b01038

Paolini, G. V., Shapland, R. H. B., Van Hoorn, W. P., Mason, J. S., and Hopkins, A. L. (2006). Global mapping of pharmacological space. *Nat. Biotechnol.* 24, 805–815. doi: 10.1038/nbt1228

PerkinElmer Informatics (1998–2015). *ChemDraw 15.0*. Available at: http://media.cambridgesoft.com/support/15/ChemDrawHelp.pdf

Peters, J. U., Hert, J., Bissantz, C., Hillebrecht, A., Gerebtzoff, G., Bendels, S., et al. (2012). Can we discover pharmacological promiscuity early in the drug discovery process? *Drug Disc. Today* 17, 325–335. doi: 10.1016/j.drudis.2012.01.001

Peters, J. U., Schnider, P., Mattei, P., and Kansy, M. (2009). Pharmacological promiscuity: dependence on compound properties and target specificity in a set of recent roche compounds. *Chemmedchem* 4, 680–686. doi: 10.1002/cmdc.200800411

R Development Core Team (2010). *R: A Language and Environment for Statistical Computing*, 3.2.2 Edn. Vienna: R Foundation for Statistical Computing.

Raies, A. B., and Bajic, V. B. (2016). In silico toxicology: computational methods for the prediction of chemical toxicity. *Wiley Interdiscip. Rev. Comput. Mol. Sci.* 6, 147–172. doi: 10.1002/wcms.1240

Rastelli, G., and Pinzi, L. (2015). Computational polypharmacology comes of age. *Front. Pharmacol.* 6:157. doi: 10.3389/fphar.2015.00157

RDKit (2015). *RDKit: Open-Source Chemoinformatics, 2015.03.1*. Available at: www.rdkit.org

Reymond, J. L. (2015). The chemical space project. *Acc. Chem. Res.* 48, 722–730. doi: 10.1021/ar500432k

Roncaglioni, A., Toropov, A. A., Toropova, A. P., and Benfenati, E. (2013). In silico methods to predict drug toxicity. *Curr. Opin. Pharmacol.* 13, 802–806. doi: 10.1016/j.coph.2013.06.001

Roth, B. L., Lopez, E., Patel, S., and Kroeze, W. K. (2000). The multiplicity of serotonin receptors: uselessly diverse molecules or an embarrassment of riches? *Neuroscientist* 6, 252–262. doi: 10.1177/107385840000600408

Rudmann, D. G. (2013). On-target and off-target-based toxicologic effects. *Toxicol. Pathol.* 41, 310–314. doi: 10.1177/0192623312464311

Silvestre, J. S., and Prous, J. R. (2007). Comparative evaluation of hERG potassium channel blockade by antipsychotics. *Methods Find. Exp. Clin. Pharmacol.* 29, 457–465. doi: 10.1358/mf.2007.29.7.1119172

Southan, C., Sharman, J. L., Benson, H. E., Faccenda, E., Pawson, A. J., Alexander, S. P. H., et al. (2016). Y The IUPHAR/BPS Guide to PHARMACOLOGY in 2016: towards curated quantitative interactions between 1300 protein targets and 6000 ligands. *Nucleic Acids Res.* 44, D1054–D1068. doi: 10.1093/nar/gkv1037

Srinivas Reddy, A., Chen, L., and Zhang, S. (2013). "Structure-based de novo drug design," in *De Novo Molecular Design*, ed. G. Schneider (Weinheim: Wiley-VCH Verlag GmbH & Co. KGaA).

The UniProt Consortium (2017). UniProt: the universal protein knowledgebase. *Nucleic Acids Res.* 45, D158–D169. doi: 10.1093/nar/gkw1099

von Grafenstein, S., Fuchs, J. E., and Liedl, K. R. (2014). "How to profit from molecular dynamics-based ensemble docking," in *Application of Computational*

Techniques in Pharmacy and Medicine, eds L. Gorb, V. Kuz'min, and E. Muratov (Dordrecht: Springer), 501–538.

Vuorinen, A., and Schuster, D. (2015). Methods for generating and applying pharmacophore models as virtual screening filters and for bioactivity profiling. *Methods* 71, 113–134. doi: 10.1016/j.ymeth.2014.10.013

Wang, X. Y., and Greene, N. (2012). Comparing measures of promiscuity and exploring their relationship to toxicity. *Mol. Inform.* 31, 145–159. doi: 10.1002/minf.201100148

Wang, Y., Bryant, S. H., Cheng, T., Wang, J., Gindulyte, A., Shoemaker, B. A., et al. (2017). PubChem BioAssay: 2017 update. *Nucleic Acids Res.* 45, D955–D963. doi: 10.1093/nar/gkw1118

Wassermann, A. M., Lounkine, E., Hoepfner, D., Le Goff, G., King, F. J., Studer, C., et al. (2015). Dark chemical matter as a promising starting point for drug lead discovery. *Nat. Chem. Biol.* 11, 958–966. doi: 10.1038/nchembio.1936

In Silico Discovery of Plant-Origin Natural Product Inhibitors of Tumor Necrosis Factor (TNF) and Receptor Activator of NF-κB Ligand (RANKL)

Georgia Melagraki[1], Evangelos Ntougkos[2], Dimitra Papadopoulou[2,3], Vagelis Rinotas[2,4], Georgios Leonis[5], Eleni Douni[2,4], Antreas Afantitis[2,5]* and George Kollias[2,3]*

[1] Hellenic Military Academy, Vari, Greece, [2] Division of Immunology, Biomedical Sciences Research Center "Alexander Fleming," Vari, Greece, [3] Department of Experimental Physiology, Medical School, National and Kapodistrian University of Athens, Athens, Greece, [4] Department of Biotechnology, Agricultural University of Athens, Athens, Greece, [5] NovaMechanics Ltd., Nicosia, Cyprus

*Correspondence:
Antreas Afantitis
afantitis@novamechanics.com
George Kollias
kollias@fleming.gr

An *in silico* drug discovery pipeline for the virtual screening of plant-origin natural products (NPs) was developed to explore new direct inhibitors of TNF and its close relative receptor activator of nuclear factor kappa-B ligand (RANKL), both representing attractive therapeutic targets for many chronic inflammatory conditions. Direct TNF inhibition through identification of potent small molecules is a highly desired goal; however, it is often hampered by severe limitations. Our approach yielded a priority list of 15 NPs as potential direct TNF inhibitors that were subsequently tested *in vitro* against TNF and RANKL. We thus identified two potent direct inhibitors of TNF function with low micromolar IC_{50} values and minimal toxicity even at high concentrations. Most importantly, one of them (A11) was proved to be a dual inhibitor of both TNF and RANKL. Extended molecular dynamics simulations with the fully automated EnalosMD suite rationalized the mode of action of the compounds at the molecular level. To our knowledge, these compounds constitute the first NP TNF inhibitors, one of which being the first NP small-molecule dual inhibitor of TNF and RANKL, and could serve as lead compounds for the development of novel treatments for inflammatory and autoimmune diseases.

Keywords: direct TNF inhibitors, RANKL inhibitors, natural products, autoimmune diseases, virtual screening, molecular dynamics

INTRODUCTION

Tumor necrosis factor (TNF) is an important human cytokine (Beutler et al., 1985) that is involved in a number of critical biological processes and diseases, including rheumatoid arthritis, Crohn's disease, multiple sclerosis, inflammatory bowel disease, psoriatic arthritis, AIDS, and cancer (Kollias et al., 1999; Apostolaki et al., 2010). Disruption of TNF binding to its principal receptor, TNFR1, has been a long-desired goal in the development of novel autoimmune therapeutics (Douni and Kollias, 1998; Kollias and Kontoyiannis, 2002). Previous *in vivo* studies from our group demonstrated that deregulated TNF production induces chronic polyarthritis in a transgenic animal model and the disease could be treated by proper anti-TNF therapy (Keffer et al., 1991). These research efforts were vital in directing the attention of the pharmaceutical industry to initial anti-TNF approaches, which eventually resulted in clinical trials that were successfully performed for a variety of chronic inflammatory diseases, including rheumatoid arthritis (Elliott et al., 1993), psoriasis, psoriatic arthritis, Crohn's disease, juvenile idiopathic arthritis, spondyloarthritis, and Behçet's disease (Sfikakis, 2010).

To date, three synthetic antibodies that block the activity of TNF have been reported, namely infliximab, adalimumab, and etanercept (Olsen and Stein, 2004). However, these expensive agents are frequently used as secondary options for patients with a poor response to regular anti-rheumatic drugs (Chaudhari et al., 2016). Moreover, biologics are associated with several other drawbacks, including high cost, inadequate clinical response, need of intravenous administration, as well as increased risk of tuberculosis and hepatitis B due to the lowered immune response. Therefore, there is a clear need for orally available, well-tolerated, inexpensive drugs that block the production of TNF associated with pathological inflammation in rheumatoid arthritis and related conditions. It has been shown that the use of small molecules in direct TNF inhibition represents an attractive alternative that offers significant benefits, such as oral administration, shorter half-lives with reduced immunosuppression, and easier manufacturing at a lower cost (Sfikakis, 2010; Lo et al., 2017; Melagraki et al., 2018).

According to a recent report (Chaudhari et al., 2016), there are no late-stage rheumatoid arthritis products targeting TNF under development. Particularly, small molecule direct inhibition of protein–protein interactions (PPIs), such as the one between TNF and its receptor, is a nontrivial approach in drug development (Sackett and Sept, 2009; Wilson, 2009; David, 2012; Arkin et al., 2014). For this purpose, successful drug design requires the identification of compounds with low molecular weight, something extremely challenging, especially when attempting to block interactions between large molecules such as proteins (Lo et al., 2017). The successful recognition of small-molecule inhibitors is also hampered by the difficulty to identify potential "hot spots" as unique binding targets that are crucial for the disruption of biomolecular interactions.

Protein–protein interactions interfaces are mostly flat, extended (approximately 1,500–2,000 Å^2), solvent-exposed, and are characterized by hydrophobic and electrostatic interactions (Jones and Thornton, 1996; Hwang et al., 2010; Sheng et al., 2015). The main difference between PPI interfaces and deep protein cavities, which usually bind small molecules, is their size, with the latter occupying a relatively small area of less than 500 Å^2 (Fuller et al., 2009). Studies on the binding energy distributions over protein interfaces by mutational analyses demonstrated that only specific residues (hot spots) at the PPI interface contribute most of the binding energy, while the majority of PPI-interface residues are not important (Arkin and Wells, 2004). It was shown that hot spots rather assemble at the middle of the interface, to form a hydrophobic region similar in size to a small molecule, and possess conformational flexibility. The location of hot spots usually coincides with the putative binding sites of the protein, and these sites consist of a number of surface residues, which favorably contribute to small-molecule binding and are also critical in stabilizing PPIs.

It has been shown that among all protein residues, these hot-spot regions contribute the major part of the binding energy in a protein–inhibitor complex. Therefore, successful identification of hot spots may offer significant advancements in the rational design of inhibitors (Kozakov et al., 2015a,b).

However, little progress has been obtained regarding fast and reliable identification of hot spots despite recent advances in high-throughput methodologies (Kouadio et al., 2005; Bakail and Ochsenbein, 2016). Various computational approaches for the recognition of hot spot areas have been developed by several research groups and include methodologies that employ dedicated energy functions (e.g., Rosetta, FoldX, and PCRPi) (Guerois et al., 2002; Kortemme et al., 2004; Guharoy et al., 2011), molecular simulations (Rajamani et al., 2004), computational alanine scanning (Kollman et al., 2000), and machine learning approaches [for instance, HSpred (Lise et al., 2011) and HotPoint (Tuncbag et al., 2010)].

Despite that PPIs vary in size and shape, the majority of inhibitors usually bind to hot spot regions that are restricted to small binding sites (<1000 Å^2) (Smith and Gestwicki, 2012; Basse et al., 2013) and partner proteins are defined by short residue sequences at the interface (Perkins et al., 2010; London et al., 2013). An effective PPI inhibitor must possess a large surface area and participate in many hydrophobic interactions with the receptor. However, such a ligand is usually accompanied by high molecular weight and low solubility; therefore, various pharmacokinetic problems may arise (Sheng et al., 2015). Moreover, identifying an adequate starting structure for successful design of small-molecule PPI inhibitors is often hampered by the lack of information about natural PPI inhibitors. To date, most of the published small molecules are indirectly targeting TNF by downregulating its expression and only a limited number of compounds is reported to directly disrupt this interaction. These include the polysulfonated naphthylurea suramin and its analogs (Alzani et al., 1993; Mancini et al., 1999) and the indole-linked chromone SPD304 (He et al., 2005), the use of which is hampered by low potency and poor selectivity with a concomitant tendency to cause adverse effects (suramin) (McGeary et al., 2008), and cell toxicity (SPD304) (Sun and Yost, 2008). Moreover, Chan et al. (2010) identified two natural product (NP)-like molecules, two FDA-approved drugs, namely darifenacin and ezetimibe (Leung et al., 2011), and a metal-based iridium(III) biquinoline complex (Leung et al., 2012), which act as direct inhibitors of TNF. Recently, our group with the aid of cheminformatics techniques identified two additional small molecules (T23 and T8) that were shown to directly inhibit TNF function (Melagraki et al., 2017). Importantly, the above compounds were also potent against receptor activator of nuclear factor kappa-B ligand (RANKL) and presented low toxicity. In 2017, another TNF small-molecule inhibitor, JNJ525, was discovered by Blevitt et al. (2017). The mechanism of PPI disruption was attributed to a change in the quaternary structure of the protein by an aggregate conglomerate of JNJ525 in a way that TNFR1 binding to TNF is blocked.

Drug discovery based on NP-like scaffolds has rapidly advanced through novel computational approaches (Baig et al., 2016; Rodrigues et al., 2016). Recent developments have demonstrated the power of computationally treating complex NP structures to recognize their protein targets and to find specific applications in rational drug design (Reutlinger et al., 2014; Rodrigues et al., 2016; Basith et al., 2018; Lima et al., 2018; Zheng et al., 2018). The abundance of NPs or compounds inspired by NPs as drugs and drug candidates (Lesney, 2004) motivated us to search for novel TNF inhibitors among them. Given the high priority of plant-origin NPs in previous and current drug development efforts (including the terpenoids, e.g., Taxol and steroids, the glycosides, e.g., digitalis and the various flavonoids, and the alkaloids, e.g., camptothecins and the opiates), we focused on identifying novel TNF small molecule inhibitors from plant sources.

MATERIALS AND METHODS

In search of plant-origin NPs as direct TNF inhibitors, we combined chemoinformatics techniques, high-throughput virtual screening, and molecular dynamics (MD) simulations with experimental evaluation, ultimately aiming at discovering potent TNF-functioning NP inhibitors. 3,573 pure NPs of plant origin were virtually screened from the MEGxp database, which is one of the largest chemical libraries of NPs available (AnalytiCon Discovery); the highest scoring compounds were then tested *in vitro* to assess their inhibitory activity against TNF.

Our strategy for identifying these novel plant-origin small molecule TNF inhibitors is presented in **Scheme 1**.

Molecular Modeling

The initial model of TNF was built from the X-ray co-crystal structure of TNF dimer with SPD304 (PDB code: 2AZ5). All structures were prepared using Molegro's Molecules and Protein Preparation Wizard (Thomsen and Christensen, 2006). Proper bond assignments, bond orders, hybridization, and

charges were calculated by Molegro Virtual Docker (MVD) software (version-5.0) (Thomsen and Christensen, 2006). Explicit hydrogen atoms were added and their hydrogen bonding (HB) patterns were also determined by MVD. Since the 3D conformation of SPD304 is known from crystallographic data, a docking template was defined. SPD304 was replaced by each ligand in TNF, and template alignment considered ligands as fully flexible: the docking algorithm recognized the optimal conformation of the ligand when fitting to the template. The MolDock score (GRID) was used as a grid-based scoring function which pre-calculates potential energy values on an evenly spaced cubic grid in order to speed up calculations. A grid resolution of 0.30 Å was set to initiate the docking process and the binding site of the protein was defined to occupy the region surrounding SPD304 in the crystal structure (including residues Ser60, Gln61, Gly121, Tyr151, and Ala156). For the pose generation, the default setting was applied (MolDock SE), namely a maximum of 1500 iterations combined with a population size of 50. If the generated pose has an energy below the predefined energy threshold (100.0 in our study), it is included into the initial population for the "simplex evolution" algorithm (Thomsen and Christensen, 2006). This algorithm performs a combined local/global search on the poses generated by the pose generator. The number of the maximum iterations of the simplex evolution algorithm (Nelder–Mead simplex minimization) was set to 300 while the neighbor distance factor, the factor which determines how close the point of the initial simplex will be to the other randomly selected individuals in the population, was set to 1.0 (causes the initial simplex to span the neighbor points evenly).

In Vitro Testing of TNF Inhibitors

Experiments included a TNF-induced death assay in L929 cells, a measurement of cytotoxicity in L929 cells, and a TNF/TNFR1

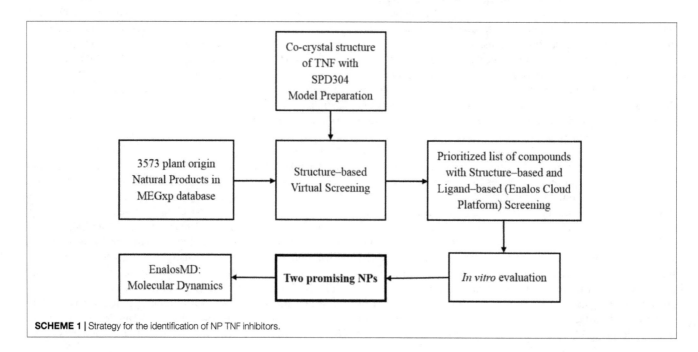

SCHEME 1 | Strategy for the identification of NP TNF inhibitors.

ELISA assay. Compounds were tested with respect to TNF using a battery of previously reported assays (Melagraki et al., 2017).

Osteoclast Differentiation and TRAP Staining

Bone marrow (BM) cells were collected after flushing out of femurs and tibiae, subjected to gradient purification using Ficoll-Paque (GE Healthcare), plated in 96-well plates at a density of 6×10^4 cells per well and cultured in AMEM medium (GIBCO) containing 10% fetal bovine serum supplemented with 40 ng/ml RANKL (Peprotech) and 25 ng/ml M-CSF (R&D Systems) for 5 days (Douni et al., 2012). Compounds A11 and A25 were pre-incubated with RANKL at various concentrations from 1 to 10 μM in AMEM medium for 1 h at room temperature and then added to cell cultures that were replenished with fresh medium every 2 days. Osteoclasts were stained for tartrate-resistant acid phosphatase (TRAP) activity using a leukocyte acid phosphatase (TRAP kit) (Sigma–Aldrich).

TRAP Activity Assay

In the TRAP activity assay, BM cells were plated in 96-well plates at a density of 6×10^4 cells per well and cultured in AMEM medium (GIBCO) containing 10% fetal bovine serum supplemented with 40 ng/ml RANKL (Peprotech) and 25 ng/ml M-CSF (R&D Systems) for 4 days. Then, cells were lysed in ice-cold phosphate buffer containing 0.1% Triton X-100. Lysates were added to 96-well plates containing phosphatase substrate (p-nitrophenol phosphate) and 40 mM tartrate acid buffer and incubated at 37°C for 30 min. The reaction was then stopped with the addition of 0.5 N NaOH. Absorbance was measured at 405 nm on a micro-plate reader (Optimax, Molecular Devices). TRAP activity was normalized to total protein which was determined using the Bradford assay (Bio-Rad).

MTT Viability Assay

Cytotoxicity was evaluated for BM cells using the 3-(4,5-dimethylthiazol-2-yl)-2,5-diphenyltetrazolium bromide (MTT) assay, which measures the ability of viable cells to reduce a soluble tetrazolium salt to an insoluble purple formazan precipitate. BM cells used for MTT assay were seeded at a density of 10^5 cells/well in 96-well plates and incubated with A11 and A25 compounds for 48 h in AMEM containing 10% fetal bovine serum supplemented with 25 ng/ml M-CSF (R&D Systems). After removal of the medium, each well was incubated with 0.5 mg/ml MTT (Sigma–Aldrich) in AMEM serum-free medium at 37°C for 2 h. At the end of the incubation period, the medium was removed and the intracellular formazan was solubilised with 200 μl DMSO and quantified by reading the absorbance at 550 nm on a micro-plate reader (Optimax, Molecular Devices). Percentage of cell viability was calculated based on the absorbance measured relative to the absorbance of the untreated control.

Molecular Dynamics with EnalosMD

Molecular dynamics simulations were performed with our in-house developed EnalosMD suite of programs (EnalosMD, NovaMechanics Ltd., 2018). A fully automated pipeline included the following steps of systems' preparation, MD runs, and analyses:

(a) Initial model structures were constructed with AmberTools16 (Case et al., 2016). Missing TNF and RANKL residues were added with Modeller 9.10 (Sali and Blundell, 1993; Fiser et al., 2000). The ff14SB force field (Maier et al., 2015) was used for the protein atoms and the general AMBER force field (GAFF) (Wang et al., 2004) represented compounds A11 and A25. Geometry optimization and AM1-BCC (Jakalian et al., 2002) charge derivation for A11 and A25 were obtained with ANTECHAMBER (Wang et al., 2006). The AM1-BCC approach is based on a fast and effective parameterization scheme that reliably reproduces the more rigorous RESP charges (Xu et al., 2013).

(b) AMBER-generated topology and coordinate files were subjected to four 1000 ns-long, all-atom, unrestrained MD simulations with the GPU version of OpenMM 7 (Eastman et al., 2017). Simulations were performed for (i) A11–TNF, (ii) A25–TNF, (iii) A11–RANKL, and (iv) A25–RANKL complexes in explicit solvent (TIP3P water model) (Jorgensen et al., 1983) and at 300 K with the GPU version of OpenMM. Periodic boundary conditions were used with a cutoff distance of 10 Å, and the Particle Mesh Ewald (PME) method (Darden et al., 1993) was employed for the treatment of long-range interactions. A Langevin thermostat with collision frequency set at 2.0 ps^{-1} regulated the temperature (Izaguirre et al., 2001).

(c) Analysis of the results (RMSD, atomic fluctuations, and hydrogen bond calculations) was performed with the cpptraj version of AmberTools.

RESULTS AND DISCUSSION

The formation of the biologically active TNF homotrimer is prevented by direct TNF inhibitors, such as SPD304, through disruption of the TNF dimer binding to the third subunit (He et al., 2005; Davis and Colangelo, 2012). TNF–inhibitor interactions are hydrophobic and shape-driven, as the inhibitor structure needs to be large enough to interact with both subunits and to prevent binding of the third subunit to the TNF dimer. We in silico explored 3,573 NPs contained in MEGxp database using a structure-based docking approach. The crystal structure of TNF dimer with SPD304 (PDB code: 2AZ5) was used as the molecular model for our investigation and the compounds were docked into the protein–protein interface. Computational molecular docking studies were performed using MVD (Thomsen and Christensen, 2006). Based on the docking score and following meticulous visual inspection of the conformations, we generated a shortlist of the top 15 commercially available NPs for in vitro validation.

Our in vitro screening strategy included one of the most commonly used assays of TNF activity. This assay exploits the

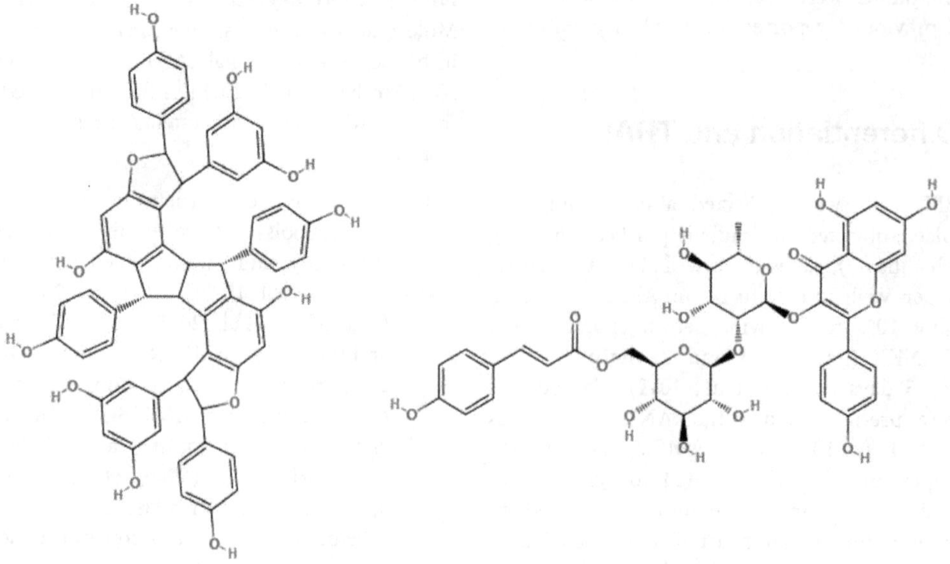

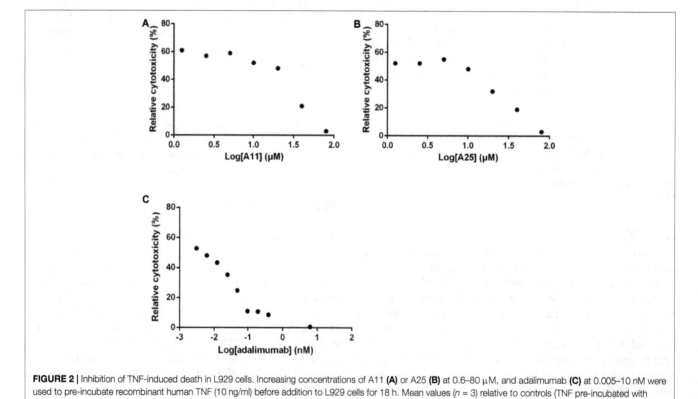

FIGURE 1 | Chemical structures of the two most promising compounds (A11 and A25).

FIGURE 2 | Inhibition of TNF-induced death in L929 cells. Increasing concentrations of A11 **(A)** or A25 **(B)** at 0.6–80 μM, and adalimumab **(C)** at 0.005–10 nM were used to pre-incubate recombinant human TNF (10 ng/ml) before addition to L929 cells for 18 h. Mean values ($n = 3$) relative to controls (TNF pre-incubated with DMSO or PBS in the adalimumab case) are shown. Data shown are representative of at least three experiments.

ability of TNF to induce death in the murine fibrosarcoma cell line L929 following sensitization by the transcription inhibitor actinomycin D. Functional inhibition of TNF by small molecules would result in reduction of the TNF-induced cytotoxicity.

Out of the 15 prioritized NPs mentioned above, two emerged as the most promising ones based on *in vitro* testing. The action of these two NPs (designated A11 and A25; structures shown in **Figure 1**) was then further characterized. In dose–response

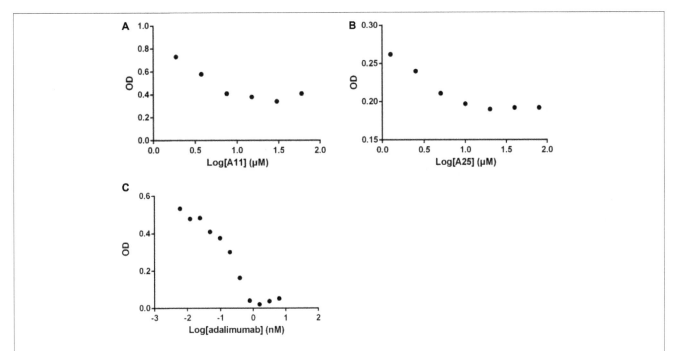

FIGURE 3 | Disruption of the TNF/TNFR1 interaction. Increasing concentrations of A11 **(A)** or A25 **(B)** at 0.6–80 µM and adalimumab **(C)** at 0.005–10 nM were used to pre-incubate human TNF (10 ng/ml) before addition on a TNFR1 substrate. Binding was measured by ELISA. Mean values ($n = 2$) of one experiment, representative of at least three replicates are shown.

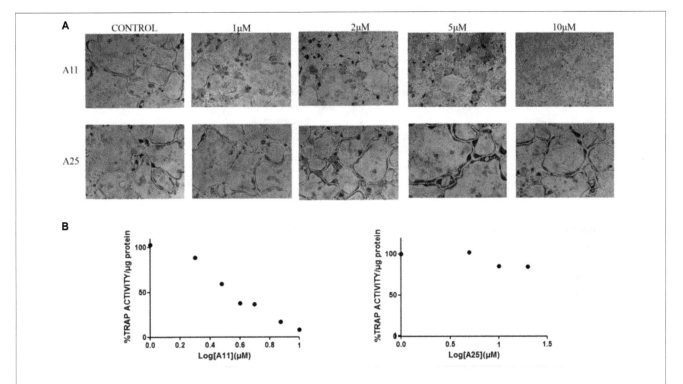

FIGURE 4 | Effects of A11 and A25 on RANKL-induced osteoclastogenesis. **(A)** TRAP staining of osteoclastogenic cultures. BMMs were treated with A11 and A25 (1, 2, 5, and 10 µM) in the presence of RANKL (50 ng/ml) and M-CSF (25 ng/ml) for 5 days. **(B)** BMMs were treated with A11 (1, 2, 3, 4, 5, 7.5, and 10 µM) and A25 (1, 5, 10, and 20 µM) in the presence of RANKL (50 ng/ml) and M-CSF (25 ng/ml) for 4 days and cell lysates were measured for TRAP activity. % TRAP activity per microgram of total protein was expressed as a percentage of the untreated control. IC_{50} values are given as mean ± SEM from three independent experiments performed in duplicate.

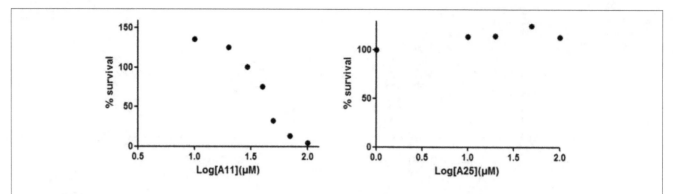

FIGURE 5 | Effects of A11 and A25 on the viability of BMMs. BMMs were treated with 10–100 μM of compounds A11 and A25, respectively, in the presence of M-CSF (25 ng/ml) for 48 h. Cytotoxicity was assessed using a MTT colorimetric assay. Cell viability (%) was expressed as a percentage of the untreated control. LC$_{50}$ values are given as mean ± SEM from three independent experiments performed in duplicate.

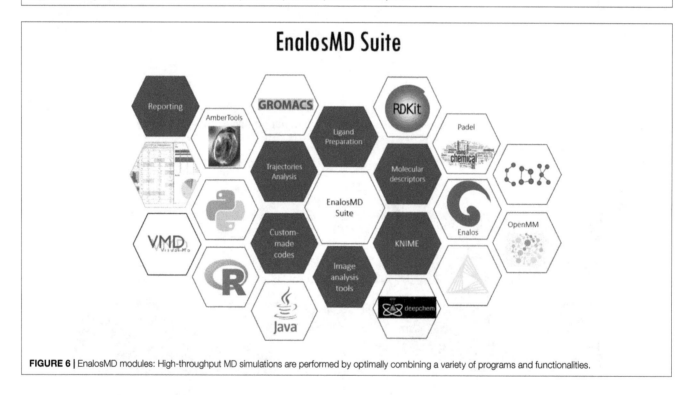

FIGURE 6 | EnalosMD modules: High-throughput MD simulations are performed by optimally combining a variety of programs and functionalities.

experiments, the small molecules were shown to inhibit human TNF-driven death in L929 cells with an IC$_{50}$ of 35 ± 3 μM (A11) and 33 ± 2 μM (A25). Both compounds were found to be minimally toxic in these cells (LC$_{50}$ > 80 μM), in contrast to the published high toxicity of SPD304 (7.5 μM) (Melagraki et al., 2017). An already approved anti-TNF biologic, adalimumab (HUMIRA, Abbott Laboratories, IL, United States), was used as a positive control of the assay. Adalimumab is a human anti-TNF monoclonal antibody approved by the U.S. Food and Drug Administration (FDA, 2002) and by the European Medicines Agency (EMEA, 2003) for RA treatment. Adalimumab inhibits TNF-driven death in L929 cells with a low IC$_{50}$ of 0.5 ± 0.1 nM, without showing any cytotoxicity (**Figure 2**).

Having established that the selected products can obstruct the function of TNF, and given that TNF exerts its functions primarily through interacting with its receptor, TNFR1, an

ELISA-based assay was used to quantify effects on this interaction. Both compounds significantly reduced binding of TNF to TNFR1, with an estimated IC$_{50}$ of 3.3 ± 0.9 μM for A11 and 4.1 ± 1.7 μM for A25. Adalimumab was again used as a positive control eliminating the TNF-TNFR1 binding with a low IC$_{50}$ of 0.2 nM (**Figure 3**).

The oligostilbenoid A11 (NP-003410, Ampelopsin H, (1R,2R,6R,6aR,7R,8R,12R,12aR)-1,7-Bis(3,5-dihydroxyphenyl)-2,6,8,12-tetrakis(4-hydroxyphenyl)-1,2,6,6a,7,8,12,12a-octahydr-ofuro[2′′,3′′:6′,7′]indeno[1′,2′:2,3]indeno [5,4-b]furan-5,11-diol) is an NP that has been isolated from *Parthenocissus tricuspidata* and the glycosyloxyflavone analog A25 (NP-008297, [(2R,3S,4S,5R,6S)-6-[(2S,3R,4R,5R,6S)-2-[5,7-dihydroxy-2-(4-hydroxyphenyl)-4-oxochromen-3-yl]oxy-4,5-dihydroxy-6-methyloxan-3-yl]oxy-3,4,5-trihydroxyoxan-2-yl]methyl(E)-3-(4-hydroxyphenyl)prop-2-enoate) is an NP that has been

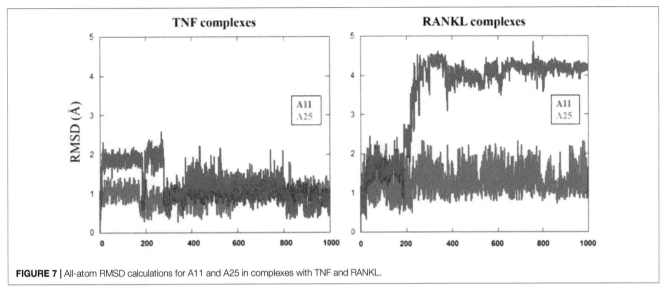

FIGURE 7 | All-atom RMSD calculations for A11 and A25 in complexes with TNF and RANKL.

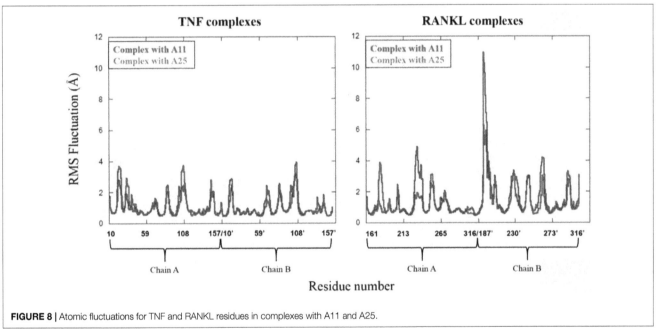

FIGURE 8 | Atomic fluctuations for TNF and RANKL residues in complexes with A11 and A25.

isolated from *Ginkgo biloba* (**Figure 1**). Except being isolated from natural sources, A11 can also be synthesized through a selective functionalization procedure as described by Rodrigues et al. (Rodrigues et al., 2016). Compounds A11 and A25 are promising PPI inhibitors as they both have large surface areas and are able to create many hydrophobic contacts at protein interfaces. Moreover, it has been observed that hydrophobic PPI hot-spot pockets tend to be excellent binders of small organic molecules, which combine a largely hydrophobic functionality with a secondary polar component (Guo et al., 2014). Indeed, the polar hydroxyl groups surrounding the hydrophobic core of A11 and A25 (**Figure 1**) constitute structures that are ideal binders to the concave hot-spot area of the protein (Mattos and Ringe, 1996; Shuker et al., 1996). It has been suggested that the ability of recognizing drug molecules (i.e., druggability) by a hot-spot

pocket depends on the balance among total surface area, and polar/nonpolar contact areas (Hajduk et al., 2005; Cheng et al., 2007; Schmidtke and Barril, 2010).

In comparison to SPD304, NPs A11 and A25 are predicted by the molecular docking study to occupy a similar region in the binding pocket, and to be relatively hydrophobic and large enough to interact with residues from both subunits of the TNF dimer. Nonpolar residues are predominant in the binding site, which mainly includes glycine, leucine, and tyrosine. Only one HB interaction is observed between compound A25 and Tyr151. Both compounds appear to be situated more closely to subunit A than subunit B and are in close contact with the Leu120-Gly121-Gly122 β-strand of subunit A. The lack of salt bridges or extended HB interactions indicates the hydrophobic character of A11 and A25 binding as also observed with SPD304.

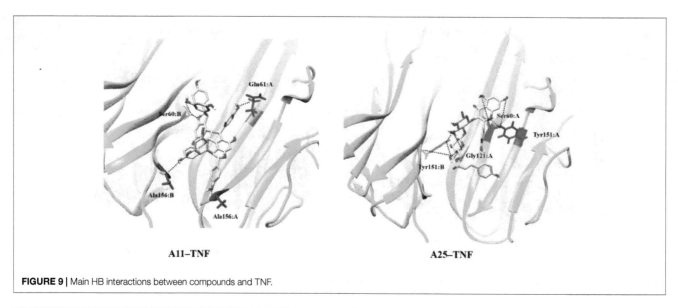

FIGURE 9 | Main HB interactions between compounds and TNF.

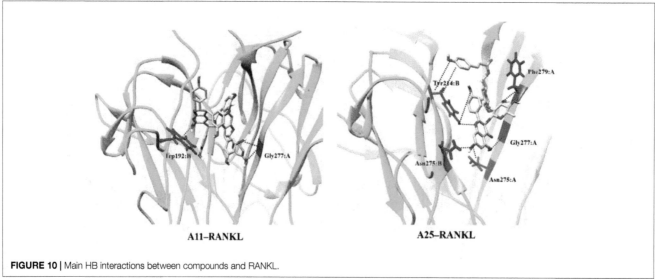

FIGURE 10 | Main HB interactions between compounds and RANKL.

The docked SPD304 conformation reproduced its crystal form, with an RMSD of 0.67 Å between the two structures. The docking score of SPD304 binding to TNF was calculated to be −171.08 (arbitrary units), and compounds A11 and A25 showed a binding score of −195.76 and −180.19, respectively, thus suggesting a strong interaction between the compounds and the TNF dimer. The high inhibitory potency of A11 and A25 against TNF was also indicated by our recently developed TNF model, released through the Enalos Cloud platform (Melagraki and Afantitis, 2014). After selecting the corresponding workflow within Enalos Cloud platform (Melagraki et al., 2017), both compounds were submitted and prediction results verified their activity. However, predictions fell out of the model's domain of applicability as expected for these complex structures.

Receptor activator of nuclear factor kappa-B ligand, another TNF superfamily member, is the main regulator of osteoclast formation and bone resorption (Fuller et al., 1998). We evaluated the effect of various concentrations of A11 and A25 on RANKL-dependent osteoclast differentiation in a culture system of BM-derived monocyte/macrophages (BMMs) stimulated with RANKL (50 ng/ml) and M-CSF (25 ng/ml) for 5 days through evaluation of the TRAP activity, an osteoclast-specific enzyme. A11 fully suppressed RANKL-induced TRAP-positive osteoclast differentiation at 10 μM, whereas A25 was ineffective even at 20 μM (**Figure 4**). Moreover, using a quantitative assay that measures TRAP activity, A11 inhibited RANKL-induced osteoclastogenesis in a dose-dependent manner, displaying an IC$_{50}$ of 3.42 $\pm$ 0.45 μM (**Figure 4B**). Furthermore, in order to exclude the possibility that inhibition of A11 on TRAP activity was due to cytotoxicity, the viability of BMMs was tested through the MTT assay. A11 displayed an LC$_{50}$ of 44.76 $\pm$ 4.61 μM (**Figure 5**), suggesting that it affects osteoclastogenesis without interfering with cell viability. On the other hand, A25 had no effect either on osteoclastogenesis or BMM viability ($LC_{50} > 100\ \mu M$) (**Figure 5**).

We subsequently investigated the binding of A11 to RANKL using the proposed molecular scaffolds in a structure-based approach. For this purpose, we employed the jFATCAT pairwise structure alignment algorithm (Ye and Godzik, 2003) to align the RANKL structure (PDB code: 1S55) to the crystal structure of TNF dimer with SPD304 (PDB code: 2AZ5). For our computational approach, we employed the murine RANKL model, which shares a 100% identity with human RANKL in the binding site, including residues Trp192, Tyr214, Asn275, Gly277, and Phe279. Also, RANKL shares a high degree of structural similarity with TNF as shown in Supplementary Figure S1. The binding conformations of both NPs and SPD304 are also depicted in the Supporting Information (Supplementary Figure S2). The docking methodology for RANKL systems was identical to the procedure followed for TNF complexes as described in the section "Materials and Methods." The docking score of SPD304 binding to RANKL was calculated to be −159.712 and compounds A11 and A25 showed a binding score of −211.79 and −146.83, respectively. For A11, the computational analysis suggests a strong binding interaction with RANKL, which is in line with the experimental results.

Additionally, we employed our recently developed EnalosMD suite to perform extended MD simulations for A11 and A25 in complexes with TNF and RANKL. EnalosMD automates the preparation of any ligand-protein system and performs MD calculations in a way that minimal effort by the user is required. This application provides a powerful way to perform robust MD calculations with unprecedented speed and easiness regarding the construction of the initial model structure. Therefore, we carried out four 1000 ns-long MD runs to identify structural and energetic properties of the complexes that may further elucidate the mode of action of the two compounds. EnalosMD offers optimal performance by combining several computational programs and functionalities (**Figure 6**).

The MD results showed that protein structures early stabilized during the simulations in all complexes with RMSD values that do not exceed 3 and 4 Å in TNF and RANKL complexes, respectively (Supplementary Figure S3). A11 and A25 appear relatively stable into either protein's cavity, with A25 showing only minor structural changes when bound to TNF after 200 ns (**Figure 7**). However, during the first 200–250 ns of A25–RANKL complex simulation, a noticeable conformational change of A25 stabilized the molecule in a new orientation with respect to the binding site of RANKL (**Figure 7**). This conformational change may have induced great flexibility to B chain terminal residues Tyr187–Asp189 as denoted by further fluctuation calculations (**Figure 8**). Therefore, the experimentally observed lower affinity of A25 against RANKL compared to A11 may be rationalized

through the A25-induced destabilization of the terminal region of monomer B. Average conformations of A11 and A25 into their protein targets, along with protein residues that are involved in dominant HB interactions with the compounds are shown in **Figures 9**, **10**. The sole interaction between A25 and Tyr151, which was shown after docking calculations in TNF complex is also observed by the MD runs, however, it is complemented by three significant interactions from chain A (**Figure 9**).

CONCLUSION

In summary, we have identified and validated experimentally the first plant-origin NPs that act as direct inhibitors of TNF by preventing the PPI between the dimer and the third subunit. Both NPs (A11 and A25) were shown to have IC_{50} values comparable to those of SPD304, but presented significantly reduced toxicity. Most importantly, A11 has been validated as the first NP dual inhibitor of TNF and RANKL. Both small molecules possess characteristics that are typical in potent PPI inhibitors, namely, large surface area and extended hydrophobic regions. Therefore, they can be explored as scaffolds representing NPs of plant origin in hit-to-lead optimization studies for the identification of direct TNF and/or RANKL inhibitors with improved pharmacological profiles and in the development of novel treatments for chronic inflammatory and autoimmune diseases.

AUTHOR CONTRIBUTIONS

AA and GK conceptualization, funding acquisition, methodology, project administration, and supervision. GM, EN, VR, DP, GL, ED, AA, and GK data curation, formal analysis, investigation, resources, validation, visualization, writing – original draft, and writing – review and editing. GM, GL, and AA software.

FUNDING

This work was funded by Greek "Cooperation" Action project TheRAlead (09SYN-21-784) co-financed by the European Regional Development Fund and NSRF 2007–2013 (http://www.gsrt.gr), the Innovative Medicines Initiative (IMI) funded project (http://www.imi.europa.eu/) BTCure (No. 115142) and Advanced European Research Council (ERC) grant (https://erc.europa.eu/funding/advanced-grants) MCs-inTEST (No. 340217) to GK. AA would like to acknowledge funding from Cyprus Research Promotion Foundation, DESMI 2008, ΕΠΙΧΕΙΡΗΣΕΙΣ/ΕΦΑΡΜ/0308/20 http://www.research.org.cy. The funders had no role in study design, data collection and analysis, decision to publish, or preparation of the manuscript.

REFERENCES

Alzani, R., Corti, A., Grazioli, L., Cozzi, E., Ghezzi, P., and Marcucci, F. (1993). Suramin induces deoligomerization of human tumor necrosis factor alpha. *J. Biol. Chem.* 268, 12526–12529.

Apostolaki, M., Armaka, M., Victoratos, P., and Kollias, G. (2010). Cellular mechanisms of TNF function in models of inflammation and autoimmunity. *Curr. Dir. Autoimmun.* 11, 1–26. doi: 10.1159/000289195

Arkin, M. R., Tang, Y., and Wells, J. A. (2014). Small-molecule inhibitors of protein-protein interactions: progressing toward the reality. *Chem. Biol.* 21, 1102–1114. doi: 10.1016/j.chembiol.2014.09.001

Arkin, M. R., and Wells, J. A. (2004). Small-molecule inhibitors of protein–protein interactions: progressing towards the dream. *Nat. Rev. Drug Discov.* 3, 301–317. doi: 10.1038/nrd1343

Baig, M. H., Ahmad, K., Roy, S., Ashraf, J. M., Adil, M., Siddiqui, M. H., et al. (2016). Computer aided drug design: success and limitations. *Curr. Pharm. Des.* 22, 572–581. doi: 10.2174/1381612822666151125000550

Bakail, M., and Ochsenbein, F. (2016). Targeting protein–protein interactions, a wide open field for drug design. *C. R. Chim.* 19, 19–27. doi: 10.1016/j.crci.2015.12.004

Basith, S., Cui, M., Macalino, S. J. Y., Park, J., Clavio, N. A. B., Kang, S., et al. (2018). Exploring G protein-coupled receptors (GPCRs) ligand space via cheminformatics approaches: impact on rational drug design. *Front. Pharmacol.* 9:128. doi: 10.3389/fphar.2018.00128

Basse, M. J., Betzi, S., Bourgeas, R., Bouzidi, S., Chetrit, B., Hamon, V., et al. (2013). 2P2Idb: a structural database dedicated to orthosteric modulation of protein–protein interactions. *Nucleic Acids Res.* 41, D824–D827. doi: 10.1093/nar/gks1002

Beutler, B., Mahoney, J., Le Trang, N., Pekala, P., and Cerami, A. (1985). Purification of cachectin, a lipoprotein lipase-suppressing hormone secreted by endotoxin-induced RAW 264.7 cells. *J. Exp. Med.* 161, 984–995. doi: 10.1084/jem.161.5.984

Blevitt, J. M., Hack, M. D., Herman, K. L., Jackson, P. F., Krawczuk, P. J., Lebsack, A. D., et al. (2017). Structural basis of small-molecule aggregate induced inhibition of a protein–protein interaction. *J. Med. Chem.* 60, 3511–3517. doi: 10.1021/acs.jmedchem.6b01836

Case, D. A., Betz, R. M., Cerutti, D. S., Cheatham, T. E. I, Darden, T. A., Duke, R. E., et al. (2016). *AMBER 2016.* San Francisco, CA: University of California.

Chan, D. S.-H., Lee, H.-M., Yang, F., Che, C.-M., Wong, C. C. L., Abagyan, R., et al. (2010). Structure-based discovery of natural-product-like TNF-α inhibitors. *Angew. Chem. Int. Ed.* 49, 2860–2864. doi: 10.1002/anie.200907360

Chaudhari, K., Rizvi, S., and Syed, B. A. (2016). Rheumatoid arthritis: current and future trends. *Nat. Rev. Drug Discov.* 15, 305–306. doi: 10.1038/nrd.2016.21

Cheng, A. C., Coleman, R. G., Smyth, K. T., Cao, Q., Soulard, P., Caffrey, D. R., et al. (2007). Structure-based maximal affinity model predicts small-molecule druggability. *Nat. Biotechnol.* 25, 71–75. doi: 10.1038/nbt1273

Darden, T., York, D., and Pedersen, L. (1993). Particle mesh ewald: an N·log(N) method for ewald sums in large systems. *J. Chem. Phys.* 98, 10089–10092. doi: 10.1063/1.464397

David, C. F. (2012). Small-molecule inhibitors of protein-protein interactions: how to mimic a protein partner. *Curr. Pharm. Des.* 18, 4679–4684. doi: 10.2174/138161212802651634

Davis, J. M., and Colangelo, J. (2012). Small-molecule inhibitors of the interaction between TNF and TNFR. *Future Med. Chem.* 5, 69–79. doi: 10.4155/fmc.12.192

Douni, E., and Kollias, G. (1998). A critical role of the p75 tumor necrosis factor receptor (p75TNF-R) in organ inflammation independent of TNF, lymphotoxin α, or the p55TNF-R. *J. Exp. Med.* 188, 1343–1352. doi: 10.1084/jem.188.7.1343

Douni, E., Rinotas, V., Makrinou, E., Zwerina, J., Penninger, J. M., Eliopoulos, E., et al. (2012). A RANKL G278R mutation causing osteopetrosis identifies a functional amino acid essential for trimer assembly in RANKL and TNF. *Hum. Mol. Genet.* 21, 784–798. doi: 10.1093/hmg/ddr510

Eastman, P., Swails, J., Chodera, J. D., McGibbon, R. T., Zhao, Y., Beauchamp, K. A., et al. (2017). OpenMM 7: rapid development of high performance algorithms for molecular dynamics. *PLoS Comput. Biol.* 13:e1005659. doi: 10.1371/journal.pcbi.1005659

Elliott, M. J., Maini, R. N., Feldmann, M., Long-Fox, A., Charles, P., Katsikis, P., et al. (1993). Treatment of rheumatoid arthritis with chimeric monoclonal antibodies to tumor necrosis factor alpha. *Arthritis Rheum.* 36, 1681–1690. doi: 10.1002/art.1780361206

EnalosMD, NovaMechanics Ltd. (2018). Available at: http://enalosmd.novamechanics.com

Fiser, A., Do, R. K., and Sali, A. (2000). Modeling of loops in protein structures. *Protein Sci.* 9, 1753–1773. doi: 10.1110/ps.9.9.1753

Fuller, J. C., Burgoyne, N. J., and Jackson, R. M. (2009). Predicting druggable binding sites at the protein–protein interface. *Drug Discov. Today* 14, 155–161. doi: 10.1016/j.drudis.2008.10.009

Fuller, K., Wong, B., Fox, S., Choi, Y., and Chambers, T. J. (1998). TRANCE is necessary and sufficient for osteoblast-mediated activation of bone resorption in osteoclasts. *J. Exp. Med.* 188, 997–1001. doi: 10.1084/jem.188.5.997

Guerois, R., Nielsen, J. E., and Serrano, L. (2002). Predicting changes in the stability of proteins and protein complexes: a study of more than 1000 mutations. *J. Mol. Biol.* 320, 369–387. doi: 10.1016/S0022-2836(02)00442-4

Guharoy, M., Pal, A., Dasgupta, M., and Chakrabarti, P. (2011). PRICE (PRotein Interface Conservation and Energetics): a server for the analysis of protein–protein interfaces. *J. Struct. Funct. Genomics* 12, 33–41. doi: 10.1007/s10969-011-9108-0

Guo, W., Wisniewski, J. A., and Ji, H. (2014). Hot spot-based design of small-molecule inhibitors for protein–protein interactions. *Bioorg. Med. Chem. Lett.* 24, 2546–2554. doi: 10.1016/j.bmcl.2014.03.095

Hajduk, P. J., Huth, J. R., and Fesik, S. W. (2005). Druggability indices for protein targets derived from NMR-based screening data. *J. Med. Chem.* 48, 2518–2525. doi: 10.1021/jm049131r

He, M. M., Smith, A. S., Oslob, J. D., Flanagan, W. M., Braisted, A. C., Whitty, A., et al. (2005). Small-molecule inhibition of TNF-α. *Science* 310, 1022–1025. doi: 10.1126/science.1116304

Hwang, H., Vreven, T., Janin, J., and Weng, Z. (2010). Protein-protein docking benchmark version 4.0. *Proteins* 78, 3111–3114. doi: 10.1002/prot.22830

Izaguirre, J. A., Catarello, D. P., Wozniak, J. M., and Skeel, R. D. (2001). Langevin stabilization of molecular dynamics. *J. Chem. Phys.* 114, 2090–2098. doi: 10.1063/1.1332990

Jakalian, A., Jack, D. B., and Bayly, C. I. (2002). Fast, efficient generation of high-quality atomic charges. AM1-BCC model: II. Parameterization and validation. *J Comput. Chem.* 23, 1623–1641. doi: 10.1002/jcc.10128

Jones, S., and Thornton, J. M. (1996). Principles of protein-protein interactions. *Proc. Natl. Acad. Sci. U.S.A.* 93, 13–20. doi: 10.1073/pnas.93.1.13

Jorgensen, W. L., Chandrasekhar, J., Madura, J. D., Impey, R. W., and Klein, M. L. (1983). Comparison of simple potential functions for simulating liquid water. *J. Chem. Phys.* 79, 926–935. doi: 10.1063/1.445869

Keffer, J., Probert, L., Cazlaris, H., Georgopoulos, S., Kaslaris, E., Kioussis, D., et al. (1991). Transgenic mice expressing human tumour necrosis factor: a predictive genetic model of arthritis. *EMBO J.* 10, 4025–4031.

Kollias, G., Douni, E., Kassiotis, G., and Kontoyiannis, D. (1999). On the role of tumor necrosis factor and receptors in models of multiorgan failure, rheumatoid arthritis, multiple sclerosis and inflammatory bowel disease. *Immunol. Rev.* 169, 175–194. doi: 10.1111/j.1600-065X.1999.tb01315.x

Kollias, G., and Kontoyiannis, D. (2002). Role of TNF/TNFR in autoimmunity: specific TNF receptor blockade may be advantageous to anti-TNF treatments. *Cytokine Growth Factor Rev.* 13, 315–321. doi: 10.1016/S1359-6101(02)00019-9

Kollman, P. A., Massova, I., Reyes, C., Kuhn, B., Huo, S., Chong, L., et al. (2000). Calculating structures and free energies of complex molecules: combining molecular mechanics and continuum models. *Acc. Chem. Res.* 33, 889–897. doi: 10.1021/ar000033j

Kortemme, T., Kim, D. E., and Baker, D. (2004). Computational alanine scanning of protein-protein interfaces. *Sci. STKE* 2004:pl2. doi: 10.1126/stke.2192004pl2

Kouadio, J.-L. K., Horn, J. R., Pal, G., and Kossiakoff, A. A. (2005). Shotgun alanine scanning shows that growth hormone can bind productively to its receptor through a drastically minimized interface. *J. Biol. Chem.* 280, 25524–25532. doi: 10.1074/jbc.M502167200

Kozakov, D., Grove, L. E., Hall, D. R., Bohnuud, T., Mottarella, S. E., Luo, L., et al. (2015a). The FTMap family of web servers for determining and characterizing ligand-binding hot spots of proteins. *Nat. Protoc.* 10, 733–755. doi: 10.1038/nprot.2015.043

Kozakov, D., Hall, D. R., Jehle, S., Luo, L., Ochiana, S. O., Jones, E. V., et al. (2015b). Ligand deconstruction: why some fragment binding positions are conserved and others are not. *Proc. Natl. Acad. Sci. U.S.A.* 112, E2585–E2594. doi: 10.1073/pnas.1501567112

Lesney, M. S. (2004). Nature's Pharmaceuticals. Natural products from plants remain at the core of modern medicinal chemistry. *Todays Chem. Work* 13, 27–32.

Leung, C.-H., Chan, D. S.-H., Kwan, M. H.-T., Cheng, Z., Wong, C.-Y., Zhu, G.-Y., et al. (2011). Structure-based repurposing of FDA-approved drugs as TNF-α inhibitors. *ChemMedChem* 6, 765–768. doi: 10.1002/cmdc.201100016

Leung, C.-H., Zhong, H.-J., Yang, H., Cheng, Z., Chan, D. S.-H., Ma, V. P.-Y., et al. (2012). A metal-based inhibitor of tumor necrosis factor-α. *Angew. Chem. Int. Ed.* 51, 9010–9014. doi: 10.1002/anie.201202937

Lima, M. N. N., Melo-Filho, C. C., Cassiano, G. C., Neves, B. J., Alves, V. M., Braga, R. C., et al. (2018). QSAR-driven design and discovery of novel compounds with antiplasmodial and transmission blocking activities. *Front. Pharmacol.* 9:146. doi: 10.3389/fphar.2018.00146

Lise, S., Buchan, D., Pontil, M., and Jones, D. T. (2011). Predictions of hot spot residues at protein-protein interfaces using support vector machines. *PLoS One* 6:e16774. doi: 10.1371/journal.pone.0016774

Lo, C. H., Vunnam, N., Lewis, A., Chiu, T.-L., Brummel, B., Schaaf, T., et al. (2017). Inhibition of tumor necrosis factor receptor 1 signaling by small molecules. *FASEB J.* 31, 611–619. doi: 10.1096/fasebj.31.1_supplement.609.11

London, N., Raveh, B., and Schueler-Furman, O. (2013). Druggable protein–protein interactions – from hot spots to hot segments. *Curr. Opin. Chem. Biol.* 17, 952–959. doi: 10.1016/j.cbpa.2013.10.011

Maier, J. A., Martinez, C., Kasavajhala, K., Wickstrom, L., Hauser, K. E., and Simmerling, C. (2015). ff14SB: improving the accuracy of protein side chain and backbone parameters from ff99SB. *J. Chem. Theory Comput.* 11, 3696–3713. doi: 10.1021/acs.jctc.5b00255

Mancini, F., Toro, C. M., Mabilia, M., Giannangeli, M., Pinza, M., and Milanese, C. (1999). Inhibition of tumor necrosis factor-α (TNF-α)/ TNF-α receptor binding by structural analogues of suramin§. *Biochem. Pharmacol.* 58, 851–859. doi: 10.1016/S0006-2952(99)00150-1

Mattos, C., and Ringe, D. (1996). Locating and characterizing binding sites on proteins. *Nat. Biotechnol.* 14, 595–599. doi: 10.1038/nbt0596-595

McGeary, R. P., Bennett, A. J., Tran, Q. B., Cosgrove, K. L., and Ross, B. P. (2008). Suramin: clinical uses and structure-activity relationships. *Mini Rev. Med. Chem.* 8, 1384–1394. doi: 10.2174/138955708786369573

Melagraki, G., Leonis, G., Ntougkos, E., Rinotas, V., Papaneophytou, C., Mavromoustakos, T., et al. (2018). Current status and future prospects of small-molecule protein-protein interaction (PPI) inhibitors of tumor necrosis factor (TNF) and receptor activator of NF-κB ligand (RANKL). *Curr. Top. Med. Chem.* 18, 1–13. doi: 10.2174/1568026618666180607084430

Melagraki, G., Ntougkos, E., Rinotas, V., Papaneophytou, C., Leonis, G., Mavromoustakos, T., et al. (2017). Cheminformatics-aided discovery of small-molecule Protein-Protein Interaction (PPI) dual inhibitors of Tumor Necrosis Factor (TNF) and Receptor Activator of NF-κB Ligand (RANKL). *PLoS Comput. Biol.* 13:e1005372. doi: 10.1371/journal.pcbi.1005372

Melagraki, G. A., and Afantitis, A. (2014). Enalos InSilicoNano platform: an online decision support tool for the design and virtual screening of nanoparticles. *RSC Adv.* 4, 50713–50725. doi: 10.1039/C4RA07756C

Olsen, N. J., and Stein, C. M. (2004). New drugs for rheumatoid arthritis. *N. Engl. J. Med.* 350, 2167–2179. doi: 10.1056/NEJMra032906

Perkins, J. R., Diboun, I., Dessailly, B. H., Lees, J. G., and Orengo, C. (2010). Transient protein-protein interactions: structural, functional, and network properties. *Structure* 18, 1233–1243. doi: 10.1016/j.str.2010.08.007

Rajamani, D., Thiel, S., Vajda, S., and Camacho, C. J. (2004). Anchor residues in protein–protein interactions. *Proc. Natl. Acad. Sci. U.S.A.* 101, 11287–11292. doi: 10.1073/pnas.0401942101

Reutlinger, M., Rodrigues, T., Schneider, P., and Schneider, G. (2014). Multi-objective molecular de novo design by adaptive fragment prioritization. *Angew. Chem. Int. Ed.* 53, 4244–4248. doi: 10.1002/anie.201310864

Rodrigues, T., Reker, D., Schneider, P., and Schneider, G. (2016). Counting on natural products for drug design. *Nat. Chem.* 8, 531–541. doi: 10.1038/nchem. 2479

Sackett, D. L., and Sept, D. (2009). Protein-protein interactions: making drug design second nature. *Nat. Chem.* 1, 596–597. doi: 10.1038/nchem.427

Sali, A., and Blundell, T. L. (1993). Comparative protein modelling by satisfaction of spatial restraints. *J. Mol. Biol.* 234, 779–815. doi: 10.1006/jmbi.1993. 1626

Schmidtke, P., and Barril, X. (2010). Understanding and predicting druggability. A high-throughput method for detection of drug binding sites. *J. Med. Chem.* 53, 5858–5867. doi: 10.1021/jm100574m

Sfikakis, P. P. (2010). The first decade of biologic TNF antagonists in clinical practice: lessons learned, unresolved issues and future directions. *Curr. Dir. Autoimmun.* 11, 180–210. doi: 10.1159/000289205

Sheng, C., Dong, G., Miao, Z., Zhang, W., and Wang, W. (2015). State-of-the-art strategies for targeting protein-protein interactions by small-molecule inhibitors. *Chem. Soc. Rev.* 44, 8238–8259. doi: 10.1039/C5CS0 0252D

Shuker, S. B., Hajduk, P. J., Meadows, R. P., and Fesik, S. W. (1996). Discovering high-affinity ligands for proteins: SAR by NMR. *Science* 274, 1531–1534. doi: 10.1126/science.274.5292.1531

Smith, M. C., and Gestwicki, J. E. (2012). Features of protein-protein interactions that translate into potent inhibitors: topology, surface area and affinity. *Expert Rev. Mol. Med.* 14:e16. doi: 10.1017/erm.2012.10

Sun, H., and Yost, G. S. (2008). Metabolic activation of a novel 3-substituted indole-containing TNF-α inhibitor: dehydrogenation and inactivation of CYP3A4. *Chem. Res. Toxicol.* 21, 374–385. doi: 10.1021/tx700294g

Thomsen, R., and Christensen, M. H. (2006). MolDock: a new technique for high-accuracy molecular docking. *J. Med. Chem.* 49, 3315–3321. doi: 10.1021/ jm051197e

Tuncbag, N., Keskin, O., and Gursoy, A. (2010). HotPoint: hot spot prediction server for protein interfaces. *Nucleic Acids Res.* 38(Suppl. 2), W402–W406. doi: 10.1093/nar/gkq323

Wang, J., Wang, W., Kollman, P., and Case, D. (2006). Automatic atom type and bond type perception in molecular mechanical calculations. *J. Mol. Graph. Model.* 25, 247–260. doi: 10.1016/j.jmgm.2005.12.005

Wang, J., Wolf, R., Caldwell, J., Kollman, P., and Case, D. (2004). Development and testing of a general amber force field. *J. Comput. Chem.* 25, 1157–1174. doi: 10.1002/jcc.20035

Wilson, A. J. (2009). Inhibition of protein-protein interactions using designed molecules. *Chem. Soc. Rev.* 38, 3289–3300. doi: 10.1039/b807 197g

Xu, L., Sun, H., Li, Y., Wang, J., and Hou, T. (2013). Assessing the performance of MM/PBSA and MM/GBSA methods. 3. The impact of force fields and ligand charge models. *J. Phys. Chem. B* 117, 8408–8421. doi: 10.1021/jp404160y

Ye, Y., and Godzik, A. (2003). Flexible structure alignment by chaining aligned fragment pairs allowing twists. *Bioinformatics* 19(Suppl. 2), ii246–ii255. doi: 10.1093/bioinformatics/btg1086

Zheng, S., Jiang, M., Zhao, C., Zhu, R., Hu, Z., Xu, Y., et al. (2018). e-Bitter: bitterant prediction by the consensus voting from the machine-learning methods. *Front. Chem.* 6:82. doi: 10.3389/fchem.2018.00082

QSAR-Based Virtual Screening: Advances and Applications in Drug Discovery

*Bruno J. Neves[1,2], Rodolpho C. Braga[1], Cleber C. Melo-Filho[1],
José Teófilo Moreira-Filho[1], Eugene N. Muratov[3,4] and Carolina Horta Andrade[1]**

[1] LabMol – Laboratory for Molecular Modeling and Drug Design, Faculdade de Farmácia, Universidade Federal de Goiás, Goiânia, Brazil, [2] Laboratory of Cheminformatics, Centro Universitário de Anápolis (UniEVANGÉLICA), Anápolis, Brazil, [3] Laboratory for Molecular Modeling, Division of Chemical Biology and Medicinal Chemistry, Eshelman School of Pharmacy, University of North Carolina at Chapel Hill, Chapel Hill, NC, United States, [4] Department of Chemical Technology, Odessa National Polytechnic University, Odessa, Ukraine

Correspondence:
Carolina Horta Andrade
carolina@ufg.br;
carolhandrade@gmail.com

Virtual screening (VS) has emerged in drug discovery as a powerful computational approach to screen large libraries of small molecules for new hits with desired properties that can then be tested experimentally. Similar to other computational approaches, VS intention is not to replace *in vitro* or *in vivo* assays, but to speed up the discovery process, to reduce the number of candidates to be tested experimentally, and to rationalize their choice. Moreover, VS has become very popular in pharmaceutical companies and academic organizations due to its time-, cost-, resources-, and labor-saving. Among the VS approaches, quantitative structure–activity relationship (QSAR) analysis is the most powerful method due to its high and fast throughput and good hit rate. As the first preliminary step of a QSAR model development, relevant chemogenomics data are collected from databases and the literature. Then, chemical descriptors are calculated on different levels of representation of molecular structure, ranging from 1D to nD, and then correlated with the biological property using machine learning techniques. Once developed and validated, QSAR models are applied to predict the biological property of novel compounds. Although the experimental testing of computational hits is not an inherent part of QSAR methodology, it is highly desired and should be performed as an ultimate validation of developed models. In this mini-review, we summarize and critically analyze the recent trends of QSAR-based VS in drug discovery and demonstrate successful applications in identifying perspective compounds with desired properties. Moreover, we provide some recommendations about the best practices for QSAR-based VS along with the future perspectives of this approach.

Keywords: cheminformatics, machine learning, molecular descriptors, computer-assisted drug design, virtual screening

INTRODUCTION

Quantitative structure–activity relationship (QSAR) analysis is a ligand-based drug design method developed more than 50 years ago by Hansch and Fujita (1964). Since then and until now, QSAR remains an efficient method for building mathematical models, which attempts to find a statistically significant correlation between the chemical structure and continuous (pIC_{50}, pEC_{50}, Ki, etc.) or categorical/binary (active, inactive, toxic, nontoxic, etc.) biological/toxicological property using regression and classification techniques, respectively (Cherkasov et al., 2014). In the last decades, QSAR has undergone several transformations, ranging from the dimensionality of the molecular descriptors (from 1D to nD) and different methods for finding a correlation between the chemical structures and the biological property. Initially, QSAR modeling was limited to small series of congeneric compounds and simple regression methods. Nowadays, QSAR modeling has grown, diversified, and evolved to the modeling and virtual screening (VS) of very large data sets comprising thousands of diverse chemical structures and using a wide variety of machine learning techniques (Cherkasov et al., 2014; Mitchell, 2014; Ekins et al., 2015; Goh et al., 2017).

This review is devoted to (i) critical analysis of advantages and disadvantages of QSAR-based VS in drug discovery; (ii) demonstration of several successful QSAR-based discoveries of compounds with desired properties; (iii) description of best practices for the QSAR-based VS; and (iv) discussion of future perspectives of this approach.

BEST PRACTICES IN QSAR MODELING AND VALIDATION

High-throughput screening (HTS) technologies resulted in the explosion of amount of data suitable for QSAR modeling. As a result, data quality problem became one of the fundamental questions in cheminformatics. As obvious as it seems, various errors in both chemical structure and experimental results are considered as major obstacle to building predictive models (Young et al., 2008; Southan et al., 2009; Williams and Ekins, 2011).

Considering these limitations, Fourches et al. (2010; 2015; 2016) developed the guidelines for chemical and biological data curation as a first and mandatory step of the predictive QSAR modeling. Organized into a solid functional process, these guidelines allow the identification, correction, or, if needed, removal of structural and biological errors in large data sets. Data curation procedures include the removal of organometallics, counterions, mixtures, and inorganics, as well as the normalization of specific chemotypes, structural cleaning (e.g., detection of valence violations), standardization of tautomeric forms, and ring aromatization. Additional curation elements include averaging, aggregating, or removal of duplicates to produce a single bioactivity result. Detailed discussion of aforementioned data curation procedures can be found elsewhere (Fourches et al., 2010, 2015, 2016).

The Organization for Economic Cooperation and Development (OECD) developed a set of guidelines that the researchers should follow to achieve the regulatory acceptance of QSAR models. According to these principles, QSAR models should be associated with (i) defined end point, (ii) unambiguous algorithm, (iii) defined domain of applicability, (iv) appropriate measures of goodness-of-fit, robustness, and predictivity, and (v) if possible, mechanistic interpretation (OECD, 2004). In our opinion, the additional rule requesting thorough data curation as a mandatory preliminary step to model development should be added there.

CONTINUING IMPORTANCE OF QSAR AS VIRTUAL SCREENING TOOL

The current pipeline to discover hit compounds in early stages of drug discovery is a data-driven process, which relies on bioactivity data obtained from HTS campaigns (Nantasenamat and Prachayasittikul, 2015). Since the cost of obtaining new hit compounds in HTS platforms is rather high, QSAR modeling has been playing a pivotal role in prioritizing compounds for synthesis and/or biological evaluation. The QSAR models can be used for both hits identification and hit-to-lead optimization. In the latter, a favorable balance between potency, selectivity, and pharmacokinetic and toxicological parameters, which is required to develop a new, safe, and effective drug, could be achieved through several optimization cycles. As no compound need to be synthesized or tested before computational evaluation, QSAR represents a labor-, time-, and cost-effective method to obtain compounds with desired biological properties. Consequently, QSAR is widely practiced in industries, universities, and research centers around the world (Cherkasov et al., 2014).

The general scheme of QSAR-based VS approach is shown in **Figure 1**. Initially, the data sets collected from external sources are curated and integrated to remove or correct inconsistent data. Using these data, QSAR models are developed and validated following OECD guidelines and best practices of modeling. Then, QSAR models are used to identify chemical compounds predicted to be active against selected endpoints from large chemical libraries (Cherkasov et al., 2014). In principle, VS is often compared to a funnel, where a large chemical library (i.e., 10^5 to 10^7 chemical structures) is reduced by QSAR models to a smaller number of compounds, which then will be tested experimentally (i.e., 10^1 to 10^3 chemical structures) (Kar and Roy, 2013; Tanrikulu et al., 2013). However, it is important to mention that modern VS workflows incorporate additional filtering steps, including: (i) sets of empirical rules [e.g., Lipinski's (Lipinski et al., 1997) rules], (ii) chemical similarity cutoffs, (iii) other QSAR-based filters (e.g., toxicological and pharmacokinetic endpoints), and (iv) chemical feasibility and/or purchasability (Cherkasov et al., 2014). Although the experimental validation of computational hits does not represent part of the QSAR methodology, this should be performed as the final important step. After experimental validation, a multi-parameter optimization (MPO) with QSAR predictions of potency, selectivity, and pharmacokinetic parameters can be conducted. This information will be crucial during hit-to lead and lead optimization design of the compound series, to find the properties balance (potency, selectivity, and PK) related with the effect of different decoration patterns to establish a new series of target compounds for *in vivo* evaluation.

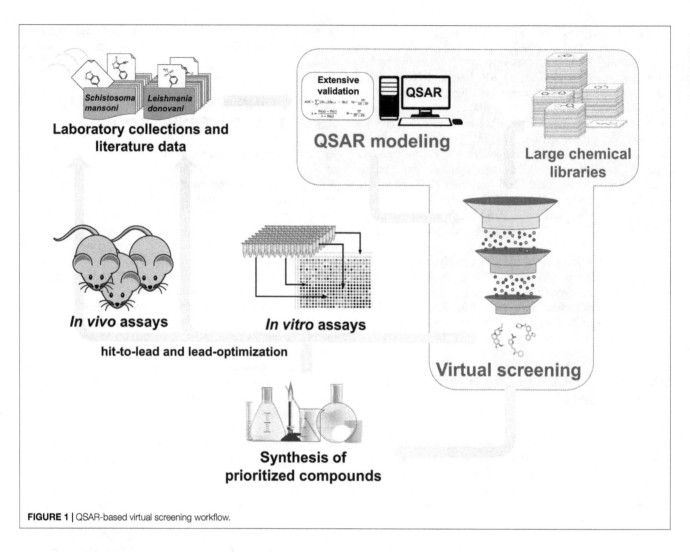

FIGURE 1 | QSAR-based virtual screening workflow.

QSAR-BASED VIRTUAL SCREENING vs. HIGH-THROUGHPUT SCREENING

High-throughput screening can rapidly identify large subsets of molecules with desired activity from large screening collections of compounds (10^5–10^6 compounds) using automated plate-based experimental assays (Mueller et al., 2012). However, the hit rate of HTS ranges between 0.01% and 0.1% and this highlights the frequently encountered limitation that most of the screened compounds are routinely reported as inactive toward the desired bioactivity (Thorne et al., 2010). Consequently, the drug discovery cost increases according to the number of tested compounds (Butkiewicz et al., 2013). On the other hand, typical hit rates from a validated VS method, including QSAR-based, typically range between 1% and 40%. Thus, VS campaigns are found to have a higher rate of biologically active compounds and at a lower cost than HTS.

In this perspective, we show that QSAR-based VS could be used to enrich hit rates of HTS campaigns. For example, Mueller et al. (2010) employed both HTS and QSAR models to search novel positive allosteric modulators for mGlu5, a G-protein coupled receptor involved in disorders like schizophrenia and

Parkinson's disease. First, the HTS of approximately 144,000 compounds resulted in a total of 1,356 hits, with a hit rate of 0.94%. Then, this dataset was used to build continuous QSAR models (combining physicochemical descriptors and neural networks), which were subsequently applied to screen a database of approximately 450,000 compounds. Finally, 824 compounds were acquired for biological testing and 232 were confirmed as active (hit rate of 28.2%) (Mueller et al., 2010). In another study, Rodriguez et al. (2010) screened approximately 160,000 compounds to identify 624 antagonists of mGlu5. Further, these data were used to develop QSAR models and, then, applied to screen near 700,000 compounds from ChemDiv database. Among them, 88 of acquired compounds were active, corresponding to a hit rate of 3.6% while the HTS had a hit rate of 0.2% (Mueller et al., 2012).

PRACTICAL APPLICATIONS OF QSAR-BASED VIRTUAL SCREENING

Despite its obvious advantages, QSAR modeling remains underestimated as a VS tool. Unfortunately, QSAR is still seen as a complementary analysis to studies of synthesis and biological evaluation, often introduced in the study without any justification or additional perspective. Despite the small number of VS applications available in the literature, most of them led to the discovery of promising hits and lead candidates. Below, we discuss some successful applications of QSAR-based VS for the discovery of new hits and hit-to-lead optimization.

Malaria

Malaria is an infectious disease caused by five different species of *Plasmodium* parasites and transmitted to humans through the bite of infected female mosquitoes of the genus *Anopheles*. The most lethal species is *P. falciparum*, which can lead to severe illness and death (Phillips et al., 2017). Malaria is a widespread disease; 91 countries and areas have ongoing transmission. According to World Health Organization (WHO), about 216 million cases and 445,000 deaths from malaria were reported in 2016 (WHO, 2018c). Furthermore, the resistance to antimalarial drugs is a common and growing issue and constitutes a substantial threat for populations in endemic regions (Gorobets et al., 2017; Menard and Dondorp, 2017). In a study reported by Zhang et al. (2013), a data set of 3,133 compounds reported as active or inactive against *P. falciparum* chloroquine susceptible strain (3D7) was used to develop QSAR models. The models were built using Dragon descriptors (0D, 1D, and 2D), ISIDA-2D fragments descriptors and support vector machines (SVM) method. During QSAR modeling and validation, the data set was randomly divided into modeling and external evaluation set. Additionally, the modeling set was divided multiple times in training and test sets using the Sphere Exclusion algorithm. Then, by using a consensus approach, the QSAR models were applied for VS of the ChemBridge database. After VS, 176 potential antimalarial compounds were identified and submitted to experimental validation along with 42 putative inactive compounds, used as negative controls. Twenty-five compounds presented antimalarial activity in *P. falciparum* growth inhibition assays and low cytotoxicity in mammalian cells. All 42 compounds predicted as inactives by the models were confirmed experimentally (Zhang et al., 2013). The confirmed experimental hits presented new chemical scaffolds against *P. falciparum* and could be promising starting points for the development of new optimized antimalarial agents.

Schistosomiasis

Schistosomiasis is a disease caused by flatworms of the genus *Schistosoma* that affects 206 million of people worldwide (WHO, 2018d). The current reliance on only one drug, praziquantel, for treatment and control of this disease calls for the urgent discovery of novel anti-schistosomal drugs (Colley et al., 2014). Aiming at discovering new drugs, our group developed binary QSAR models for *Schistosoma mansoni* thioredoxin glutathione reductase (*Sm*TGR), a validated target for schistosomiasis (Kuntz et al., 2007), to find new structurally dissimilar compounds with antischistosomal activity (Neves et al., 2016). To achieve this goal, we designed a study with the following steps: (i) curation of the largest possible data set of *Sm*TGR inhibitors, (ii) development of rigorously validated and mechanistically interpretable models,

and (iii) application of generated models for VS of ChemBridge library. Using the QSAR models, we prioritized 29 compounds for further experimental evaluation. As a result, we found that the QSAR models were efficient for discovery of six novel hit compounds active against schistosomula and three hits active against adult worms (hit rate of 20.6%). Among them, 2-[2-(3-methyl-4-nitro-5-isoxazolyl)vinyl]pyridine and 2-(benzylsulfonyl)-1,3-benzothiazole, two compounds representing new chemical scaffolds have activity against schistosomula and adult worms at low micromolar concentrations and therefore represent promising antischistosomal hits for further hit-to-lead optimization (Neves et al., 2016).

In another study, we developed continuous QSAR models for a data set of oxadiazoles inhibitors of *sm*TGR (Melo-Filho et al., 2016). Using a combi-QSAR approach, we built a consensus model combining the predictions of individual 2D- and 3D-QSAR models. Then, the model was used for VS of ChemBridge database and the 10 top ranked compounds were further evaluated *in vitro* against schistosomula and adult worms. Additionally, we applied five highly predictive in-house QSAR models for prediction of important pharmacokinetics and toxicity properties of the new hits. The experimental results showed that 4-nitro-3,5-bis(1-nitro-1H-pyrazol-4-yl)-1H-pyrazole (LabMol-17) and 3-nitro-4-{[(4-nitro-1,2,5-oxadiazol-3-yl)oxy]methyl}-1,2,5-oxadiazole (LabMol-19), two compounds containing new chemical scaffolds (hit rate of 20.6%), were highly active in both life stages of the parasite at low micromolar concentrations (Melo-Filho et al., 2016).

Tuberculosis

Mycobacterium tuberculosis, the causative agent of tuberculosis (TB), kills about 1.6 million people every year (WHO, 2018e). The current treatment of this disease takes approximately 9 months, which normally leads to noncompliance and, hence, the emergence of multidrug-resistant bacteria (AlMatar et al., 2017). Aiming the design of new anti-TB agents, our group used QSAR models to design new series of chalcone (1,3-diaryl-2-propen-1-ones) derivatives. Initially, we retrieved from the literature all chalcone compounds with *in vitro* inhibition data against *M. tuberculosis* H37Rv strain. After rigorous data curation, these chalcones were subject to structure–activity relationships (SAR) analysis. Based on SAR rules, bioisosteric replacements were employed to design new chalcone derivatives with optimized anti-TB activity. In parallel, binary QSAR models were generated using several machine learning methods and molecular fingerprints. The fivefold external cross-validation procedure confirmed the high predictive power of the developed models. Using these models, we prioritized series of chalcone derivatives for synthesis and biological evaluation (Gomes et al., 2017). As a result, five 5-nitro-substituted heteroaryl chalcones were found to exhibit MICs at nanomolar concentrations against replicating mycobacteria, as well as low micromolar activity against nonreplicating bacteria. In addition, four of these compounds were more potent than standard drug isoniazid. The series also showed low cytotoxicity against commensal bacteria and mammalian cells. These results suggest that designed heteroaryl chalcones, identified with the help of QSAR models, are promising anti-TB lead candidates (Gomes et al., 2017).

Viral Infections

Yearly, influenza epidemics can seriously affect all populations in the world. These annual epidemics are estimated to result in about 5 million cases and 650,000 deaths (WHO, 2018b). Influenza virus is mutating constantly, resulting in novel resistant strains, and hence, the development of new anti-influenza drugs active against these new strains is important to prevent pandemics (Laborda et al., 2016). Aiming the discovery of new anti-influenza A drugs, Lian et al. (2015) built binary QSAR models, using SVM and Naïve Bayesian methods, to predict neuraminidase inhibition, a validated protein target for influenza. Then, four different combinations of machine learning methods and molecular descriptors were applied to screen 15,600 compounds from an in-house database, among which 60 compounds were selected to experimental evaluation on neuraminidase activity. Nine inhibitors were identified, five of which were oseltamivir derivatives exhibiting potent neuraminidase inhibition at nanomolar concentrations. Other four active compounds belonged to novel scaffolds, with potent inhibition at low micromolar concentrations (Lian et al., 2015).

According to WHO, approximately 35 million people are infected with HIV (WHO, 2018a). The treatment for HIV infections requires a lifelong antiretroviral therapy, targeting different stages of HIV replication cycle. Consequently, because of the emergence of resistance and the lack of tolerability, development of novel anti-HIV drugs is of high demand (Cihlar and Fordyce, 2016; Garbelli et al., 2017). With the purpose of discovering new anti-HIV-1 drugs, Kurczyk et al. (2015) developed a two-step VS approach to prioritize compounds against HIV integrase, an important target to viral replication cycle. The first step was based on binary QSAR models, and the second on privileged fragments. Then, 1.5 million of commercially available compounds were screened, and 13 compounds were selected to be tested *in vitro* for inhibiting HIV-1 replication. Among them, two novel chemotypes with moderate anti-HIV-1 potencies were identified, and therefore, represent new starting points for prospective structural optimization studies.

Mood and Anxiety Disorders

The 5-hydroxytryptamine 1A (5-HT$_{1A}$) serotonin receptor has been an attractive target for treating mood and anxiety disorders such as schizophrenia (Nichols and Nichols, 2008; Lacivita et al., 2012). However, the currently marketed drugs targeting 5-HT$_{1A}$ receptor possess severe side effects. To address this, Luo et al. (2014) developed a QSAR-based VS workflow to find new hit compounds targeting 5-HT$_{1A}$ receptor. First, binary QSAR models were generated using Dragon descriptors and several machine learning methods. Then, developed QSAR models were rigorously validated and applied in consensus for VS four commercial chemical databases. Fifteen compounds were selected for experimental testing, and nine of them have proven to be active at low nanomolar concentrations. One

of the confirmed hits, [(8α)-6-methyl-9,10-didehydroergolin-8-yl]methanol), showed very high binding affinity (Ki) of 2.3 nM against 5-HT$_{1A}$ receptor.

Future Directions and Conclusion

To summarize, we would like to emphasize that QSAR modeling represents a time-, labor-, and cost-effective tool to discover hit compounds and lead candidates in the early stages of drug discovery process. Analyzing the examples of QSAR-based VS available in the literature, one can see that many of them led to the identification of promising lead candidates. However, along with success stories, many QSAR projects fail on the model building stage. This is caused by the lack of understanding that QSAR is highly interdisciplinary and application field as well as general ignorance of the best practices in the field (Tropsha, 2010; Ban et al., 2017). Earlier, we have explained this by the undesirably high population of "button pushers," that is, researchers who conduct modeling without understanding and analyzing the data and modeling process itself (Muratov et al., 2012). This was also explained by the elusive ease of obtaining computational model and making even advanced calculations without understanding of the sense and limitations of the approach (Bajorath, 2012). In addition to this, a lot of even experienced researchers target their efforts to a "vicious statistical cycle," which main goal is to validate models using as many metrics as possible. In this case, the QSAR modeling is restricted to a single simple question: "What is the best metrics or the best statistical method"? Although we recognize that the right choice of statistical approach and especially rigorous external validation are necessary and represent an essential step in any computer-aided drug discovery study, we want to reinforce that QSAR modeling is useful only if it is applied for the solution of a formulated problem and results in development of new compounds with desired properties.

As future directions, we would like to point out that the era of big data has just started, and it is still in the chemical/biological data accumulation stage. Therefore, to avoid the situation that the number of assayed compounds available on literature exceeds the modeling capability, the development, and implementation of new machine learning algorithms and data curation methods capable of handling millions of compounds are urgently needed. Finally, the overall success of any QSAR-based VS project depends on the ability of a scientist to think critically and prioritize the most promising hits according to his experience. Moreover, the success rate of collaborative drug discovery projects, where the final selection of computational hits is done by both a modeler and an expert in a given field, is much higher than success rate of the projects driven solely by computational or experimental scientists.

AUTHOR CONTRIBUTIONS

All authors listed have made a substantial, direct and intellectual contribution to the work, and approved it for publication.

FUNDING

This work was partially funded by the Grant No. 1U01CA207160 from NIH and Grant No. 400760/2014-2 from CNPq. CHA is Research Fellow in productivity of CNPq.

ACKNOWLEDGMENTS

The authors would like to thank Brazilian funding agencies, CNPq, CAPES, and FAPEG, for financial support and fellowships.

REFERENCES

AlMatar, M., AlMandeal, H., Var, I., Kayar, B., and Köksal, F. (2017). New drugs for the treatment of *Mycobacterium tuberculosis* infection. *Biomed. Pharmacother.* 91, 546–558. doi: 10.1016/j.biopha.2017.04.105

Bajorath, J. (2012). Computational chemistry in pharmaceutical research: at the crossroads. *J. Comput. Aided. Mol. Des.* 26, 11–12. doi: 10.1007/s10822-011-9488-z

Ban, F., Dalal, K., Li, H., LeBlanc, E., Rennie, P. S., and Cherkasov, A. (2017). Best practices of computer-aided drug discovery: lessons learned from the development of a preclinical candidate for prostate cancer with a new mechanism of action. *J. Chem. Inf. Model.* 57, 1018–1028. doi: 10.1021/acs.jcim.7b00137

Butkiewicz, M., Lowe, E. W., Mueller, R., Mendenhall, J. L., Teixeira, P. L., Weaver, C. D., et al. (2013). Benchmarking ligand-based virtual high-throughput screening with the pubchem database. *Molecules* 18, 735–756. doi: 10.3390/molecules18010735

Cherkasov, A., Muratov, E. N., Fourches, D., Varnek, A., Baskin, I. I., Cronin, M., et al. (2014). QSAR modeling: where have you been? Where are you going to? *J. Med. Chem.* 57, 4977–5010. doi: 10.1021/jm4004285

Cihlar, T., and Fordyce, M. (2016). Current status and prospects of HIV treatment. *Curr. Opin. Virol.* 18, 50–56. doi: 10.1016/j.coviro.2016.03.004

Colley, D. G., Bustinduy, A. L., Secor, W. E., and King, C. H. (2014). Human schistosomiasis. *Lancet* 383, 2253–2264. doi: 10.1016/S0140-6736(13)61949-2

Ekins, S., Lage de Siqueira-Neto, J., McCall, L.-I., Sarker, M., Yadav, M., Ponder, E. L., et al. (2015). Machine learning models and pathway genome data base for *Trypanosoma cruzi* drug discovery. *PLoS Negl. Trop. Dis.* 9:e0003878. doi: 10.1371/journal.pntd.0003878

Fourches, D., Muratov, E., and Tropsha, A. (2010). Trust, but verify: on the importance of chemical structure curation in cheminformatics and QSAR modeling research. *J. Chem. Inf. Model.* 50, 1189–1204. doi: 10.1021/ci100176x

Fourches, D., Muratov, E., and Tropsha, A. (2015). Curation of chemogenomics data. *Nat. Chem. Biol.* 11, 535–535. doi: 10.1038/nchembio.1881

Fourches, D., Muratov, E., and Tropsha, A. (2016). Trust, but verify II: a practical guide to chemogenomics data curation. *J. Chem. Inf. Model.* 56, 1243–1252. doi: 10.1021/acs.jcim.6b00129

Garbelli, A., Riva, V., Crespan, E., and Maga, G. (2017). How to win the HIV-1 drug resistance hurdle race: running faster or jumping higher? *Biochem. J.* 474, 1559–1577. doi: 10.1042/BCJ20160772

Goh, G. B., Hodas, N. O., and Vishnu, A. (2017). Deep learning for computational chemistry. *J. Comput. Chem.* 38, 1291–1307. doi: 10.1002/jcc.24764

Gomes, M. N. M. N., Braga, R. C. R. C., Grzelak, E. M. E. M., Neves, B. J. B. J., Muratov, E., Ma, R., et al. (2017). QSAR-driven design, synthesis and discovery of potent chalcone derivatives with antitubercular activity. *Eur. J. Med. Chem.* 137, 126–138. doi: 10.1016/j.ejmech.2017.05.026

Gorobets, N. Y., Sedash, Y. V., Singh, B. K., Poonam, A., and Rathi, B. (2017). An overview of currently available antimalarials. *Curr. Top. Med. Chem.* 17, 2143–2157. doi: 10.2174/1568026617666170130123520

Hansch, C., and Fujita, T. (1964). ρ -σ-π analysis. A method for the correlation of biological activity and chemical structure. *J. Am. Chem. Soc.* 86, 1616–1626. doi: 10.1021/ja01062a035

Kar, S., and Roy, K. (2013). How far can virtual screening take us in drug discovery? *Expert Opin. Drug Discov.* 8, 245–261. doi: 10.1517/17460441.2013.761204

Kuntz, A. N., Davioud-Charvet, E., Sayed, A. A., Califf, L. L., Dessolin, J., Arnér, E. S. J., et al. (2007). Thioredoxin glutathione reductase from *Schistosoma mansoni*: an essential parasite enzyme and a key drug target. *PLoS Med.* 4:e206. doi: 10.1371/journal.pmed.0040206

Kurczyk, A., Warszycki, D., Musiol, R., Kafel, R., Bojarski, A. J., and Polanski, J. (2015). Ligand-based virtual screening in a search for novel anti-HIV-1 chemotypes. *J. Chem. Inf. Model.* 55, 2168–2177. doi: 10.1021/acs.jcim.5b00295

Laborda, P., Wang, S. Y., and Voglmeir, J. (2016). Influenza neuraminidase inhibitors: synthetic approaches, derivatives and biological activity. *Molecules* 21, 1–40. doi: 10.3390/molecules21111513

Lacivita, E., Di Pilato, P., De Giorgio, P., Colabufo, N. A., Berardi, F., Perrone, R., et al. (2012). The therapeutic potential of 5-HT1A receptors: a patent review. *Expert Opin. Ther. Pat.* 22, 887–902. doi: 10.1517/13543776.2012.703654

Lian, W., Fang, J., Li, C., Pang, X., Liu, A.-L., and Du, G.-H. (2015). Discovery of influenza A virus neuraminidase inhibitors using support vector machine and Naïve Bayesian models. *Mol. Divers.* 20, 439–451. doi: 10.1007/s11030-015-9641-z

Lipinski, C. A., Lombardo, F., Dominy, B. W., and Feeney, P. J. (1997). Experimental and computational approaches to estimate solubility and permeability in drug discovery and development settings. *Adv. Drug Deliv. Rev.* 23, 3–25. doi: 10.1016/S0169-409X(96)00423-1

Luo, M., Wang, X. S., Roth, B. L., Golbraikh, A., and Tropsha, A. (2014). Application of quantitative structure-activity relationship models of 5-HT1A receptor binding to virtual screening identifies novel and potent 5-HT1A ligands. *J. Chem. Inf. Model.* 54, 634–647. doi: 10.1021/ci400460q

Melo-Filho, C. C., Dantas, R. F., Braga, R. C., Neves, B. J., Senger, M. R., Valente, W. C. G., et al. (2016). QSAR-driven discovery of novel chemical scaffolds active against *Schistosoma mansoni*. *J. Chem. Inf. Model.* 56, 1357–1372. doi: 10.1021/acs.jcim.6b00055

Menard, D., and Dondorp, A. (2017). Antimalarial drug resistance: a threat to malaria elimination. *Cold Spring Harb. Perspect. Med.* 7:a025619. doi: 10.1101/cshperspect.a025619

Mitchell, J. B. O. (2014). Machine learning methods in chemoinformatics. *Wiley Interdisc. Rev. Comput. Mol. Sci.* 4, 468–481. doi: 10.1002/wcms.1183

Mueller, R., Dawson, E. S., Meiler, J., Rodriguez, A. L., Chauder, B. A., Bates, B. S., et al. (2012). Discovery of 2-(2-Benzoxazoyl amino)-4-Aryl-5-cyanopyrimidine as negative allosteric modulators (NAMs) of metabotropic glutamate receptor5 (mGlu 5): from an artificial neural network virtual screen to an in vivo tool compound. *ChemMedChem* 7, 406–414. doi: 10.1002/cmdc.201100510

Mueller, R., Rodriguez, A. L., Dawson, E. S., Butkiewicz, M., Nguyen, T. T., Oleszkiewicz, S., et al. (2010). Identification of metabotropic glutamate receptor subtype 5 potentiators using virtual high-throughput screening. *ACS Chem. Neurosci.* 1, 288–305. doi: 10.1021/cn9000389

Muratov, E. N., Varlamova, E. V., Artemenko, A. G., Polishchuk, P. G., and Kuz'min, V. E. (2012). Existing and developing approaches for QSAR analysis of mixtures. *Mol. Inform.* 31, 202–221. doi: 10.1002/minf.201100129

Nantasenamat, C., and Prachayasittikul, V. (2015). Maximizing computational tools for successful drug discovery. *Expert Opin. Drug Discov.* 10, 321–329. doi: 10.1517/17460441.2015.1016497

Neves, B. J., Dantas, R. F., Senger, M. R., Melo-Filho, C. C., Valente, W. C. G., de Almeida, A. C. M., et al. (2016). Discovery of new anti-schistosomal hits by integration of QSAR-based virtual screening and high content screening. *J. Med. Chem.* 59, 7075–7088. doi: 10.1021/acs.jmedchem.5b02038

Nichols, D. E., and Nichols, C. D. (2008). Serotonin receptors. *Chem. Rev.* 108, 1614–1641. doi: 10.1021/cr078224o

OECD (2004). *OECD Principles for the Validation, for Regulatory Purposes, of (Quantitative) Structure-Activity Relationship Models.* Available at: https://www.oecd.org/chemicalsafety/risk-assessment/37849783.pdf [accessed September 20, 2018]

Phillips, M. A., Burrows, J. N., Manyando, C., van Huijsduijnen, R. H., Van Voorhis, W. C., and Wells, T. N. C. (2017). Malaria. *Nat. Rev. Dis. Prim.* 3:17050. doi: 10.1038/nrdp.2017.50

Rodriguez, A. L., Grier, M. D., Jones, C. K., Herman, E. J., Kane, A. S., Smith, R. L., et al. (2010). Discovery of novel allosteric modulators of metabotropic glutamate receptor subtype 5 reveals chemical and functional diversity and in vivo activity in rat behavioral models of anxiolytic and antipsychotic activity. *Mol. Pharmacol.* 78, 1105–1123. doi: 10.1124/mol.110.067207

Southan, C., Várkonyi, P., and Muresan, S. (2009). Quantitative assessment of the expanding complementarity between public and commercial databases of bioactive compounds. *J. Cheminform.* 1:10. doi: 10.1186/1758-2946-1-10

Tanrikulu, Y., Krüger, B., and Proschak, E. (2013). The holistic integration of virtual screening in drug discovery. *Drug Discov. Today* 18, 358–364. doi: 10.1016/j.drudis.2013.01.007

Thorne, N., Auld, D. S., and Inglese, J. (2010). Apparent activity in high-throughput screening: origins of compound-dependent assay interference. *Curr. Opin. Chem. Biol.* 14, 315–324. doi: 10.1016/j.cbpa.2010.03.020

Tropsha, A. (2010). Best practices for QSAR model development, validation, and exploitation. *Mol. Inform.* 29, 476–488. doi: 10.1002/minf.201000061

WHO (2018a). *HIV/AIDS.* Available at: http://www.who.int/news-room/fact-sheets/detail/hiv-aids [accessed September 20, 2018].

WHO (2018b). *Influenza (Seasonal).* Available at: http://www.who.int/news-room/fact-sheets/detail/influenza-(seasonal) [accessed September 20, 2018].

WHO (2018c). *Malaria.* Available at: http://www.who.int/news-room/fact-sheets/detail/malaria [accessed September 20, 2018].

WHO (2018d). *Schistosomiasis.* Available at: http://www.who.int/news-room/fact-sheets/detail/schistosomiasis [accessed September 20, 2018].

WHO (2018e). *Tuberculosis.* Available at: http://www.who.int/news-room/fact-sheets/detail/tuberculosis [accessed September 20, 2018].

Williams, A. J., and Ekins, S. (2011). A quality alert and call for improved curation of public chemistry databases. *Drug Discov. Today* 16, 747–750. doi: 10.1016/j.drudis.2011.07.007

Young, D., Martin, T., Venkatapathy, R., and Harten, P. (2008). Are the chemical structures in your QSAR correct? *QSAR Comb. Sci.* 27, 1337–1345. doi: 10.1002/qsar.200810084

Zhang, L., Fourches, D., Sedykh, A., Zhu, H., Golbraikh, A., Ekins, S., et al. (2013). Discovery of novel antimalarial compounds enabled by QSAR-based virtual screening. *J. Chem. Inf. Model.* 53, 475–492. doi: 10.1021/ci300421n

Targets Fishing and Identification of Calenduloside E as Hsp90AB1: Design, Synthesis and Evaluation of Clickable Activity-Based Probe

Shan Wang [1†], Yu Tian [1†], Jing-Yi Zhang [1], Hui-Bo Xu [2], Ping Zhou [1], Min Wang [1],
Sen-Bao Lu [3], Yun Luo [1], Min Wang [4], Gui-Bo Sun [1*], Xu-Dong Xu [1*] and Xiao-Bo Sun [1*]

[1] Beijing Key Laboratory of Innovative Drug Discovery of Traditional Chinese Medicine (Natural Medicine) and Translational Medicine, Institute of Medicinal Plant Development, Chinese Academy of Medical Sciences & Peking Union Medical College, Beijing, China, [2] Academy of Chinese Medical Sciences of Jilin Province, Changchun, China, [3] Department of Bioengineering, Santa Clara University, Santa Clara, CA, United States, [4] Life and Environmental Science Research Center, Harbin University of Commerce, Harbin, China

*Correspondence:
Gui-Bo Sun
gbsun@implad.ac.cn
Xu-Dong Xu
xdxu@implad.ac.cn
Xiao-Bo Sun
sun_xiaobo163@163.com

†These authors have contributed equally to this work.

Calenduloside E (CE), a natural triterpenoid compound isolated from *Aralia elata*, can protect against ox-LDL-induced human umbilical vein endothelial cell (HUVEC) injury in our previous reports. However, the exact targets and mechanisms of CE remain elusive. For the sake of resolving this question, we designed and synthesized a clickable activity-based probe (CE-P), which could be utilized to fish the functional targets in HUVECs using a gel-based strategy. Based on the previous studies of the structure-activity relationship (SAR), we introduced an alkyne moiety at the C-28 carboxylic group of CE, which kept the protective and anti-apoptosis activity. Via proteomic approach, one of the potential proteins bound to CE-P was identified as Hsp90AB1, and further verification was performed by pure recombinant Hsp90AB1 and competitive assay. These results demonstrated that CE could bind to Hsp90AB1. We also found that CE could reverse the Hsp90AB1 decrease after ox-LDL treatment. To make our results more convincing, we performed SPR analysis and the affinity kinetic assay showed that CE/CE-P could bind to Hsp90AB1 in a dose-dependent manner. Taken together, our research showed CE could probably bind to Hsp90AB1 to protect the cell injury, which might provide the basis for the further exploration of its cardiovascular protective mechanisms. For the sake of resolving this question, we designed and synthesized a clickable activity-based probe (CE-P), which could be utilized to fish the functional targets in HUVECs using a gel-based strategy.

Keywords: Calenduloside E, clickable activity based protein profiling, computational chemistry, HUVECs, Hsp90AB1

INTRODUCTION

Natural products represent an enormous source of pharmacologically useful compounds and are often used as the starting point in modern drug discovery. However, many biologically interesting natural products are not being pursued as potential drug candidates, partly due to the lack of well-defined mechanisms of action. The identification of drug targets is very important in the process of drug discovery, which allows researchers to clarify the mechanisms of drug action

(Krysiak and Breinbauer, 2012; Yue et al., 2012). Activity-based protein profiling (ABPP) is a chemical proteomic method that uses active site-directed chemical probes to selectively target subsets of proteins in the proteome based on shared mechanistic and/or structural features (Barglow and Cravatt, 2007; Cravatt et al., 2008; Pichler et al., 2016). This technique has been widely used in enzyme proteomes with quantitative proteomics development; this technique has been used to identify unknown target compounds (Chen et al., 2017). The basic chemical structure of the molecular probe consists of three parts: a reactive group, a binding group, and a reporter tag. The ABPP probe targets a large number of proteins via the reactive group, providing researchers with a global view of the proteome profile. Then, target proteins are identified by quantitative proteomics analysis (Hunerdosse and Nomura, 2014; Wright and Sieber, 2016). However, most tags are relatively bulky compared with the small molecule probe, which influences cell permeability and may prevent the reactive group from entering the active site. With the development of click chemistry, CC-ABPP strategies using a biorthogonal reaction with a label-free probe have been increasingly applied to circumvent this issue (Speers and Cravatt, 2009; Li et al., 2012). The reporter group is substituted with a small, latent chemical handle (alkyne or azide), which does not impede cell permeability, and can be simultaneously diversified with a variety of reporter groups without the need to develop new synthetic routes (Martell and Weerapana, 2014). The CC-ABP probe has advanced the ABPP field by expanding the enzyme classes targeted by ABPs, enabling cellular and *in vivo* studies and providing technological platforms to quantitatively monitor protein activities in complex biological systems. Currently, the CC-ABPP technology has become an effective method for the discovery of functional targets of small molecules (Lapinsky and Johnson, 2015).

Aralia elata (Miq) Seem (AS), which is used extensively in traditional Chinese medicine (TCM), has been used as a tonic herb due to its anti-arrhythmic, anti-arthritic, anti-hypertensive and anti-diabetic effects (Baranov, 1982). Moreover, as a main component of *A. elata* Xinmaitong capsules (Clinical Trial Approval Number 2003L01111 by the China Food and Drug Administration), AS was developed for the treatment of coronary heart disease and has successfully completed Phase III clinical trials in China. According to our previous studies, AS exhibited anti-myocardial ischemia and anti-hypoxia activities (Wang et al., 2014, 2015, 2017). The total saponins from AS are considered the main pharmacologically active ingredients of AS. Various oleanane-type triterpene saponins were extracted from AS and identified. Calenduloside E (CE, **Figure 1**) is one of the natural triterpene saponins extracted from AS. Calenduloside E was previously shown to protect endothelial cells from injury

and reduce apoptotic endotheliocytes and it could protect against H_2O_2-induced H9c2 cardiomyocytes apoptosis (Tian et al., 2017a,b). Using the ABPP probe, we identified 587 proteins as the most likely targets of CE. In our previous paper, our ABPP probe was the basic probe, but the biotin tag on the probe may have interfered with the binding of CE to the targets. In our present research, for the first time, we designed and synthesized a clickable probe CE-P, which could be introduced the biotin tag via click chemistry to avoid the interference of bulk molecule. Utilizing this CC-ABPP strategy, we identified and confirmed potential targets of CE.

MATERIALS AND METHODS

Materials

ox-LDL was obtained from Union-Biotechnology. Annexin-V/Propidium iodide (FITC/PI) staining kit (V13241) was Molecular Probes™. MTT [3-(4, 5-dimethylthiazol-2-yl)-2, 5-diphenyltetrazoliumbromide, 0973] was the products of Amresco. JC-1 (C2005) was purchased from Beyotime biotechnology. Caspase-3 fluorometric assay kit (K105-200) was acquired from BioVision. VascuLife® VEGF Endothelial Cell Culture Medium (LL-0003) was the products of Lifeline cell technology. TBTA (Tris[(1-benzyl-1H-1, 2, 3-triazol-4-yl)methyl]-amineT2993), TCEP (Tris(2-carboxyethyl)phosphine, T1656) were purchased from Tokyo Chemical Industry. Biotin-azide was provided from the Institute of Medicinal Plant Development (Beijing, China) (Tian et al., 2017b). HOBt (N-Hydroxybenzotriazole), EDCI (1-Ethyl-(3-dimethylaminopropyl) carbodiimide hydrochloride), TEMPO (2, 2, 6, 6-Tetramethylpiperidine1-oxyl) were purchased from Energy Chemical Industry. Pierce™ Streptavidin Agarose (20347), Pierce™ Silver Stain for Mass Spectrometry (24600) was from Thermo Fisher Scientific. The primary antibody against Hsp90AB1, Bcl2, Cytochrome C was obtained from Santa Cruz Biotechnology (Santa Cruz, CA, USA). Lox1 primary antibody was from Abcam (Cambridge, UK).Recombinant human Hsp90AB1 protein was from Abcam (Cambridge, UK).

Chemistry

Glycosyl donor **compound i** was prepared from galactose, and the reaction conditions were reported previously by Schmidt (Sun et al., 2014).

Synthesis of Compound I

To a solution of ursolic acid (10.0 g, 21.8 mmol) in dry DCM (300 mL), TBAB (0.8 g, 2.5 mmol) and K_2CO_3 (7.4 g, 53.6 mmol) in water (50 mL) were added, and benzyl bromide (3.2 mL, 26.8 mmol) was dropped at 0°C. Then the reaction mixture was stirred at room temperature for 18 h. Reaction was monitored by TLC. The crude mixture was separated and the water layer was extracted with DCM (3 × 100 mL). The combined organic layer was washed with 0.1 mol/L HCl aqueous solution, $NaHCO_3$ saturated aqueous solution and NaCl saturated aqueous solution in sequence, and then dried over Na_2SO_4 and purified through column chromatography (eluent: PE-EtOAc, 8:1) to offer pure white solid **compound I** (11.1 mg, 93% yield). ¹H-NMR (600

Abbreviations: CE, Calenduloside E; CE-P, Calenduloside E Probe; HUVEC, human umbilical vein endothelial cell; ABPP, Activity-based protein profiling; CC-ABPP, click chemistry-Activity-based protein profiling; SAR, structure-activity relationship; BnBr, benzyl bromide; K₂CO₃, potassium carbonate solution; TBAB, tetrabutylammonium bromide; DCM, dichloromethane; TMSOTf, trimethylsilyl trifluoromethanesulfonate; ox-LDL, Oxidized Low density lipoprotein; PI, propidium iodide; 1DGE, one-dimensional gel electrophoresis; LC-MS/MS, liquid chromatography/tandem mass spectrometry; Hsp90, Heat shock protein.

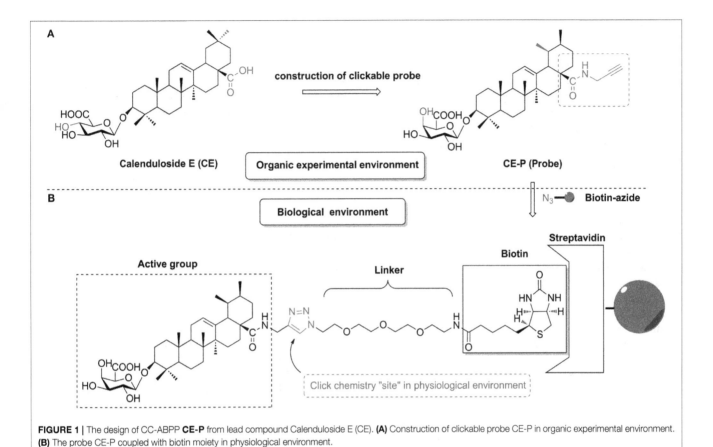

FIGURE 1 | The design of CC-ABPP **CE-P** from lead compound Calenduloside E (CE). **(A)** Construction of clickable probe CE-P in organic experimental environment. **(B)** The probe CE-P coupled with biotin moiety in physiological environment.

MHz, pyridine-d_5) δ: 7.36–7.29 (m, 5H, OPh-H), 5.23 (t, $J =$ 3.3 Hz, 1H, H-12), 5.10 (d, $J = 12.5$ Hz, 1H, CH_2OPh), 4.98 (d, $J = 12.5$ Hz, 1H, CH_2OPh), 3.23–3.19 (m, 1H, H-3), 2.26 (d, $J =$ 11.1 Hz, 1H, H-18), 1.07 (s, 3H, CH_3), 0.98 (s, 3H, CH_3), 0.93 (d, $J = 6.3$ Hz, 3H, CH_3), 0.89 (s, 3H, CH_3), 0.85 (d, $J = 6.5$ Hz, 3H, CH_3), 0.77 (s, 3H, CH_3), 0.64 (s, 3H, CH_3); ^{13}C-NMR (150 MHz, pyridine-d_5) δ: 177.5, 138.2, 136.5, 128.5, 128.3, 128.1, 125.8, 79.2, 77.4, 77.2, 76.9, 66.1, 55.3, 53.0, 48.2, 47.7, 42.2, 39.6, 39.2, 39.0, 38.9, 38.7, 37.1, 36.8, 33.1, 30.8, 28.3, 28.1, 27.3, 24.4, 23.7, 23.4, 21.3, 18.4, 17.1, 15.8, 15.6.

Synthesis of Compound II

To a solution of **compound I** (3.3 g, 6.0 mmol) in dry DCM (50 mL), glycosyl donor **compound i** (5.8 g, 7.9 mmol) and 4Å molecular sieve 0.5 g were added and stirred at room temperature for 1 h under N_2 air. Then lewis acid TMSOTf (60 μg, 0.3 mmol) was dropped and reacted for 2–4 h. When complete, triethylamine 1.0 mL was added to quench the reaction. Then the suspension was filtered out and the filtrate was evaporated and the crude product was subjected to column chromatography (eluent: PE-EtOAc, 10:1) to gain pure **compound II** (4.7 g, 70% yield) as white solid. ^{1}H-NMR (600 MHz, pyridine-d_5) δ: 8.25–8.22 (m, 4H, OBz-H), 8.16–8.15 (m, 2H, OBz-H), 8.01–8.00 (m, 2H, OBz-H), 7.56–7.52 (m, 3H, OBz-H), 7.49–7.41 (m, 6H, OBz-H), 7.38–7.34 (m, 3H, OBz-H), 7.29–7.27 (m, 3H, OBz-H), 7.10–7.08 (m, 2H, OBz-H), 6.55–6.54 (m, 1H, Gal-H), 6.48–6.45 (m,

1H, Gal-H), 6.40–6.38 (m, 1H, Gal-H), 5.43 (d, $J = 7.9$ Hz, 1H, Glc-H-1'), 5.41 (t, $J = 3.3$ Hz, 1H, H-12), 5.34 (d, $J = 12.5$ Hz, 1H, OBn-H), 5.22 (d, $J = 12.4$ Hz, 1H, OBn-H), 5.16–5.13 (m, 1H, Gal-H), 4.96–4.94 (m, 1H, Gal-H), 4.80–4.77 (m, 1H, Gal-H), 3.39 (dd, $J = 11.9$ Hz, 4.4 Hz, 1H, H-3), 2.47 (d, $J = 11.3$ Hz, 1H, H-18), 1.15 (s, 3H, CH_3), 0.97 (d, $J = 6.5$ Hz, 3H, CH_3), 0.93 (s, 6H, 2×CH_3), 0.79 (s, 3H, CH_3), 0.77 (s, 3H, CH_3), 0.73 (s, 3H, CH_3); ^{13}C-NMR (150 MHz, pyridine-d_5) δ: 176.8, 166.1, 166.0, 165.8, 165.7, 138.5, 137.1, 133.8, 133.6, 133.5, 133.4, 130.3, 130.1, 130.0, 129.9, 129.8, 129.5, 129.0, 128.8, 128.7, 128.5, 128.3, 125.9, 103.8, 90.2, 72.6, 71.7, 71.1, 69.3, 66.1, 62.7, 55.5, 53.3, 48.2, 47.7, 42.2, 39.7, 39.2, 39.0, 38.9, 38.5, 36.9, 36.6, 33.2, 30.7, 28.2, 27.9, 26.4, 24.5, 23.7, 23.4, 21.2, 18.2, 17.2, 17.1, 16.6, 15.3.

Synthesis of Compound III

A mixture of **compound II** (3.0 g, 2.6 mmol) and 10% Pd/C (1.5 mg) was hydrogenated at 1 atm for 4–6 h in refluxing EtOAc (30 mL). The mixture was filtered and concentrated, the residue was purified by silica gel column chromatography (eluent: PE-EtOAc, 3:1) to get pure **compound III** (2.4 g, 91% yield) as white solid. ^{1}H-NMR (600 MHz, pyridine-d_5) δ: 8.24–8.21 (m, 4H, OBz-H), 8.14–8.13 (m, 2H, OBz-H), 8.00–7.98 (m, 2H, OBz-H), 7.56–7.53 (m, 1H, OBz-H), 7.48–7.45 (m, 2H, OBz-H), 7.43–7.41 (m, 2H, OBz-H), 7.38–7.35 (m, 2H, OBz-H), 7.28–7.26 (m, 3H, OBz-H), 7.10–7.07 (m, 2H, OBz-H), 6.54–6.53 (m, 1H, Gal-H), 6.46–6.43 (m, 1H, Gal-H), 6.39–6.36 (m, 1H, Gal-H), 5.50 (t, J

= 3.3 Hz, 1H, H-12), 5.42 (d, J = 7.9 Hz, 1H, Glc-H-1′), 5.15–5.12 (m, 1H, Gal-H), 4.96–4.93 (m, 1H, Gal-H), 4.79–4.76 (m, 1H, Gal-H), 3.38 (dd, J = 11.7 Hz, 4.3 Hz, 1H, H-3), 2.65 (d, J = 11.3 Hz, 1H, H-18), 1.22 (s, 3H, CH$_3$), 1.05 (d, J = 6.4 Hz, 3H, CH$_3$), 0.98–0.97 (m, 6H, 2×CH$_3$), 0.92 (s, 3H, CH$_3$), 0.76 (s, 3H, CH$_3$), 0.72 (s, 3H, CH$_3$); ^{13}C-NMR (150 MHz, pyridine-d_5) δ: 179.8, 166.1, 166.0, 165.8, 165.7, 139.1, 133.8, 133.6, 133.6, 133.4, 130.3, 130.0, 130.0, 130.0, 129.8, 129.4, 129.4, 129.0, 128.8, 128.8, 128.6, 125.4, 103.7, 90.2, 72.5, 71.7, 71.0, 69.3, 62.7, 55.7, 53.4, 47.9, 47.8, 43.3, 42.3, 39.7, 39.4, 39.3, 38.9, 38.5, 37.3, 36.6, 33.3, 30.9, 28.5, 27.8, 26.4, 24.8, 23.8, 23.4, 21.3, 18.2, 17.4, 17.2, 16.6, 15.3.

Synthesis of Compound IV

To a solution of compound **III** (1.0 g, 0.98 mmol) in dry DCM (15 mL), HOBt (0.2 g, 1.46 mmol) and EDCI (0.28 g, 1.46 mmol) were added and stirred at room temperature for 1 h. To this mixture, propargylamine (0.22 g, 3.92 mmol) was added respectively at 0°C and the reaction mixture was stirred until its completion for 8 h. The solvent was washed with 0.1 mol/L HCl aqueous solution, NaHCO$_3$ saturated aqueous solution and NaCl saturated aqueous solution in sequence, and then dried over Na$_2$SO$_4$. The suspension was filtered and the filtrate was concentrated and purified through column chromatography (eluent: DCM-CH$_3$OH, 100:1) to offer pure white solid compound **IV** as white solid, 79% yield. ^{1}H-NMR (600 MHz, pyridine-d_5) δ: 8.24–8.22 (m, 4H, OBz-H), 8.14–8.13 (m, 2H, OBz-H), 7.99–7.98 (m, 2H, OBz-H), 7.94 (t, 1H, CON$\underline{H}$), 7.53–7.52 (m, 1H, OBz-H), 7.47–7.46 (m, 2H, OBz-H), 7.43–7.40 (m, 2H, OBz-H), 7.37–7.35 (m, 2H, OBz-H), 7.28–7.26 (m, 3H, OBz-H), 7.09–7.07 (m, 2H, OBz-H), 6.54 (m, 1H, Gal-H), 6.46–6.37 (m, 2H, Gal-H), 5.47–5.42 (m, 2H, H-12, Glc-H-1′), 5.15–5.12 (m, 1H, Gal-H), 4.95 (m, 1H, Gal-H), 4.79–4.77 (m, 1H, Gal-H), 4.33 (m, 2H, CONHC$\underline{H}_2$), 3.39 (m, 1H, H-3), 3.13 (m, 1H, CCH), 2.47 (d, J = 10.3 Hz, 1H, H-18), 1.19 (s, 3H, CH$_3$), 1.00 (d, J = 5.2 Hz, 3H, CH$_3$), 0.97–0.92 (m, 9H, 3×CH$_3$), 0.78–0.77 (m, 6H, 2×CH$_3$); ^{13}C-NMR (150 MHz, pyridine-d_5) δ: 177.1, 166.1, 166.0, 165.8, 165.7, 139.2, 133.8, 133.6, 133.6, 133.4, 130.3, 130.0, 130.0, 130.0, 129.8, 129.4, 129.4, 129.0, 128.8, 128.8, 128.6, 125.8, 103.7, 90.2, 81.9, 72.5, 71.9, 71.7, 71.0, 69.3, 62.7, 55.5, 53.1, 47.8, 47.7, 43.3, 42.3, 39.8, 39.7, 39.2, 38.9, 38.5, 37.7, 36.6, 33.1, 31.0, 29.9, 29.1, 28.1, 27.8, 26.4, 24.7, 23.7, 23.5, 21.3, 18.2, 17.5, 17.4, 16.6, 15.3.

Synthesis of Compound V

To a solution of compound **IV** in MeOH/DCM (8 mL, 3:1) was added 1 mol/L NaOMe/NaOH solvent (1.6 mL). The reaction mixture was stirred for 2 h until its completion, after that Amberlite IR-120 was added to acidate PH 7. The suspension was filtered out and the filtrate was evaporated and purified through column chromatography (eluent: DCM-CH$_3$OH, 10:1) to offer pure white solid compound **V** as white solid, 93% yield. ^{1}H-NMR (600 MHz, pyridine-d_5) δ: 7.84 (t, J = 5.4 Hz, 1H, N-H), 5.45 (t, J = 3.3 Hz, 1H, H-12), 4.89 (d, J = 7.7 Hz, 1H, H-1′), 4.60–4.59 (m, 1H, Gal-H), 4.52–4.46 (m, 3H, Gal-H), 4.40–4.28 (m, 2H, H-31), 4.19 (dd, J = 3.4 Hz, 9.4 Hz, 1H, Gal-H), 4.13 (t, J = 6.2 Hz, 1H, Gal-H), 3.43 (dd, J = 11.8 Hz, 4.5 Hz, 1H, H-3), 3.10 (t, J =

2.4 Hz, 1H, H-33), 2.44 (d, J = 10.8 Hz, 1H, H-18), 1.34 (s, 3H, CH$_3$), 1.24 (s, 3H, CH$_3$), 1.02 (s, 3H, CH$_3$), 1.00 (s, 3H, CH$_3$), 0.97 (d, J = 6.5 Hz, 3H, CH$_3$), 0.94 (s, 3H, CH$_3$), 0.90 (s, 3H, CH$_3$); ^{13}C-NMR (150 MHz, pyridine-d_5) δ: 177.2, 139.4, 126.0, 107.5, 88.8, 81.9, 76.8, 75.4, 73.1, 71.9, 70.3, 62.5, 55.9, 53.3, 47.9, 47.8, 42.5, 40.0, 39.8, 39.5, 39.3, 38.9, 37.8, 36.8, 33.3, 31.1, 29.2, 28.3, 26.7, 24.8, 23.8, 23.6, 21.3, 18.4, 17.6, 17.4, 17.0, 15.6; HRMS (ESI): Calcd for [M + H]$^+$ C$_{39}$H$_{62}$NO$_7$: 656.4526, found 656.4516.

Synthesis of Compound VI (CE-P)

To a solution of compound **V** (200.0 mg, 305.14 mmol) in DCM (1 mL), KBr (7.26 mg, 61.03 mmol), TEMPO (0.95 mg, 6.1 mmol) and TBAB (19.67 mg, 61.03 mmol) were added at room temperature. To a solution of this mixture was added Na$_2$CO$_3$/NaHCO$_3$ (3 mL, PH 9.5). To this mixture, Ca(ClO)$_2$ (87.26 mg, 610.28 mmol) was added at 0°C and the reaction mixture was stirred violently until its completion. The Na$_2$SO$_3$ 20 mg was added to quench the reaction, and then 6N HCl was dropped to acidate PH 3. The crude mixture was extracted with DCM (3 × 15 mL) and the combined organic layer was dried over Na$_2$SO$_4$ and purified through column chromatography (eluent: CH$_2$Cl$_2$-CH$_3$OH-H$_2$O, 50:10:1) to offer pure compound **VI** as white solid. (63.4 mg, 31% yield). ^{1}H-NMR (600 MHz, pyridine-d^5) δ: 7.91 (t, J = 5.4 Hz, 1H, N-H), 5.48 (t, J = 3.4 Hz, 1H, H-12), 4.87 (d, J = 7.7 Hz, 1H, H-1′), 4.65–4.58 (m, 1H, Gal-H), 4.56–4.46 (m, 1H, Gal-H), 4.46–4.28 (m, 3H, H-31, Gal-H), 4.24–4.12 (m, 1H, Gal-H), 3.43 (m, 1H, H-3), 3.11 (s, 1H, H-33), 2.48 (m, 14H, H-18), 1.36 (s, 3H, CH$_3$), 1.25 (s, 3H, CH$_3$), 1.02 (s, 3H, CH$_3$), 0.99 (s, 3H, CH$_3$), 0.97 (s, 6H, 2×CH$_3$), 0.89 (s, 3H, CH$_3$); ^{13}C-NMR (150 MHz, pyridine-d^5) δ: 177.1, 175.9, 139.3, 125.8, 107.0, 88.3, 81.9, 76.1, 75.9, 72.7, 72.5, 71.9, 55.8, 53.2, 47.8, 47.7, 42.4, 39.9, 39.9, 39.7, 39.4, 39.2, 37.7, 36.8, 33.4, 31.1, 29.9, 29.2, 28.9, 28.2, 24.7, 23.8, 23.6, 21.3, 18.4, 17.5, 17.5, 16.9, 15.6; HRMS calcd mass for C$_{39}$H$_{59}$NNaO$_8$ [M+Na]$^+$ 692.4138, found 692.4145. The spectrograms of the compounds I–VI were shown in Electronic Supplementary Material (ESI).

Biological Studies

Cell Preparation and Culture

HUVECs were isolated from fresh human umbilical veins using 0.1% collagenase I, as previously described (Qin et al., 2015). After dissociation, the cells were collected and cultured in VascuLife® VEGF Endothelial Cell Culture Medium (Lifeline Cell Technology, MD, USA) supplemented with 100 U/mL penicillin and 100 μg/mL streptomycin. All cell cultures were maintained in a humidified 37°C incubator with 5% CO2, and the media were refreshed every 3 days. Cells at passages 3–7 were used in subsequent experiments. Neonatal umbilical cords were donated by the Maternal and Child Care Service Center in Beijing, China.

Cell Viability Assay

Cell viability was determined using the MTT (3-(4, 5-dimethylthiazol-2-yl)-2, 5-diphenyl tetrazolium, Amresco, 0973) assay as previously described (Tian et al., 2017b). Briefly, HUVECs were plated on 96-well plates at a density of 8 × 10^4 cells/well and then grown at 37°C for 24 h. The treatment group cells were pretreated with CE-P/CE for 8 h, followed by treatment with ox-LDL (80 μg/mL, 24 h), the control group was pretreated with vehicle for 8 h then exposed without ox-LDL. Twenty microliters of MTT (5 mg/mL) were added to each well and incubated for 4 h. The medium was removed and the formazan crystals were dissolved with dimethyl sulfoxide (DMSO). The absorbance was measured at 570 nm on a microplate reader (TECAN Infinite M1000, Austria).

Assessments of Cell Apoptosis

HUVECs were incubated with ox-LDL (70 μg/mL, 24 h) and pretreated with BCEA for 8 h prior to the apoptosis assay. Double fluorescence staining was performed using an Annexin V-FITC/PI apoptosis staining kit (Molecular Probes™, V13241) according to the manufacturer's instructions to detect early apoptotic and necrotic cells. Cellular fluorescence was measured using flow cytometry with a FACS Calibur Flow Cytometer (BD Biosciences, USA).

Determination of ΔΨm

We used JC-1 (5, 5′, 6, 6′-tetrachloro-1, 1′, 3, 3′-tetraethyl benzimidazolyl carbocyanine iodide, Beyotime Biotechnology, (C2005) to analyze ΔΨm. HUVECs were cultured on coverslips, the ox-LDL was removed, and the cells were washed twice with warm PBS and incubated with JC-1 (2 μM final concentration) for 30 min in the dark. The cells were finally washed twice with PBS, and images were captured using an EVOS® FL fluorescence microscope (Thermo Fisher Scientific, USA).

Analysis of Caspase-3 Activation

Caspase-3 activity was measured using a Fluorometric Assay Kit (BioVision, USA) according to the manufacturer's instructions. The samples were measured in a Fluoroskan Ascent FL fluorometer (Thermo Fisher Scientific, USA) using a 400 nm excitation wavelength and a 505 nm emission wavelength. The results are expressed as fold changes compared to the control.

Biotin–Neutravidin Pull-Down Assay

HUVECs were cultured in a T75 culture flask. HUVECs at 100% confluence were lysed in PBS buffer, and the protein concentration was adjusted to 2 mg/mL. For each experimental and control sample, 2 × 0.5 mL aliquots of the 2 mg/mL cell homogenate were transferred into microcentrifuge tubes. The experimental and control samples were incubated with 5 μL of 10 mg/mL CE-P or 5 μL of DMSO at room temperature for 1 h. Then, the proteomes were labeled with biotin-azide (100 μM), TCEP, 1 mM), TBTA, 100 μM), and CuSO4·5H2O (1 mM) for 1 h. Seven hundred fifty microliters of cold MeOH were added and sonicated for 3–4 sec using a probe sonicator (~30% power level) at 4°C to re-suspend the protein. The samples were then centrifuged for 4 min at 6,500 × g at 4°C and the supernatant was removed. The pellets were dissolved in PBS containing 1.2% SDS via sonication and then diluted with PBS containing 0.2% SDS. The samples were incubated with streptavidin beads for 2 h at room temperature and washed with PBS several times. Samples were denatured by heating in 2 × SDS-loading buffer and analyzed by SDS-PAGE. The resulting bands were visualized with Coomassie blue staining (Lee et al., 2014). Next, trypsin digestion was performed on selected visible protein bands.

Western Blot

Cell extracts were lysed in RIPA lysis buffer (Beyotime, Shanghai, China) containing a 1% protease inhibitor cocktail (Roche, Basel, Switzerland) (Sun et al., 2012). The protein content was measured with a BCA Protein Assay Kit (CWBiotech, Beijing, China). Approximately 30–50 μg of protein were resolved using 10 or 12% SDS-PAGE and then transferred to polyvinylidene difluoride membranes. The membranes were incubated with 1:500-diluted primary antibodies overnight at 4°C, followed by horseradish peroxidase-conjugated secondary antibodies at room temperature. Then, the proteins were developed with an enhanced chemiluminescence detection system and imaged using a Bio-Rad imaging system (Bio-Rad, Hercules, CA, USA).

CE-P Binds to Recombinant Hsp90AB1

CE-P was incubated with the recombinant Hsp90AB1 protein at room temperature for 1 h. The protein was pulled down as the same as the previous described methods (**Biotin–neutravidin pull-down assay**), then was detected by silver staining (Thermo Fisher Scientific, USA).

Targets Predicted by Discovery Studio 2016

The molecular targets of CE-P were predicted using Discovery Studio 2016 (BIOVIA Software Inc., San Diego, CA, USA), a software suite for performing computational analysis of data relevant to Life Sciences research. To determine the probable target of CE-P, we employed the Ligand Profiler protocol which maps a set of pharmacophores, including Pharma DB by default. The ligand CE-P was prepared by the Specifying Ligands parameter protocol. After inputting all parameters, the job was run and the results were monitored from the Jobs Explorer.

Molecular Docking

To explore the potential interacting mode of CE/CE-P with the Hsp90AB1 protein (PDB code: 3NMQ), a molecular modeling study was performed using the docking program named Induced-Fit, a refinement method in another software MOE. To eliminate any bond length and bond angle biases, the ligand (CE/CE-P) was subjected to an "energy minimize" prior to docking. The binding affinities (S-values) in MOE were used to evaluate the interactions between Hsp90AB1 and CE/CE-P. The scores (binding affinities) were obtained based on the virtual calculation of various interactions of the ligands with the targeted receptor.

Surface-Plasmon Resonance (SPR)

The molecule/protein interaction detection and kinetic constant measurement were studied using the Biacore System. CM5 Sensor Chip was activated using sulpho-NHS/EDC chemistry in a buffer consisting of 2.7 mM KCl 137 mM NaCl, 0.05% (v/v) surfactant P20, pH 7.4. The chip was subsequently immobilized with the recombinant human Hsp90AB1 protein at a concentration of 37 μg/ml in sodium acetate, pH 4.5 and then blocked with 1 M ethanolamine, pH 8.0. Compounds were dissolved to 10 mM in 100% DMSO and then 50-fold into running buffer without DMSO then diluted two-fold by running buffer into 12.5, 6.25, 3.125, 1.56, 0.78, and 0 μM before injection. The optical interference pattern was recorded as a change in optical path difference in units of nm. Data were analyzed with Biacore T200 Evaluation Software.

Statistical Analysis

Data are presented as the means ± standard deviation (SD) of three independent experiments. The groups were compared using one-way ANOVA followed by Tukey's multiple comparison tests using the statistics module of Graph Pad Prism 5.0. A value of $P < 0.05$ was considered statistically significant.

RESULTS

Design and Synthesis of the CC Activity-Based Protein Profiling Probe CE-P Based on CE

According to previous studies, the biotinylated probe BCEA, which maintains the active moiety of the parental compound CE, exhibits similar protective effects against ox-LDL-induced human umbilical vein endothelial cell (HUVEC) damage and identified 128 proteins related to cell survival signaling pathways as the targets (Tian et al., 2017b). Based on studies of the structure-activity relationship (SAR), amide derivatives of CE containing ursane and galactoside scaffolds maintained similar activity to the parental compound CE (Tian et al., 2017a,b). In the current study, we describe the design and construction of the CC-Activity-Based Protein Profiling Probe CE-P (CC-ABPP CE-P, **Figure 1**) and its subsequent use in identifying the targets of CE. An alkynyl group was introduced at the C-28 carboxylic moiety of the saponin scaffold, which enabled the hydrophilic PEG chain to link to biotin through a Cu(I)-catalyzed Huisgen 1,3-dipolar cycloaddition reaction.

As illustrated in **Scheme 1**, naturally abundant ursolic acid was treated with benzyl bromide (BnBr), a potassium carbonate solution (K_2CO_3), and tetrabutylammonium bromide (TBAB) in dry dichloromethane (DCM) to obtain a good yield of compound **I**. The glycosyl donor **i** was prepared from galactose using the conditions reported by Schmidt (Schmidt and Michel, 1980). Compound **I** was reacted with glycosyl donor **i** under Lewis acidic conditions in the presence of trimethylsilyl trifluoromethanesulfonate (TMSOTf) to produce compound **II**, which was subjected to hydrogenation to obtain compound **III** in the presence of a catalytic amount of 10% Pd-C at atmospheric pressure. The above reaction conditions were reported in our previous paper. Compound **IV** was attained via amidation of the C-28 carboxyl group of saponin scaffold with propargylamine, followed by deprotection of the glycosyl groups in the presence of a NaOMe/MeOH solution to obtain compound **V**. In the final step, an oxidation reaction was performed using compound **V** and TEMPO/Ca(ClO)$_2$ in the presence of KBr and a TBAB catalyst in an Na_2CO_3/NaHCO$_3$ solution, yielding the CC-ABPP **CE-P** (compound **VI**).

CE-P Protects Against ox-LDL-Induced Endothelial Cell Injury

As shown in our previous study, CE protected against ox-LDL-induced endothelial cell injury (Tian et al., 2017b). In this context, we introduced a very small alkyne group into CE to create a click chemistry activity-based probe. We first measured cell viability using the MTT assay to investigate the activity of CE-P. The cytotoxicity of CE-P was measured, and the results shown in **Figure 2A** did not reveal obvious changes in cell viability. Then, we determined whether CE-P protects cells from ox-LDL-induced injury. As shown in **Figure 2B**, the control group was pretreated for 8h with vehicle then exposed without ox-LDL, the other groups exposed to ox-LDL exhibited dramatically decreased cell viability, whereas pretreatment with CE or CE-P (0.625 or 1.25 μg/mL) for 8 h significantly ameliorated cell injury. We found that there were no significant differences between the two compounds at the same doses for sustaining the cell viability. CE-P retained the ability of inhibiting ox-LDL induced HUVECs damage, and the presence of the small alkyne moiety does not affect the biological activity of CE.

CE-P Attenuates ox-LDL-Induced HUVEC Apoptosis

CE has been shown to protect against cell apoptosis (Tian et al., 2017b). We first detected the phosphatidylserine (PS) levels using Annexin V/propidium iodide (PI) double staining and flow cytometry to explore whether the effects of CE-P on protecting cells from ox-LDL-induced injury involved the inhibition of cell apoptosis. During the early stage of apoptosis, phosphatidylserine is exposed on the extracellular side of the cell membrane, and Annexin V specifically binds PS (Qin et al., 2015). As shown in **Figure 3A**, the protective effect of CE-P on ox-LDL-induced cell death following PS exposure was investigated using Annexin V/PI double staining and flow cytometry. An 8 h CE-P pretreatment decreased the percentage of Annexin V(+)/PI(−) cells. Mitochondrial damage is closely related to cell apoptosis, and a change in the mitochondrial membrane potential ($\Delta\Psi$m) is one of the main functional markers of mitochondrial injury (Yu et al., 2016). JC-1 is an indicator of the mitochondrial transmembrane potential. As indicated by the JC-1 staining shown in **Figure 3B**, red fluorescence represents the normal mitochondria, and green fluorescence indicates HUVECs in which the mitochondrial membrane potential was depolarized. The ox-LDL-treated group exhibited a decrease in the intensity of red fluorescence and an increase of green signal. In contrast, the CE-P-pretreated group reversed this change by decreasing the green signal and increasing red fluorescence intensity, indicating that CE-P mitigated $\Delta\Psi$m. Caspase-3, one of the critical enzymes involved in apoptosis, the active form cleaved capase-3 is induced at the late stage of apoptosis. DEVD-AFC is used to detect cleaved caspase-3 activity (Sun et al., 2014). As shown in **Figure 3C**, the CE-P pretreatment remarkably reduced cleaved caspase-3 activation. We evaluated the expression of apoptosis-related proteins using western blot analyses to further confirm the anti-apoptotic effects of CE-P on HUVECs. As shown in **Figure 3D**, CE-P increased the levels of Bcl2 and pro-caspase-3

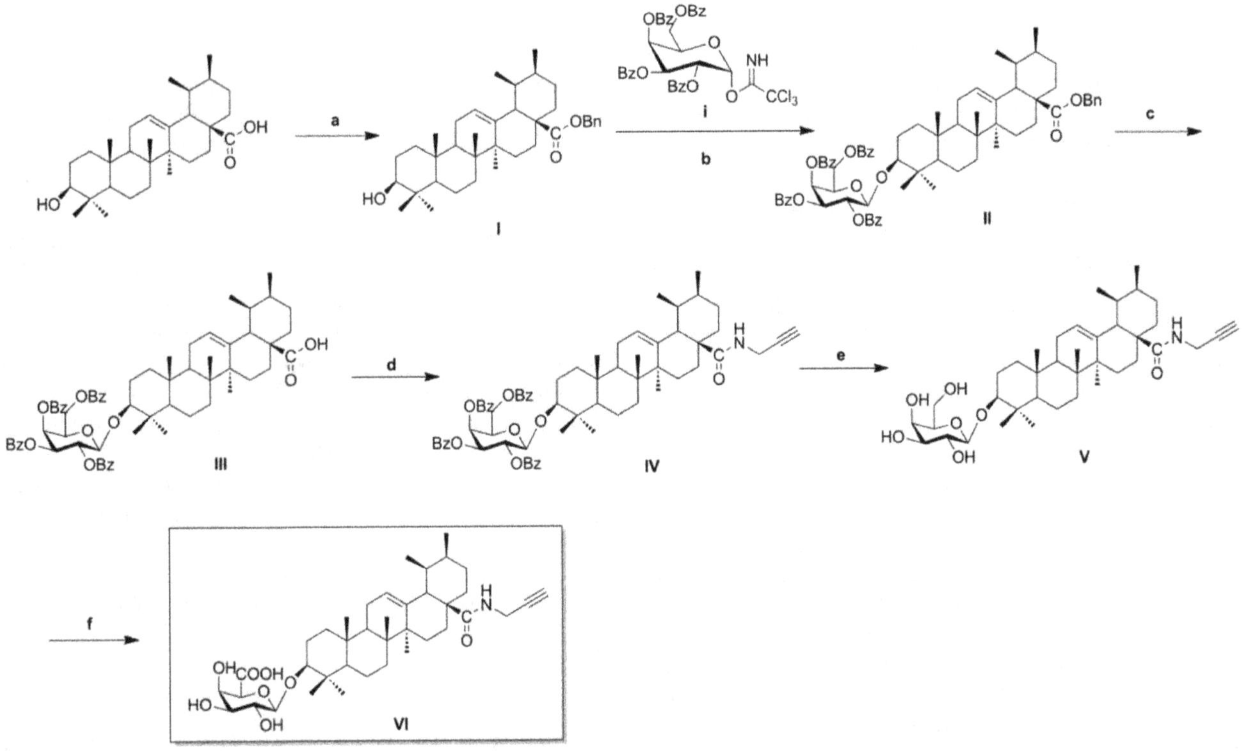

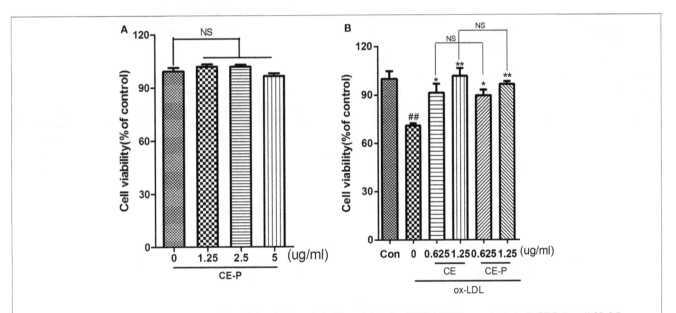

SCHEME 1 | Synthesis of biotinylated probe CE-P. Reagents and conditions: (a) BnBr, K_2CO_3, TBAB, DCM–H_2O, rt, 18 h; (b) glycosyl donor **i**, TMSOTf, 4Å MS, DCM, rt, 2–4 h; (c) H_2, Pd–C (10%), EtOAc, reflux, 4–6 h; (d) HOBt, EDCI, propargylamine, rt, 6–8 h; (e) NaOMe, MeOH, rt, 2–3 h; (f), KBr, TEMPO, TBAB, Na_2CO_3/NaHCO$_3$, Ca(ClO)$_2$, 0°C, 8 h.

FIGURE 2 | CE-P protects ox-LDL-induced endothelial cell injury. **(A)** To evaluated the cytotoxicity of CE-P, HUVECs were treated with CE-P alone (1.25, 2.5, 5 μg/mL) for 24 h and then the cell viability was measured by MTT assay. **(B)** HUVECs were pretreated with CE or CE-P (0.625, 1.25 μg/mL) for 8 h, then were incubated with or without ox-LDL for another 24 h and finally cell viability was assayed by MTT. The data are expressed as means ± SD. from three independent experiments. ##$P < 0.01$ vs. control group, *$P < 0.05$, **$P < 0.01$ versus ox-LDL treatment group. NS is no significance.

and decreased the levels of Cytochrome C, consistent with our previous results showing the anti-apoptosis activity of CE. Lox-1 is the main ox-LDL receptor in HUVECs, and ox-LDL has been shown to induce the Lox-1 expression, which triggers cell apoptosis (Li et al., 2003; Li and Mehta, 2009). In our study, the CE-P pretreatment remarkably attenuated Lox-1 expression during ox-LDL-induced injury. Based on these results, CE-P protected HUVECs from ox-LDL-induced cell apoptosis.

Profiling of CE-P Target Proteins in HUVEC Cell Lysates Using Click Chemistry

With the effective chemical probe in hands, we performed pull-down experiments followed by proteomics analysis to identify the cellular targets of CE (**Figure 4A**). CE-P was first incubated with a cell lysate to identify the potential targets of CE. Proteomes were obtained from lysates incubated with DMSO and CE-P with a biotin-azide linker using a click reaction, after which the labeled proteins were enriched by an affinity pull-down method using streptavidin beads. The enriched proteomes were eluted and separated by one-dimensional gel electrophoresis (1DGE). As shown in **Figure 4B**, we observed a single labeled protein band in the cell lysate in the CE-P lane (band A, indicated by an arrow). We also examined the washes from the CE-P reaction to exclude non-specific binding of CE-P. After extensive washing with the binding buffer, the unbound proteins were eluted. In **Figure 4C**, lane 1 is the cell lysate, lane 2 is the first elution solution, and lane 3 is the final washing solution. Thus, band A represents proteins that specifically bound to CE-P (Yi et al., 2012). Next, we cut band A from the DMSO lane and CE-P lane for the liquid chromatography/tandem mass spectrometry (LC-MS/MS) analysis. The Mascot search algorithm was used to identify proteins from the resulting peptides identified by LC-MS/MS. A large number of proteins were identified from each LC/MS run. The proteins which got the scores > 100, were considered as reliable hits (Table S1) (Weerapana et al., 2010; Shi et al., 2011). Some of these proteins were inevitably non-specific proteins, many of which were "sticky" and/or highly abundant proteins. These proteins were automatically removed. "False" hits that appeared in control pull-down/LC/MS experiments were also eliminated to generate the final complete list of proteins (Table S1). Consequently, we identified 37 proteins as specific targets of CE-P.

Hsp90AB1 as a Potential Target of CE-P

The molecular targets of CE-P were predicted using Discovery Studio 2016 software. Nineteen potential targets were found and shown to have probable relationships with the pharmacological effects of CE-P. Among these candidates, we selected targets with scores > 0.5 for the subsequent investigations and finally identified 9 proteins, as shown in **Figure 5A**. Moreover, Hsp90 which was predicted with a higher score 0.848264, was also identified by gel proteomic with the high score 217 in Table S1 and **Figure 5B**. Comparing these above results we thought Hsp90AB1 might be one of potential targets and be critical for cell apoptosis (Cohen-Saidon et al., 2006; Lanneau et al., 2007; Didelot et al., 2008; Chen et al., 2009). To further

validate Hsp90AB1 as the direct binding target of CE-P, we confirmed the identity of the proteins that were pulled down using immunoblotting with their respective antibodies. As shown in **Figure 5C**, the CE-P pull-down precipitated Hsp90AB1, but almost no signal was observed in the control group. To verify the interaction of CE-P with Hsp90AB1, we incubated recombinant Hsp90AB1 protein with CE-P. As shown in **Figure 5D**, Hsp90AB1 was obviously pulled down by CE-P, which was detected by silver staining. We also found that CE-P can pull down Hsp90AB1 in dose-dependent manner as shown in **Figure 5E**. We incubated HUVEC cell lysates with CE-P in the absence or the presence of an excess amount of CE for competitive binding. As shown in **Figure 5F**, Hsp90AB1 was obviously pulled down by CE-P, moreover, an excess amount of CE effectively blocked the binding of Hsp90AB1 to CE-P, which were detected by Western blot. Taken together, the above results unequivocally confirmed a direct interaction between CE-P and Hsp90AB1. To further investigate the potential biological role of CE about Hsp90AB1, we then detected the effects of CE on Hsp90AB1 expression levels in ox-LDL induced HUVEC damage. **Figures 5G,H** showed that CE pretreatment significantly inhibited the down-regulation of the ox-LDL-induced Hsp90AB1 expression.

Molecular Docking Between CE/CE-P and Hsp90AB1

Based on the predicted molecular targets, we analyzed the possible interaction between CE/CE-P and the 3D Hsp90AB1 receptor binding sites (PDBID: 3NMQ) using Molecular Operating Environment (MOE) software package. The S-values (CE: −8.70 and CE-P: − 8.78) were obtained based on the virtual calculation of the interaction of CE/CE-P with the targeted Hsp90 AB1 protein. Molecular modeling of CE/CE-P showed that both two compounds could bind to the N-terminal domain of Hsp90AB1 and participated in important hydrogen bonds with key amino acid residues Asp 93 and Asn 51 (**Figures 6A,B**). As shown in **Figure 6C**, the glycosyl moieties of CE (gray) and CE-P (green) are responsible important for binding with the key amino acid residuces of Hsp90AB1 with amino acid residues, and the propargyl group (red frame) that exposing on the edge of the pockets were designed for "clicking" conveniently with biotin tag.

SPR Analysis of CE/CE-P Binding to Hsp90AB1

Surface plasmon resonance (SPR) biosensors are most commonly applied for real-time dynamic analysis and measurement of interactions in bio-molecular studies and compounds analysis without the need for labeling processes. In our research, we applied this system to confirm the interaction of CE/CE-P with Hsp90AB1 and explore its binding affinity. As shown in **Figures 7A,B**, SPR data analysis revealed that both CE and CE-P could bind to Hsp90AB1 in a dose-dependent manner. The KD-value of CE-P binding to Hsp90AB1 was 23.4 μM (**Figure 7D**), and CE was 2.34 μM (**Figure 7C**).

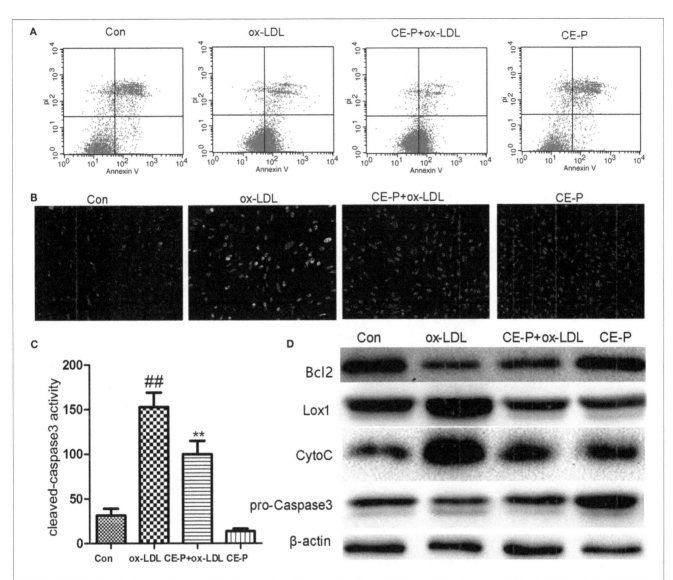

FIGURE 3 | CE-P attenuates the ox-LDL induced HUVECs apoptosis. The protective effect of CE-P on ox-LDL-induced apoptosis was determined via AnnexinV/PI double staining, JC-1 staining, cleaved-caspase3 activity, and western blot assay. HUVECs were pretreated with CE-P (1.25 μg/mL) for 8 h and then incubated with or without ox-LDL for additional 24 h for associated measures. **(A)** After cell treatment, cell early apoptosis was measured via AnnexinV/PI double staining by flow cytometry. **(B)** The mitochondria damage during apoptosis was detected by JC-1 staining through fluorescence microscope. **(C)** At the final stage of apoptosis, the cleaved caspase3 activity was measured by fluorometric assay. **(D)** Apoptosis associated proteins Bcl2, Caspase3, Cytochrome C were evaluated by western blot. The data are expressed as means ± SD from three independent experiments. ##$P < 0.01$ vs. control group, **$P < 0.01$ vs. ox-LDL treatment group.

DISCUSSION

The design and synthesis of potential probes represents a major challenge for target identification. In our previous study, the introduction of a substituent at the C-28 position of CE maintained its protective effects. Based on the results of preliminary SAR studies, amide derivatives of CE that containing ursane and galactoside scaffolds maintained similar activity to the parental compound CE. In the current study, the *N*-propargylamide derivative CE-P was chosen as the clickable activity-based probe in which the biotin tag was introduced using a Cu (I)-catalyzed Huisgen 1, 3-dipolar cycloaddition reaction. According to the results of the MTT assay, the CE-P probe

exhibited promising protective effects against ox-LDL-induced HUVEC damage. We also confirmed that CE-P protects against apoptosis using Annexin V/PI staining, JC-1 staining, caspase-3 activity assays and western blotting. Based on these results, CE-P maintains its anti-apoptosis activity and is suitable for use in further research.

In this context, we introduced a very small alkyne group into CE to create a clickable activity-based probe. Unlike the bulky biotin tag, the small alkyne group does not affect the interaction of this compound with the potential targets *in vitro* or its ability to penetrate the plasma membrane. In our previous reports, we utilized an ABPP probe and identified ~750 potential targets, however, with this probe, we identified 37 proteins as the most

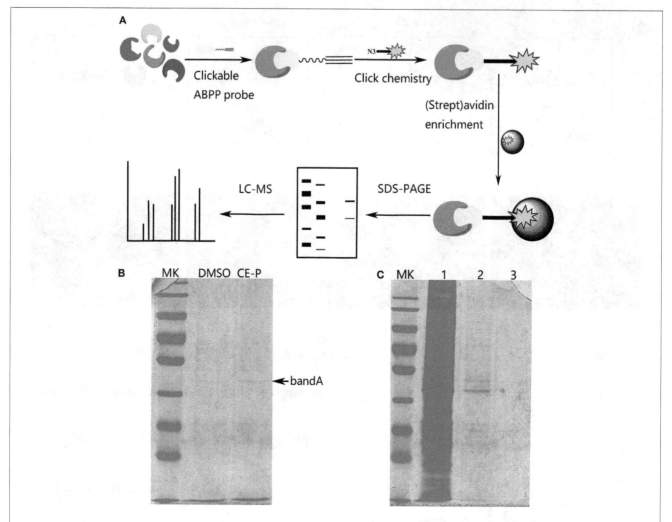

FIGURE 4 | Protein Profiling of CE-P by click chemistry in HUVEC cell lysate. **(A)** Schematic image of proteome profiling of potential cellular targets of CE-P in HUVEC cell lysate. **(B)** The binding proteins was separated by SDS-PAGE and stained by coomassie blue staining. **(C)** The washing solution of CE-P was assayed by coomassie blue staining. Lane 1 is the whole cell lysate, lane 2 is the first washing solution, and lane 3 is the final washing solution.

promising targets using the gel-based strategy. The clickable probe excluded a significant number of non-specific proteins and increased the possibility of identifying potential targets to prevent further injury. The probe will also be used to explore potential targets *in vivo* in future studies.

The ability to predict and interpret the mechanisms of action and biological targets of drugs has become feasible with the development of computational chemistry. Using DS 2016 software, we screened 9 proteins as potential targets that modulate a number of biological functions. Among these candidates, we focused on Hsp90AB1 because it had higher scores both in DS vital prediction and proteomics identification of the pull-down targets with CE-P. To rule out the interference of others, we used Hsp90AB1 pure proteins to repeat the binding experiments. The SPR results also revealed the affinity characters between them. By affinity analysis, we found CE-P (23.4 μM) had a relatively weaker affinity than CE (2.43 μM), but still maintained the property

to bind the Hsp90AB1 in a dose-dependent manner. To explore their mode of action, we performed virtual assay and found both ligands could bind with Hsp90AB1, maybe it was the way that CE could influence the target function. However, this binding site was speculative and based only on molecular modeling. To confirm its exact binding domain of CE with Hsp90AB1, it needs more powerful researches such as ATP/ADP site mutation and cocrystallization to prove this.

The Hsp90s are a family of molecular chaperones that function in the cellular stabilization, regulation, and activation of a range of "client" protein. The human isoforms of Hsp90 include Hsp90α and Hsp90β (also named Hsp90AA1 and Hsp90AB1) which are 85% identical (Li and Buchner, 2013; Synoradzki and Bieganowski, 2015). Their distinct functions have been identified (Lamoth et al., 2016). Hsp90α correlates with tumor invasiveness, angiogenesis and metastasis (Tsutsumi et al., 2008; Song et al., 2010). In contrast, Hsp90β appears to have specific

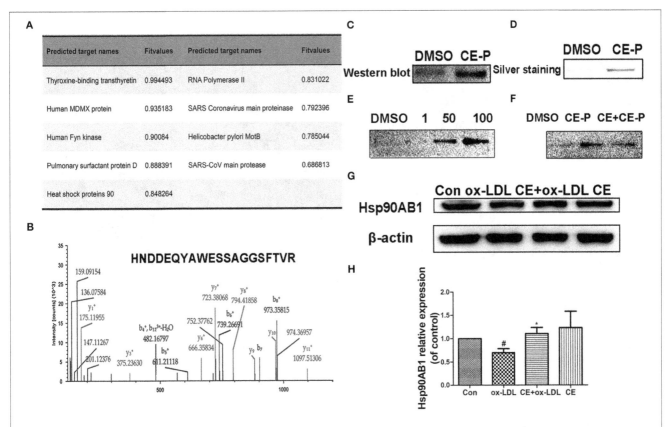

FIGURE 5 | Hsp90ab1 as potential target of CE-P. **(A)** The predicted proteins by Discovery Studio 2016 software. **(B)** Identified peptide of Hsp90ab1 by LC/MS **(C)** Western-blotting validation of the CE-P target Hsp90ab1 by whole cell lysate pull-down assay. **(D)** The pull-down assay of the recombinant Hsp90AB1 by CE-P. **(E)** CE-P could pull down Hsp90AB1 in dose-dependent manner. **(F)** CE could inhibit the binding to Hsp90AB1 and then the proteins bound to CE-P were detected by Western blot. **(G)** Effects of CE on Hsp90AB1 expression levels in ox-LDL induced HUVEC damage. Cell lysates were harvested, and Western blot analysis was performed. β-actin expression was examined as the protein loading control. **(H)** Densitometric analysis was used to quantify the levels of Hsp90AB1. Values are expressed as the mean ± SD $^{#}p < 0.05$ ox-LDL group vs. control group; $^{*}p < 0.05$, vs. ox-LDL group.

role in the anti-apoptitic functions of Bcl2 and cIAP1 (Cohen-Saidon et al., 2006; Lanneau et al., 2007; Didelot et al., 2008; Chen et al., 2009). Hsp90α and Hsp90β were also recently found to have differing effects on the activity of endothelial nitric oxide synthase (Cortes-González et al., 2010; Fismen et al., 2012). In our research, the specific domains of Hsp90AB1 were identified by LC/MS of pull-down proteins. CE could protect ox-LDL induced apoptosis and this coincides with the function of Hsp90AB1, so we mainly focused on Hsp90AB1. Indeed, we also identified one non-specific sequence (HFSVEGQLEFR) of Hsp90AA1 and Hsp90AB1 except most of the specific sequences. Might it was also a possible insight for other Hsp90s such as Hsp90AA1 as the potential target of CE, but was still need a lot of experimental results to prove it. Hsp90AB1, as molecular chaperone, interact with a lot of clients to form complexes to regulate its activity. In our research, we have confirmed CE could directly bind to Hsp90AB1 by SPR assay, if CE binds Hsp90AB1 clients still need more exploration (Hartson and Matts, 2012).

Post-translation modification (PTM) is central to biology by expanding and modulating the function of a large number of proteins. PTM contains a lot of styles such as attachment of small moieties cofactors, phosphorylation, acetylation, methylation, ubiquitylation (Hartley et al., 2015). Hsp90 undergoes extensive post-translational modifications, such as posphorylation, acetylation, S-nitrosylation, and ubiquitination (Mollapour and Neckers, 2012). Each of these factors can impact significantly on protein structure and function thus influencing and even enabling inherent protein activity. In our research, we confirmed CE binds Hsp90AB1 to interfere its function. If there is some other post-translation modifications involved in their interaction need more exploration.

Taken together all these results, we have focused our attention on Hsp90AB1 as one potential target of CE in HUVECs for further studies. The other candidates in this report should still be considered as potential targets, but their roles must be confirmed in additional experiments. In our future studies, we will perform *in vivo* experiments to further examine all the candidates.

CONCLUSION

In summary, our present researches employed chemical proteomics and click chemistry approaches for the first time to

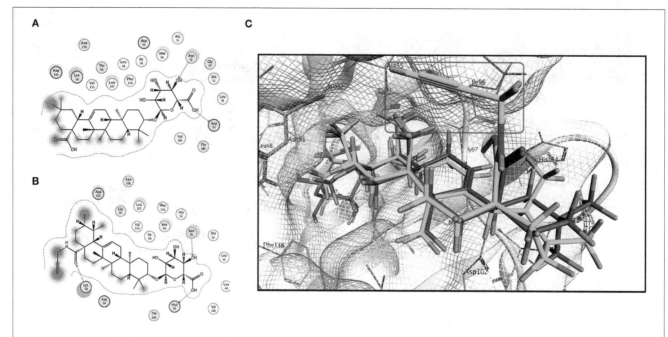

FIGURE 6 | Modeling study of the structure of CE/CE-P binding to Hsp90AB1 protein. **(A)** Two-dimensional ligand interaction diagram of CE and Hsp90AB1. **(B)** Two-dimensional ligand interaction diagram of CE-P and Hsp90AB1. **(C)** Three-dimensional modeling of CE/CE-P binding with Hsp90AB1.

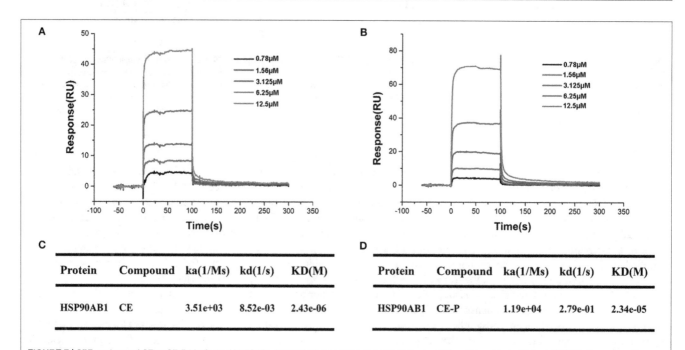

FIGURE 7 | SPR analyses of CE or CE-P binding to Hsp90AB1. Hsp90AB1 immobilized to a CM5 Sensor Chip was provided with the CE/CE-P at concentrations varying from 0.75 to 12.5 μM. **(A,B)** Representative binding curves of CE **(A)** and CE-P **(B)** binding to Hsp90AB1. **(C,D)** Kinetic binding constants of CE **(C)**/CE-P **(D)** with Hsp90AB1.

explore the targets of CE in HUVECs and identified Hsp90AB1 as possible molecular target. In our report, we designed and synthesized the clickable CE-P probe and showed that it exhibited similar activity to CE by inhibiting ox-LDL-induced cell injury. For the sake of fishing its targets, we pulled down the proteins in HUVECs cell lysate with CE-P and identified 37 potential targets using the gel-based proteomic strategy. Combining fishing data by DS 2016, we finally focused on Hsp90AB1 protein on account of the higher scores both in the pull-down assay and virtual assay. To confirm the target, we firstly detected its existence in whole cell lysate by western blotting. The probe CE-P performed the same mode of interaction and had the same binding site with Hsp90AB1, which were proved by the competitive inhibition experiment and molecular docking software respectively. To further confirm the interactions of CE-P with Hsp90AB1, we used the recombinant Hsp90AB1 protein to exclude the interference of others protein in cell lysate. Moreover, the SPR analysis revealed that both CE/CE-P could bind to Hsp90AB1 with the similar protein affinity which proved that both CE and CE-P could direct bind to protein Hsp90AB1. Based on upon reliable data, we believe that Hsp90AB1 is the potential target of CE, and will be a more promising target for future explorations.

AUTHOR CONTRIBUTIONS

G-BS, X-DX, and X-BS conducted the study. SW and YT designed the detailed experiments, performed the study, and

collected and analyzed data. J-YZ, H-BX, PZ, MW (sixth author), S-BL, YL and MW (ninth author) took part in the experiments in this study. All Authors commented the study and approved the final manuscript.

ACKNOWLEDGMENTS

This work was supported by the National Natural Sciences Foundation of China (Grant Nos. 81473380, 81302656, and 81502929), the Natural Sciences Foundation of Beijing (Grant No. 7144225, 7152102), the National Science and Technology Major Project (Grant No.2015ZX09501004-001-003), Peking Union Medical College Graduate Student Innovation Fund (Grant No. 2016-1007-06), and the CAMS Innovation Fund for Medical Science (CIFMS) (Grant No. 2016-I2M-1-012).

REFERENCES

Baranov, A. I. (1982). Medicinal uses of ginseng and related plants in the soviet union: recent trends in the soviet literature. *J. Ethnopharmacol.* 6, 339–353. doi: 10.1016/0378-8741(82)90055-1

Barglow, K. T., and Cravatt, B. F. (2007). Activity-based protein profiling for the functional annotation of enzymes. *Nat. Methods* 4, 822–827. doi: 10.1038/nmeth1092

Chen, H., Xia, Y., Fang, D., Hawke, D., and Lu, Z. (2009). Caspase-10-mediated heat shock protein 90 beta cleavage promotes UVB irradiation-induced cell apoptosis. *Mol. Cell. Biol.* 29, 3657–3664. doi: 10.1128/MCB.01640-08

Chen, X., Wong, Y. K., Wang, J., Zhang, J., Lee, Y. M., Shen, H. M., et al. (2017). Target identification with quantitative activity based protein profiling (ABPP). *Proteomics* 17:1600212. doi: 10.1002/pmic.201600212

Cohen-Saidon, C., Carmi, I., Keren, A., and Razin, E. (2006). Antiapoptotic function of Bcl-2 in mast cells is dependent on its association with heat shock protein 90β. *Blood* 107, 1413–1420. doi: 10.1182/blood-2005-07-2648

Cortes-González, C., Barrera-Chimal, J., Ibarra-Sánchez, M., Gilbert, M., Gamba, G., Zentella, A., et al. (2010). Opposite effect of Hsp90α and Hsp90β on eNOS ability to produce nitric oxide or superoxide anion in human embryonic kidney cells. *Cell. Physiol. Biochem.* 26, 657–668. doi: 10.1159/000322333

Cravatt, B. F., Wright, A. T., and Kozarich, J. W. (2008). Activity-based protein profiling: from enzyme chemistry to proteomic chemistry. *Annu. Rev. Biochem.* 77, 383–414. doi: 10.1146/annurev.biochem.75.101304.124125

Didelot, C., Lanneau, D., Brunet, M., Bouchot, A., Cartier, J., Jacquel, A., et al. (2008). Interaction of heat-shock protein 90 beta isoform (HSP90 beta) with cellular inhibitor of apoptosis 1 (c-IAP1) is required for cell differentiation. *Cell Death Differ.* 15, 859–866. doi: 10.1038/cdd.2008.5

Fismen, L., Hjelde, A., Svardal, A. M., and Djurhuus, R. (2012). Differential effects on nitric oxide synthase, heat shock proteins and glutathione in human endothelial cells exposed to heat stress and simulated diving. *Eur. J. Appl. Physiol.* 112, 2717–2725. doi: 10.1007/s00421-011-2241-4

Hartley, A. M., Zaki, A. J., McGarrity, A. R., Robert-Ansart, C., Moskalenko, A. V., Jones, G. F., et al. (2015). Functional modulation and directed assembly of an enzyme through designed non-natural post-translation modification. *Chem. Sci.* 6, 3712–3717. doi: 10.1039/C4SC03900A

Hartson, S. D., and Matts, R. L. (2012). Approaches for defining the Hsp90-dependent proteome. *Biochim. Biophys. Acta* 1823, 656–667. doi: 10.1016/j.bbamcr.2011.08.013

Hunerdosse, D., and Nomura, D. K. (2014). Activity-based proteomic and metabolomic approaches for understanding metabolism. *Curr. Opin. Biotechnol.* 28, 116–126. doi: 10.1016/j.copbio.2014.02.001

Krysiak, J., and Breinbauer, R. (2012). Activity-based protein profiling for natural product target discovery. *Top. Curr. Chem.* 324, 43–84. doi: 10.1007/128_2011_289

Lamoth, F., Juvvadi, P. R., and Steinbach, W. J. (2016). Heat shock protein 90 (Hsp90): A novel antifungal target against *Aspergillus fumigatus. Crit. Rev. Microbiol.* 42, 310–321. doi: 10.3109/1040841X.2014.947239

Lanneau, D., de Thonel, A., Maurel, S., Didelot, C., and Garrido, C. (2007). Apoptosis versus cell differentiation role of heat shock proteins HSP90, HSP70 and HSP27. *Prion* 1, 53–60. doi: 10.4161/pri.1.1.4059

Lapinsky, D. J., and Johnson, D. S. (2015). Recent developments and applications of clickable photoprobes in medicinal chemistry and chemical biology. *Future Med. Chem.* 7, 2143–2171. doi: 10.4155/fmc.15.136

Lee, J. S., Yoo, Y. H., and Yoon, C. N. (2014). Small-molecule probes elucidate global enzyme activity in a proteomic context. *BMB Rep.* 47, 149–157. doi: 10.5483/BMBRep.2014.47.3.264

Li, D., Liu, L., Chen, H., Sawamura, T., and Mehta, J. L. (2003). LOX-1, an oxidized LDL endothelial receptor, induces CD40/CD40L signaling in human coronary artery endothelial cells. *Arterioscler. Thromb. Vasc. Biol.* 23, 816–821. doi: 10.1161/01.ATV.0000066685.13434.FA

Li, D., and Mehta, J. L. (2009). Intracellular signaling of LOX-1 in endothelial cell apoptosis. *Circ. Res.* 104, 566–568. doi: 10.1161/CIRCRESAHA.109.194209

Li, J., and Buchner, J. (2013). Structure, function and regulation of the hsp90 machinery. *Biomed. J.* 36, 106–117. doi: 10.4103/2319-4170.113230

Li, N., Overkleeft, H. S., and Florea, B. I. (2012). Activity-based protein profiling: an enabling technology in chemical biology research. *Curr. Opin. Chem. Biol.* 16, 227–233. doi: 10.1016/j.cbpa.2012.01.008

Martell, J., and Weerapana, E. (2014). Applications of copper-catalyzed click chemistry in activity-based protein profiling. *Molecules* 19, 1378–1393. doi: 10.3390/molecules19021378

Mollapour, M., and Neckers, L. (2012). Post-translational modifications of Hsp90 and their contributions to chaperone regulation. *Biochim. Biophys. Acta* 1823, 648–655. doi: 10.1016/j.bbamcr.2011.07.018

Pichler, C. M., Krysiak, J., and Breinbauer, R. (2016). Target identification of covalently binding drugs by activity-based protein profiling (ABPP). *Bioorg. Med. Chem.* 24, 3291–3303. doi: 10.1016/j.bmc.2016.03.050

Qin, M., Luo, Y., Meng, X. B., Wang, M., Wang, H. W., Song, S. Y., et al. (2015). Myricitrin attenuates endothelial cell apoptosis to prevent atherosclerosis: an insight into PI3K/Akt activation and STAT3 signaling pathways. *Vasc. Pharmacol.* 70, 23–34. doi: 10.1016/j.vph.2015.03.002

Schmidt, R. R., and Michel, J. (1980). Facile synthesis of a- and P-0-Glycosyl imidates preparation of glycosides and disaccharides. *Angew. Chem. Inr. Ed. Engl.* 9, 731–732. doi: 10.1002/anie.198007311

Shi, H., Cheng, X., Sze, S. K., and Yao, S. Q. (2011). Proteome profiling reveals potential cellular targets of staurosporine using a clickable cell-permeable probe. *Chem. Commun.* 47, 11306–11308. doi: 10.1039/c1cc14824a

Song, X., Wang, X., Zhuo, W., Shi, H., Feng, D., Sun, Y., et al. (2010). The regulatory mechanism of extracellular Hsp90{alpha} on matrix metalloproteinase-2 processing and tumor angiogenesis. *J. Biol. Chem.*

285, 40039–40049. doi: 10.1074/jbc.M110.181941

Speers, A. E., and Cravatt, B. F. (2009). Activity-based protein profiling (ABPP) and click chemistry (CC)-ABPP by MudPIT mass spectrometry. *Curr. Protoc. Chem. Biol.* 1, 29–41. doi: 10.1002/9780470559277.ch090138

Sun, G. B., Sun, X., Wang, M., Ye, J. X., Si, J. Y., Xu, H. B., et al. (2012). Oxidative stress suppression by luteolin-induced heme oxygenase-1 expression. *Toxicol. Appl. Pharmacol.* 265, 229–240. doi: 10.1016/j.taap.2012.10.002

Sun, X., Chen, R. C., Yang, Z. H., Sun, G. B., Wang, M., Ma, X. J., et al. (2014). Taxifolin prevents diabetic cardiomyopathy *in vivo* and *in vitro* by inhibition of oxidative stress and cell apoptosis. *Food Chem. Toxicol.* 63, 221–232. doi: 10.1016/j.fct.2013.11.013

Synoradzki, K., and Bieganowski, P. (2015). Middle domain of human Hsp90 isoforms differentially binds Aha1 in human cells and alters Hsp90 activity in yeast. *Biochim. Biophys. Acta* 1853, 445–452. doi: 10.1016/j.bbamcr.2014.11.026

Tian, Y., Du, Y. Y., Shang, H., Wang, M., Sun, Z. H., Wang, B. Q., et al. (2017a). Calenduloside E analogues protecting H9c2 cardiomyocytes against H2O2-Induced apoptosis: design, synthesis and biological evaluation. *Front. Pharmacol.* 8:862. doi: 10.3389/fphar.2017.00862

Tian, Y., Wang, S., Shang, H., Wang, M., Sun, G., Xu, X., et al. (2017b). The proteomic profiling of calenduloside E targets in HUVEC: design, synthesis and application of biotinylated probe BCEA. *RSC Adv.* 7, 6259–6265. doi: 10.1039/C6RA25572H

Tsutsumi, S., Scroggins, B., Koga, F., Lee, M. J., Trepel, J., Felts, S., et al. (2008). A small molecule cell-impermeant Hsp90 antagonist inhibits tumor cell motility and invasion. *Oncogene* 27, 2478–2487. doi: 10.1038/sj.onc.1210897

Wang, M., Meng, X. B., Yu, Y. L., Sun, G. B., Xu, X. D., Zhang, X. P., et al. (2014). Elatoside C protects against hypoxia/reoxygenation-induced apoptosis in H9c2 cardiomyocytes through the reduction of endoplasmic reticulum stress partially depending on STAT3 activation. *Apoptosis* 19, 1727–1735. doi: 10.1007/s10495-014-1039-3

Wang, M., Sun, G. B., Zhang, J. Y., Luo, Y., Yu, Y. L., Xu, X. D., et al. (2015). Elatoside C protects the heart from ischaemia/reperfusion injury through the modulation of oxidative stress and intracellular Ca(2)(+) homeostasis. *Int. J. Cardiol.* 185, 167–176. doi: 10.1016/j.ijcard.2015.03.140

Wang, M., Tian, Y., Du, Y. Y., Sun, G. B., Xu, X. D., Jiang, H., et al. (2017). Protective effects of Araloside C against myocardial ischaemia/reperfusion injury: potential involvement of heat shock protein 90. *J. Cell. Mol. Med.* 21, 1870–1880. doi: 10.1111/jcmm.13107

Weerapana, E., Wang, C., Simon, G. M., Richter, F., Khare, S., Dillon, M. B., et al. (2010). Quantitative reactivity profiling predicts functional cysteines in proteomes. *Nature* 468, 790–795. doi: 10.1038/nature09472

Wright, M. H., and Sieber, S. A. (2016). Chemical proteomics approaches for identifying the cellular targets of natural products. *Nat. Prod. Rep.* 33, 681–708. doi: 10.1039/C6NP00001K

Yi, X., Zhong, B., Smith, K. M., Geldenhuys, W. J., Feng, Y., Pink, J. J., et al. (2012). Identification of a class of novel tubulin inhibitors. *J. Med. Chem.* 55, 3425–3435. doi: 10.1021/jm300100d

Yu, Y., Sun, G., Luo, Y., Wang, M., Chen, R., Zhang, J., et al. (2016). Cardioprotective effects of Notoginsenoside R1 against ischemia/reperfusion injuries by regulating oxidative stress- and endoplasmic reticulum stress-related signaling pathways. *Sci. Rep.* 6:21730. doi: 10.1038/srep21730

Yue, R., Shan, L., Yang, X., and Zhang, W. (2012). Approaches to target profiling of natural products. *Curr. Med. Chem.* 19, 3841–3855. doi: 10.2174/092986712801661068

Improving Docking Performance Using Negative Image-Based Rescoring

Sami T. Kurkinen[1], Sanna Niinivehmas[1], Mira Ahinko[1], Sakari Lätti[1], Olli T. Pentikäinen[1,2] and Pekka A. Postila[1*]

[1] Department of Biological and Environmental Science and Nanoscience Center, University of Jyvaskyla, Jyväskylä, Finland,
[2] Institute of Biomedicine, Integrative Physiology and Pharmacy, University of Turku, Turku, Finland

*Correspondence:
Pekka A. Postila
pekka.a.postila@jyu.fi

Despite the large computational costs of molecular docking, the default scoring functions are often unable to recognize the active hits from the inactive molecules in large-scale virtual screening experiments. Thus, even though a correct binding pose might be sampled during the docking, the active compound or its biologically relevant pose is not necessarily given high enough score to arouse the attention. Various rescoring and post-processing approaches have emerged for improving the docking performance. Here, it is shown that the very early enrichment (number of actives scored higher than 1% of the highest ranked decoys) can be improved on average 2.5-fold or even 8.7-fold by comparing the docking-based ligand conformers directly against the target protein's cavity shape and electrostatics. The similarity comparison of the conformers is performed without geometry optimization against the negative image of the target protein's ligand-binding cavity using the negative image-based (NIB) screening protocol. The viability of the NIB rescoring or the R-NiB, pioneered in this study, was tested with 11 target proteins using benchmark libraries. By focusing on the shape/electrostatics complementarity of the ligand-receptor association, the R-NiB is able to improve the early enrichment of docking essentially without adding to the computing cost. By implementing consensus scoring, in which the R-NiB and the original docking scoring are weighted for optimal outcome, the early enrichment is improved to a level that facilitates effective drug discovery. Moreover, the use of equal weight from the original docking scoring and the R-NiB scoring improves the yield in most cases.

Keywords: molecular docking, docking rescoring, negative image-based rescoring (R-NiB), benchmarking, consensus scoring

INTRODUCTION

Molecular docking is an *in silico* technique that samples potential binding poses of ligands flexibly against the ligand-binding cavities of receptor protein structures. This ability to mimic ligand-receptor recognition at the atom level can yield valuable insight on complex and experimentally difficult to approach phenomena such as enzyme reaction mechanics or ligand-receptor association especially when it is coupled to atomistic simulations.

The main interest for docking comes from its use in computer-aided drug discovery and virtual screening experiments that aim to discover novel drug compounds from vast compound libraries—a process that ideally lowers the amount of costly experimental testing. On the one hand, the docking algorithms reproduce experimentally verified ligand binding geometries with remarkable accuracy (Kitchen et al., 2004; Warren et al., 2006; Kolb and Irwin, 2009; Meng et al., 2011). On the other hand, anybody who has used docking on routine basis can confirm that these successes are case-specific and the methodology often fails to produce sufficient enrichment (Ferrara et al., 2004; Mohan et al., 2005; Sousa et al., 2006; McGaughey et al., 2007; Plewczynski et al., 2011). In part, this hit-or-miss nature of docking is caused by the lack of relevant 3D structure data on the target proteins (Schapira et al., 2003) or inadequacies of the ligand conformer sampling (Sastry et al., 2013), but the other fundamental problem is the failure in scoring the sampled docking solutions (Wang et al., 2003; Warren et al., 2006; Plewczynski et al., 2011; Pagadala et al., 2017).

In other words, although the conformational space of the ligand binding might be sampled exhaustively, the best binding poses or the most potent compounds are not necessarily put to the top of the ranking lists by the default scoring functions (Wang et al., 2003; Ferrara et al., 2004; Cross et al., 2009; Plewczynski et al., 2011). An experienced researcher might be able to select the best pose out of 10 different conformers, but the situation becomes quickly unattainable when dealing with hundreds or thousands of compounds. The docking scoring functions put a certain weight on the specific ligand-receptor interactions such as hydrogen bonding, halogen bonding and π-π stacking but also the internal energies of the ligand conformers are considered. Despite the undeniable merits, these binding favorability or energy assessments do not always work (Chen et al., 2006; Cross et al., 2009), which means that the best pose or, more relevantly, the active compound is frequently ignored in the docking screening.

The docking solutions can be rescored after the fact to increase the yield. This is done by reassessing the favorability of the solutions utilizing a set of empirical binding descriptors that put weight on different binding characteristics. In the consensus scoring, a set of different scoring functions are employed and together they produce better enrichment than any of the functions accomplish alone (Charifson et al., 1999; Clark et al., 2002; Oda et al., 2006). Tasking more than one scoring methodology should in theory cover all the bases and, furthermore, a mix of dissimilar functions should facilitate the discovery of active hits from vast compound pools. The inherent problem with the consensus rescoring, however, is that the optimal settings are specific for each target. Accordingly, their successful use with novel targets lacking benchmark test sets is difficult to ascertain beforehand (Cheng et al., 2009).

In addition, performance enhancement might be produced by docking the ligands with different software to improve the sampling (Houston and Walkinshaw, 2013) or by optimizing and estimating the binding poses using the Poisson–Boltzmann or generalized Born and surface area continuum solvation (MM/PBSA or MM/GBSA), free energy perturbation (FEP) or solvated interaction energy (SIE) calculations (Bash et al., 1987; Kollman et al., 2000; Onufriev et al., 2004; Naïm et al., 2007; Guimarães and Cardozo, 2008; Sulea et al., 2011, 2012;

Genheden and Ryde, 2015; Virtanen et al., 2015; Juvonen et al., 2016). Because these post-processing steps require a lot of extra computing, it limits their applicability in the real-world screening studies involving potentially hundreds of thousands of compounds. In addition, the success-rates of the post-processing methods vary on a case-by-case basis (Virtanen et al., 2015) and, beforehand, there is no way to tell whether the extra investment will pay out. In short, there is a genuine need for reliable rescoring methodologies that do not require a lot of extra computing resources or experiment-based tinkering.

The aim of the study was to demonstrate that by focusing solely on the shape/electrostatics complementarity between the docked ligand poses and the receptor protein's ligand-binding site, the yield of the small-molecule docking could be improved.

In the negative image-based (NIB) screening (Virtanen and Pentikäinen, 2010; Niinivehmas et al., 2011, 2015), a negative image or a NIB model is generated by inverting the shape and electrostatics of a ligand-binding cavity using a specifically tailored software PANTHER (Niinivehmas et al., 2015). The resulting NIB model is used by similarity comparison algorithms such as ShaEP (Vainio et al., 2009) the same way as ligand 3D structures extracted from the X-ray crystal structures are used in the ligand-based screening. The ligand 3D conformers, used in the similarity comparison, are generated from scratch using software such as BALLOON (Vainio and Johnson, 2007); but, notably, the conformers could also originate from molecular docking sampling.

To explore this idea further and to improve docking enrichment, the NIB screening methodology was repurposed for rescoring multiple explicit docking solutions output by the docking software PLANTS (Korb et al., 2009). The main difference between the established NIB methodology and the here introduced NIB rescoring or the R-NiB (**Figure 1**) is that it is performed as is. The coordinates of the cavity-based negative image and the docked ligand conformers are not superimposed or optimized for a better match. The rescoring was performed with 11 target proteins ranging from nuclear receptors such as progesterone receptor (PR) to neuraminidase (NEU) using established virtual screening benchmark libraries containing both known active and inactive decoy ligands (Huang et al., 2006; Mysinger et al., 2012). Altogether 22 different benchmark sets were used to validate the new methodology (**Table 1**).

As a whole, the results show that the R-NiB produces moderate or excellent early enrichment improvements using the basic settings in the NIB model generation and similarity screening. In most cases, the early enrichment of the docking can be improved also by consensus scoring, in which the original PLANTS docking scoring and the PANTHER/ShaEP-based R-NiB scoring are given an optimal weight ratio. What is more, the rescoring indicates that the hit rate is typically enhanced even when both of these scoring functions are bluntly given equal (50/50%) weight in the consensus scoring.

In summary, the success of the R-NiB approach in sorting out the active ligands from the inactive molecules is directly related to the fact that the shape/electrostatics complementarity between the ligand and the receptor is an essential part of the complex formation.

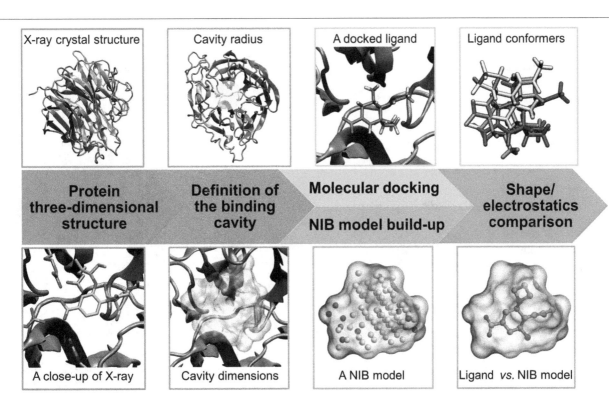

FIGURE 1 | Negative image-based rescoring workflow. Firstly, the protein 3D structure (neuraminidase; gray cartoon; PDB: 1B9V) (Finley et al., 1999) and ligand 3D structures for molecular docking are prepared (e.g., protonation). Secondly, the ligand-binding cavity is outlined using a detection radius for docking (yellow transparent circle above) and NIB model generation (yellow transparent surface below). If there exist a bound ligand in the PDB entry (BANA206 as a stick model with cyan backbone in the close-up below), it can be used in defining the cavity center and/or dimensions. Thirdly, the docking of ligands into the cavity is performed using a standard docking software and multiple docking solutions or conformers are outputted for rescoring. Fourthly, a cavity-based NIB model, composed of explicit cavity points (white neutral; blue positive; red negative) is generated with PANTHER (Niinivehmas et al., 2015) for the same cavity. Fifthly, the NIB model shape/electrostatics (transparent surface with charge potential) are compared directly against the docking solutions using a similarity comparison algorithm ShaEP (Vainio et al., 2009) without geometry optimization. Those solutions matching the cavity information are given higher scores than the ones that differ.

MATERIALS AND METHODS

Ligand Set Preparation

The ligand sets, including the active and inactive decoy compounds, were acquired from the DUD (A Directory of Useful Decoys) (Huang et al., 2006) and DUD-E (A Database of Useful (Docking) Decoys -Enhanced) (Mysinger et al., 2012) databases for the target proteins (**Table 1**). The initial 3D coordinates for the DUD ligands were converted to the SMILES (Simplified Molecular-Input Line-Entry System) format using STRUCTCONVERT in MAESTRO 2017-1 (Schrödinger, LLC, New York, NY, USA, 2017). LIGPREP in MAESTRO was used to generate OPLS3 charges and tautomeric states for both the DUD and DUD-E ligand sets at pH 7.4. Next, both of the ligand sets were converted to the SYBYL MOL2 format using MOL2CONVERT in MAESTRO. The back-and-forth conversion between MOL2 and SMILES formats was done with the DUD ligands to avoid potential bias of the original 3D conformations for the molecular docking (Zoete et al., 2016).

Protein Preparation

The 3D structures of the target proteins, which were used in the molecular docking and the NIB model generation, were acquired

from the Protein Data Bank (PDB) (Berman et al., 2000; Burley et al., 2017). All of the used PDB entries are listed in **Table 1**. The benchmarking was done mainly using the PDB entries listed for the DUD and DUD-E datasets and, thus, both the docking and rescoring could work better or worse using different structures. The necessary PDB entry editing (**Figure 1**) such as the removal of bound ligands from the active sites was done in the BODIL Molecular Modeling Environment (Lehtonen et al., 2004). The protein residues were protonated with the default settings in REDUCE3.24 (Word et al., 1999). The X-ray crystal structure waters were left in the deprotonated state for NIB model building.

Molecular Docking

The molecular docking of the DUD and DUD-E compound sets (**Figure 1**) into the ligand-binding sites of the target proteins was performed using PLANTS1.2 (Korb et al., 2009). The default settings were used in the docking screenings. Accordingly, the initial docking scoring was performed with the ChemPLP that combines the PLP (Piecewise Linear Potential) with GOLD's Chemscore (Korb et al., 2009). The centroid coordinates of ligands bound in the target protein structures were used as the binding site centers in the docking. A relatively large binding

TABLE 1 | Target protein 3D structures used in the virtual screening.

Target protein[a]	DUD				DUD-E			
	PDB code	Resolution (Å)	Ligs[b]	Decs[c]	PDB code	Resolution (Å)	Ligs[b]	Decs[b]
ER-agonist	1L2I	1.95	67	2,352	–	–	–	–
ER-antagonist	3ERT	1.9	39	1,394	–	–	–	–
ER-mixed[c]	–	–	106	3,746	1SJ0	1.9	383	20,663
AR	2AO6	1.89	74	2,628	2AM9	1.64	269	14,343
GR	1M2Z	2.5	78	2,797	3BQD	2.5	258	14,986
MR	2AA2	1.95	15	535	2AA2	1.95	94	5,146
PPARγ	1FM9	2.1	81	2,906	2GTK	2.1	484	25,256
RXRα	1MVC	1.9	20	706	1MV9	1.9	131	6,935
COX2	1CX2	3.0	348	12,462	3LN1	2.4	435	23,136
PDE5	1XP0	1.79	51	1,808	1UDT	2.3	398	27,520
	1UDT[d]	2.3	–	–	1XOZ[d]	1.37	–	–
PR	1SR7	1.46	27	967	3KBA	2.0	293	15,642
NEU	–	–	–	–	1B9V	2.35	98	6,197
CYP3A4	–	–	–	–	3NXU	2.0	170	11,797

[a]AR, androgen receptor; COX2, cyclo-oxygenase 2; CYP3A4, cytochrome P450 3A4; ER, estrogen receptor alpha; GR, glucocorticoid receptor; MR, mineralocorticoid receptor; NEU, neuraminidase; PPARγ, peroxisome proliferator activated receptor gamma; PR, progesterone receptor; RXRα, retinoid X receptor alpha; PDE5, phosphodiesterase type 5. ER-agonist, ER-antagonist and ER-mixed refer to ligand sets containing ER-specific agonists, antagonists or both, respectively.
[b]Number of active ligands (Ligs) and decoy (Decs) molecules after preprocessing with LIGPREP.
[c]In the DUD database, ER agonists and antagonists are separated into two separate datasets, but in the case of the DUD-E the ligands are mixed. For comparison, the ER datasets in the DUD were also mixed.
[d]Used in the NIB model generation.

site radius of 10 Å was generally used in the docking. The radius was slightly reduced for glucocorticoid receptor (GR; 9 Å) based on the size of the ligand-binding site. Altogether 10 docking solutions were output for each compound for the purpose of NIB rescoring. The idea is to provide enough different docking solutions for the rescoring.

Negative Image-Based Model Generation

The negative images or the NIB models of the target proteins' ligand-binding cavities (**Figure 1**) were prepared using the default settings in PANTHER0.18.15 (Niinivehmas et al., 2015). The centroids used in the NIB model generation were based on the centroid coordinates of the ligand compounds bound in the original protein 3D structures the same way as was done with the docking. The NIB models were prepared in three different ways: (1) the NIB model size and dimensions were adjusted using the box radius option (6–10 Å); (2) the cavity size was limited to a certain radius (1.5–3.0 Å) from the bound ligand in the original structure using the ligand distance limit option; (3) when available and producing better results, a model (referred as PANTHER model) was taken also from a prior NIB screening study (Niinivehmas et al., 2015). The NIB model coordinates for all new NIB models are included in the Supplementary Material.

Negative Image-Based Rescoring

The NIB rescoring (or the R-NiB; **Figure 1**) of the original docking solutions was performed using ShaEP1.0.7.915 (Vainio et al., 2009). The shape and electrostatics of each docking solution was compared directly against the template NIB models

without superimposing or optimizing their coordinates (– noOptimization option). Both the shape and electrostatics were given equal amount of weight (ESP = 0.5) in the ShaEP similarity scoring (default option). Because altogether 10 conformers were outputted for each docked compound, even those solutions given lower scores by PLANTS (Korb et al., 2009) could be later considered in the PANTHER/ShaEP-based (Virtanen and Pentikäinen, 2010; Niinivehmas et al., 2011, 2015) NIB rescoring.

Rescoring With Alternative Methodologies

The docking poses initially scored by PLANTS using ChemPLP scoring function were also rescored using an alternative scoring function PLP in PLANTS. Otherwise, default options were used in the PLANTS-based rescoring. In addition, the docking solutions were also re-ranked using the default settings of XSCORE1.2.1 (Wang et al., 2002) for comparison. The XSCORE has three empirical scoring functions HPSCORE, HMSCORE and HSSCORE that can be fine-tuned on case-by-case basis to improve the docking yield. None of the scoring functions produced markedly better early enrichment separately for the docking results at least without special adjustments; thus, the software's default option of using X-CSCORE consensus scoring with all three functions was utilized.

Consensus Scoring

The R-NiB relies heavily on the initial success of the docking software used to generate the multiple docking poses for the rescoring phase, because no coordinate optimization or extra sampling is performed (**Figure 1**). Essentially, this means that the used PLANTS scoring is intrinsically influencing the R-NiB yield in this study. The consensus scoring takes this aspect further by directly incorporating the initial ChemPLP docking scoring with the R-NiB scoring. All possible combinations, in which both PLANTS- and ShaEP-based scoring were given different weights, were considered with 5% interval and those consensus scoring settings producing the highest early enrichment are discussed. The scores for each docked conformer outputted by PLANTS and ShaEP were normalized to fit into the scale from 1 to 0 and then combined for a consensus score.

Table and Figure Preparation

Figures 1, **4**, **5** were prepared using BODIL (Lehtonen et al., 2004), MOLSCRIPT2.1.2 (Kraulis, 1991), RASTER3D3.0.2 (Merritt and Murphy, 1994), and VMD1.9.2 (Humphrey et al., 1996). The area under curve (AUC) values (**Tables 2**, **3**), the early enrichment values (**Tables 4**, **5**) were calculated with ROCKER0.1.4 (Lätti et al., 2016). The enrichment factors were calculated as true positive rate when 1 or 5% of the decoy molecules have been found (EFn%$_{DEC}$; see equation below) in order to make future comparison reliable against other methodologies (Lätti et al., 2016).

$$EF_{n\%DEC} = \frac{Ligs_{n\%DEC}}{Ligs_{all}} \times 100 \qquad (1)$$

In Equation (1), Ligs$_{n\%DEC}$ is the number of ligands ranked higher than n % of the decoys whereas Ligs$_{all}$ is the total number of all ligands in the dataset. The receiver operating characteristics (ROC) curves were plotted using ROCKER with the semi-log10 scale (only x axis logarithmic) in **Figures 2**, **3** to highlight the very early enrichment of the actives. The standard deviation for the AUC is acquired in ROCKER utilizing the derived error for the Wilcoxon statistic (Hanley and McNeil, 1982). The Wilcoxon statistic estimates the probability of ranking a random ligand higher than a random decoy, which is equivalent to the value of AUC; thus, making the errors also equal.

RESULTS

Negative Image-Based Rescoring of Docking Solutions

The aim of the negative image-based rescoring or R-NiB (**Figure 1**) is to rescore existing molecular docking solutions and, by doing so, enrich active hits from a vast pool of compounds. The enrichment is achieved by comparing the shape/electrostatics similarity between the ligand conformers and the negative image of the target protein's ligand-binding cavity. The established NIB methodology (Virtanen and Pentikäinen, 2010; Niinivehmas et al., 2011, 2015) is employed in building the cavity-based NIB models of the target proteins' ligand-binding sites (PANTHER) and in comparing them against each docking solution (ShaEP). The starting point of the R-NiB workflow (**Figure 1**) is that the ligands are docked into the same target protein's cavity using a standard docking algorithm and, preferably, multiple solutions that roughly fit into the cavity are outputted for the rescoring.

Molecular Docking Produces Moderate or High Enrichment in the Benchmarking

The AUC and early enrichment values (**Tables 2**, **3**) show that the molecular docking, performed with PLANTS (Korb et al., 2009), worked relatively well with both the DUD and DUD-E datasets (Huang et al., 2006; Mysinger et al., 2012). With the DUD, the AUC values ranged from 0.60 to 0.95 indicating either moderate or substantial enrichment of actives with a majority of the targets (**Tables 3**). Markedly, the docking for the estrogen receptor alpha agonists (ER-agonist; AUC = 0.81), PR (AUC = 0.63) and the peroxisome proliferator activated receptor gamma (PPARγ; AUC = 0.95) worked so well that the AUC values were not improved by the R-NiB (**Table 2**). A side note, the DUD sets are small, containing 15–348 actives (**Table 1**) and, accordingly, a difference of a few active ligands in the ranking can sometimes have disproportionate effects on the AUC values. The docking worked also with the more demanding DUD-E ligand sets, containing a lot more of actives and decoys (**Table 1**), as the AUC values were typically well above 0.50 (**Table 3**). The AUC values could not be improved with the ER-mixed (AUC = 0.74), PPARγ (AUC = 0.85), phosphodiesterase type 5 (PDE5; AUC = 0.78) and cytochrome P450 3A4 (CYP3A4; AUC = 0.61) DUD-E sets using the R-NiB (**Table 3**).

Instead of the AUC values, it is often more practical to concentrate on the early enrichment when estimating the success of the virtual screening. That is to say, paradoxically, a high AUC value does not necessarily guarantee that the very top results contain active hits despite the fact that it is a good metric for estimating the overall success-rate of the screening. By large, the docking struggled in ranking the actives to the very top of the list, when inspecting the EF1%$_{DEC}$ or EF5%$_{DEC}$ values with the DUD and DUD-E datasets (**Tables 4**, **5**). Accordingly, the very early enrichment or EF1%$_{DEC}$ was improved by the R-NiB with all of the DUD sets (**Table 4**). With the DUD-E, the R-NiB could not produce improvement for the ER-mixed (EF1%$_{DEC}$ = 21.7%), PPARγ (EF1%$_{DEC}$ = 24.2%), retinoid X receptor alpha (RXRα; EF1%$_{DEC}$ = 11.5%), cyclo-oxygenase 2 (COX2; EF1%$_{DEC}$ = 5.7%), and PDE5 (EF1%$_{DEC}$ = 11.3%; **Table 5**), however, in the remaining six datasets the early enrichment was improved notably (discussed below). The ROC curves, which were plotted using the semi-log10 scale to highlight the very early enrichment, corroborate the numerical trends for both of the benchmark datasets (**Figures 2**, **3**).

Negative Image Generation for Rescoring Is a Straightforward Process

The NIB model has to contain key features of the target protein's ligand-binding cavity in order to produce enrichment by the R-NiB (**Figure 1**). Firstly, the shape and size of the model should be limited to the cavity area that facilitates the ligand binding. Secondly, if the cavity contains vital hydrogen bond acceptor or donor groups, the NIB model must reflect those features in its charge properties. Each data point in the NIB model can be tested and adjusted iteratively using validated ligand sets that include both active and inactive compounds. This sort of "trial-and-error" refinement is generally

TABLE 2 | The AUC values for the DUD datasets.

	Docking	Rescoring				
Target protein	PLANTS ChemPLP	R-NiB: Ligand distance[a]	R-NiB: Box radius[b]	R-NiB: prior models[c]	XSCORE	PLANTS PLP
ER-agonist	0.81 ± 0.03	0.78 ± 0.03	0.76 ± 0.03	0.79 ± 0.03	0.82 ± 0.03	0.78 ± 0.03
ER-antagonist	0.81 ± 0.04	0.85 ± 0.04	0.77 ± 0.04	0.82 ± 0.04	0.71 ± 0.05	0.83 ± 0.04
ER-mixed	0.64 ± 0.03	**0.77 ± 0.03**	**0.70 ± 0.03**	**0.74 ± 0.03**	0.66 ± 0.03	0.61 ± 0.03
AR	0.80 ± 0.03	**0.84 ± 0.03**	0.81 ± 0.03	–	0.79 ± 0.03	0.78 ± 0.03
GR	0.60 ± 0.03	**0.80 ± 0.03**	**0.83 ± 0.03**	**0.84 ± 0.03**	**0.75 ± 0.03**	0.53 ± 0.03
MR	0.80 ± 0.07	**0.93 ± 0.05**	**0.91 ± 0.05**	0.82 ± 0.07	**0.92 ± 0.05**	0.78 ± 0.07
PPARγ	0.95 ± 0.02	0.92 ± 0.02	0.87 ± 0.03	–	0.81 ± 0.03	0.94 ± 0.02
PR	0.63 ± 0.06	0.52 ± 0.06	0.50 ± 0.06	0.50 ± 0.06	0.51 ± 0.06	0.58 ± 0.06
RXRα	0.78 ± 0.06	**0.89 ± 0.05**	0.84 ± 0.06	**0.90 ± 0.05**	**0.97 ± 0.02**	0.76 ± 0.06
COX2	0.81 ± 0.01	**0.93 ± 0.01**	**0.92 ± 0.01**	**0.95 ± 0.01**	0.65 ± 0.02	**0.85 ± 0.01**
PDE5	0.71 ± 0.04	0.67 ± 0.04	0.67 ± 0.04	0.72 ± 0.04	0.54 ± 0.04	0.66 ± 0.04

If the rescoring produced higher AUC value in comparison to the initial docking (no overlapping standard error ranges), those numbers are shown in bold.
[a] The ligand distance limit used in PANTHER varied between the targets due to the size/shape differences of the binding cavities and the screened ligand sets. Limits included 1.5 Å (ER, AR, MR, PPARγ, PR RXRα, and COX2), 2.0 Å (GR), and 3.0 Å (PDE5).
[b] The box radius varied between the targets due to the size/shape differences of the binding cavities and screened ligand sets. The radiuses included 6.0 Å (GR, PR and COX2), 7.0 Å (ER-mixed, MR and RXRα), and 8.0 Å (ER-agonist, ER-antagonist, AR, PPARγ and PDE5).
[c] The previously published PANTHER models, optimized for regular NIB screening, were taken from a prior study (Niinivehmas et al., 2015).

TABLE 3 | The AUC values for the DUD-E datasets.

	Docking	Rescoring				
Target protein	PLANTS ChemPLP	R-NiB: Ligand distance[a]	R-NiB: Box radius[b]	R-NiB: Prior models[c]	XSCORE	PLANTS PLP
ER-mixed	0.74 ± 0.01	0.66 ± 0.02	0.65 ± 0.02	–	0.71 ± 0.01	0.70 ± 0.02
AR	0.54 ± 0.02	**0.76 ± 0.02**	**0.73 ± 0.02**	**0.75 ± 0.02**	**0.65 ± 0.02**	0.53 ± 0.02
GR	0.54 ± 0.02	**0.74 ± 0.02**	**0.76 ± 0.02**	**0.70 ± 0.02**	**0.69 ± 0.02**	0.51 ± 0.02
MR	0.55 ± 0.03	**0.74 ± 0.03**	**0.76 ± 0.03**	**0.68 ± 0.03**	**0.69 ± 0.03**	0.53 ± 0.03
PPARγ	0.85 ± 0.01	0.77 ± 0.01	0.75 ± 0.01	–	0.66 ± 0.01	0.84 ± 0.01
PR	0.63 ± 0.02	**0.74 ± 0.02**	**0.75 ± 0.02**	0.63 ± 0.02	**0.67 ± 0.02**	0.61 ± 0.02
RXRα	0.77 ± 0.02	**0.83 ± 0.02**	**0.81 ± 0.02**	**0.81 ± 0.02**	**0.85 ± 0.02**	0.70 ± 0.03
COX2	0.66 ± 0.01	**0.75 ± 0.01**	0.65 ± 0.01	–	0.62 ± 0.01	0.67 ± 0.01
PDE5	0.78 ± 0.01	0.72 ± 0.02	0.70 ± 0.02	–	0.58 ± 0.02	0.74 ± 0.01
NEU	0.85 ± 0.02	**0.89 ± 0.02**	**0.89 ± 0.02**	–	0.68 ± 0.03	0.56 ± 0.03
CYP3A4	0.61 ± 0.02	0.60 ± 0.02	0.60 ± 0.02	–	0.53 ± 0.02	0.60 ± 0.02

If the rescoring produced higher AUC value in comparison to the initial docking (no overlapping standard error ranges), those numbers are shown in bold.
[a] The ligand distance limit used in PANTHER varied between the targets due to the size/shape differences of the binding cavities and screened ligand sets. Limits included 1.5 Å (ER-mixed, AR, PPARγ, PR, and COX2), 2.0 Å (MR, RXRα, NEU, PDE5, and CYP3A4) and 3.0 Å (GR).
[b] The box radius varied between the targets due to the size/shape differences of the binding cavities and screened ligand sets. The radiuses included 6.0 Å (AR, GR, MR, COX2, NEU, and PR), 7.0 Å (PDE5, RXRα, and CYP3A4) and 9.0 Å (PPARγ) and 10.0 Å (ER-mixed).
[c] The previously published PANTHER models, optimized for regular NIB screening, were taken from a prior study (Niinivehmas et al., 2015).

not feasible and, accordingly, the R-NiB methodology was applied here using default easy-to-replicate PANTHER/ShaEP settings (Vainio et al., 2009; Niinivehmas et al., 2015). Effective models were acquired by simply adjusting the cavity detection box radius or by limiting the cavity dimensions with the ligand distance limit in PANTHER (Niinivehmas et al., 2015). The model generation relied solely on the PDB entry used also in the docking and generally the first-tried basic settings were enough to improve the enrichment (**Tables 2–5**; **Figures 2**, **3**). For comparison, the rescoring was also performed with prior PANTHER models (**Tables 2–5**)

optimized for the standard NIB screening (Niinivehmas et al., 2015).

Negative Image-Based Rescoring Improves the Early Enrichment With Most Targets

The R-NiB (**Figure 1**) does not rely on superimposing or geometry optimization prior to the similarity comparison of the docking solutions against the cavity-based NIB models. In a nutshell, either the docked ligand poses outputted by the docking

TABLE 4 | The enrichment given as true positive rates for the DUD datasets.

		Docking			Rescoring			
Target protein	EF %$_{DEC}$	PLANTS ChemPLP	R-NiB: ligand distance[a]	R-NiB: box radius[b]	R-NiB: prior models[c]	XSCORE	PLANTS PLP
ER-agonist	1%	17.9	**37.3**	**31.3**	23.9	19.4	10.4
	5%	44.8	52.2	58.2	59.7	52.2	26.9
ER-antagonist	1%	15.4	**28.2**	7.7	12.8	15.4	12.8
	5%	33.3	43.6	25.6	38.5	25.6	35.9
ER-mixed	1%	0.0	**11.3**	**1.9**	**2.8**	**2.8**	0.0
	5%	20.8	23.6	5.7	8.5	6.6	7.5
AR	1%	17.6	27.0	12.2	–	9.5	14.9
	5%	40.5	45.9	45.9	–	31.1	39.2
GR	1%	6.4	**11.5**	**16.7**	**12.8**	29.5	3.8
	5%	15.4	28.2	28.2	29.5	50.0	14.1
MR	1%	26.7	33.3	13.3	0.0	0.0	33.3
	5%	60.0	73.3	40.0	26.7	40.0	60.0
PPARγ	1%	69.1	79.0	22.2	–	21.0	66.7
	5%	84.0	86.4	65.4	–	48.1	85.2
PR	1%	3.7	**33.3**	**33.3**	**29.6**	**18.5**	3.7
	5%	11.1	**40.7**	**40.7**	**40.7**	**22.2**	7.4
RXRα	1%	5.0	**35.0**	**20.0**	**20.0**	**70.0**	0.0
	5%	30.0	**80.0**	**45.0**	**80.0**	**85.0**	30.0
COX2	1%	13.5	**43.7**	**40.5**	**62.6**	9.2	**20.1**
	5%	35.3	**70.4**	**64.1**	**83.0**	20.1	44.8
PDE5	1%	13.7	**31.4**	**31.4**	13.7	3.9	9.8
	5%	25.5	**37.3**	**39.2**	23.5	5.9	25.5

Those EF%$_{DEC}$ values that are at least 1.5-fold compared to the initial docking are shown in bold.

[a] The ligand distance limit used in PANTHER varied between the targets due to the size/shape differences of the binding cavities and the screened ligand sets. Limits included 1.5 Å (ER-agonist, ER-mixed, AR, MR, PPARγ, RXRα, and COX2) and 2.0 Å (GR and PR), 3.0 Å (ER-antagonist) and 4.0 Å (PDE5).

[b] The box radius varied between the targets due to the size/shape differences of the binding cavities and screened ligand sets. The radiuses included 6.0 Å (MR and COX2), 7.0 Å (AR and PR) and 8.0 Å (ER's, GR, PPARγ and RXRα) and 9.0 Å (PDE5).

[c] The previously published PANTHER models, optimized for regular NIB screening, were taken from a prior study (Niinivehmas et al., 2015).

software match the cavity-based NIB models or they do not—the similarity score (from 1 to 0) of ShaEP reflects this reality. Therefore, it is crucial that the initial docking has sampled the ligand conformers thoroughly and produces "correct" ligand poses that can be discovered by the R-NiB. Understandably, the rescoring cannot enrich active compounds, if they are docked completely outside the cavity space that was used in the NIB model generation.

With the DUD datasets (Huang et al., 2006), the AUC values from docking were improved somewhat or greatly with most of the target proteins using the R-NiB (**Table 2**). The AUC improvement was sizeable with the GR (0.60 vs. 0.84), RXRα (0.78 vs. 0.90), mineralocorticoid receptor (MR; 0.80 vs. 0.93) and COX2 (0.81 vs. 0.95) to name a few examples (**Table 2**). Moreover, the R-NiB could improve the AUC values substantially even with the more demanding DUD-E sets (Mysinger et al., 2012) where the docking scoring started to falter (**Table 3**). This positive effect in favor of the R-NiB was seen with a multitude of target proteins, including the androgen receptor (AR; 0.54 vs. 0.76), GR (0.54 vs. 0.74), MR, (0.55 vs. 0.74), PR (0.63 vs. 0.74), RXRα (0.77 vs. 0.83), and COX2 (0.66 vs. 0.75). The AUC values worsened or improved marginally for the CYP3A4 (0.61

vs. 0.60) and NEU (0.85 vs. 0.89), respectively, but in these cases the results remained within the margin of error (**Table 3**). The R-NiB clearly could not improve the AUC values for the PDE5, PPARγ and ER-mixed with the DUD-E datasets (**Table 3**). The PDE5 and ER-mixed datasets are particularly demanding, because they both contain two distinct ligand groups for which one cannot build a single satisfactory NIB model (Niinivehmas et al., 2011).

As stated above, it is more important that the virtual screening produces the highest possible early enrichment rather than the best AUC value. To this end, the R-NiB was able to improve the early enrichment somewhat or substantially with most of the target proteins included in the DUD datasets (**Table 4**). The EF1%$_{DEC}$ improvement ranged from 1.9 to 49.1% between the different targets. On average the EF1%$_{DEC}$ or EF5%$_{DEC}$ improvement was 3.3-fold or 1.8-fold, respectively, but, alas, the EF1%$_{DEC}$ of PR improved 9.0-fold using the R-NiB. A close inspection of the semi-logarithmic ROC curves (**Figure 2**) indicates that the very early enrichment produced by the R-NiB was always as good or better than that of the original docking scoring (well above the random rate; **Figure 2**). This suggests that the rescoring generally has a positive effect for the yield with the

TABLE 5 | The enrichment given as true positive rates for the DUD-E datasets.

| Target protein | EF%$_{DEC}$ | Docking | | | Rescoring | | | |
		PLANTS ChemPLP	R-NiB: ligand distance[a]	R-NiB: box radius[b]	R-NiB: prior models[c]	XSCORE	PLANTS PLP
ER-mixed	1%	21.7	18.3	5.5	–	6.3	12.8
	5%	36.6	32.6	20.1	–	24.8	28.7
AR	1%	1.5	**13.0**	**5.6**	**8.9**	1.9	0.4
	5%	7.1	**23.0**	**15.2**	**22.3**	7.8	5.2
GR	1%	1.2	**4.7**	**3.5**	**5.8**	1.2	1.2
	5%	12.0	**22.5**	12.8	**17.4**	10.5	10.1
MR	1%	3.2	**11.7**	**6.4**	3.2	1.1	1.1
	5%	19.1	25.5	19.1	18.1	8.5	11.7
PPARγ	1%	24.2	4.5	10.3	–	5.0	19.6
	5%	57.0	24.4	32.4	–	13.8	48.3
PR	1%	2.0	**4.4**	**3.8**	**3.8**	2.0	2.4
	5%	17.1	17.1	11.6	17.4	11.6	15.0
RXRα	1%	11.5	6.9	1.5	10.7	15.3	1.5
	5%	37.4	25.2	12.2	23.9	45.8	19.8
COX2	1%	5.7	2.3	0.5	–	2.1	**9.9**
	5%	21.6	19.1	4.1	–	6.4	25.1
PDE5	1%	11.3	10.6	3.8	–	1.5	8.8
	5%	28.1	25.9	14.1	–	7.0	24.4
NEU	1%	4.1	**13.3**	**6.1**	–	1.0	0.0
	5%	32.7	42.9	35.7	–	4.1	4.1
CYP3A4	1%	7.1	7.6	5.3	–	2.4	6.5
	5%	12.9	**18.8**	15.3	–	6.5	13.5

Those EF%$_{DEC}$ values that are at least 1.5-fold compared to the initial docking are shown in bold.

[a] The ligand distance limit used in PANTHER varied between the targets due to the size/shape differences of the binding cavities and screened ligand sets. Limits included 1.5 Å (ER-mixed, AR, PDE5, GR, MR, PR and COX2), 2.0 Å (RXRα, NEU and CYP3A4) and 3.0 Å (PPARγ).

[b] The box radius varied between the targets due to the size/shape differences of the binding cavities and screened ligand sets. The radiuses included 6.0 Å (AR, GR, MR and NEU), 7.0 Å (RXRα, PR, PDE5 and CYP3A4), 8.0 Å (COX2), 9.0 Å (PPARγ) and 11.0 Å (ER-mixed).

[c] The previously published PANTHER models, optimized for regular NIB screening, were taken from a prior study (Niinivehmas et al., 2015).

tested DUD datasets. The EF1%$_{DEC}$ improvement (**Table 4**) was most prominent with the COX2 (13.5 vs. 62.6 %), but the R-NiB worked exceptionally well also based on the EF5%$_{DEC}$ for example with the RXRα (30.0 vs. 80.0%), COX2 (35.3 vs. 83.0%), PDE5 (25.5 vs. 39.2%) and ER-agonist (44.8 vs. 59.7%).

Based on the early enrichment values (**Table 4**) and the plotted ROC curves (**Figure 3**), the overall performance of the R-NiB with the DUD-E dataset showed similar trends as with the DUD (**Table 3**; **Figure 2**). The improvement over the original docking was on average 2.5-fold for the EF1%$_{DEC}$ (**Table 5**) despite the fact that the DUD-E ligand sets are much larger than the smaller but better curated DUD datasets (**Table 1**). For example, the EF1%$_{DEC}$ improvement of 2.1% (from 2.0 to 4.1%) with PR might seem minor at the first glance, but in terms of absolute compound numbers it is a marked uptick from the discovery of six to 13 actives over the original docking. The EF1%$_{DEC}$ (**Table 5**) was improved by the R-NiB substantially with the AR (1.5 vs. 13.0%), MR (3.2 vs. 11.7%) and NEU (4.1 vs. 13.3%). Although in the case of the RXRα the EF1%$_{DEC}$ values suggested that the docking scoring worked better than the R-NiB (**Table 5**), a close inspection of the semi-logarithmic ROC plot shows that the rescoring actually produced higher very early enrichment (EF0.5%$_{DEC}$ 6.1 vs. 3.8%; **Figure 3**). The EF5%$_{DEC}$ was improved

on average 1.3-fold for these targets (**Table 5**) and, for example, the GR (12.0 vs. 22.5%) received a 1.9-fold improvement.

Negative Image-Based Rescoring Is Both Ultrafast and Efficient

For the purpose of comparison, the original docking solutions were also re-evaluated using empirical rescoring algorithm XSCORE (Wang et al., 2002) and the PLP scoring function in PLANTS. Target-specific settings for ligand-receptor interactions such as hydrogen bonding or hydrophobicity are considered via multivariate analysis in XSCORE. Although the R-NiB generally produced better enrichment than XSCORE, the latter algorithm excelled with both the DUD and DUD-E datasets for the RXRα (**Tables 2–5**). The rescoring with the PLP function in PLANTS could only in some cases (e.g., COX2) improve the original ChemPLP-based ranking and, generally, the R-NiB produced substantially better results (**Tables 2–5**).

The use of non-default XSCORE settings could have produced higher early enrichment; however, similar fine-tuning of the R-NiB models or even PLANTS settings could likely have improved the enrichment as well. By adjusting the assortment of the cavity charge points capable of hydrogen bonding and/or lowering/increasing the weight of the electrostatics in

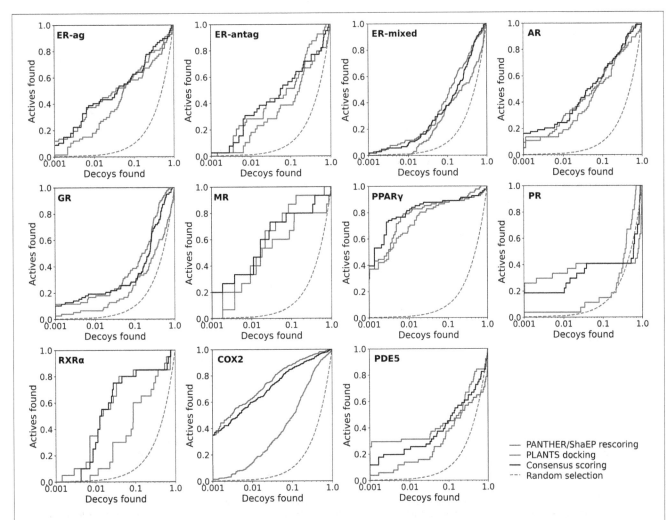

FIGURE 2 | The semi-logarithmic receiver operating characteristics plots for the docking and negative image-based rescoring with the DUD dataset. Only those R-NiB results with the highest early enrichment were plotted (EF1%$_{DEC}$ in **Table 5**). The red line shows the original docking enrichment by PLANTS, the blue line gives the result after PANTHER/ShaEP-based rescoring, and the black line gives the result from consensus scoring where both of them are given equal weight (50/50%). The dashed line outlines the random selection (AUC = 0.50). The semi-log10 scale is used only for the x axis to highlight the very early enrichment or lack thereof.

the similarity screening generally improves the enrichment. For example, in our test runs the R-NiB produced notably better early enrichment (EF1%$_{DEC}$ 12.2–23.0%) for the DUD set of the AR with the box radius option when only a few cavity points were added or removed instead of using the default NIB model (data not shown). In fact, one could even over-emphasize certain properties (e.g., charge) artificially in the NIB model to produce better enrichment in the rescoring than what the default settings would otherwise allow. Because this kind of rescoring bias does not alter the actual ligand poses, the preferred docking solutions remain within the realm of possible. The situation can be entirely different, if the original docking scoring function, affecting the ligand conformer sampling, is altered radically; i.e., unrealistic conformations could be put forward.

Excluding the time taken for the NIB model generation, the actual rescoring performed with ShaEP is computationally very inexpensive; spending only a fraction of the time required for

the initial docking. This is possible, because no ligand conformer sampling or even geometry optimization between the NIB model and docked ligand conformers is done. In fact, the ShaEP-based scoring with the DUD sets for the ER-agonist (1.94 ms/comp. vs. ∼24.4 ms/comp.), PDE5 (3.81 ms/comp. vs. ∼35.7 ms/comp.), and COX2 (2.43 ms/comp. vs. ∼54.0 ms/comp.) was at least 10 times faster than the XSCORE rescoring, which is already very fast. Similarly, rescoring with PLP function in PLANTS took roughly double the time with the ER-agonist (1.94 ms/comp. vs. ∼3.21 ms/comp.), PDE5 (3.81 ms/comp. vs. ∼7.15 ms/comp.), and COX2 (2.43 ms/comp. vs. ∼4.54 ms/comp.) datasets, when compared to the R-NiB. These benchmark numbers vary depending on the computer set-up. Here, the software were run using a single Intel Xeon CPU (W3670 3.2 GHz) and RAM 12 GB DDR 1333 MHz in a LINUX desktop. The absolute size of the NIB model and that of the compounds being rescored affect the R-NiB performance; however, the differences in the wall time are minor.

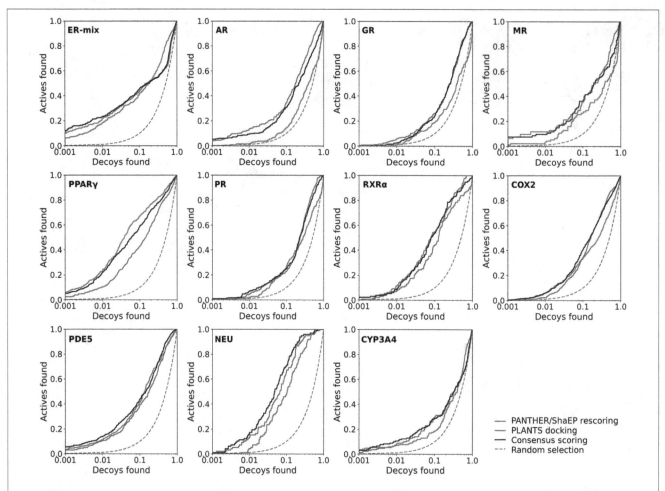

FIGURE 3 | The semi-logarithmic receiver operating characteristics plots for the docking and negative image-based rescoring with the DUD-E dataset. Only those R-NiB results with the highest very early enrichment were plotted (EF1%$_{DEC}$ in **Table 6**). With retinoid X receptor alpha (RXRα), the results are shown for the model (ligand exclusion of 2.0 Å; **Table 6**) producing the highest very early enrichment, which is visible in the plotted curve. For interpretation see **Figure 2**.

DISCUSSION

The negative image-based rescoring or the R-NiB is a truly novel way of rescoring docking solutions, because it does not rely on the use molecular mechanics force fields, empirical or knowledge-based descriptors in evaluating the favorability of the ligand binding. For example, the binding free energy is not considered in any shape or form during the rescoring. Although the selected atom charges and van der Waals radiuses affect the NIB model generation profoundly, the ShaEP-based rescoring itself is a simple matter of shape/electrostatics comparison. No force field-based sampling or even coordinate superimposition is needed. The NIB models can be trained for optimal effect using experimental ligand sets with the "trial-and-error" approach, but generally this is not needed.

Applicability of Negative Image-Based Rescoring

A NIB model can be built for virtually any target protein as long as there is a solid idea where the potential small-molecule binding

or initial docking should happen. The target pocket can be a well-defined and enclosed cavity (see CYP3A4 in **Figures 4A–D** and GR in **Figures 4E–H**), an opening on the protein surface (see NEU in **Figures 4I–L**), a sub-cavity, a groove or even a small dent on the protein surface (**Figure 4**). The R-NiB results with the benchmark sets confirm this hypothesis, because the method improves docking enrichment with a variety of different target proteins (**Tables 2–5**; **Figures 2, 3**) and, more importantly, with physically different kind of ligand-binding cavities (**Figure 4**). The enrichment values (**Tables 2–4**) and semi-logarithmic ROC curves (**Figures 2, 3**) show that the R-NiB (**Figure 1**) clearly improves the yield with a multitude of DUD-E datasets, including the nuclear receptors AR, GR, MR, and PR, but also with entirely different kind of target protein NEU.

Overall, the R-NiB results (**Tables 2–5**; **Figures 2, 3**) show that a satisfactory enrichment can be acquired in most cases by building NIB models by simply adjusting the cavity detection radius or by limiting the cavity search area using a receptor-bound ligand included in the PDB entry (**Figures 1, 4**). Having protrusions outside this cavity space do not necessarily worsen

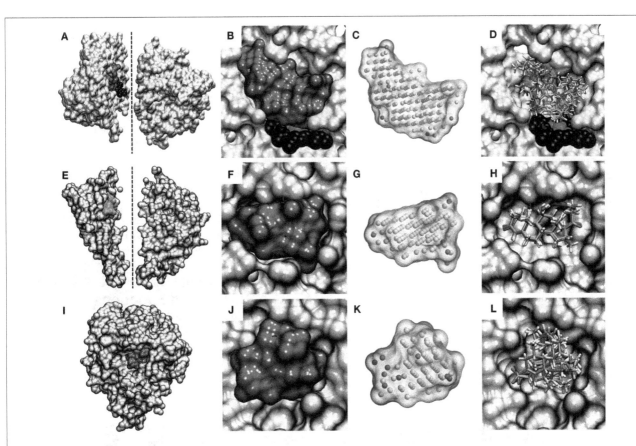

FIGURE 4 | The cavity-based NIB models and the docking solutions are aligned. The protein 3D structures of **(A)** cytochrome P450 3A4 (CYP3A4; lime; PDB: 3NXU) (Sevrioukova and Poulos, 2010), **(E)** glucocorticoid receptor (GR; white; PDB: 1M2Z) (Bledsoe et al., 2005) and **(I)** neuraminidase (NEU; yellow; PDB: 1B9V) (Finley et al., 1999) are shown as opaque surfaces on the far left. With CYP3A4 and GR, the X-ray crystal structures are shown in two sections to highlight the buried locations of their active sites (mauve opaque surfaces) at the center. The dotted lines indicate the cutting planes for the cross-sections chosen for the illustration. The prosthetic heme group is shown as a CPK model (black backbone) for CYP3A4. With NEU, the enzyme's active which opens directly from the protein surface, is only partially buried and, thus, no cross-sectioning was done. The contours of the active sites of **(B,C)** CYP3A4, **(F,G)** GR, and **(J,K)** NEU are shown both as opaque surfaces and finalized NIB models (transparent surfaces with charge potential) in the cross-section close-ups. The red, blue, and white dots in the NIB model indicate the negative, positive and neutral cavity dots (or filler atoms) constituting the negative image. The docked poses of five known active compounds (stick models with orange backbone) for **(D)** CYP3A4, **(H)** GR, and **(L)** NEU from PLANTS are shown stacked in the far right.

any ligand's similarity score a lot (a marginal penalty inflicted in the ShaEP scoring); however, it is important to understand that those ligand segments outside the cavity will be effectively ignored in the rescoring.

So, the emphasis of R-NiB is resolutely on the cavity's negative image (**Figure 4**) and it is recommended that unpractically large ligands for the cavity in question are filtered away before docking and/or rescoring. Essentially, docking sizable ligands with a lot of rotatable bonds (e.g., PPARγ datasets) or with particularly large cavities (e.g., PDE5) is likely to produce errors or difficult ascertain alternative poses that cannot be reliably rescored using the R-NiB. Despite this, in theory, the R-NiB could be used to rescore even docked peptides (not tested here) as long as their binding is dependent on the shape/electrostatics complementarity with the cavity. This narrow focus on the area designated by the NIB model for the ligand binding makes the R-NiB (**Figure 1**) truly a precision technique.

The downside of this narrow focus is that it also limits the usability of different benchmark test sets in evaluating the R-NiB (**Figure 1**). If the test set contains active compounds that bind into completely different or only partially connected ligand-binding sites in the target protein, the R-NiB cannot possibly rank all those ligands high up in the list using a single NIB model (**Figure 4**). Moreover, when dealing with large ligand-binding cavities such as the active site of PDE5, where inhibitors can have very different binding locations and poses, with very little overlap, and/or water molecules play a big role in coordinating the ligand binding, a single NIB model simply cannot provide all the necessary information needed for the enrichment. One can try to solve this issue by curating the ligand sets better, limiting the search radius for docking or by applying multiple NIB models to the task. Naturally, this level of focus is not a problem when working in an actual screening project, in which the efforts are centered on a specific binding site or subcavity.

Recognizing Biologically Relevant Ligand-Binding Poses

The R-NiB is not optimizing the ligand positioning inside the protein's ligand-binding pocket, but merely comparing the earlier produced docking poses against the cavity's shape/electrostatics (**Figure 1**). The highest scored poses for the active compounds might not differ from the original docking; however, the enrichment can improve due to lower ranking of the inactives by the R-NiB. In fact, improvement in the enrichment values is not an absolute guarantee that the "correct" conformers are discovered during the rescoring. With certain ligand-binding pockets and compounds it is very difficult to conclude what is the actual binding pose and there might even exist more than one valid pose (Mobley and Dill, 2009). One can attempt to address this issue by looking at the individual docking solutions, their exact binding interactions and, ultimately, compare them against the experimentally validated data for the same compound or its closely-related structural analogs (**Figure 5**). For example, the R-NiB seems to be able to recognize the biologically relevant binding pose of hydrocortisone with the MR whereas the original docking scoring fails (**Figure 5**).

Because the R-NiB can only reorder the docking solutions and if all of the ligand conformers are docked in a completely "wrong" way or even outside the ligand-binding pocket, the "correct" pose

or ligand cannot emerge on top of the results list. This is true for all rescoring methodologies as they mainly reshuffle existing solutions. To a certain extent, this is the case even for force field-based post-processing methodologies, because the initial ligand-receptor complex is crucial for the sampling as well. In certain cases even a partial shape/electrostatics match with the cavity-based NIB model can give the docked compound a substantially higher ranking and improve the enrichment. By docking the decoys mostly outside the binding cavity, one could also improve the enrichment as long as the actives reside at the site. Here, it was made sure that the docked compounds and the generated NIB models occupied roughly the same 3D space in relation to the protein. The match between the cavity space and the outputted docking solutions is highlighted for the CYP3A4 (**Figure 4C** vs. **Figure 4D**), GR (**Figure 4G** vs. **Figure 4H**), and NEU (**Figure 4K** vs. **Figure 4L**) in **Figure 4**.

Consensus Scoring—Finding the Balance Between the Scoring Functions

If the initial docking produced the "correct" or at least reasonable pose for the active compound but it was not favored by the docking software, in theory one should be able recognize it from the multiple outputted poses using a superior scoring method. In reality, all of the scoring methodologies excel on some targets and

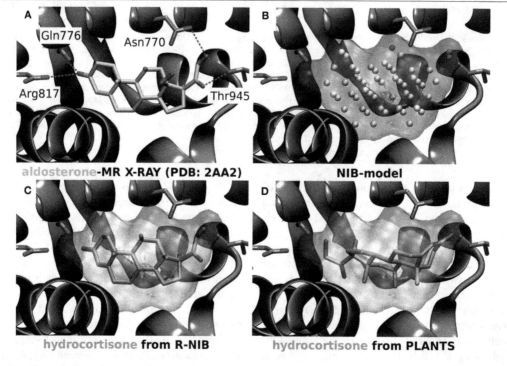

FIGURE 5 | A negative image-based rescoring example with mineralocorticoid receptor. **(A)** The X-ray crystal structure of mineralocorticoid receptor (MR; silver cartoon model; PDB: 2AA2) (Bledsoe et al., 2005) and the amino acid residues (stick models) making hydrogen bonds (magenta dotted lines) with the inhibitor aldosterone (stick model with cyan backbone) are shown. **(B)** The negative image or NIB model (transparent surface) of the MR active site was build using the same PDB entry (Bledsoe et al., 2005) and the 1.5 Å ligand distance limit option in PANTHER. The red and blue dots depict the negatively and positively charged cavity points, respectively, whereas the white dots are neutral. **(C)** The rescored pose (rank #13) of hydrocortisone (stick model with orange backbone) reminds closely the experimentally verified pose of its structural analog aldosterone (**A** vs. **C**). **(D)** Hence, the pose of hydrocortisone given the highest score by PLANTS (rank #17), showing a reversed pose in comparison to the aldosterone (**A** vs. **D**), is likely erroneous **(D)**.

TABLE 6 | The consensus scoring of the DUD Datasets.

Target protein			Optimal weight				Equal weight			
	ShaEP weight[a]	AUC	$EF1\%_{DEC}$	$\Delta EF1\%_{DEC}$[b]	$EF5\%_{DEC}$	$\Delta EF5\%_{DEC}$[b]	$EF1\%_{DEC}$	$\Delta EF1\%_{DEC}$[b]	$EF5\%_{DEC}$	$\Delta EF5\%_{DEC}$[b]
ER-agonist	0.70	0.81 ± 0.03 (↔)	41.8	4.5	56.7	4.5	40.3	3.0	53.7	1.5
ER-antagonist	0.55	0.78 ± 0.04 (↓)	35.9	7.7	43.6	0.0	35.9	7.7	43.6	0.0
ER-mixed	0.90	0.77 ± 0.03 (↑)	11.3	0.0	26.4	2.8	7.5	−3.8	29.2	5.6
AR	0.25	0.85 ± 0.03 (↑)	32.4	5.4	47.3	1.4	28.4	1.4	50.0	4.1
GR	0.60	0.76 ± 0.03 (↑)	19.2	2.5	26.9	−1.3	19.2	2.5	25.6	−2.6
MR	1.0	0.93 ± 0.05 (↑)	33.3	0.0	73.3	0.0	33.3	0.0	73.3	0.0
PPARγ	0.35	0.93 ± 0.02 (↓)	84.0	5.0	87.7	1.3	81.5	2.5	87.7	1.3
PR	0.60	0.53 ± 0.06 (↓)	33.3	0.0	40.7	0.0	22.2	−11.1	40.7	0.0
RXRα	1.0	0.89 ± 0.05 (↑)	35.0	0.0	80.0	0.0	25.0	−10.0	80.0	0.0
COX2	0.80	0.95 ± 0.01 (↑)	65.2	2.6	82.8	−0.2	59.8	−2.8	77.6	−5.4
PDE5	0.85	0.64 ± 0.04 (↓)	31.4	0.0	43.1	3.8	23.5	−7.9	33.3	−5.9

*The NIB model producing the highest EF1%$_{DEC}$ (**Table 4**) was used in the consensus scoring with PLANTS. When optimal and equal (50/50%) weight is used, all datasets produced better EF1%$_{DEC}$ and EF5%$_{DEC}$ enrichments than the docking.*
[a] If the ShaEP weight is 1.0, the consensus score comes entirely from ShaEP rescoring, and, vice versa, if the weight is 0, only the PLANTS score is used. The value of 0.50 corresponds to the situation in which PLANTS docking and ShaEP rescoring effect have equal weight in the results. Both the ShaEP and PLANTS scores were normalized to fit the scale from 0 to 1 before combining them. The consensus scoring was not done to acquire the best AUC enrichment possible and, accordingly, upon a rare occasion the value could decrease (downward arrow) instead improving it (upward arrow).
[b] ΔEF%$_{DEC}$ corresponds to the EF%$_{DEC}$ difference between the consensus scoring and the original ShaEP rescoring of the same NIB-model.

TABLE 7 | The consensus scoring of the DUD-E datasets.

Target protein			Optimal weight				Equal weight			
	ShaEP weight	AUC	$EF 1\%_{DEC}$	$\Delta EF1\%_{DEC}$	$EF5\%_{DEC}$	$\Delta EF5\%_{DEC}$	$EF1\%_{DEC}$	$\Delta EF1\%_{DEC}$	$EF5\%_{DEC}$	$\Delta EF5\%_{DEC}$
ER-mixed	0.35	0.69 ± 0.02 (↓)	24.5	6.2	37.9	5.3	23.0	4.7	36.8	4.2
AR	1.0	0.76 ± 0.02 (↑)	13.0	0.0	23.0	0.0	9.3	−3.7	19.0	−4.0
GR	1.0	0.70 ± 0.02 (↑)	5.8	0.0	17.4	0.0	2.3	−3.5	16.7	−0.7
MR	1.0	0.70 ± 0.03 (↑)	11.7	0.0	25.5	0.0	9.6	−2.1	21.3	−4.2
PPARγ	0.20	0.85 ± 0.01 (↔)	27.7	17.4	58.1	25.7	21.9	11.2	46.7	14.3
PR	0.55	0.72 ± 0.02 (↑)	6.8	2.4	18.4	1.3	6.8	2.4	18.1	1.3
RXRa	0.25	0.82 ± 0.02 (↑)	19.1	8.4	46.6	22.7	14.5	3.8	29.0	5.1
COX2	0.10	0.69 ± 0.01 (↑)	7.6	5.3	25.5	6.4	6.0	3.7	23.4	4.3
PDE5	0.25	0.82 ± 0.01 (↑)	17.6	7.0	36.4	10.5	13.8	3.2	31.7	5.8
NEU	0.50	0.91 ± 0.02 (↑)	16.3	3.0	52.0	9.1	16.3	3.0	52.0	9.1
CYP3A4	0.50	0.61 ± 0.02 (↔)	10.6	3.0	21.2	2.4	10.6	3.0	21.2	2.4

*The NIB model producing the highest EF1%$_{DEC}$ (**Table 5**) was used in the consensus scoring with PLANTS. When optimal weight is used, all datasets produced better EF1%$_{DEC}$ and EF5%$_{DEC}$ enrichments than the docking. In the case of equal (50/50%) weight, only the PPARγ dataset produced weaker early enrichment than the original docking. See **Table 6** for further details.*

ligand sets for different and sometimes even conflicting reasons. Because both the original docking software PLANTS (Korb et al., 2009) and the similarity comparison algorithm ShaEP (Vainio et al., 2009) output their own scores for each ligand conformer, it is possible to normalize and combine the results and adjust their relative weight with different targets (**Tables 6, 7**).

This score weighting or consensus scoring (**Tables 6, 7**) was performed to determine, if the ranking benefitted more from either of the scoring functions and if there is a generally applicable weight ratio that could be routinely used. Because the emphasis in the consensus scoring was put on the EF1%$_{DEC}$ improvement, the AUC values of the DUD datasets were

not necessarily improved (e.g., PPARγ; **Table 2** vs. **Table 6**). Similarly, with the ER-mixed, plagued also by the dualistic nature of the included agonist/antagonist ligands, the AUC values were not improved for the DUD-E (**Table 3** vs. **Table 7**). Moreover, focusing on the early enrichment indicates that the consensus scoring worked almost without an exception better than the docking for both the DUD (**Table 4** vs. **Table 6**) and DUD-E datasets (**Table 5** vs. **Table 7**). Even a relatively tiny push by the R-NiB (e.g., 10–35% weight from ShaEP) was enough to help the early enrichment (**Tables 6, 7**).

Dealing with a completely new target protein cavity or heterogeneous ligand set is likely to require re-weighting and careful optimization upon the arrival of experimental results. Despite this, the yield was in most cases improved by simply giving both scoring functions an equal weight in the consensus scoring (**Tables 6, 7**) instead of using the default PLANTS scoring or the R-NiB alone (**Tables 4, 5**). With the DUD datasets, the equal weight consensus scoring produced always better early enrichment than the docking, but the non-weighted R-NiB could sometimes work slightly better (see the negative ΔEF values in **Table 6**; **Figure 2**). Similarly, the equal weighting produced better early enrichment than docking scoring alone with the DUD-E datasets; however, the yield for the PPARγ did not benefit from this arrangement. Regardless, with a multitude of targets, the non-weighted R-NiB produced higher early enrichment than the equal weight consensus scoring (see the negative ΔEF values in **Table 7**; **Figure 3**).

Although the equal weighting in the consensus scoring could reduce the early enrichment marginally in certain cases, the tradeoff was that in general it produced better early enrichment; making it a viable option for future docking screening experiments.

CONCLUSIONS

This study demonstrates that by simply focusing on the shape/electrostatics complementarity between the ligand and the receptor protein's binding cavity, the docking performance regarding the early enrichment can be improved across the board. The rescoring is done by generating a negative image of the protein's ligand-binding cavity that is then used directly in the similarity comparison of the docking solutions (**Figure 1**). The results show that the negative image-based rescoring (or the R-NiB) can enhance the success-rate of docking screenings to a level that facilitates effective drug discovery. Moreover, the R-NiB can be used in unison with other docking scoring functions in consensus scoring to improve the early enrichment yet further.

AUTHOR CONTRIBUTIONS

STK performed the docking and rescoring assays with the assistance from SN and MA. PAP wrote the manuscript with the help from the co-authors. OTP and PAP designed the experiments based on the original concept by OTP and SL. PAP supervised the study.

ACKNOWLEDGMENTS

The Finnish IT Center for Science (CSC) is acknowledged for generous computational resources (OTP; Project Nos. jyy2516 and jyy2585).

REFERENCES

Bash, P. A., Field, M. J., and Karplus, M. (1987). Free energy perturbation method for chemical reactions in the condensed phase: a dynamic approach based on a combined quantum and molecular mechanics potential. *J. Am. Chem. Soc.* 109, 8092–8094. doi: 10.1021/ja00260a028

Berman, H. M., Westbrook, J., Feng, Z., Gilliland, G., Bhat, T. N., Weissig, H., et al. (2000). The protein data bank. *Nucleic Acids Res.* 28, 235–242. doi: 10.1093/nar/28.1.235

Bledsoe, R. K., Madauss, K. P., Holt, J. A., Apolito, C. J., Lambert, M. H., Pearce, K. H., et al. (2005). A ligand-mediated hydrogen bond network required for the activation of the mineralocorticoid receptor. *J. Biol. Chem.* 280, 31283–31293. doi: 10.1074/jbc.M504098200

Burley, S. K., Berman, H. M., Kleywegt, G. J., Markley, J. L., Nakamura, H., and Velankar, S. (2017). Protein Data Bank (PDB): the single global macromolecular structure archive. *Methods Mol. Biol.* 1607, 627–641. doi: 10.1007/978-1-4939-7000-1_26

Charifson, P. S., Corkery, J. J., Murcko, M. A., and Walters, W. P. (1999). Consensus scoring: a method for obtaining improved hit rates from docking databases of three-dimensional structures into proteins. *J. Med. Chem.* 42, 5100–5109. doi: 10.1021/jm990352k

Chen, H., Lyne, P. D., Giordanetto, F., Lovell, T., and Li, J. (2006). On evaluating molecular-docking methods for pose prediction and enrichment factors. *J. Chem. Inf. Model.* 46, 401–415. doi: 10.1021/ci0503255

Cheng, T., Li, X., Li, Y., Liu, Z., and Wang, R. (2009). Comparative assessment of Sscoring functions on a diverse test set. *J. Chem. Inf. Model.* 49, 1079–1093. doi: 10.1021/ci9000053

Clark, R. D., Strizhev, A., Leonard, J. M., Blake, J. F., and Matthew, J. B. (2002). Consensus scoring for ligand/protein interactions. *J. Mol. Graph. Model.* 20, 281–295. doi: 10.1016/S1093-3263(01)00125-5

Cross, J. B., Thompson, D. C., Rai, B. K., Baber, J. C., Fan, K. Y., Hu, Y., et al. (2009). Comparison of several molecular docking programs: pose prediction and virtual screening accuracy. *J. Chem. Inf. Model.* 49, 1455–1474. doi: 10.1021/ci900056c

Ferrara, P., Gohlke, H., Price, D. J., Klebe, G., and Brooks, C. L. (2004). Assessing scoring functions for protein-ligand interactions. *J. Med. Chem.* 47, 3032–3047. doi: 10.1021/jm030489h

Finley, J. B., Atigadda, V. R., Duarte, F., Zhao, J. J., Brouillette, W. J., Air, G. M., et al. (1999). Novel aromatic inhibitors of influenza virus neuraminidase make selective interactions with conserved residues and water molecules in the active site. *J. Mol. Biol.* 293, 1107–1119. doi: 10.1006/jmbi.1999.3180

Genheden, S., and Ryde, U. (2015). The MM/PBSA and MM/GBSA methods to estimate ligand-binding affinities. *Expert Opin. Drug Discov.* 10, 449–461. doi: 10.1517/17460441.2015.1032936

Guimarães, C. R., and Cardozo, M. (2008). MM-GB/SA rescoring of docking poses in structure-based lead optimization. *J. Chem. Inf. Model.* 48, 958–970. doi: 10.1021/ci800004w

Hanley, A. J., and McNeil, J. B. (1982). The meaning and use of the area under a Receiver Operating Characteristic (ROC) Curve. *Radiology* 143, 29–36. doi: 10.1148/radiology.143.1.7063747

Houston, D. R., and Walkinshaw, M. D. (2013). Consensus docking: improving the reliability of docking in a virtual screening context. *J. Chem. Inf. Model.* 53, 384–390. doi: 10.1021/ci300399w

Huang, N., Shoichet, B. K., and Irwin, J. J. (2006). Benchmarking sets for molecular docking. *J. Med. Chem.* 49, 6789–6801. doi: 10.1021/jm0608356

Humphrey, W., Dalke, A., and Schulten, K. (1996). VMD: visual molecular dynamics. *J. Mol. Graph.* 14, 33–38, 27–28. doi: 10.1016/0263-7855(96)00018-5

Juvonen, R. O., Kuusisto, M., Fohrgrup, C., Pitkänen, M. H., Nevalainen, T. J., Auriola, S., et al. (2016). Inhibitory effects and oxidation of 6-methylcoumarin, 7-methylcoumarin and 7-formylcoumarin *via* human

CYP2A6 and its mouse and pig orthologous enzymes. *Xenobiotica* 46, 14–24. doi: 10.3109/00498254.2015.1048327

Kitchen, D. B., Decornez, H., Furr, J. R., and Bajorath, J. (2004). Docking and scoring in virtual screening for drug discovery: methods and applications. *Nat. Rev. Drug Discov.* 3, 935–949. doi: 10.1038/nrd1549

Kolb, P., and Irwin, J. (2009). Docking screens: right for the right reasons? *Curr. Top. Med. Chem.* 9, 755–770. doi: 10.2174/156802609789207091

Kollman, P. A., Massova, I., Reyes, C., Kuhn, B., Huo, S., Chong, L., et al. (2000). Calculating structures and free energies of complex molecules: combining molecular mechanics and continuum models. *Acc. Chem. Res.* 33, 889–897. doi: 10.1021/ar000033j

Korb, O., Stützle, T., and Exner, T. E. (2009). Empirical scoring functions for advanced protein-ligand docking with PLANTS. *J. Chem. Inf. Model.* 49, 84–96. doi: 10.1021/ci800298z

Kraulis, P. J. (1991). MOLSCRIPT: a program to produce both detailed and schematic plots of protein structures. *J. Appl. Crystallogr.* 24, 946–950. doi: 10.1107/S0021889891004399

Lätti, S., Niinivehmas, S., and Pentikäinen, O. T. (2016). Rocker: open source, easy-to-use tool for AUC and enrichment calculations and ROC visualization. *J. Cheminform.* 8, 1–5. doi: 10.1186/s13321-016-0158-y

Lehtonen, J. V., Still, D.-J., Rantanen, V.-V., Ekholm, J., Björklund, D., Iftikhar, Z., et al. (2004). BODIL: a molecular modeling environment for structure-function analysis and drug design. *J. Comput. Aided. Mol. Des.* 18, 401–19. doi: 10.1007/s10822-004-3752-4

McGaughey, G. B., Sheridan, R. P., Bayly, C. I., Culberson, J. C., Kreatsoulas, C., Lindsley, S., et al. (2007). Comparison of topological, shape, and docking methods in virtual screening. *J. Chem. Inf. Model.* 47, 1504–1519. doi: 10.1021/ci700052x

Meng, X.-Y., Zhang, H.-X., Mezei, M., and Cui, M. (2011). Molecular docking: a powerful approach for structure-based drug discovery. *Curr. Comput. Aided. Drug Des.* 7, 146–157. doi: 10.2174/157340911795677602

Merritt, E. A., and Murphy, M. E. (1994). Raster3D Version 2.0. A program for photorealistic molecular graphics. *Acta Crystallogr. Sect. D Biol. Crystallogr.* 50, 869–873. doi: 10.1107/S0907444994006396

Mobley, D. L., and Dill, K. A. (2009). Binding of small-molecule ligands to proteins: "What You See" is not Always "What You Get." *Structure* 17, 489–498. doi: 10.1016/j.str.2009.02.010

Mohan, V., Gibbs, A. C., Cummings, M. D., Jaeger, E. P., and Renee, L. (2005). Docking : successes and challenges. *Curr. Pharm. Des.* 11, 323–333. doi: 10.2174/1381612053382106

Mysinger, M. M., Carchia, M., Irwin, J. J., and Shoichet, B. K. (2012). Directory of useful decoys, enhanced (DUD-E): Better ligands and decoys for better benchmarking. *J. Med. Chem.* 55, 6582–6594. doi: 10.1021/jm300687e

Naïm, M., Bhat, S., Rankin, K. N., Dennis, S., Chowdhury, S. F., Siddiqi, I., et al. (2007). Solvated Interaction Energy (SIE) for scoring protein-ligand binding affinities. 1. Exploring the parameter space. *J. Chem. Inf. Model.* 47, 122–133. doi: 10.1021/ci600406v

Niinivehmas, S. P., Salokas, K., Lätti, S., Raunio, H., and Pentikäinen, O. T. (2015). Ultrafast protein structure-based virtual screening with Panther. *J. Comput. Aided. Mol. Des.* 29, 989–1006. doi: 10.1007/s10822-015-9870-3

Niinivehmas, S. P., Virtanen, S. I., Lehtonen, J. V., Postila, P. A., and Pentikäinen, O. T. (2011). Comparison of virtual high-throughput screening methods for the identification of phosphodiesterase-5 inhibitors. *J. Chem. Inf. Model.* 51, 1353–1363. doi: 10.1021/ci1004527

Oda, A., Tsuchida, K., Takakura, T., Yamaotsu, N., and Hirono, S. (2006). Comparison of consensus scoring strategies for evaluating computational models of protein-ligand complexes. *J. Chem. Inf. Model.* 46, 380–391. doi: 10.1021/ci050283k

Onufriev, A., Bashford, D., and Case, D. A. (2004). Exploring protein native states and large-scale conformational changes with a modified generalized born model. *Proteins Struct. Funct. Genet.* 55, 383–394. doi: 10.1002/prot.20033

Pagadala, N. S., Syed, K., and Tuszynski, J. (2017). Software for molecular docking: a review. *Biophys. Rev.* 9, 91–102. doi: 10.1007/s12551-016-0247-1

Plewczynski, D., Łazniewski, M., Augustyniak, R., and Ginalski, K. (2011). Can we trust docking results? evaluation of seven commonly used programs on PDBbind database. *J. Comput. Chem.* 32, 742–755. doi: 10.1002/jcc.21643

Sastry, M. G., Adzhigirey, M., Day, T., Annabhimoju, R., and Sherman, W. (2013). Protein and ligand preparation: parameters, protocols, and influence

on virtual screening enrichments. *J. Comput. Aided. Mol. Des.* 27, 221–234. doi: 10.1007/s10822-013-9644-8

Schapira, M., Abagyan, R., and Totrov, M. (2003). Nuclear hormone receptor targeted virtual screening. *J. Med. Chem.* 46, 3045–3059. doi: 10.1021/jm0300173

Sevrioukova, I. F., and Poulos, T. L. (2010). Structure and mechanism of the complex between cytochrome P4503A4 and ritonavir. *Proc. Natl. Acad. Sci.U.S.A.* 107, 18422–18427. doi: 10.1073/pnas.1010693107

Sousa, S. F., Fernandes, P. A., and Ramos, M. J. (2006). Protein-ligand docking: Current status and future challenges. *Proteins Struct. Funct. Bioinforma.* 65, 15–26. doi: 10.1002/prot.21082

Sulea, T., Cui, Q., and Purisima, E. O. (2011). Solvated interaction energy (SIE) for scoring protein-ligand binding affinities. 2. benchmark in the CSAR-2010 scoring exercise. *J. Chem. Inf. Model.* 51, 2066–2081. doi: 10.1021/ci2000242

Sulea, T., Hogues, H., and Purisima, E. O. (2012). Exhaustive search and solvated interaction energy (SIE) for virtual screening and affinity prediction. *J. Comput. Aided. Mol. Des.* 26, 617–633. doi: 10.1007/s10822-011-9529-7

Vainio, M. J., and Johnson, M. S. (2007). Generating conformer ensembles using a multiobjective genetic algorithm. *J. Chem. Inf. Model.* 47, 2462–2474. doi: 10.1021/ci6005646

Vainio, M. J., Puranen, J. S., and Johnson, M. S. (2009). ShaEP: Molecular overlay based on shape and electrostatic potential. *J. Chem. Inf. Model.* 49, 492–502. doi: 10.1021/ci800315d

Virtanen, S. I., Niinivehmas, S. P., and Pentikäinen, O. T. (2015). Case-specific performance of MM-PBSA, MM-GBSA, and SIE in virtual screening. *J. Mol. Graph. Model.* 62, 303–318. doi: 10.1016/j.jmgm.2015.10.012

Virtanen, S. I., and Pentikäinen, O. T. (2010). Efficient virtual screening using multiple protein conformations described as negative images of the ligand-binding site. *J. Chem. Inf. Model.* 50, 1005–1011. doi: 10.1021/ci100121c

Wang, R., Lai, L., and Wang, S. (2002). Further development and validation of empirical scoring functions for structure-based binding affinity prediction. *J. Comput. Aided. Mol. Des.* 16, 11–26. doi: 10.1023/A:1016357811882

Wang, R., Lu, Y., and Wang, S. (2003). Comparative evaluation of 11 scoring functions for molecular docking. *J. Med. Chem.* 46, 2287–2303. doi: 10.1021/jm0203783

Warren, G. L., Andrews, C. W., Capelli, A. M., Clarke, B., LaLonde, J., Lambert, M. H., et al. (2006). A critical assessment of docking programs and scoring functions. *J. Med. Chem.* 49, 5912–5931. doi: 10.1021/jm050362n

Word, J. M., Lovell, S. C., Richardson, J. S., and Richardson, D. C. (1999). Asparagine and glutamine: using hydrogen atom contacts in the choice of side-chain amide orientation. *J. Mol. Biol.* 285, 1735–1747. doi: 10.1006/jmbi.1998.2401

Zoete, V., Schuepbach, T., Bovigny, C., Chaskar, P., Daina, A., Röhrig, U. F., et al. (2016). Attracting cavities for docking. Replacing the rough energy landscape of the protein by a smooth attracting landscape. *J. Comput. Chem.* 37, 437–447. doi: 10.1002/jcc.24249

Permissions

All chapters in this book were first published by Frontiers; hereby published with permission under the Creative Commons Attribution License or equivalent. Every chapter published in this book has been scrutinized by our experts. Their significance has been extensively debated. The topics covered herein carry significant findings which will fuel the growth of the discipline. They may even be implemented as practical applications or may be referred to as a beginning point for another development.

The contributors of this book come from diverse backgrounds, making this book a truly international effort. This book will bring forth new frontiers with its revolutionizing research information and detailed analysis of the nascent developments around the world.

We would like to thank all the contributing authors for lending their expertise to make the book truly unique. They have played a crucial role in the development of this book. Without their invaluable contributions this book wouldn't have been possible. They have made vital efforts to compile up to date information on the varied aspects of this subject to make this book a valuable addition to the collection of many professionals and students.

This book was conceptualized with the vision of imparting up-to-date information and advanced data in this field. To ensure the same, a matchless editorial board was set up. Every individual on the board went through rigorous rounds of assessment to prove their worth. After which they invested a large part of their time researching and compiling the most relevant data for our readers.

The editorial board has been involved in producing this book since its inception. They have spent rigorous hours researching and exploring the diverse topics which have resulted in the successful publishing of this book. They have passed on their knowledge of decades through this book. To expedite this challenging task, the publisher supported the team at every step. A small team of assistant editors was also appointed to further simplify the editing procedure and attain best results for the readers.

Apart from the editorial board, the designing team has also invested a significant amount of their time in understanding the subject and creating the most relevant covers. They scrutinized every image to scout for the most suitable representation of the subject and create an appropriate cover for the book.

The publishing team has been an ardent support to the editorial, designing and production team. Their endless efforts to recruit the best for this project, has resulted in the accomplishment of this book. They are a veteran in the field of academics and their pool of knowledge is as vast as their experience in printing. Their expertise and guidance has proved useful at every step. Their uncompromising quality standards have made this book an exceptional effort. Their encouragement from time to time has been an inspiration for everyone.

The publisher and the editorial board hope that this book will prove to be a valuable piece of knowledge for researchers, students, practitioners and scholars across the globe.

List of Contributors

Leonardo L. G. Ferreira and Adriano D. Andricopulo
Laboratory of Medicinal and Computational Chemistry, Center for Research and Innovation in Biodiversity and Drug Discovery, São Carlos Institute of Physics, University of São Paulo, São Carlos, Brazil

Tamir Dingjan and Elizabeth Yuriev
Medicinal Chemistry, Monash Institute of Pharmaceutical Sciences, Monash University, Melbourne, VIC, Australia

Anne Imberty
Centre de Recherches sur les Macromolécules Végétales, Centre National de la Recherche Scientifique UPR5301, Université Grenoble Alpes, Grenoble, France

Serge Pérez
Département de Pharmacochimie Moléculaire, Centre National de la Recherche Scientifique, UMR5063, Université Grenoble Alpes, Grenoble, France

Paul A. Ramsland
School of Science, RMIT University, Melbourne, VIC, Australia
Department of Surgery Austin Health, University of Melbourne, Melbourne, VIC, Australia
Department of Immunology, Central Clinical School, Monash University, Melbourne, VIC, Australia
Burnet Institute, Melbourne, VIC, Australia

Veronica Salmaso and Stefano Moro
Molecular Modeling Section, Department of Pharmaceutical and Pharmacological Sciences, University of Padova, Padova, Italy

Yuwei Wang, Huanling Lai, Xingxing Fan, Lianxiang Luo, Fugang Duan, Zebo Jiang, Qianqian Wang, Liang Liu and Xiaojun Yao
State Key Laboratory of Quality Research in Chinese Medicine, Macau University of Science and Technology, Macau, China

Marcelo D. Polêto and Hugo Verli
Grupo de Bioinformática Estrutural, Centro de Biotecnologia, Universidade Federal do Rio Grande do Sul, Porto Alegre, Brazil

Victor H. Rusu
Swiss National Supercomputing Centre, Lugano, Switzerland

Bruno I. Grisci and Marcio Dorn
Instituto de Informática, Universidade Federal do Rio Grande do Sul, Porto Alegre, Brazil

Roberto D. Lins
Instituto Aggeu Magalhães, Fundação Oswaldo Cruz, Recife, Brazil

Qianqian Wang, Jiahui Xu, Ying Li, Jumin Huang, Zebo Jiang, Yuwei Wang and Liang Liu
State Key Laboratory of Quality Research in Chinese Medicine, Macau Institute for Applied Research in Medicine and Health, Macau University of Science and Technology, Taipa, Macau

Elaine Lai Han Leung
State Key Laboratory of Quality Research in Chinese Medicine, Macau Institute for Applied Research in Medicine and Health, Macau University of Science and Technology, Taipa, Macau
State Key Laboratory of Respiratory Diseases, Guangzhou Institute of Respiratory Disease, The First Affiliated Hospital of Guangzhou Medical College, Guangzhou, China
Department of Respiratory Medicine, Taihe Hospital, Hubei University of Medicine, Hubei, China

Xiaojun Yao
State Key Laboratory of Quality Research in Chinese Medicine, Macau Institute for Applied Research in Medicine and Health, Macau University of Science and Technology, Taipa, Macau
State Key Laboratory of Applied Organic Chemistry, Department of Chemistry, Lanzhou University, Lanzhou, China

Elaine Lai Han Leung
State Key Laboratory of Quality Research in Chinese Medicine, Macau University of Science and Technology, Macau, China
Department of Thoracic Surgery, Guangzhou Institute of Respiratory Health and State Key Laboratory of Respiratory Disease, The First Affiliated Hospital of Guangzhou Medical University, Guangzhou, China
Respiratory Medicine Department Taihe Hospital, Hubei University of Medicine, Hubei, China

Kiminori Hori and Natsuko Goda
Laboratory of Structural Molecular Pharmacology, Graduate School of Pharmaceutical Sciences, Nagoya University, Nagoya, Japan

Kasumi Ajioka
Department of Biological Science, School of Science, Nagoya University, Nagoya, Japan

Asako Shindo
Division of Biological Science, Graduate School of Science, Nagoya University, Nagoya, Japan

Maki Takagishi
Department of Pathology, Graduate School of Medicine, Nagoya University, Nagoya, Japan

Takeshi Tenno
Laboratory of Structural Molecular Pharmacology, Graduate School of Pharmaceutical Sciences, Nagoya University, Nagoya, Japan
BeCellBar LLC, Business Incubation Center, Nagoya University, Nagoya, Japan

Hidekazu Hiroaki
Laboratory of Structural Molecular Pharmacology, Graduate School of Pharmaceutical Sciences, Nagoya University, Nagoya, Japan
Department of Biological Science, School of Science, Nagoya University, Nagoya, Japan
BeCellBar LLC, Business Incubation Center, Nagoya University, Nagoya, Japan

Manuel Pastor, Jordi Quintana and Ferran Sanz
Research Programme on Biomedical Informatics (GRIB), Institut Hospital del Mar d'Investigacions Mèdiques (IMIM), Department of Experimental and Health Sciences, Universitat Pompeu Fabra, Barcelona, Spain

Sugunadevi Sakkiah, Bohu Pan, Wenjing Guo, Weigong Ge, Weida Tong and Huixiao Hong
Division of Bioinformatics and Biostatistics, National Center for Toxicological Research, U.S. Food and Drug Administration, Jefferson, AR, United States

Rebecca Kusko
Immuneering Corporation, Cambridge, MA, United States

Samuel Lampa, Jonathan Alvarsson, Staffan Arvidsson Mc Shane, Arvid Berg and Ola Spjuth
Pharmaceutical Bioinformatics Group, Department of Pharmaceutical Biosciences, Uppsala University, Uppsala, Sweden

Ernst Ahlberg
Predictive Compound ADME and Safety, Drug Safety and Metabolism, AstraZeneca IMED Biotech Unit, Mölndal, Sweden

Hector E. Sanchez-Ibarra, Luisa M. Reyes-Cortes, Claudia M. Luna-Aguirre, Dionicio Aguirre-Trevino and Ivan A. Morales-Alvarado
Molecular Genetics Laboratory, Vitagénesis, S.A. de C.V., Monterrey, Mexico

Xian-Li Jiang
Evolutionary Information Laboratory,Department of Biological Sciences, University of Texas at Dallas, Richardson, TX, United States

Rafael B. Leon-Cachon
Departamento de Ciencias Básicas, Centro de Diagnóstico Molecular y Medicina Personalizada, Vicerrectoría de Ciencias de la Salud, Universidad de Monterrey, Monterrey, Mexico

Fernando Lavalle-Gonzale
Servicio de Endocrinología, Hospital Universitario Dr. José E. González, Universidad Autónoma de Nuevo León, Monterrey, Mexico

Faruck Morcos
Center for Systems Biology, University of Texas at Dallas, Richardson, TX, United States
Evolutionary Information Laboratory, Department of Biological Sciences, University of Texas at Dallas, Richardson, TX, United States

Hugo A. Barrera-Saldaña
Molecular Genetics Laboratory, Vitagénesis, S.A. de C.V., Monterrey, Mexico
Tecnológico de Monterrey, Monterrey, Mexico

Isabella A. Guedes, Felipe S. S. Pereira and Laurent E. Dardenne
Grupo de Modelagem Molecular em Sistemas Biológicos, Laboratório Nacional de Computação Científica, Petrópolis, Brazil

Richard P. I. Lewis and Andreas Bender
Department of Chemistry, Centre for Molecular Informatics, University of Cambridge, Cambridge, United Kingdom

Daniel J. Mason
Department of Chemistry, Centre for Molecular Informatics, University of Cambridge, Cambridge, United Kingdom
Healx Ltd., Cambridge, United Kingdom

Richard T. Eastman and Rajarshi Guha
Division of Preclinical Innovation, National Center for Advancing Translational Sciences, National Institutes of Health, Rockville, MD, United States

Ian P. Stott
Unilever Research and Development, Wirral, United Kingdom

Stefania Monteleone, Julian E. Fuchs and Klaus R. Liedl
Institute of General, Inorganic and Theoretical Chemistry, Center of Molecular Biosciences, University of Innsbruck, Innsbruck, Austria

Georgia Melagraki
Hellenic Military Academy, Vari, Greece

Evangelos Ntougkos
Division of Immunology, Biomedical Sciences Research Center "Alexander Fleming," Vari, Greece

George Kollias and Dimitra Papadopoulou
Division of Immunology, Biomedical Sciences Research Center "Alexander Fleming," Vari, Greece
Department of Experimental Physiology, Medical School, National and Kapodistrian University of Athens, Athens, Greece

Vagelis Rinotas and Eleni Douni
Division of Immunology, Biomedical Sciences Research Center "Alexander Fleming," Vari, Greece
Department of Biotechnology, Agricultural University of Athens, Athens, Greece

Sen-Bao Lu
Department of Bioengineering, Santa Clara University, Santa Clara, CA, United States

Antreas Afantitis
Division of Immunology, Biomedical Sciences Research Center "Alexander Fleming," Vari, Greece
NovaMechanics Ltd., Nicosia, Cyprus

Rodolpho C. Braga, Cleber C. Melo-Filho, José Teófilo Moreira-Filho and Carolina Horta Andrade
LabMol – Laboratory for Molecular Modeling and Drug Design, Faculdade de Farmácia, Universidade Federal de Goiás, Goiânia, Brazil

Bruno J. Neves
LabMol – Laboratory for Molecular Modeling and Drug Design, Faculdade de Farmácia, Universidade Federal de Goiás, Goiânia, Brazil
Laboratory of Cheminformatics, Centro Universitário de Anápolis (UniEVANGÉLICA), Anápolis, Brazil

Eugene N. Muratov
Laboratory for Molecular Modeling, Division of Chemical Biology and Medicinal Chemistry, Eshelman School of Pharmacy, University of North Carolina at Chapel Hill, Chapel Hill, NC, United States
Department of Chemical Technology, Odessa National Polytechnic University, Odessa, Ukraine

Shan Wang, Yu Tian, Jing-Yi Zhang, Ping Zhou, Min Wang, Gui-Bo Sun, Xu-Dong Xu, Yun Luo and Xiao-Bo Sun
Beijing Key Laboratory of Innovative Drug Discovery of Traditional Chinese Medicine (Natural Medicine) and Translational Medicine, Institute of Medicinal Plant Development, Chinese Academy of Medical Sciences & Peking Union Medical College, Beijing, China

Hui-Bo Xu
Academy of Chinese Medical Sciences of Jilin Province, Changchun, China

Georgios Leonis
NovaMechanics Ltd., Nicosia, Cyprus

Min Wang
Life and Enviromental Science Research Center, Harbin University of Commerce, Harbin, China

Sami T. Kurkinen, Sanna Niinivehmas, Mira Ahinko, Sakari Lätti and Pekka A. Postila
Department of Biological and Environmental Science and Nanoscience Center, University of Jyvaskyla, Jyväskylä, Finland

Olli T. Pentikäinen
Department of Biological and Environmental Science and Nanoscience Center, University of Jyvaskyla, Jyväskylä, Finland
Institute of Biomedicine, Integrative Physiology and Pharmacy, University of Turku, Turku, Finland

Index

A

Activation Loop, 181

Adverse Drug Reactions, 118, 168

Amastigotes, 5-9

Androgen Receptor, 104, 114-116, 220, 223

Antibiotics, 13, 48, 87, 167, 172-173

Antileishmanial Activity, 4-8, 10

Antimalarial Properties, 167-168

Antiparasitic Activity, 6, 8-9

B

Bicalutamide, 104-116

Binding Affinity Prediction, 141, 145, 148, 153, 155-156, 158, 231

Bioavailability, 5, 8, 93

C

Cancer Stem Cells, 82, 94

Cell Apoptosis, 44, 46-47, 207-208, 210, 215-216

Cell Culture, 48, 73, 204, 206

Cell Migration, 44, 46

Cell Viability Assay, 206

Central Nervous System, 165

Cheminformatics, 70, 118, 128, 153-154, 171, 182, 185, 194-197, 201

Chemotherapy, 1, 44, 51, 82-83

Chemscore, 30, 86, 143-145, 150, 152, 219

Computer-aided Drug Design, 10, 29, 40, 43, 69, 141, 153

Coronary Heart Disease, 204

Cytotoxic, 75, 77

D

Dihydroergotamine, 159, 164-168, 173

Drug Resistance, 1, 26, 45, 105, 160, 201

E

Electrophoresis, 7, 50, 204, 210

Epidermal Growth Factor Receptor, 44, 50-51, 116

Equilibration, 15-16, 56, 74

Ergotamine, 165-166, 173

Estrogen Receptor, 104, 115-116, 220-221

F

Flow Cytometer, 46, 49, 207

G

Goldscore, 29, 86, 150

Gossypol, 44-51

Guanethidine, 163-166, 168, 170

H

Hydrophobic Interactions, 18, 44, 68, 112, 150

Hydroxyzine, 159, 164-166, 170-171

I

Inhibition Mechanism, 44, 78, 81

Ischemia, 173, 204, 216

L

Leishmaniasis, 1-5, 7, 9-11

Ligand-based Drug Design, 1, 3, 196

Ligand-based Virtual Screening, 7, 201

M

Machine Learning, 30, 96, 102-103, 117-119, 121, 128, 141, 145, 148, 153-154, 158-159, 161-162, 171, 173, 185, 196-197, 199-201

Macrolides, 168, 173

Mass Spectrometry, 7, 204, 210, 216

Medicinal Chemistry, 1, 11-12, 52-53, 70, 154, 156-157, 182, 195-196, 215

Methylation, 68, 73, 77, 80-81, 213

Miltefosine, 1, 8, 10-11

Molecular Docking, 2-4, 6-7, 10, 22, 24, 26-29, 31, 33-34, 39, 41-44, 47, 49, 73, 86, 104, 106, 116, 141, 154-156, 158, 187, 191, 195, 207, 210, 215, 217, 219, 221, 230-231

Molecular Dynamics Simulation, 43, 72, 74, 115-116

Molecular Modeling, 1, 15, 28, 32, 35, 105, 186, 196, 207, 210, 212, 219, 231

N

Neglected Tropical Disease, 1

Non-small Cell Lung Cancer, 44, 50-51, 72-73, 76

P

Pathogenesis, 44-45, 51

Phenotype, 26, 94, 134-135, 138, 140, 168

Plasmodium Falciparum, 159-160, 172-174

Principal Component Analysis, 7, 156

Promastigotes, 4-9

Protein Arginine Methyltransferases, 72, 81

Q

Quorum Sensing, 165-166

R

Random Forest, 118, 156, 158, 170

Reperfusion Injury, 216

Root Mean Square Deviation, 13, 108

Root Mean Square Fluctuation, 108-109

S

Scoring Function, 29-30, 40, 43, 83-84, 92, 141-158, 186, 220, 224-225

Stabilization, 194, 212

Structure-based Drug Design, 1, 4-6, 10-11, 29, 41-42, 69, 115, 141, 154-155

Symmetric Dimethylation, 72-73, 77

T

Teratogenicity, 1

Thiosemicarbazone Hybrids, 8

Triazole, 8, 62-63

Trifluoperazine, 164-165, 167, 170-172

Triple Negative Breast Cancer, 82, 92, 94-95

Tyrosine Kinase Inhibitor, 45, 51, 165, 167

V

Virtual Screening, 2-3, 5, 7, 10-11, 13, 26, 29, 31, 33, 41-43, 70, 72-74, 79, 81-84, 86, 88, 94, 114, 116, 141-142, 153-158, 172, 176, 182-184, 186, 195-198, 201-202, 217-218, 220-221, 223, 230-231

W

Western Blot Analysis, 47, 49, 74, 76-77, 213